AF772539

Toxicology and Pesticide Chemistry

Toxicology and Pesticide Chemistry

Editor:

Gonzalo Delgado, Ph.D.

ArclerPress

www.arclerpress.com

Toxicology and Pesticide Chemistry

Editor: Gonzalo Delgado, Ph.D.

© 2017 Arcler Press LLC

708 3rd Avenue, 6th Floor
New York
NY 10017
United States of America
www.arclerpress.com

ISBN: 978-1-68094-425-9

Library of Congress Control Number: 2016951167

This book contains information obtained from highly regarded resources. Reprinted material sources are indicated. Copyright for individual articles remains with the authors as indicated. A Wide variety of references are listed. Reasonable efforts have been made to publish reliable data and views articulated in the chapters are those of the individual contributors, and not necessarily those of the editors or publishers. Editors or publishers are not responsible for the accuracy of the information in the published chapters or consequences of their use. The publisher believes no responsibility for any damage or grievance to the persons or property arising out of the use of any materials, instructions, methods or thoughts in the book. The editors and the publisher have attempted to trace the copyright holders of all material reproduced in this publication and apologize to copyright holders if permission has not been obtained. If any copyright holder has not been acknowledged, please write to us so we may rectify.

Notice: Registered trademark of products or corporate names are used only for explanation and identification without intent of infringement.

Arcler Press LLC publishes wide variety of books and eBooks. For more information about Arcler Press and its products, visit our website at www.arclerpress.com

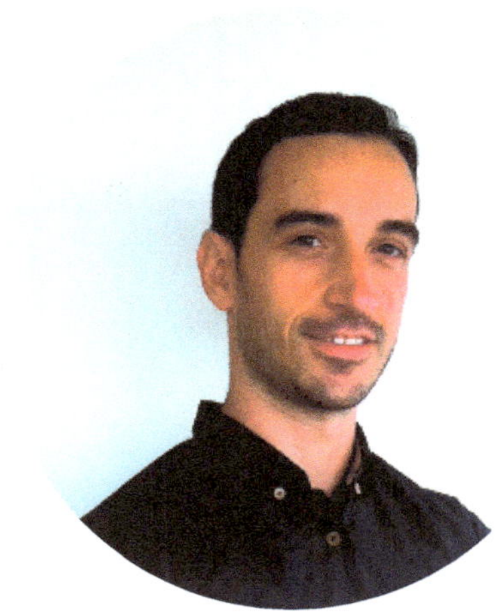

About the Editor

Gonzalo Delgado, Ph.D.

Gonzalo Delgado is graduated in Chemistry and Biochemistry and obtained his PhD in Biomedicine from the University of Barcelona (Spain) in 2014. His interests range from oncology and molecular medicine to toxicology and organic production. He is currently scientific and biomedical advisor for biotech companies and startups.

Contents

List of Contributors

Natalia TG
Federal University of Ceara – Fortaleza, Ceara, Brazil

Robert MH
Sustainable Futures Institute, Michigan Technological University, Houghton, MI, USA

Hoda M. Nasr
Department of plant protection, Faculty of Agriculture, Damanhour University, Damanhour, Egypt`

Suresh Kumar
Division of Biochemistry, Indian Agricultural Research Institute, New Delhi-110012, India

Archana Singh
Division of Biochemistry, Indian Agricultural Research Institute, New Delhi-110012, India

Nagappan Raja
Department of Biology, College of Natural and Computational Sciences, University of Gondar, Ethiopia

Getinet Masresha
Department of Biology, College of Natural and Computational Sciences, University of Gondar, Ethiopia

Anupama Pradhan
Department of Chemistry, T.S.S. Govt College Pathalgaon, Dist. -Jashpur (C.G.) India.

S. K. Markande
Department of Botony, T.S.S. Govt College Pathalgaon, Dist. -Jashpur (C.G.) India.

Rakesh Kumar Kurre
Department of Physics, T.S.S. Govt College Pathalgaon, Dist. -Jashpur (C.G.) India.

Francisco Sánchez-Bayo
Centre for Ecotoxicology, University of Technology Sydney, Lidcombe NSW 2141, Australia

Richard Ortega
University of Bordeaux, CENBG, UMR 5797, F-33170 Gradignan, France

Shivani Jaggi
Maya Institute of Technology & Management Selaqui, Dehradun, Uttarakhand, India

Bikram Singh
Institute of Himalayan Bioresource Technology (IHBT), Council of Scientific & Industrial Research, Palampur (Himachal Pradesh), India

Adarsh Shanker
Institute of Himalayan Bioresource Technology (IHBT), Council of Scientific & Industrial Research, Palampur (Himachal Pradesh), India

Juan D. López Jr
USDA-ARS, Aerial Application Technology Research Unit, College Station, USA

Mohamed A. Latheef
USDA-ARS, Aerial Application Technology Research Unit, College Station, USA

Wesley C. Hoffmann
USDA-ARS, Aerial Application Technology Research Unit, College Station, USA

Abida Bibi
Department of Microbiology, Quaid-i-Azam University, Islamabad, Pakistan

Khalique Ahmed
KarakuramUniversity, Gilgit, Pakistan

Najma Ayub
Department of Microbiology, Quaid-i-Azam University, Islamabad, Pakistan

Sadia Alam
Departmentof Microbiology, University of Haripur, Haripur, Pakistan

Zining Cui
Key Laboratory of Pesticide Chemistry and Application, Ministry of Agriculture, Department of Applied Chemistry, College of Science, China Agricultural University, Beijing 100193, China

Yun Ling
Key Laboratory of Pesticide Chemistry and Application, Ministry of Agriculture, Department of Applied Chemistry, College of Science, China Agricultural University, Beijing 100193, China

Baoju Li
Institute of Vegetables and Flowers, Chinese Academy of Agricultural Science, Beijing 100081, China

Yongqiang Li
Key Laboratory of Pesticide Chemistry and Application, Ministry of Agriculture, Department of Applied Chemistry, College of Science, China Agricultural University, Beijing 100193, China

Changhui Rui
Key Laboratory of Pesticide Chemistry and Application, Ministry of Agriculture, Department of Applied Chemistry, College of Science, China Agricultural University, Beijing 100193, China

Jingrong Cui
State Key Laboratory of Natural and Biomimetic Drugs, School of Pharmaceutical Science, Peking University, Beijing 100083, China

Yanxia Shi
Institute of Vegetables and Flowers, Chinese Academy of Agricultural Science, Beijing 100081, China

Xinling Yang
Key Laboratory of Pesticide Chemistry and Application, Ministry of Agriculture, Department of Applied Chemistry, College of Science, China Agricultural University, Beijing 100193, China

M Balali-Mood
Medical Toxicology Research Centre, Faculty of Medicine, Mashhad University of Medical Sciences, Mashhad, Iran

K Balali-Mood
NextDocs Corporation, Compass House, Vision Park, Chivers Way, Histon, Cambridge, UK

M Moodi
Dept. of Health Education, Birjand University of Medical Sciences, Birjand, Iran

B Balali-Mood
Institute of Chemical Biology, Imperial College London, England, UK

Elisa Sauer
Laboratory of Toxicology (LATOX), Department of Clinical and Toxicology Analysis, Federal University of Rio Grande do Sul, Porto Alegre, RS 90610000, Brazil
Institute of Cardiology, University Foundation of Cardiology, Porto Alegre, RS 90040371, Brazil

Angela M. Moro
Laboratory of Toxicology (LATOX), Department of Clinical and Toxicology Analysis, Federal University of Rio Grande do Sul, Porto Alegre, RS 90610000, Brazil
Laboratory of Toxicology, Center of Biological and Health Sciences University of Caxias do Sul, Caxias do Sul, RS, 96815900, Brazil
Post-Graduate Program Pharmaceutical Sciences, Federal University of Rio Grande do Sul, Porto Alegre, RS 90610000, Brazil

Natália Brucker
Laboratory of Toxicology (LATOX), Department of Clinical and Toxicology Analysis, Federal University of Rio Grande do Sul, Porto Alegre, RS 90610000, Brazil
Post-Graduate Program Pharmaceutical Sciences, Federal University of Rio Grande do Sul, Porto Alegre, RS 90610000, Brazil
Department of Clinical and Toxicology Analysis, Federal University of Santa Maria, RS 97105900, Brazil

Sabrina Nascimento
Laboratory of Toxicology (LATOX), Department of Clinical and Toxicology Analysis, Federal University of Rio Grande do Sul, Porto Alegre, RS 90610000, Brazil
Post-Graduate Program Pharmaceutical Sciences, Federal University of Rio Grande do Sul, Porto Alegre, RS 90610000, Brazil

Bruna Gauer
Laboratory of Toxicology (LATOX), Department of Clinical and Toxicology Analysis, Federal University of Rio Grande do Sul, Porto Alegre, RS 90610000, Brazil

Rafael Fracasso
Laboratory of Toxicology (LATOX), Department of Clinical and Toxicology Analysis, Federal University of Rio Grande do Sul, Porto Alegre, RS 90610000, Brazil
Post-Graduate Program Pharmaceutical Sciences, Federal University of Rio Grande do Sul, Porto Alegre, RS 90610000, Brazil

Adriana Gioda
Department of Chemistry, Pontifical Catholic University of Rio de Janeiro (PUC-Rio), Rio de Janeiro, RJ 22453900, Brazil

Ruy Beck
Department of Production and Drug Control, Federal University of Rio Grande do Sul, Porto Alegre, RS 90610000, Brazil

José C. F. Moreira
Department of Biochemistry, Federal University of Rio Grande do Sul, Porto Alegre, RS 90035003, Brazil

Vera Lucia Eifler-Lima
Department of Production of Source-Material, Federal University of Rio Grande do Sul, Porto Alegre, RS 90610000, Brazil

Solange Cristina Garcia
Laboratory of Toxicology (LATOX), Department of Clinical and Toxicology Analysis, Federal University of Rio Grande do Sul, Porto Alegre, RS 90610000, Brazil

Institute of Cardiology, University Foundation of Cardiology, Porto Alegre, RS 90040371, Brazil
Department of Clinical and Toxicology Analysis, Federal University of Santa Maria, RS 97105900, Brazil

Yi-hua Gu
Obstetrics & Gynecology Hospital, Institute of Reproduction & Development, Fudan University, Shanghai, P. R. of China
Shanghai Institute of Planned Parenthood Research, Institute of Reproduction & Development, Fudan University, Shanghai, P. R. of China

Yan Li
Reproductive Medical Center, the First Affiliated Hospital of Wenzhou Medical University, Wenzhou, Zhejiang, P. R. of China

Xue-feng Huang
Obstetrics & Gynecology Hospital, Institute of Reproduction & Development, Fudan University, Shanghai, P. R. of China
Reproductive Medical Center, the First Affiliated Hospital of Wenzhou Medical University, Wenzhou, Zhejiang, P. R. of China

Ju-fen Zheng
Shanghai Institute of Planned Parenthood Research, Institute of Reproduction & Development, Fudan University, Shanghai, P. R. of China

Jun Yang
Shanghai Institute of Planned Parenthood Research, Institute of Reproduction & Development, Fudan University, Shanghai, P. R. of China

Hua Diao
Obstetrics & Gynecology Hospital, Institute of Reproduction & Development, Fudan University, Shanghai, P. R. of China
Shanghai Institute of Planned Parenthood Research, Institute of Reproduction & Development, Fudan University, Shanghai, P. R. of China

Yao Yuan
Shanghai Institute of Planned Parenthood Research, Institute of Reproduction & Development, Fudan University, Shanghai, P. R. of China

Yan Xu
Obstetrics & Gynecology Hospital, Institute of Reproduction & Development, Fudan University, Shanghai, P. R. of China

Miao Liu
Obstetrics & Gynecology Hospital, Institute of Reproduction & Development, Fudan University, Shanghai, P. R. of China

Hui-juan Shi
Obstetrics & Gynecology Hospital, Institute of Reproduction & Development, Fudan University, Shanghai, P. R. of China
Shanghai Institute of Planned Parenthood Research, Institute of Reproduction & Development, Fudan University, Shanghai, P. R. of China

Wen-ping Xu
School of Pharmacy, East China University of Science and Technology, Shanghai, P. R. of China
State Key Laboratory of Reproductive Biology, Institute of Zoology, Chinese Academy of Sciences, China

Sahdeo Prasad
Proteomics Laboratory, Indian Institute of Toxicology Research, Mahatma Gandhi Marg, Lucknow 226001, India

Smita Srivastava
Proteomics Laboratory, Indian Institute of Toxicology Research, Mahatma Gandhi Marg, Lucknow 226001, India

Madhulika Singh
Proteomics Laboratory, Indian Institute of Toxicology Research, Mahatma Gandhi Marg, Lucknow 226001, India

Yogeshwer Shukla
Proteomics Laboratory, Indian Institute of Toxicology Research, Mahatma Gandhi Marg, Lucknow 226001, India

Nagat Aly
Department of Mammalian Toxicology, Pesticides Central Laboratory, Agricultural Research Center, Alexandria, Egypt

Kawther El-Gendy
Department of Pesticide Chemistry& Toxicology, Faculty of Agriculture, Alexandria University, Alexandria, Egypt

Devanur R.M.M. Prasad
Department of Forensic Medicine and Toxicology, Government of Karnataka, District Hospital, Chamarajanagar, Karnataka, India

Prasanna S. Jirli
Department of Forensic Medicine and Toxicology, Karnataka Lingayath Education Society University, Jawaharlal Nehru Medical College, Belgaum, Karnataka, India

Mahadevaiah Mahesh
Department of General Medicine, JSS University, JSS Medical College, Mysore, Karnataka, India

Shivanagappa Mamatha
Department of Obstetrics and Gynaecology, JSS University, JSS Medical College, Mysore, Karnataka, India

Antonio F. Hernández
Department of Legal Medicine and Toxicology, University of Granada School of Medicine, Granada 18016, Spain

Pablo Menéndez
Department of Biomedicine, Josep Carreras Leukemia Research Institute, School of Medicine, University of Barcelona, Barcelona 08036, Spain
Instituciò Catalana de Recerca i Estudis Avançats (ICREA), Barcelona 08010, Spain

Gasnier C
Laboratory of Biochemistry EA2608, Institute of Biology, University of Caen, France.

Benachour N
Laboratory of Biochemistry EA2608, Institute of Biology, University of Caen, France.

Clair E
Laboratory of Biochemistry EA2608, Institute of Biology, University of Caen, France.

Travert C
Laboratory of Biochemistry EA2608, Institute of Biology, University of Caen, France.

Langlois F
Laboratory of Biochemistry EA2608, Institute of Biology, University of Caen, France.

Laurant C
Laboratory of Biochemistry EA2608, Institute of Biology, University of Caen, France.

Decroix-Laporte C
Laboratory of Biochemistry EA2608, Institute of Biology, University of Caen, France.

Séralini GE
Laboratory of Biochemistry EA2608, Institute of Biology, University of Caen, France.

Nobonita Deb
Department of Life Science and Bioinformatics Assam University, Silchar, India-788011

Suchismita Das
Department of Life Science and Bioinformatics Assam University, Silchar, India-788011

Swale DR
University of Florida, Emerging Pathogens Institute, Department of Entomology and Nematology, Gainesville, Florida, United States of America.

Sun B
University of Florida, Emerging Pathogens Institute, Department of Entomology and Nematology, Gainesville, Florida, United States of America.

Tong f and
University of Florida, Emerging Pathogens Institute, Department of Entomology and Nematology, Gainesville, Florida, United States of America.

Bloomquist JR
University of Florida, Emerging Pathogens Institute, Department of Entomology and Nematology, Gainesville, Florida, United States of America.

Rashid Ahmed Khan
Key Laboratory of Plant Protection Resources and Pest Management, Ministry of Education, College of Plant Protection, Northwest A&F University, Yangling 712100, Shaanxi, China

Ji Yuan Liu
Key Laboratory of Plant Protection Resources and Pest Management, Ministry of Education, College of Plant Protection, Northwest A&F University, Yangling 712100, Shaanxi, China

Maryam Rashid
Key Laboratory of Plant Protection Resources and Pest Management, Ministry of Education, College of Plant Protection, Northwest A&F University, Yangling 712100, Shaanxi, China

Dun Wang
Key Laboratory of Plant Protection Resources and Pest Management, Ministry of Education, College of Plant Protection, Northwest A&F University, Yangling 712100, Shaanxi, China
Institute of Entomology, Northwest A&F University, Yangling 712100, Shaanxi, China

Ya Lin Zhang
Key Laboratory of Plant Protection Resources and Pest Management, Ministry of Education, College of Plant Protection, Northwest A&F University, Yangling 712100, Shaanxi, China

Suchismita Das
Assistant professor, Department of Life Science and Bioinformatics, Assam University, Silchar, India-788011

Brandon D. Gaytán
Department of Nutritional Science and Toxicology, University of California, Berkeley, Berkeley, California, United States of America

Alex V. Loguinov
Department of Nutritional Science and Toxicology, University of California, Berkeley, Berkeley, California, United States of America

Xenia Peñate
Departamento de Genética, Universidad de Sevilla and Instituto de Biomedicina de Sevilla, Hospital Universitario Virgen del Rocío/CSIC/Universidad de Sevilla, Seville, Spain

Jan-Michael Lerot
Department of Nutritional Science and Toxicology, University of California, Berkeley, Berkeley, California, United States of America

Sebastián Chávez
Departamento de Genética, Universidad de Sevilla and Instituto de Biomedicina de Sevilla, Hospital Universitario Virgen del Rocío/CSIC/Universidad de Sevilla, Seville, Spain

Nancy D. Denslow
Department of Physiological Sciences and Center for Environmental and Human Toxicology, University of Florida, Gainesville, Florida, United States of America

Chris D. Vulpe
Department of Nutritional Science and Toxicology, University of California, Berkeley, Berkeley, California, United States of America

Mark J. Miles
Dow AgroSciences, Abingdon, UK

Anne Alix
Dow AgroSciences, Abingdon, UK

Chloe Bourgouin
Dow AgroSciences France, Saint Quentin en Yvelines, France

Stephan Schmitzer
IBACON, Rossdorf, Germany

Michael D. Coleman
School of Life and Health Sciences, Aston University, Birmingham, United Kingdom

John D. O'Neil
School of Life and Health Sciences, Aston University, Birmingham, United Kingdom

Elizabeth K. Woehrling
School of Life and Health Sciences, Aston University, Birmingham, United Kingdom

Oscar Bate Akide Ndunge
School of Life and Health Sciences, Aston University, Birmingham, United Kingdom

Eric J. Hill
School of Life and Health Sciences, Aston University, Birmingham, United Kingdom

Andre Menache
Antidote Europe, Perpignan, France National Institutes of Health, United States of America

Claude J. Reiss
Antidote Europe, Perpignan, France National Institutes of Health, United States of America

Andrew H. Dawson
South Asian Clinical Toxicology Research Collaboration, Faculty of Medicine, University of Peradeniya, Peradeniya, Sri Lanka
School of Medicine and Public Health, University of Newcastle, Newcastle, Australia
Professorial Medicine Unit, POW Clinical School, University of New South Wales, Sydney, Australia

Michael Eddleston
South Asian Clinical Toxicology Research Collaboration, Faculty of Medicine, University of Peradeniya, Peradeniya, Sri Lanka
National Poisons Information Service - Edinburgh, Royal Infirmary of Edinburgh, Edinburgh, United Kingdom, Clinical Pharmacology Unit, Centre for Cardiovascular Science, University of Edinburgh, Edinburgh, United Kingdom

Lalith Senarathna
South Asian Clinical Toxicology Research Collaboration, Faculty of Medicine, University of Peradeniya, Peradeniya, Sri Lanka

Fahim Mohamed
South Asian Clinical Toxicology Research Collaboration, Faculty of Medicine, University of Peradeniya, Peradeniya, Sri Lanka

Indika Gawarammana
South Asian Clinical Toxicology Research Collaboration, Faculty of Medicine, University of Peradeniya, Peradeniya, Sri Lanka

Steven J. Bowe
School of Medicine and Public Health, University of Newcastle, Newcastle, Australia

Gamini Manuweera
Office of the Pesticide Registrar, Government Department of Agriculture, Peradeniya, Sri Lanka

Nicholas A. Buckley
South Asian Clinical Toxicology Research Collaboration, Faculty of Medicine, University of Peradeniya, Peradeniya, Sri Lanka
Professorial Medicine Unit, POW Clinical School, University of New South Wales, Sydney, Australia

Martins JB
REQUIMTE (Rede de Química e Tecnologia), Laboratório de Toxicologia, Departamento de Ciências Biológicas, Faculdade de Farmácia, Universidade do Porto, Rua de Jorge Viterbo Ferreira 228, 4050-313 Porto, Portugal.

Bastos Mde L
REQUIMTE (Rede de Química e Tecnologia), Laboratório de Toxicologia, Departamento de Ciências Biológicas, Faculdade de Farmácia, Universidade do Porto, Rua de Jorge Viterbo Ferreira 228, 4050-313 Porto, Portugal.

Carvalho F
REQUIMTE (Rede de Química e Tecnologia), Laboratório de Toxicologia, Departamento de Ciências Biológicas, Faculdade de Farmácia, Universidade do Porto, Rua de Jorge Viterbo Ferreira 228, 4050-313 Porto, Portugal.

Capela JP
REQUIMTE (Rede de Química e Tecnologia), Laboratório de Toxicologia, Departamento de Ciências Biológicas, Faculdade de Farmácia, Universidade do Porto, Rua de Jorge Viterbo Ferreira 228, 4050-313 Porto, Portugal.

Zhang J
Cyrus Tang Hematology Center, Soochow University, Suzhou, China.

Tang J
Cyrus Tang Hematology Center, Soochow University, Suzhou, China.

Cao B
Cyrus Tang Hematology Center, Soochow University, Suzhou, China.

Zhang Z
Cyrus Tang Hematology Center, Soochow University, Suzhou, China.

Li J
Cyrus Tang Hematology Center, Soochow University, Suzhou, China.

Schimmer AD
Cyrus Tang Hematology Center, Soochow University, Suzhou, China.

He S
Cyrus Tang Hematology Center, Soochow University, Suzhou, China.

Mao X
Cyrus Tang Hematology Center, Soochow University, Suzhou, China.

Roni A Neff
Center for a Livable Future, Johns Hopkins Bloomberg School of Public Health, 615 N. Wolfe St. Suite W7010, Baltimore, MD 21205-2179, USA.
Department of Environmental Health Sciences, Johns Hopkins Bloomberg School of Public Health, 624 N. Broadway, Baltimore, MD 21205-2179, USA.

Jennifer C Hartle
Center for a Livable Future, Johns Hopkins Bloomberg School of Public Health, 615 N. Wolfe St. Suite W7010, Baltimore, MD 21205-2179, USA.
Department of Environmental Health Sciences, Johns Hopkins Bloomberg School of Public Health, 624 N. Broadway, Baltimore, MD 21205-2179, USA.

Linnea I Laestadius
Center for a Livable Future, Johns Hopkins Bloomberg School of Public Health, 615 N. Wolfe St. Suite W7010, Baltimore, MD 21205-2179, USA.
Department of Health Policy & Management, Johns Hopkins Bloomberg School of Public Health, 615 N. Wolfe St., Baltimore, MD 21205-2179, USA.

Kathleen Dolan
Center for a Livable Future, Johns Hopkins Bloomberg School of Public Health, 615 N. Wolfe St. Suite W7010, Baltimore, MD 21205-2179, USA.
Association of State and Territorial Health Officials, 2231 Crystal Drive, Suite 450, Arlington, Virginia 22202, USA.

Anne C Rosenthal
Center for a Livable Future, Johns Hopkins Bloomberg School of Public Health, 615 N. Wolfe St. Suite W7010, Baltimore, MD 21205-2179, USA.

Fulbright Scholar, Center for Studies on Sustainable Development, CP 130/02, 50 av. F. Roosevelt, 1050 Brussels, Belgium.

Keeve E Nachman
Center for a Livable Future, Johns Hopkins Bloomberg School of Public Health, 615 N. Wolfe St. Suite W7010, Baltimore, MD 21205-2179, USA.
Department of Environmental Health Sciences, Johns Hopkins Bloomberg School of Public Health, 624 N. Broadway, Baltimore, MD 21205-2179, USA.

Preface

Pesticides are used to control pests, such as insects, weeds, and rodents, which negatively affect and sometimes ruin agriculture production. Pesticides types improved with the development of synthetic chemistry in the 1950's century, and as the demand for food production increased, so did pesticide use. With little understanding of environmental impact or health risks, pesticide use continued for years without regulation.

In the last decades, research of these implications has led to the restriction and banning of many pesticides. Nowadays, regulatory agencies such as the FDA and EC establish the maximum limit of pesticide residue on produce that's considered safe for human consumption. The growth in the demand of organic food demonstrates society's increasing awareness of health risks associated with pesticide consumption. Pest management strategies have advanced significantly, scientists develop safer and more targeted methods to replace broad-spectrum pesticides that had long-lasting and harmful environmental impact. Toxicology and Pesticide Chemistry explains the major chemical aspects of the most widely used pesticides, as well as those banned and newly developed. The types are grouped by target species: insecticides, acaricides, nematocides, rodenticides, fungicides and herbicides. The organic syntheses are explained, as are the biochemical mechanism of action and their effectiveness. The toxicity effects are discussed in detail. This book is referenced with a wide selection of published studies, and is aimed at professionals in agriculture and regulatory bodies and researchers in the field of pesticides, food and agricultural sciences.

Editor

Gonzalo Delgado, Ph.D.

INTRODUCTION

Pesticides are biocides especially designed to kill, repel, attract and mitigate the organisms, which are nuisance to humans and their agricultural and hygiene activities. The pesticides may be the organic molecules or inorganic synthetic molecules or the biopesticides. The toxicological activities on pests depend on their chemical structure and different life stages. These pesticides can be classified as organ chlorine compounds, organ phosphorus compounds, carbonates, pyrethroids and neonicotenoids. In organochlorinc compounds, the number and position of CI in molecule decides the toxicity. They are nonpolar and lipophilic in nature. Organ phosphorous pesticides (OP) are neutral ester or amide derivatives of phosphorous acids carrying a phosphoryl (P-O) or thiophosphoryl (P-S) group. OP pesticides are identified by single characteristic i.e., they act by inhibiting cholinesterase enzyme. Carbamates are anticholinesterase inhibitor pesticides and are synthetic derivative of physostigmine, also known as eserine, which is a principle alkaloid of plant, *Physcssfigma venenosum*, Calabar bean. Chemically, they are esters of carbamic acid, $HOOC.NH_2$, with insecticidal (and related) properties. Pyrethroids are esters formed by the combination of two acids *i.e.* Chrysenthemic acid and Pyrethric acid, with three alcohols namely Pyrethrolone, Cinerolone and Jasmolone. They are nerve poisons and affect the nerve axon, causing repetitive discharge of nerves which results in eventual paralysis. The neonicotinoids, are the newest major class of insecticides, derived synthetically from nicotinoids. Mode of action of neonicotinoids is that they act as agonists at the insect nicotinic acetylcholine receptor (nAChR).

Pesticide control involves killing pest organisms or otherwise preventing them from destructive behavior. Pesticides are either natural or synthetic and are applied to target pests in a myriad of formulations (EC,WP, SP, FP, G etc.) and application technology systems (sprays, baits, slow-release diffusion, dust, etc.). In recent years, the bacterial genes coding for insecticidal proteins have been incorporated into various crops that dealt with the mortality of the pests feeding on them. Many other eco-friendly methods for insect pest control such as Integrated Pest Management (IPM), use of bio-pesticides etc., are becoming popular. Bio-pesticides and IPM should show good growth in the future, as there is growing concern for the eco-friendly organic agriculture and could be achieved through Good Agriculture Practices (GAP).

Pesticides are chemicals that kill pests, and are categorized by the types of pests they kill. For example, insecticides kill insects, herbicides kill weeds, bactericides kill bacteria, fungicides kill fungi, and algaecides kill algae.

History of Pesticides

Throughout history, various types of pests, such as insects, weeds, bacteria, rodents, and other biological organisms, have bothered humans or threatened human health. People have been using pesticides for thousands of years to try to control these pests. The Sumerians used sulfur to control insects and mites 5,000 years ago. The Chinese used mercury and arsenic compounds to control body lice and other pests. The Greeks and Romans used oil, ash, sulfur, and other materials to protect themselves, their livestock, and their crops from various pests. And people in various cultures have used smoke, salt, spices, and insect-repelling plants to preserve food and keep pests away.

Classes of Pesticides

Although the use of pesticides is not new, the types of substances people have used as pesticides have changed over time. The earliest pesticides were inorganic substances such as sulfur, mercury, lead, arsenic, and ash. Some of these inorganic pesticides are still used today. For example, sulfur is still used as a fungicide, copper is used as an algicide, lead and arsenic were used as insecticides until World War II, and chromium, copper, and arsenic have been used as wood preservatives to prevent microorganisms from causing wood decay. Even though many of these substances are effective pesticides, the use of some of these materials has been banned or restricted because of health and environmental concerns. Lead and arsenic are no longer used as insecticides, the use of mercury as a fungicide has been restricted, and the U.S. Environmental Protection Agency (EPA) is phasing out the use of arsenic as a wood preservative.

The modern era of chemical pest control began around the time of World War II, when the synthetic organic chemical industry began to develop. The first synthetic organic pesticides were organochlorine compounds, such as dichlorodiphenyltrichloroethane (DDT). Commercial production of DDT began in 1943. At that time, DDT was considered to be a wonderful invention. It was cheap to produce, very toxic to insects, and much less toxic to mammals. DDT and other organochlorine insecticides were used for many years to control mosquitoes and as a broad-spectrum insecticide against insect pests that damaged food and crops. Unfortunately, scientists learned later that many organochlorine insecticides were persistent in the environment (they did not degrade readily) and were bioaccumulation in birds, humans, and other animals. In 1962 Rachel Carson wrote the book *Silent Spring,* in which she reported that DDT was causing eggshell thinning in bird eggs and thus was leading to the near extinction of bird species such as peregrine falcons and bald eagles. Today most of the organochlorine pesticides have been banned in the United States by the EPA because of the tendency of these compounds to persist in the environment and bioaccumulate in animals.

Other classes of insecticides include the organophosphates, carbamates, pyrethroids, and biopesticides. These other classes of pesticides are not as persistent in the environment as the organochlorine pesticides. The organophosphate and carbamate pesticides affect the nervous system by disrupting the enzyme that regulates acetylcholine, a neurotransmitter. However, carbamate pesticides are less toxic to humans because their interactions with important enzymes are reversible. As a group, the organophosphate and carbamate pesticides are probably the most widely used insecticides, although many are being restricted by the EPA because of their toxicity.

Pyrethroid pesticides were developed as synthetic versions of the naturally occurring pesticide pyrethrin, which is found in chrysanthemums. Most pyrethroids are safer than the organochlorines, organophosphates, and carbamates, although some synthetic pyrethroids are toxic to the nervous system. Pyrethroids have been modified to increase their stability in the environment, and many different pyrethroids are being used today.

Pesticide Residues

Pesticide residues are the materials that remain on plants and food when a crop is treated with a pesticide. The U.S. government establishes safe residue levels, called tolerances or maximum residue levels, for each food commodity. However, the presence of pesticide residues in food has been a public concern. There has also been a concern about pesticide residues in water, air, and soil. In response to this concern, the U.S. Congress passed the Food Quality Protection Act in 1996, which has had an impact on safety standards for pesticides.

Approaches to pest management have changed significantly since the 1950s and will continue to change as scientists learn more about the toxicity and environmental behavior of pesticides. Scientists will continue to develop newer approaches to insect pest management that are considered to be safer than the use of broad-spectrum pesticides. The most effective strategy for controlling pests may be to combine methods in an approach known as integrated pest management (IPM), which emphasizes preventing pest damage. In IPM information about pests and available pest control methods is used to manage pest damage by the most economical means and causing the least possible hazard to people, property, and the environment. Methods for pest management will continue to evolve as scientists conduct research and develop new information.

Identity of pesticides

How can pesticides be identified?

Many of the pesticides that we use in our crops, gardens or domestic animals, are often a mixture of several chemicals mixed together in desired proportions suspended in appropriate carrier or diluent materials. These chemicals are called active ingredients that are responsible for killing or otherwise affecting the pests. Apart from the active ingredients, there are other chemicals that are formulated together with the active ingredients that usually do not kill pests. These are called inert ingredients that serve as carriers, diluents, binders, dispersants, prolong the shelf life of active ingredients or make the pesticide smell better. It is often the case that active ingredients on the container labels are named using common names. However, common names are not the only way to identify pesticides and in fact common names do not give complete information on the chemical nature of the pesticides. When chemists want to give a specific and unambiguous name to a chemical, they use what is called "systematic name". These names are usually long and complicated, but they are necessary for naming the millions of known chemicals. There are two main systems for deriving the systematic names of chemicals, one from the International Union of Pure and Applied Chemistry (IUPAC) and the other from the Chemical Abstracts Service (CAS). As an example of the two systematic naming described above, the following insecticide is names respective as; IUPAC systematic name: (E)-1-(6-chloro-3-pyridylmethyl)-N-nitroimidazolidin-2- ylideneamine The same insecticide has the following CAS systematic name: (2E)-1-[(6-chloro-3-pyridinyl) methyl]-N-nitro-2-imidazolidinimine In addition to a systematic name, CAS assigns a registry number to each chemical which is different from one chemical to another. For example the insecticide just described above has a CAS registry number of 138261-41-3 As pointed out earlier, systematic names are long and complicated for a mere user of pesticides (layman). For that matter, systematic names are more used by experts in the field of pesticides who pursue specific researches in which a proper identification of the chemical is needed. For many purposes, a relatively short and simple name would be helpful than a systematic name or registry number, and that is the role of common names.

How are the common names of pesticides derived?

What most people need when reading, writing or talking about a pesticides is a short, fairly simple and reasonably memorable name. Common names are approved by the International Organization for Standardization (ISO) based on given guidelines. For example the common name for the insecticide (E)-1-(6-chloro-3-pyridylmethyl)-N-nitroimidazolidin-2- ylideneamine is given as "imidacloprid" derived from parts of the systematic name. The process of registering common names usually starts with the pesticides manufacturers submitting proposals for names to ISO and the ISO committee checks that the proposed names comply with the rules, not misleading, and are not likely to be confused with the existing names of pesticides or drugs. Once common names are approved by ISO, they no longer belong to the company, but rather they can be used in other countries.

Classification of pesticides

The word "pesticide" is an umbrella term for all insecticides, herbicides, fungicides, rodenticides, wood preservatives, garden chemicals and household disinfectants that may be used to kill some pests. Since pesticides varies in identity, physical and chemical properties, it`s therefore logical to have them classified and their properties studied under their respective groups. Synthetic pesticides are classified based on various ways depending on the needs. However, there are three most popular ways of classifying pesticides which are; classification based on the mode of action, classification based on the targeted pest species and classification based on the chemical composition of the pesticide.

Classification of pesticides based on the mode of action

Under this type of classification, pesticides are classified based on the way in which they act to bring about the desired effect. In this way pesticides are classified as contact (nonsystemic) and systemic pesticides. The non-systemic pesticides are those that do not appreciably penetrate plant tissues and consequently not transported within the plant vascular system. The non-systemic pesticides will only bring about the desired effect when they come in contact with the targeted pest, hence the name contact pesticides. Examples of contact pesticides are parquet and piquet bromide. On the other hand, the systemic pesticides are those which effectively penetrate the plant tissues and move through the plant vascular system in order to bring about the desired effect. Examples of systemic pesticides include 2, 4-D and glyphosate. Under this classification, also are stomach poisons that bring about the desired effect after being eaten eg. Rodenticides. Fumigants are those pesticides that produce vapor which kills the pests

Classification of pesticides based on the targeted pest species

In this type of classification, pesticides are named after the name of the corresponding pest in target as shown in table

Type of pesticide	Target organism/pest
Insecticides	Insects
Herbicides	Weeds
Rodenticides	Rodents
Fungicides	Fungi
Acaricides and Miticides	Arachnids of the order Acarina such as ticks and Mites
Molluscicides	Mollusks
Bactericides	Bacteria
Avicides	Bird pests
Virucides	Virus
Algicides	Algae

Classification of pesticides based on the chemical composition

Under chemical classification, pesticides are categorized according to the chemical nature of the active ingredients. The chemical classification of pesticides is by far the most useful classification to researchers in the field of pesticides and environment and to those who search for details. This is because, it is from this kind of classification that gives the clue of the efficacy, physical and chemical properties of the respective pesticides, the knowledge of which is very important in the mode of application, precautions that need to be taken during application and the application rates. Based on chemical classification, pesticides are classified into four main groups namely; organ chlorines, organ phosphorous, carbamates and pyrethrin and pyrethroids. Organ chlorines pesticides are organic compounds with five or more chlorine atoms. Organochlorines were the first synthetic organic pesticides to be used in agriculture and in public health. Most of them were widely used as insecticides for the control of a wide range of insects, and they have a long-term residual effect in the environment since them are resistant to most chemical and microbial degradations. Organochlorine insecticides act as nervous system disruptors leading to convulsions and paralysis of the insect and its eventual death. Some of the commonly used representative examples of organochlorine pesticides are DDT, lindane, endosulfan, aldrin, dieldrin and chlordane and their chemical structures are presented hereunder.

Other minor classes of pesticides

Activity spectrum of the pesticide

In this system of classification, pesticides are classified into two groups as broad spectrum pesticides and selective pesticides. Broad spectrum pesticides are those pesticides that are designed to kill a wide range of pests and other no target organisms. They are nonselective and are often lethal to reptiles, fish, pets and birds. Some examples of broad spectrum pesticides are chlorpyrifos and chlordane. Selective pesticides on the other hand are those pesticides which kill only a specific or group of pests leaving other organisms with a little or no effect at all. A good example in this case is a herbicide 2,4-D which affects broad-leaved plants leaving the grassy crops unaffected.

Mode of formulation

Emulifiable concentrates (EC) are fine suspensions of oil droplets in water and appears milky in color. They do not require constant agitation prior to each application. Wet table Powders (WP) are suspensions of fine particles suspended in water. These suspension require constant agitation prior to each application. Granules (G). Granules are obtained by mixing the active ingredient with clay for outdoor applications. Baits. These are obtained by mixing the active ingredient with food base especially used for the control of rodents. Dusts (D). Dusts cannot be mixed with water and they must be applied dry. The common carriers for dusts are clay, talc, silica gel or diatomacious earth. Fumigants. These are gaseous insecticides usually packaged under pressure and stored as liquids. Some are tablets or pellets that release gas when mixed with water.

Toxicity level

The World Health Organization (WHO) has developed a classification system that group pesticides according to the potential risks to human health caused by accidental contact to human being and they are grouped into the following classes;

- Class Ia = extremely hazardous
- Class Ib = highly hazardous
- Class II = moderately hazardous
- Class III = slightly hazrdous
- Class IV = products unlikely to present acute hazard in normal use

Pesticide control involves killing pest organisms or otherwise preventing them from destructive behavior. Pesticides are either natural or synthetic and are applied to target pests in a myriad of formulations (EC,WP, SP, FP, G etc.) and application technology systems (sprays, baits, slow-release diffusion, dust, etc.). In recent years, the bacterial genes coding for insecticidal proteins have been incorporated into various crops that dealt with the mortality of the pests feeding on them. Many other eco-friendly methods for insect pest control such as Integrated Pest Management (IPM), use of bio-pesticides etc., are becoming popular. Bio-pesticides and IPM should show good growth in the future, as there is growing concern for the eco-friendly organic agriculture and could be achieved through Good Agriculture Practices (GAP).

Use of pesticides requires a proper understanding of the chemistry, their handling and their use in crop protection or hygiene. These are toxic chemicals and require a good understanding of therapy and antidotes at the time of poisoning. This e-book covers pesticide chemistry, metabolic/degradation pathways, biochemical toxicology, therapy and antidotes, nano-pesticides and terminologies associated with pesticide toxicology. The book should serve as a text book for academia, or as a reference work for agriculturists, environmentalists and industry professionals.

Pesticides: Toxicity, Formulations, Use & Safety

Rationale: Despite trends of trying to significantly reduce pesticide use, pesticides are still a major necessity for crop protection, managing disease vectors, and managing pests in our urban habitats. Sooner or later you will have to deal with an insect or mite pest and you will likely have to resort to a pesticide of some sort. There is no doubt that pesticides are designed and used to kill things! Therefore, there is always the risk that these same pesticides may kill other living things though we are intending to only kill a target pest. In this exercise, we will review some basic toxicological principles, learn how to select the best pesticide for our purposes and learn how to interpret a pesticide label.

Toxicology

Toxicology is the study of poisons and their effects, both intended and unintended. A pesticide is a chemical (synthetic or natural) that is used to kill a pest. Virtually all chemicals are poisonous at some level, even water! So, one of the first principles in toxicology is, "The Dose Makes the Poison!" Every day, you eat or drink things that have toxins in them, but you ingest minute quantities and your body either breaks the toxins down (metabolizes them – usually in the liver) or excretes them.

Pesticide Types – We have developed many kinds of pesticides and most are named for the pest group for which they are intended. We use herbicides to kill plants, insecticides to kill insects, and miticides to kill mites. Associate the pesticide names below with the target pests:

_____ Avicide		A. Algae
_____ Rodenticide		B. Bacteria
_____ Nematicide		C. Birds
_____ Fungicide		D. Fungi
_____ Bactericide (antibiotic)		E. Nematodes
_____ Algicide		F. Rats & Mice

Lethal Doses: Toxicologists often talk about how toxic a chemical is by determining how much toxin is needed to kill a living organism. These are called lethal doses. Pesticides can be ingested (oral), applied to the surface of the pest (dermal or contact), or inhaled by a pest. Lethal doses are determined for the pest in the laboratory, but comparing a plant, insect or fungal lethal dose to a human lethal dose doesn't make much sense. Therefore, to get a RELATIVE idea of how toxic these chemicals are, we test pesticides against a standard animal, usually the poor rat or mouse. While it is obvious that rats and mice are not humans, they are mammals and have fairly similar physiologies to humans.

The term used to give us an idea of the relative toxicity of chemicals is generally called the LD50 (lethal dose that would kill 50% of the individuals in the test population). When a new chemical is identified to have pesticide properties (actually, all chemicals have to undergo this procedure in order to be approved for use by the government!), groups of rats are given a range of doses. These rats are then watched to see how many die at each dose. A graph is constructed and the amount of the chemical that would theoretically kill 50% is calculated. This is the LD50. For oral and dermal LD50s, the units are given in milligrams of toxicant per kilogram of body weight (mg/kg). Therefore, a chemical that has an LD50 of 10.5 mg/kg is very toxic, but a chemical that has an LD50 of 2300 mg/kg is low in toxicity. In short, the smaller the LD50 number, the MORE TOXIC a chemical is! This can be confusing!

Looking up some LD_{50}s – Go to the Internet and look up the LD_{50}s for the following chemicals. Just enter in the chemical name followed by "LD_{50}" and see what your search engine finds. In science, we often use the Chemical Handbook which lists the attributes of thousands of chemicals

________ Asprin	________ Acetaminophen
________ Caffeine	________ Sugar
________ Ethyl Alcohol	________ Bleach (sodium hypochlorite)
________ Joy Dishwashing Detergent	________ Table Salt (sodium chloride)
________ DDT	________ Delta-endotoxin (*Bacillus thuringiensis*)
________ Carbaryl (Sevin insecticide)	________ Imidacloprid (Merit insecticide)
________ Fipronil (flea & ant insecticide)	________ Azadirachtin (botanical insecticide)
________ Clothianidin (Arena insecticide)	________ Chlorantraniliprole (Acelepryn)

DDT was banned in the United States in the 1970s, Sevin is one of the most commonly used home and garden insecticides, Fipronil is in Frontline pet topical flea and tick control, Merit is the most commonly used grub insecticide, and Acelepryn is the new insecticide for urban landscape use.

While LD50 helps us determine relative, acute (single dose) toxicity, there are other issues with pesticides (and chemicals). Most chemicals are taken into the body over time in small, sub-acute doses. Studies are performed (again with rats or mice) where the chemical is fed to the animals at low doses over time. The blood or tissues are sampled to see if the chemical is building up (to lethal levels) or is being eliminated. Chemicals can also cause tumors, cancer and birth defects, so they are also evaluated for these effects. So, where can you find this information? You need to look at the Material Safety Data Sheet (MSDS). You probably already saw some of these sheets while looking up the LD50s. The MSDS sheets present data on other attributes, corrosiveness, eye irritation, skin irritation, inhalation effects, and etc.

U.S. Environmental Protection Agency Pesticide Categories – In order to make availability, use and proper handling of pesticides a more simple process, the US-EPA has set up four pesticide categories:

	Signal Word	Symbol	Oral LD_{50}	Relative Toxicity
Category I	Danger-Poison!	Skull & CB	<50 mg/kg	highly toxic
Category II	Warning	none	51-500	moderately toxic
Category III	Caution	none	501-5000	low toxicity
Category IV	Caution (or none)	none	>5000	practically non-toxic

CHAPTER 1

LIFE-CYCLE ASSESSMENT OF NEONICOTINOID PESTICIDES

Natalia TG and Robert MH

Keywords: Neonicotinoid; Pesticide; Imidacloprid; Thiamethoxam

INTRODUCTION

Insecticides are a class of pesticides used to kill, harm, or repel different species of insects. They act in different ways in organisms based on their active ingredients. For instance, corn plantations commonly use insecticides that have organophosphates and carbamate as the active ingredient, which acts on the enzyme acetylcholinesterase within an insect nervous system. In many cases, these standard insecticide products are being phased out for a new class of insecticide known as neonicotinoids, which use nicotine as the active ingredient. Neonicotinoid compounds interact with nicotinic acetylcholine receptors (nAChR) of the central nervous systems of insects [1]. Nicotine acts in an insect's system in the same way that it acts in the human body. However, neonicotinoids are more toxic for invertebrates than they are to mammals, birds and other higher organisms. Neonicotinoids became popular because of their high water solubility, which makes their soil application travel through the entire plant. Nowadays, neonicotinoids are one of the most widely used class of insecticides for controlling sucking insects and soil insects. In 2004, the worldwide annual usage of neonicotinoids was approximately 11-15% of the total insecticides in the market [2]. Different generations of neonicotinoids have been created over time. They have the same principle of action in the nervous system; however, the specific active ingredients are different. The first generation of this pesticide class used was 1-(6-chloro-1,3-thiazol- 5-ylmethyl)-1,3,5-oxadiazinan-4-ylidenene(nitro)amine, known as Imidacloprid. It was first registered for use in the United States by the United States Environmental Protection Agency in 1994. It is the most widely used generation of neonicotinoids, and there are several hundred Imidacloprid-based products for sale in U.S. In 2006, the worldwide sales of those products were near $1.6 billion [3]. In 2009, Imidacloprid was applied to hundreds of thousands of acres in California, one of the most used pesticides that time [4]. Some commercial examples of this class of insecticide are Gaucho® (seed treatment), Admire® (soil application), Provado® (foliar application), Merit® (turf and ornamental use) and Premise® (termite control). Most are produced by Bayer Company [5]. The second generation of neonicotinoids is known as Thiamethoxam. The most active ingredient is 1-(6-chloro-1,3-thiazol- 5-ylmethyl)-1,3,5-oxadiazinan-4-ylidenene(nitro)amine. It was first approved in 1999 for use as an antimicrobial wood preservative and as a pesticide. The main products of this generation are produced

Citation: Natalia TG, Robert MH (2016) Life-Cycle Assessment of Neonicotinoid Pesticides. J Fertil Pestic 7:165. doi:10.4172/2471-2728.1000165

by Syngenta Company, including Platinum®, Actara®, Centric®, Cruiser®. Flagship® and Helix® among others [6]. Those products were introduced in the US market in 2001 [5]. Even though neonicotinoids have different effects in mammals and insects, they are a source of large concerns in the world. Many countries in the EU and around the world have banned the use of these chemicals. This is primarily because some classes of neonicotinoids have been demonstrated to be quite toxic for bees and other beneficial insects. Many studies show that bee disorders are being caused by the contamination of this type of insecticide in plant nectars that feed bees (A review of Research into the Effects of Neonicotinoids Insecticides on Bees, with Recommendations for Actions by The Xerces Society for Invertebrate Conservation) [7]. These beneficial insects are responsible for more than $15 billion in crop production in United States annually [8]. Many studies are being developed to analyze the actual risk of neonicotinoids in those insects. Also, neonicotinoids can persist in the soil for years, so it may contaminate other plants and nontarget species over time. Pesticides may contaminate water, soil, fish, and other living species [9,10]. One important study method used to assess the potential environmental impacts of products and systems is Life Cycle Assessment (LCA). This technique has been applied to many different products throughout many different industries, but the generally accepted best practices for LCA consist of [11] rigorously defining the goal, scope, and system boundary of the study, [12] compiling an inventory of the important flows of materials and energy throughout the product life cycle system boundary, [5] assessing the environmental impacts of this inventory data with a transparent and replicable impact assessment method, and [4] interpreting data to define new study conditions or suggest improvements to the product life cycle (ISO, 2006). Ideally, an LCA study should be cradle-to-grave, examining environmental impacts throughout the product life cycle, from extraction of raw materials, to product assembly, use, and finally to disposal of wastes. In this article, a life cycle assessment method is used to quantify the environmental impacts of production, transport, and usage of the active ingredients in two common neonicotinoids, Imidacloprid and Thiamethoxam. SimaPro 8.0 LCA software was used in conjunction with the Ecoinvent life cycle inventory database [13] to construct product life cycles for both pesticide active ingredients and assess the impacts, in terms of regards of human health and ecosystem quality. Additional discussions regarding the toxicity and persistence in the environmental after their application, and how this would impact the environmental impacts of these products, are also offered based on a literature review of their use in typical cultivation systems.

STUDY METHODS

Goal and Scope

The goal of this study is to determine the environmental impacts of two different generations of neonicotinoids, Imidacloprid and Thiamethoxam, resulting from their production, transport, and ultimate application in the environment. The environmental impacts being assessed are terrestrial ecotoxicity, aquatic ecotoxicity, and human health impacts. The functional unit used in this experiment is 1 kg of insecticide applied to land. The system boundary includes production and transport of materials and energy used in the production, transport, and application stages of each pesticides life cycle. Figure 1 displays the system boundary along with key inputs that are described in more detail below. In each scenario for the two different pesticides, the application stage is assumed to take place on a farm in the State of Ceará, Brazil, as a common point of reference.

Life Cycle Inventory

To accomplish this life cycle assessment study, information on the inputs of materials and energy related to the full product life cycles was collected from a variety of peer-reviewed publications, government reports, and other sources. The following sections summarize the key inputs of materials and energy that have been considered in each stage of the insecticide life cycle, along with key assumptions relating to the development of this input data.

Production stage: Imidacloprid production was summarized in a 2006 article originating from the Institut fur Lebensmittelchemie in Germany [14], and this information is utilized in this study to model the production of this pesticide. There are alternate routes to production [15], but few studies include as much detail on the synthesis as the Schippers and Schwack work [14]. The synthesis is divided in five steps with an overall yield of 10%. In the beginning, ammonia is used to react with coumalic acid methyl ester to form the hydroxyl nicotinic acid. This is the cheapest way to start the production of the insecticide. All products and their amounts are specified in Table 1, with an estimated production of 1.01 grams of Imidacloprid. These amounts were scaled up proportionally to the reported yield in order to model a production of 1 kg in the life cycle model. In the synthesis procedure, some reactions need heating and cooling as part of the process. In order to estimate the energy usage required for these steps in a commercial application, an assumption was made that heat can be provided or removed from the system via a heat exchange system with an efficiency of 80%, using water as the exchange fluid. Some reagents utilized in this synthesis method were not available in the Ecoinvent database, and in these cases similar products were used or the creation of the required reagents was modeled using required inputs when present within the Ecoinvent database. These assumptions have been noted in Table 1. Reagents used just to wash or extract a chemical were assumed to require 50 mL per washing step in this production process, unless otherwise indicated in Table 1. Thiamethoxam synthesis was modeled according to the route described in a paper from Syngenta Crop Protection researchers [16]. The materials and energy requirements for synthesis of 220 g of Thiamethoxam at 98% purity are presented in Table 2, and are scaled up to a production of 1 kg with our LCA model to be consistent with the functional unit of this study. Similar assumptions are used in this production unit operation as were used for Imidacloprid, namely that heat exchangers can or remove heat from the system while operating at an efficiency of 80%, and the specific heat of water is used to represent the solution heat capacity and working heat exchange fluid. The main compound used in this production system is dimethyl carbonate. It is used in the production in different steps, however in Table 2 it is shown in a single amount. Transportation stage: Inputs and assumptions for the transportation stage can be seen in Table 3, where 1 kg of the pesticide was moved according to the following multi-modal transportation scheme. Each of the neonicotinoid pesticides are produced in commercial quantities at locations far away from the farm field in Ceará where the pesticides are used in this scenario, which reflects the global supply chains that many chemicals currently have. For each pesticide, the predominant production facility was assumed according to available public information. Transportation from the production facilities in India (Imidacloprid) and Germany (Thiamethoxam) to the nearest local commercial scale port facility was accomplished with truck transportation profiles available in the Ecoinvent database, followed by shipping from the ports in the respective countries to the city of Fortaleza. Final truck transportation to a farm field in central Ceará was assumed to be equivalent in each scenario.

Application stage: In the application stage, this LCA study attempts to quantify the impacts associated with the actual application activity required to spread the pesticides on a farm field, along with the resultant impacts of that soil application. The use of machinery to apply insecticides to the field is included in the study. The most common way to apply neonicotinoids in the environment is using the in-furrow method with tractors, which is faster and safer for workers. This is possible because both pesticides area able to translocate throughout the plants from the roots. AmTide Imidacloprid 2F, a commercial product of Imidacloprid, is applied in a maximum rate in of 0.35 kg / ha in potatoes and other tuber-based agricultural cultivation systems (Amtide). Thiamethoxam needs to be applied in a rate of 0.14 kg/ ha of soil [10] in for cultivation of potatoes and other tubers. Using a consistent tractor fuel usage rate of 2.6 L diesel/ha of soil [11], it is possible to calculate the tractor fuel requirements for spreading 1 kg of each pesticide. To account for the other inputs of materials and energy (tractor production, equipment use) and other engine emissions, a pesticide application process profile in Ecoinvent was modified to include the appropriate level of fuel consumption and fuel combustion per hectare as indicated in Ref. [11], and used to model the overall application process. After being applied in the environment, pesticides generally move into soil and water at variable rates, where they may interact with several different non-target species, and this is a subject of much recent research interest. The half-life of Imidacloprid in soil has been reported in different conditions. On average, it is 130 days, but it can increase with the pH or absence of light [17]. For Thiamethoxam, the half-life is 47-54 days in presence of light [6]. It means that both pesticides persist in the soil for a long time so it can interact with other plants or living species in the soil. The study of hydrolysis of those insecticides is a useful method to analyze their persistence and potential contamination of water bodies. After application, neonicotinoids can reach either lakes or groundwater. Sunlight makes the hydrolysis faster, however Imidacloprid can persist in the water for more than 30 days in pH 7 [18] and Thiamethoxam can be stable at pH 5 and persist for 580 days in pH 7 [19]. As insecticides are persistent in the soil and water, they can interact with different living species. Neonicotinoids act in different ways in mammals and insects, but they can be toxic to humans and mammals in general. Many studies show the lethal dose in rats or rabbits as model species. Once in the environment, Imidacloprid and Thiamethoxam can get in human bodies from different routes, such as oral, dermal, and inhalation, with potentially different toxic effects from different routes of exposure. Using rats as an example, the lethal dose for 50% of exposed animals (LD50, a common toxicity metric) via oral exposure is 450 mg/kg for Imidacloprid [20]. For Thiamethoxam, the LD50 is 100 mg/kg [21]. They are classified as moderately toxic. Some signs of toxicity with Imidacloprid in humans are drowsiness, dizziness, vomiting, disorientation, increased heart and respiratory rates, and fever. However, when neonicotinoids contaminate foods, they generally do not represent a risk for human health due to the low dosage and relatively rapid excretion. In regards to carcinogenicity, Imidacloprid has been classified into Group E, meaning there is no evidence of carcinogenicity in studies with rats [22]. However, a study of human lymphocytes exposed to greater than 5200 μg/ml of Imidacloprid demonstrated a slight increase in chromosome abnormalities in vitro [23]. Studies for Thiamethoxam show that it does not have a carcinogen risk for humans and rats too [24]. In bees or other insects, the impacts can be more serious. Since bees are more similar to the target insects of neonicotinoids, the lethal dose for them is smaller. Because of it, many disorders are being caused in different cultivations around the world. Pesticides can affect bees though direct contact or though ingestion of pollen or nectar. The lethal dose needed to kill 50% of bees is 0.0037 μg/bee of Imidacloprid via oral and 0.0179 μg/bee via contact [25]. For Thiamethoxam, the LD50 for honey bees is 0.005 μg/bee via oral and 0.024 μg/bee via contact [26]. Thus, both classes of insecticides are classified as highly toxic to honey bees. Since Imidacloprid and Thiamethoxam are not present within the set of pesticides available within the current Ecoinvent database or the environmental impact assessment methods available to quantify the ecosystem or human health impacts, a similar insecticide available within the LCA modeling platform was used as a proxy. Relative toxicity values between the three pesticides were then used to simulate the appropriate exposure impact in land, water, and air. Fenvalerate is a pyrethrin insecticide, and is considered moderately toxic to mammals and highly toxic to insects, including bees. The LD50 for Fenvalerate in rats is 451 mg/kg, which is very similar to Imidacloprid and 4.5-fold higher than Thiamethoxam. The assumption used for this study followed the guidance of available rat exposure data, that 1 kg of Imidacloprid emission to the environment could be reasonably represented by 1 kg of Fenvalerate emissions, while 4.5 kg of Fenvalerate emissions would have to be used to represent 1 kg of Thiamethoxam emissions to the environment. Fenvalerate is classified as highly toxic to bees with a reported LD50 of 0.017 μg / bee, similar to the neonicotinoid pesticides [27].

Impact Assessment

To analyze different environmental impacts, the SimaPro LCA tool includes several established impact assessment methods that characterize different aspects of environmental impact. The method used in this experiment is Impact 2002+. This methodology proposes a feasible implementation a combined midpoint/damage approach, linking all types of life cycle inventory results via 14 midpoint categories to 4 damage categories [28-30], which is explained in greater detail in other resources. For this study, the two endpoint damage categories being assessed are ecosystem quality and human health impacts. Ecosystem quality is quantified by combining multiple midpoint indicators and is expressed in terms of Potentially

Disappeared Fraction (PDF) of species ovre a certain area per year, in this case PDF/m2/yr. Human Health impacts are also quantified by combining several midpoint indicators, and are cumulatively expressed in terms of Disability-adjusted Life Years (DALY), accounting for human health in terms of changing mortality and morbidity related to environmental impacts [31-36].

RESULTS AND DISCUSSION

A summary of endpoint results for the life cycle Human Health and Ecosystem Quality impacts of each pesticide can be seen in Table 4. Results are separated into each stage of the life cycle, and several of the most impactful items in each stage are shown as well. Figures 2 and 3 display the results of the midpoint indicators that contribute to the ultimate quantification of the two endpoint categories. Because each of the midpoint categories are assessed using different units, a normalization procedure was performed in order to display them on the same Figures with each other. Life cycle results for Imidacloprid in each of the midpoint categories were normalized to a value of 1.0, to remove the influence of different units. Life cycle results for Thiamethoxam were also normalized on the same basis, in order to facilitate comparison between the two pesticides across a range of midpoint categories.

Imidacloprid Life Cycle

The production stage of the imidacloprid life cycle is a significant source of environmental impacts, especially concerning Human Health, where roughly 90% of the life cycle impacts occur (7.11 × 10-4 DALY). These large impacts at the production stage stem from the reliance of pesticide production on organic chemicals such as ethyl acetate or acetone to serve as solvents or washing agents for various parts of the production process. In addition to these organic agents, the NaCl used in the production stage also contributes strongly to the overall Ecosystem Quality damage of the life cycle. The small amounts of heating and cooling required for the various steps of the production stage did not contribute a significant fraction of the overall impact in either endpoint category, less than 1% of the total environmental impact in each category. Transportation of Imidacloprid from its production location in Germany to the farm field in Brazil contributes a negligible amount of impact to both the Human Health and Ecosystem Quality impact metrics. Despite the long voyage, transportation of these products is done on a large scale where 1 kg of pesticide constitutes a trivial portion of the payload in every transport step. Pesticide application is an important part of the life cycle, contributing ~8% of the overall Human Health impact, and 42% of the Ecosystem Quality impact. Interestingly, in both of these impact metrics, the contribution of the tractor use and associated infrastructure for the application of the pesticide was ~30-40X more impactful than the resulting environmental impacts associated with emission of the pesticide into the environment, as modeled by our fenvalerate proxy in the SimaPro modeling tool. Midpoint indicators from the LCA study are presented below in Figures 2 and 3 for indicators contributing to the overall Human Health and Ecosystem Quality results, respectively. In regards to the Human Health impact of Imidacloprid, the production stage was responsible for over 95% of the impacts in 5 of 6 midpoint categories, the only exception being exposure to Non-carcinogenic air pollutants. For the midpoint indicators leading to the Ecosystem Quality result, the impacts were also primarily attributable to the production stage. For Terrestrial ecotoxicity, however, impacts were split roughly evenly between production and application stages, which illustrate the impact on terrestrial organisms from pesticide application to the landscape.

Thiamethoxam Life Cycle

The LCA results for the Thiamethoxam life cycle (Table 4) illustrate some important differences from Imidacloprid. The production stage of the Thiamethoxam life cycle results in Human Health impacts that are roughly 10X smaller than the Imidacloprid system and Ecosystem Quality impacts that are roughly 20X smaller. The items responsible for the largest impact in the Thiamethoxam life cycle in both impact categories are actual regents or building blocks of reagents in the production system (coumalic acid), as opposed to the organic solvents and washing agents in the Imidacloprid system. Heating and cooling requirements were also shown to contribute less than 1% of the environmental impacts associated with the production stage, similar to the Imidacloprid case. Also similarly, the transportation stage for moving Thiamethoxam from India to Brazil was negligible in the overall product life cycle, compared to impacts associated with production or application. In the application stage, the Thiamethoxam system used more tractor transport and associated materials and energy to spread the pesticide, because the reported dosage per unit land area was lower. Most of the environmental impact at the application stage was again due to the usage of the tractor for pesticide application, as opposed to the impacts associated with Thiamethoxam exposure on the landscape, as modeled by the fenvelarate proxy compound in this study. Overall, the Thiamethoxam life cycle had Human Health impacts that were 70% lower than Imidacloprid (2.40 × 10-4 DALY vs. 7.75 × 10-4 DALY). This general result can be seen in most of the midpoint indicators that contribute to the Human Health impact (Figure 2), where the Thiamethoxam life cycle impacts are generally less than 25% of the comparable midpoint indicator score for Imidacloprid. Non-carcinogenic air pollution is the one midpoint indicator that does not follow this trend, with a higher score for Thiamethoxam that is primarily due to emissions from the production stage, which makes sense due to the higher tractor use assumed for this scenario in our 1 kg functional unit comparison, and engine exhaust is an important source of these air emissions in this life cycle. Total Ecosystem Quality impacts are 11% higher for the Thiamethoxam (189.73 vs. 170.24 PDF / m2 / yr). In the comparison of midpoint indicators contributing to the Ecosystem Quality impact score (Figure 3), very clear differences are observed between the two pesticides. In the Thiamethoxam life cycle, the production stage is the primary contributor to all Ecosystemrelated midpoint indicators, and for Aquatic and Terrestrial Ecotoxicity, the total impacts are equivalent or higher than Imidacloprid.

Alternative Functional Unit COMPARISON

When conducting an LCA study of a product or process, it is important to keep in mind the function for which that product or system is intended. For a product such as a pesticide, the ultimate service being provided is plant protection from insects. As an alternative to comparing equivalent masses of pesticide over a comparable life cycle, it may also be advisable to make comparisons between pesticides based on an equivalent level of plant protection. To illustrate this alternative comparison, the life cycle scenarios for both pesticides are represented in Table 5 on the basis of 1 ha of field protection, using the same input data and assumptions that have been outlined previously in the article. Because the reported dosage rate for Imidacloprid (the first-generation neonicotinoid pesticide) is 2.48X higher than Thiamethoxam, less Thiamethoxam is needed to provide the same level of plant protection. When the life cycles for each pesticide are normalized to 1 ha of plant protection, the inherent advantage of this lower pesticide requirement is illustrated more clearly. On a 1 ha equivalent basis, the Thiamethoxam life cycle is 87% lower in Human Health impact and 45% lower in Ecosystem Quality, compared to the Imidacloprid life cycle. As opposed to the data presented in Table 4, in this alternative LCA scenario the impacts associated with pesticide application are nearly equivalent, because each case assumes tractor usage for 1 ha of pesticide application, with minor differences due to toxicity impacts of the pesticides after application. Many of the same general points about the two pesticide life cycles made in the preceding sections about individual life cycle stages and the important factors within each stage are still true in this alternative LCA scenario, however, such as the importance of individual ingredients in each pesticide production stage, the minor contribution of pesticide transport, and the importance of the tractor usage in comparison to effects due to emissions of pesticide onto the landscape in contributing to the overall life cycle impacts calculated here.

CONCLUSION

This study represents an illustration of a method for comparing environmental impacts of pesticides across their life cycles of production, transportation, and application. This LCA method has been applied to 2 neonicotinoid pesticides, using the best available data, to compare the environmental impacts of each life cycle and offer guidance on potential areas for improvement, both for future studies and the ultimate pesticide life cycle designs. In this study, Thiamethoxam appears to offer considerable advantages over the first generation Imidacloprid pesticide, on the basis of Human Health and Ecosystem Quality. Production data for commercial products made by private industry is always difficult to acquire for the purposes of public LCA studies, but due to the importance of the production stage in this LCA, efforts should be made to continually improve the understanding of how these pesticides are made on a commercial scale, in order to reduce the uncertainly associated with modeling this stage. Once the commercial processes are better understood, more guidance can be offered in terms of how best to reduce environmental impacts of concern through eliminating certain synthesis routes, reducing use of impactful chemicals and solvents, and other approaches. The life cycles of these pesticides are likely to involve global supply chains that link production and consumption locations, but initial efforts at modeling life cycles that involve significant transportation steps reveal that these transport modes appear to influence the overall life cycle in a minimal fashion. Pesticide application should be performed as efficiently as possible, and the ability to use less pesticide when protecting a given quantity of agricultural land can have positive repercussions throughout the supply chain, as less material needs to be produced, transported, and applied to yield the same impact. Although the neonicotinoid pesticides under study here have come under considerable scrutiny for their potential impacts on bee populations, the initial attempts here to model what the Human Health and Ecosystem Quality impacts would be for pesticide application seem to indicate that the impacts associated with operating the tractor have a larger ultimate impact than the actual emissions of the pesticide itself onto the land. This toxicity modeling was performed by relating the available common toxicity metrics for the neonicotinoid pesticide and a third proxy pesticide in the SimaPro LCA modeling platform. This approach has been described in detail, but additional toxicity data for the neonicotinoid pesticides should ultimately be verified by multiple research teams and made publicly available within life cycle inventory databases and modeling platforms to facilitate the study of these environmental impacts. In addition to focusing on the toxic impact of the pesticides as they are released in the environment, this initial study suggests that the environmental impacts associated with tractor usage during pesticide application are actually a larger source of environmental harm in multiple impact categories, and this should be one large focus of the goal of achieving life-cycle reductions in the impact of pesticide use in agricultural systems.

REFERENCES

1. Yamamoto I, Casida JE (1999) Nicotinoid insecticides and the nicotinic acetylcholine receptor. p: 300.
2. Tomizawa M, Casida JE (2005) Neonicotinoid insecticide toxicology: mechanisms of selective action. Annu Rev Pharmacol Toxicol 45: 247-268.
3. Jeschke P, Nauen R (2008) Neonicotinoids-from zero to hero in insecticide chemistry. Pest Manag Sci 64: 1084-1098.
4. California Department of Pesticide Regulation (CA DPR) (2010)Summary of Pesticide Use Report Data 2009.
5. Fisher DL, Chalmers A (2007) Neonicotinoid Insecticides and Honey Bees: Technical Answers to FAQs. Ecotoxicology Section, Bayer CropScience LP.
6. Syngenta Crop Protection Group (2005) Thiamethoxam Envirofacts.
7. Hopwood J, Vaughan M, Shepherd M, Biddinger D, Mader E, et al.(2012) Are Neonicotinoids Killing Bees? A Review of Research into the Effects of Neonicotinoid Insecticides on Bees, with Recommendations for Action. The Xerces Society for Invertebrate Conservation, Portland.
8. Morse RA, Calderone NW (2000) The value of honey bees as pollinators of US crops in 2000. Bee culture 3: 1-15.
9. Hladik ML, Kolpin DW, Kuivila KM (2014) Widespread occurrence of neonicotinoid insecticides in streams in a high corn and soybean producing region, USA. Environ Pollut 193: 189-196.
10. Huseth AS, Groves RL (2014) Environmental fate of soil applied neonicotinoid insecticides in an irrigated potato

agroecosystem. PLoS One 9: e97081.

11. Adler PR, De Grosso SJ, Parton WJ (2007) Life-cycle assessment of net greenhouse-gas flux for bioenergy cropping systems. Ecol Appl 17: 675-691.
12. Amtide Imidacloprid 2F, Insecticide Informational Label. Amtide, LLC.
13. Weidema BP, Bauer C, Hischier R, Mutel C, Nemecek T,et al. (2013) Overview and methodology: Data quality guideline for the ecoinvent database version 3. Swiss Centre for Life Cycle Inventories.
14. Schippers N,Schwack W (2006)Synthesis of the 15N-labelled insecticide imidacloprid. Journal of Labelled Compounds and Radiopharmaceuticals 3: 305-310.
15. Moriya K, Shibuya K, Hattori Y, Tsuboi SI, Shiokawa K,et al. (1992) 1-(6-Chloronicotinyl)-2-nitroimino-imidazolidines and related compounds as potential new insecticides. Bioscience, biotechnology, and biochemistry 56: 364-365.
16. Maienfisch P (2006) Synthesis and properties of thiamethoxam and related compounds. Zeitschrift für Naturforschung B 61: 353-359.
17. Krohn J, Hellpointner E (2002) Environmental fate of Imidacloprid. Pflanzenschutz-Nachr 55: 1-25.
18. Kollman W, Segawa R (1995) Interim Report Of The Pesticide Chemistry Database 1995. California Department of Pesticide Regulation.
19. Karmakar R, Singh SB, Kulshrestha G (2009) Kinetics and mechanism of the hydrolysis of thiamethoxam. J Environ Sci Health B 44: 435-441.
20. Meister RT (1995) Farm Chemicals Handbook. Meister Publishing Company. pp: 120-125.
21. Food and Agriculture Organization (2014) United Nations. FAO specifications and evaluations for agricultural pesticides: Thiamethoxam.
22. US Environmental Protection Agency (1995) Pesticide Tolerance and Raw Agricultural commodities: Imidacloprid. 40 CFR Part 180 Section 472.
23. World Health Organization (WHO) (2004) Toxicological Evaluations: Imidacloprid. International Programme on Chemical Safety, Roland Solecki.
24. Green T, Toghill A, Lee R, Waechter F, Weber E, et al. (2005) Thiamethoxam induced mouse liver tumors and their relevance to humans part 1: Mode of action studies in the mouse. Toxicological Sciences 86: 36-47.
25. European Food Safety Authority (EFSA) (2013) Conclusion on the peer review of the pesticide risk assessment for bees for the active substance thiamethoxam. EFSA J 11: 3067.
26. Laurino D, Manino A, Patetta A, Porporato M (2013) Toxicity of neonicotinoid insecticides on different honey bee genotypes. Bulletin of Insectology 66: 119-126.
27. US Environmental Protection Agency (EPA) (1991) Asana: Honey Bee Data Memorandum. Office of Pesticides and Toxic Substances.
28. Jolliet O, Margni M, Charles R, Humbert S, Payet J, et al. (2003) IMPACT 2002+: a new life cycle impact assessment methodology. The International Journal of Life Cycle Assessment 8: 324-330.
29. Decker M (2001) US Patent No. 6,214,998. Washington, DC: US Patent and Trademark Office.
30. International Organization for Standardization (ISO) (2006) 14044: environmental management—life cycle assessment—requirements and guidelines.
31. Mathiesen K, Goldenburg S (2016) US government says widely used pesticide could harm honeybees. The Guardian.
32. Smith NR,WileyRH (1963) Isodehydroacetic acid and ethyl isodehydroacetate. Organic Syntheses. pp: 76-76.
33. Syngenta (2016) Company History.
34. The Economic Times (2004) Bayer Crop invests Rs 15 cr in insecticide plant via JV.
35. Tundo P, Selva M (2002) The chemistry of dimethyl carbonate. Acc Chem Res 35: 706-716.
36. Walker J, Johnston J (1905) C—Tetramethylammonium hydroxide. Journal of the Chemical Society, Transactions 87: 955-961.

CHAPTER 2

TOXICITY AND BIOCHEMICAL EFFECT OF ORGANOPHOSPHATES AND BIO-PESTICIDES AGAINST ROOT-KNOT NEMATODE, MELOIDOGYNE INCOGNITA

Hoda M. Nasr

INTRODUCTION

Plant–parasitic nematodes are recognized as the causes of serious yield losses on a wide range of crops [1]. The most destructive species is Meloidogyne incognita which cause serious problem in various agricultural crops. Root–knot nematode, Meloidogyne incognita Kofoid and White Chitwood (Tylenchida: Heteroderidae) is a major plant parasitic nematodes affecting quantity and quality of the crop production in many annual and perennial crops. Infected plants show typical symptoms including root galling stunting and nutrient deficiency, particularly nitrogen deficiency [2]. M. incognita causing an estimated yearly crop loss of $100 billion worldwide [3]. Nematodes are difficult to control because of their wide host range and high rate of reproduction, with females capable of producing up to thousandeggs/ female [4]. Chemical control is expensive and is economically viable only for high value crops and creates a potential hazard to the environment and human health [5]. Biopesticides currently are integrated into many diverse agricultural production schemes. These materials can be effective and safe, but their use requires more sophistication than chemical pesticides on the part of the user. Many of these products have specific requirements for storage and application, and to treat them like a chemical pesticide often results in failure. As biological organisms they require appropriate biotic as well as abiotic conditions for success. Users would benefit from learning how to maximize efficacy before or after the organisms have been applied. Among microorganisms regulating nematode densities in soil, fungi hold an important position due to their parasitic, antagonistic or predatory behaviors. Some species have potentials in biocontrol and exhibit a range of antagonistic activities, including production of nematotoxic compounds [2,6,7]. Nematophagous fungi directly parasitize nematodes or secrete nematicidal metabolites affecting viability of one or more stages. The search for nematotoxic or antagonistic compounds in culture filtrates hasgreatly intensified in recent years, due to the number of toxins, enzymes or compounds derivable from their metabolites [8-10]. Inhibition of ChE activity is one of the best characterized biomarkers and has been intensively used in environmental studies, showing a specific response to organophosphate (OP) and carbamate pesticides [11,12]. Abamectin is a macrocyclic lactone derived from the soil bacterium Streptomyces avermitilis that has been shown to have nematicidal properties [13]. And a different mode of action than the other currently available nematicides

Citation: Nasr HM (2015) Toxicity and Biochemical Effect of Organophosphates and Bio-pesticides against Root-knot Nematode, Meloidogyne incognita. J Pollut Eff Cont 4:151. doi:10.4172/2375-4397.1000151

[14]. It is suitable compound for seed treatment since it can be stored for several months while maintaining its nematicide properties. It can be applied to seeds at high concentrations, does not bio-accumulate and is not taken up by plants [15]. Cadusafos is an organophosphorus nematicide under the trade name "Rugby, Cadusafos controls a wide range of plant parasitic nematodes, such as Tylenchulus semipenetrans [16]. ChE stands out as an ideal biomarker to evaluate agriculture-related pollution effects in the area. Further, it would be useful to trace a link between pesticide use, detection of residues in the environment and their toxic effects AChE has been widely studied in many different species because it can be inhibited by Ops and CAs. ATP ase is a group of enzymes that play an important role in intracellular functions and that are considered to be a sensitive indicator of toxicity [17]. It can be target for many groups of pesticides. The aim of this is to investigates the effect of Organophosphates (cadusafos , fenitrothion) and the Biopesticides (abamectin, biofly) against root knot nematode Meloidogyne incognita also The potency of these pesticides to inhibit acetylcholine esterase (AChE) and adenosine triphosphatase (ATPase) activity of such root knot nematode.

MATERIALS AND METHODS

Nematode Cultures

The root-knot nematode M. incognita was isolated from infected roots of eggplant (Solanum melongena L.) obtained from El-Nubaria region, Behera Governorate, Egypt. Eggs and second-stage juveniles (J2) were extracted from infected roots by the sodium hypochlorite method [18].

Synthetic Insecticides

Abamectin: Group name: Avermectin (Biopesticide) Common name: Abamectin Trade name: Vabcomic Empirical formula: $C_{48}H_{72}O_{14}$ (80% avermectin B1a); $C_{47}H_{70}O_{14}$ (20% avermectin B1b) Molecular weight: 873.1 (avermectin B1a); 860.1 (avermectin B1b) Formulation: 1.8% E.C. Source: Hebei Veyong Bio-Chemical Co, ltd, china).

Biofly: Group name: Biological insecticide Common name: Beauveria bassiana Used and applied rate: Entomopathogenic fungus used for control of a wide range of coleopteran, homopteran and heteropteran pests. Fungus applied at rate of 100cm3/100liter water Trade name: Biofly Source: E1-Nasr Bio insecticides and Fertilizers Company, E1-Sadaat, Egypt.

Cadusafos: Group name: Organophosphorus, Common name. cadusafos Trade name: Rugby.Chemical name (IUPAC): S,S-di-secbutyl O-ethyl phosphorodithioate Empirical formula: $C_{10}H_{23}O_2PS_2$ Molecular weight: 270.4 Formulation: 20% E.C a Use: Agricultural Nematicide / Insecticide .Source: FMC Australasia Pty Ltd.

Fenitrothion: Group name: Organophosphorus Common name: Fenitrothion Trade name: Fentro Chemical name (IUPAC): O,Odimethyl O-4-nitro-m-tolyl phosphorothioate Empirical formula: $C_9H_{12}NO_5PS$ Molecular weight: 277.2 Formulation: 50% E.C applied at rate of 250 cm3/100 liter water Use: insecticides Source: Agrochem, Alwatneia Company, Alex., Egypt.

Nematicidal Assay on Eggs

M. incognita was cultured in the greenhouse on tomato plants (New L-402, nematode susceptible) inoculated with a single nematode egg mass [18]. After 55 days, egg masses were hand-picked from galls of tomato roots and surface sterilized in 0.5% sodium hypochlorite for 3 min and washed with sterile water 3 Times. J2 were hatched from the egg masses, collected daily and Stored at 4°C. 2ml of egg masses of nearly uniform size were transferred to a 6cm-diameter autoclaved Petri dishes containing 2ml filtrate of different dilutions of (1.8% abamectins, 100% biofly 20% cadusafos and 50% fentrothion) the series of concentration were around recommended dose of each pesticides ,eggs maintained at the same volume of disteled water served as controls; three replicates of each treatment and control were included. Plate lids were sealed with parafilm and the plates were kept at 25°C. After 7 days hatched J2 were counted with the use of an inverted microscope and egg hatched reduction for a treatment was calculated as: average % of non-hatched J2 in the filtrate/average % non-hatch in control with sterilized water × 100.

Nematicidal Assay Second Stage Juveniles (J2)

2ml of the above solutions as previously described from each concentration was added to 2ml of nematode suspensions M. incognita second stage juveniles & in 50 ml glass capsule. A control treatment was made by adding 2ml of distilled water plus 2ml of the nematode suspension. Each treatment was replicated three times. The number oviable and dead nematodes was counted with the aid of a light microscope after 24, 48 and 72hrs at 25 ± 1°C and the nematode mortality was calculated for each treatment. Only the nematodes which did not regain motility were considered "dead". The mortality percentage was calculated according to the Abbott's [19] formula:

Whereas: m and n percentages mortality in treated sample and control.

Enzyme Preparation

1ml, of nematode suspension or egg filtrate of each pesticides mixture stoked for 48 hrs from bioassay test were homogenized with ice cold buffer for 30 s and a small amount of glass beads (<106 1 m, Sigma) were adding during homogenization with cooling to obtain at least 95% breakage. Homogenate was centrifuged. The clear supernatant was collected and kept frozen at -20°C until assayed.

Enzyme Determination

Acetylcholinesterse (AChE) activity: The AChE was determined by the colorimetric method of Ellman et al. [20]. The suspension was homogenized in 0.1M phosphate buffer (pH 7.0). The homogenates were then centrifuged at 5,000 rpm for 20 min at 0°C. The supernatants were used as enzyme source for assay of AChE activity. Enzyme (150 uL), 100ul DTNB (0.01 M), and 30 uL ATChI (0.075 M) were added to 2.8 mL 0.1 M phosphate buffer (pH 8.0). The mixture was incubated at 37°C for 15 min. The absorbance was measured at 412 nm using Unico 1200 spectrophotometer. All of the treatments were done in triplicate. The specific activity of AChE was expressed as nmoles of acetylthiocholine iodide hydrolyzed/mg protein/min. Inhibition percentages of the activities against control were estimated in the enzymatic assay. Total protein assay: Total protein was determined according to Lowry et al. [21]. This method was used to determine the protein content in nematode extract Protein extract (100 uL) was added to 2 mL alkaline copper reagent [48 of 2% (w/v) sodium carbonate in 0.1N sodium hydroxide 1 mL 1% (w/v) sodium-potassium tartrate 1 mL 0.5% (w/v) copper sulfate] and immediately mixed. After 10 min, 0.2 mL Folin-Ciocalteu phenol reagent was added and the samples were thoroughly mixed, then the absorbance of the developed blue color was measured at 600 nm using a Unico 1200 spectrophotometer. The protein content of the sample was determined by comparing to the standard curve of BSA.

Adenosine triphosphatase (ATPase) activity assay: ATPase activity was determined according to Koch [22]. After 48 h of bioassay test on the tested concentration, the nematode suspension was homogenized in Tris-HCl buffer (pH 7.4). The homogenates were centrifuged at 5,000 rpm for 10 min at -4°C. The supernatant was then centrifuged at 17,000 rpm for 30 min at -4°C. The pellets were resuspended in the same buffer. This suspension was used as enzyme source for the assay of ATPase activity. The enzyme activity was determined colorimetrically according to. Enzyme suspension was added to the reaction mixture that contained 100 mM NaCl, 20 mM KCl, 5 mM Mg2Cl, and 5 mM ATP and the volume was adjusted to 8501 L with Tris-HCl buffer (pH 7.4). This mixture was incubated at 37°C for 15 min and then stopped with 150 uL TCA. Four milliliters of fresh color reagent (5 g ferrous sulfate in 10 mL ammonium molybdate solution prepared in 10 N sulfuric acid) was added and absorbance was measured at 740 nm by using a Unico 1200 spectrophotometer. The enzyme activity was represented as micromoles inorganic phosphorus (Pi/mg protein/h). Inhibition percentages of the activities compared with control were considered in the enzymatic assay.

Statistical Analysis

Data obtained were statistically analyzed according to SAS software program [23] Statistical analysis was performed using the SPSS 12.0 software program (Statistical Package for Social Sciences, USA). The log dose–response curves allowed determination of the LC50 values for the nematode bioassay according to probit analysis [24]. The 95% confidence limits for the range of LC50 were determined by leastsquare regression analysis of the relative growth rate (percentage of control) against the logarithm of the compound concentration. The data for AChE and ATPase activities were analyzed by one-way analysis of variance (ANOVA).

RESULTS

Toxicity of the tested pesticides to M .incognita

Results in (Tables 1a-1c and Table 2) indicated that all tested pesticides have toxic effect against M. incognita second-stage juveniles (J2) after 24 hrs of application while abamectin was the most toxic one with LC50 value 2.94 mg/L followed by 147.44 mg/L for fenitrothion, 976.77 mg/L for cadusafos while biofly was the least toxic one with LC50 value of3190.18 mg/L. The toxicity increased after 48 hrs of treatment and the LC50 value were (1.68 & 34.69 & 163.13 and 877.98) respectively for abamectin, fenitrothion, cadusafos and biofly. The same trend of toxicity observed after 72 hrs of treatment abamectin was most toxic one followed by, fentirothion & cadusafos and biofly was least toxic with LC50 value (1.07, 20.64, 47.6 and 386.48) mg/L respectively. On the other hand the effect of the same tested solutions on Percentage of egg hatched reduction was calculated as: average % of non-hatched J2 in the filtrate/ average % non-hatch in control with sterilized water × 100. Result in Table 2 indicated that abamectin was most effective in hatching reducing of M. incognita followed by cadusafos, fenitrothion and biofly was the least effective one with the LC50value (1.102. 308.04, 577.69, 620.62)mg/L, respectively.

The in vivo inhibitory effect of abamectin, biofly, cadusafos and fentrothion to M. incognita Acetylcholinesterase (AChE) activity

The in vivo inhibitory effect of the above pesticides on AChE activity isolated from culture filtrate of M. incognita second stage juveniles (J2) and eggs filtrates was examined and the results are presented in Tables 3 and 4. Specific activity calculated as (n moles of acetylthiocholine iodide hydrolyzed/mg protein/min). Percentage of inhibition was calculated. It was observed that pesticides induced decrease in AChE activity compared with the control. Cadusafos was tested at concentration ranged between 300 to 6000 mg/L all concentration had inhibitory effect on AChE activity and the high inhibitory effect was found at 6000 mg/L it induced 94.81 inhibition the inhibition percentage are dose dependent (Table 3). Abamectin at concentrations ranged from 4.5 to 0,25 mg/ L decreases the activity of nematode second stage juveniles AChE in all tested concentration and the most inhibitory effect was 73.93 at 4.5 mg/L followed by biofly it decreased the activity of larval second stage enzyme to 68.28 at 2000 mg/L. It was observed that fenitrothion had least inhibitory effect on AChE activity and the percentage of inhibition was 57.19 at 1250 mg/L. data a (Table 4), illustrate the inhibition of AChE activity in M. incognita egg filtrates abamectin at 4.5 mg/L induced 73.93 while Cadusafos at 6000 mg/L induced 64.81 inhibition followed by biofly at 2000/mg L induced 62.73 inhibition fenitrothion induced only 44.34 inhibition at 1250 mg/L it was least effective on the in vivo effect inhibition of AChE activity in M. incognita egg filtrates than second stage juveniles (J2) It was observed that all the tested pesticides has an inhibitory effect on AChE activity and the inhibitory effect increased when the pesticides applied at the juveniles more than egg filtrates.

The in vivo effect of abamectin, biofly, cadusafos and fenitrothion to M. incognita ATPase activity.

Result indicated that abamectin was more effective than other pesticides on ATPase activity and the inhibition increase in case of egg filtrates than second stage juveniles (J2) it was 90.44 with egg filtrates at 4.5 mg/L of abamectin while it was 81.95 at the same concentration in case of juveniles (Tables 5 and 6). Biofly had the same inhibitory effect on ATPase activity and it was 81.98 at 2000 mg/L with egg filtrates and 78.80 at the same concentration with juveniles. Cadusafos and fentrothion had low inhibitory effect on ATPase activity in nematode egg filtrates and second stages juveniles comparing with abamectin and biofly.

DISCUSSION

This study illustrated the possibility of using abamectin and biofly (biological pesticides) in controlling M. incognita instead of using the chemical pesticides to decrease the environmental pollutants of organophosphates, carbamates and other group of pesticides because the excessive use of organophosphates in agriculture has originated serious problems in the environment [25]. Although, these pesticides degrade quickly in water, there is always the possibility that residues and byproducts will remain, in relatively harmful levels in the organisms [26]. So this work indicates that abamectin the Bioproducts which based on pathogenic micro-organisms often referred as microbial pesticides; they are host specific and are potential candidates with regard to integrated pest management [27]. It has to be effective in controlling root knot nematode as cadusafos and more toxic than fenitrothion the organophosphate pesticides this result was in agreement with El-Nagdi and Youssef [28] who found that Abamectin significantly reduced the population density of M. incognita with increasing the measured plant growth. Also Nwadinobi et al. [29] reported that Abamectin is biocides reduced galling and delayed invasion and development of Meloidogyne spp. for 20 days when roots of 14 day old tomato seedlings were dipped in a low concentration of abamectin. The present study also investigates the toxicity of biofly the (biological pesticides) to nematode it act as the nematicides on its toxicity although it is less toxic than the other pesticides used but it had an inhibitory effect on both tested enzymes , it has an chemicals are inherently toxic. Therefore, alternative environment friendly measures are needed to be developed also biopesticides are often considered as one of the lowest impact on many beneficial organisms compared with other pesticides. They have attracted considerable attention recently for their inclusion in Integrated Pest Management (IPM) programs, but effects are highly variable depending on the species and studied developmental stage [30,31]. AChE activity is not due exclusively to organophosphates and carbamates, but those other classes of environmental contaminants such as complex mixtures of pollutants, detergents, and they also involved in AChE reduction [32-35]. There is general agreement that the toxic action of organophosphate and carbamate pesticides upon nematodes, insects and vertebrates is caused by their ability to inhibit acetylcholinesterase (AChE) in various parts of the nervous system, and thereby, disrupt nervoys transmission at that location [36]. So this illustrate why Cadusafos and fenitrothion had an inhibitory effect on AChE activity and why this enzyme used as biomarker for cadusafous and fenitrothion toxicity in nematode It was accepted that the mode of action of organophosphate (cadusafos) was reasonably certain that these compounds acted by the inhibition of acetylcholinesterase (AChE) at cholinergic synapses in the nematode nervous system. Inhibition of ACHE was most likely explanation for the observed effect of organosphosphate and carbamate nematicides on the orientation behavior of nematodes [37,38]. These chemicals perform their action by impairing nematode neuromuscular activity, thereby, reducing their movement, invasion, feeding and consequentially the rate of development and reproduction [39]. Bunt [40] suggested that these chemicals acted against the root-knot nematode by inhibiting egg hatching, their movement and host invasion by infective juveniles and checked further development of second stage juveniles that had penetrated the roots. Using AChE and ATP ase as biomarkers for the biofly and abamectin is considered to be a new trail to show whether this pesticides can follow this mode of action in nematode or not while results indicated that abamectin and biofly had an inhibitory effect on both enzymes this result was in agreement with Turner and Schaeffer [14] who indicated that although Abamectin is a macrocyclic lactone derived from the soil bacterium Streptomyces avermitilis that has been shown to have nematicidal properties and a different mode of action than the other currently available nematicides. Also Radwan [41] reported that Abamectin studied are needed in more precisely molecular level to strictly detect the mode of action of these pesticides. An explanation of this decrease of AchE activity could refer to the new mode of action of this biopesticides, which seem to work in a similar manner of other closely related compound (i.e., metabolites of actinomycetes) our result in agreement. This hyperactivity was different insect control agent which all of them caused either no change or a reduction in AchE activity. It seem as if it works in a reversible manner, producing an extra release of AchE which may prevents principally any message to be sent to the receptor and thus the insect become without neural orientation. Although the previously used Abamectin was believed to be of noncholinergic role, it seems that in the present study does. A hypothesis was offered to explain this decrease in AchE during the use of a closely related actinomycete derived compound Spinosad where Salgado [42] demonstrated that the receptors do so by mimicking the action of Ach at its binding site. Since Ach cannot then bind, such compounds don't enhance and usually antagonize the response to currently applied Ach. Spinosad, instead of depressing the Ach response, greatly prolongs its duration. The ability of spinosad to prolong the action of AchE indicates that it and Ach can act simultaneously and therefore that studied are needed in more precisely molecular level to strictly detect the mode of action of biopesticides as abamectin and biofly which holds much promise to control insects in a novel mode of action. ATP ase is a group of enzymes that play an important role in intracellular functions and that are considered to be a sensitive indicator of toxicity [17]. Detection of ATPase inhibition could prove to be an important index for tolerable levels of a large group of environmental contaminants [43]. In the present study, the statistical tests performed on the data represent that biofly the biological pesticides and abamectin as biopesticides has modern mode of action on inhibiting such enzyme in nematode while the organophosphates pesticides cadusafos and fenitrothion had low inhibitory effect on ATP ase this related to their mode of action as an organophosphates and their action related to the inhibition acetylcholinesterase (ACHE) at cholinergic synapses in the nematode nervous system [37,38]. Inhibition of ACHE was most likely explanation for the observed effect of organosphosphate and carbamate nematicides on the orientation behavior of nematodes. Finally, it could be concluded that the results from this study indicated that using of both organophosphates and biopesticides achieved a highly activity against the root-knot nematode, M. incognita. Therefore, the results imply that it should focus on using biological agents as a safety method for human and environment to management the root-knot nematode in Egypt.

REFERENCES

1. Javad N, Gowmen SR, Ulhaq MI, Abdullah K, Shahina F (2006) Systemic and persistent effect of neem (Azardirachtaindica) formulations against root knot nematodes, Meloidogynejavanicaand their storage life. Crop Protection 26: 911-916.
2. Siddiqui ZA, Mahmood I (1999) Role of bacteria in the management of plant parasitic nematodes: A review. Bioresource Technol. 69: 167-179.
3. Oka Y, Yermiyahu U (2002) Suppressive effect of composts against the root-knot nematode Meloidogynejavanicaon tomato. Nematology 4: 891-898.
4. Natarajan N, Cork A, Boomathi N, Pandi R, Velavan S, Dhaskshanamoorthy G (2006) Cold aqueous extracts of African marigold, Tageteserectafor control tomato root-knot nematode, Meloidogyne incognita.Crop Protection25:1210-1213.
5. Tsay TT, Wu TS, Lin YY (2004) Evaluation of asteraceae plant for control of Meloidogyne incognita. Journal of Nematology 36: 36-41.
6. Kerry BR (2000) Rhizosphere interactions and the exploitation of microbial agents for the biological control of plant-parasitic nematodes. Annu Rev Phytopathol 38: 423-441.
7. Lopez-Llorca LV, Jansson HB (2006) In: Robson GD, van West P, Gadd GM (eds.) Fungal parasites of invertebrates: multimodal biocontrol agents. Exploitation of Fungi. Cambridge University Press, Cambridge 310-335.
8. Ciancio A (1995) Observations on the nematicidal properties of some mycotoxins. Fund ApplNematol 18: 451-454.
9. Liu T, Wang L, Duan YX, Wang X (2008) Nematicidal activity of culture filtrate of Beauveriabassiana against Meloidogynehapla. World J Micro Biotec 24:113-118.
10. Lopez-Llorca LV, Macia´-Vicente JG, Jansson H-B (2008) In: Ciancio A, Mukerji KG (eds.) Mode of action and interactions of nematophagous fungi. Integrated management and biocontrol of vegetable and grain crops nematodes. Springer, NL 49-74.
11. Gruber S, Munn D (1998) Organophosphate and Carbamate insecticides in agricultural waters and Cholinesterase (ChE) inhibition in common carp (Cyprinuscarpio). Arch Environ ContamToxicol 35: 391-396.
12. Thompson H (1999) Esterases as markers of exposure to organophosphates and carbamates. Ecotoxicology 8: 369-384.
13. Putter I, Mac connell JG, Preiser FA, Haidri AA, Ristich SS et al. (1981) Avermectins: novel insecticides, acaricides and nematicides from a soil microorganism. Experientia37: 963-964.
14. Turner MJ, Schaeffer JM (1989) In: W.C. Campbell (ed.) Mode of action of ivermectin. Ivermectin and Abamectin, Springer-Verlag, New York. 73-88.
15. Dybas RA (1989) Abamectin use in crop protection. In: Ivermectinand Abamectin(ed. W.C. Campbell) Springer, New York. 287-310.
16. McCutchen WF, Flexner L (1999) In: Hall DR &Menn JJ (Eds.) Join Action of Baculovirus and Other Control Agents, Biopesticides Use and Delivery. Humana Press, ISBN 0-89603-515-8, New Jersey, USA 341-355.
17. Yadwad VB, Kallapur VL, Basalingappa S (1990) Inhibition of gill Na+ K+-ATPase activity in dragonfly larva, Pantalaflavesens, by endosulfan. Bull Environ ContamToxicol 44: 585-589.
18. Khan TA, Nasir S, Ashraf MS (2004) Effect of population levels of Meloidogynejavanicaon plant growth and nematode multiplication on cucurbits. Pak J Nematol22: 83-87.
19. Abbot WS (1925) A method of computing the effectiveness of an insecticide. J Econ Entomol18: 267-267.
20. Ellman GL, Courtney D, Andres V, Featherstone RM (1961) A newand rapid colorimetric determination of acetylcholinesterase activity. Biochem Pharm 7: 88-95.
21. Lowry OH, Rosebrough NJ, Farr AL, Randall RJ (1951) Protein measurement with the folin phenol reagent. J BiolChem 193: 265-275.
22. Koch RB (1969) Chlorinated hydrocarbon insecticides: inhibition of rabbit brain ATPase activities. J Neurochem 16: 269-271.
23. SAS Institute (1998) SAS / STAT User›s Guide. 6th Ed. SAS Institute Inc. Carry, NC, USA. 1028.
24. Finney DJ (1971) Probit analysis, 3rd edn. Cambridge University Press, London.
25. Singh BK, Walker A (2006) Microbial Degradation of Organophosphorus Compounds, FEMS Microbiology Review 30: 428-471.
26. Ragnarsdottir K (2000) Environmental Fate and Toxicology of Organophosphate Pesticides. Journal of the Geological Society London. 157: 859-876.
27. Arora R, Battu GS, Ramakrishnan N (2000)In: Dhaliwal GS and Singh B (eds.) Microbial pesticides: current status and future outlook. Pesticides and Environment. Commonwealth Publishers, New Delhi 344- 395.
28. El-Nagdi WMA, Youssef MM (2004) A soaking faba bean seed in some bio-agents as prophylactic treatment for controlling Meloidogyne incognitaroot-knot nematode infection. J of Pest Sci 77: 75-78.
29. Nwadinobi EI, Hague NGM, Gowen SR, Badmin (1989) The control of Meloidogyne incognitaon tomato using avermectin B1 as a root dip. Tests of Agrochemicals and Cultivars 10: 18-19.
30. Darvas B, Polgar LA (1998) In: Ishaaya I, Degheele D (eds.) Novel type insecticides: specificity and effects on non-target organisms. Insecticides with novel modes of action. Springer, Berlin 188-259.
31. Schneider M, Smagghe G, Vin˜uela E (2003) Susceptibility of Hyposoterdidymator (Hymenoptera: Ichenumonidae) adults to several IGRs pesticides and spinosad by different exposure methods. IOBC/wprs Bull 26:111-122.
32. Payne JF, Mathieu A, Melvin W, Fancy LL (1996) Acetylcholinesterase, an old biomarker with a new future? Fields trials in association with two urban rivers

and a paper mill in Newfounfland. Physiol 97: 275-281.

33. Bendahou N, Bounias M, Fleche C (1999) Toxicity of cypermethrin and fenitrothion on the hemolymph carbohydrates, head acetylcholinesterase, and thoracic muscle Na, K.ATPase of emerging honey bees (Apismellifera L). Ecotoxicol Environ Saf 44:139-146.

34. Frasco MF, Fournier D, Carvalho F, Guilhermino L (2005) Do metals inhibit acetylcholinesterase (AChE)? Implementation of assay conditions for the use of AChE activity as a biomarker of metal toxicity. Biomarkers 10: 360-375.

35. Guilhermino L, Barros P, Silva MC, Soares AMVM (1998) Should the use of inhibition of cholinesterases as a specific biomarker for organophosphate and carbamate pesticides be questioned? Biomarkers 3:157-163.

36. Corbett JR, Wright K, Baillie AC (1984) The Biochemical Mode of Action of Pesticides. 2nd ed. London, Academic Press, 382.

37. Wright DJ (1981) In: Zuckerman BM, Rohde RA (eds.) Nematicides: Mode of action and new approaches to chemical control. Plant parasiticnematodes.Academic Press, New York 3: 421-449.

38. Opperman CH, Chang S (1990) Plant-parasitic nematode acetylcholinesterase inhibition by carbamate and organophosphate nematicides. J Nematol22: 481-488.

39. Nelmes AJ, Trudgill DL, Corbett DCM (1973) In: Taylor AR, Muller R (Eds.) Chemotherapy in the study of plant parasitic nematodes. Chemotherapeutic Agents in the Study of Parasites. ProcSymp., British Society of Parasitology, Oxford, England 2: 95-112.

40. Bunt JA (1987)In: VeechJA, DicksonDW(eds.) Mode of action of nematicides. Vistas on Nematology: a commemorationof the 25th anniversary of the Society of NematologistSociety of Nematologist, Inc. Hyattsiville, MD. 461-468.

41. Radwan EMA (2001) Biological and Biochemical effects of certain insecticides on the spiny bollworm, Eariasinsulana(Biosd.) Ph. D. Thesis, Fac., Sci., Ain Shams Univ.

42. Salgado VL (1997) The mode of action of spinosad and other insect control Products. Down to Earth, 52: 35-34.

43. OzcanOruc E, Uner N, Tamer L (2002) Comparison of Na, K-ATPase activities and malondialdehyde contents in liver tissue for three fish species exposed to azinphosmethyl. Bull Environ ContamToxicol 69: 271-277.

CHAPTER 3

BIOPESTICIDES: PRESENT STATUS AND THE FUTURE PROSPECTS

Suresh Kumar and Archana Singh

Keywords: fertilizers; pesticides; agricultural

Agriculture is adversely affected by numerous pests like bacteria, fungi, weeds and insects, leading to reduced yield and poor quality of the produce [1]. Since 1960s, the most common method for pest control has been the intensive use of synthetic pesticides. Such pesticide was adopted in 1940s with the use of dichloro-diphenyl-trichloroethane (DDT), followed by other organophosphate and carbamate pesticides [2]. Thereafter, Green Revolution technology of crop production could increase food production in developing countries through the intensive use of inputs like chemical fertilizers and pesticides etc. Albeit, the use of the agrochemicals helped a lot in increasing agricultural productivity; they have caused adverse effects on soil health, water quality, produce quality and developed problems like insect resistance, genetic variation in plants, toxic residues food and feed. Moreover dependence on chemical pesticides and their indiscriminate use caused several detrimental effects on the. Recognizing the ill effects of the agrochemicals such as pesticide resistance, pest resurgence, outbreak of secondary pests, pesticide residues in the produce, soil, air and water [3], it has become important now to develop alternatives of these synthetic agro-inputs. The need of the day is to produce maximum from the diminishing natural resources and protect the produce from post-harvest loses without adversely affecting the environment. Use of biofertilizers and biopesticides can play major role in dealing with these challenges in a sustainable manner.

Biopesticides and biofertilizers, the naturally occurring formulations made from the substances that control pests by non toxic mechanisms and in ecofriendly manner, are not newer technologies. They have been used in various forms since human civilization. Biopesticides being a living organisms (natural enemies) or products there of pose less threat to the environment and to human health, hence can be used for the management of pests. One of the most widely used microbial biopesticides is Bacillus thuringiensis, popularly known as Bt. Potential benefits of the use of biopesticides to agriculture and public health programmes are considerable.

ADVANTAGES OF BIOPESTICIDE

Biopesticide is gaining interest because of its advantages associated with the environmental safety, target-specificity, efficacy, biodegradability and suitability in the integrated pest management (IPM) programs. Thus, biopesticide is one of the promising alternatives to manage environmental pollutions.

Citation: Kumar S, Singh A (2015) Biopesticides: Present Status and the Future Prospects. J Biofertil Biopestici 6:e129. doi:10.4172/2155-6202.1000e129

Though potential application of biopesticides in environmental safety is well known, it has gained interest in view of the growing demands for organic food. Although use of agrochemicals is indispensable to meet the ever growing demands of food, feed and fodder, opportunities do exist in selected crops and niche areas where biopesticides can be used as a component of IPM. Through wider application of biopesticides in agriculture and health programs, environmental safety can be beneficially affected.

PRESENT STATUS

Presently, biopesticides cover only 2% of the plant protectants used globally; however its growth rate shows an increasing trend in past two decades. Global production of biopesticides has been estimated to be over 3,000 tons per year, which is increasing rapidly. Increasing demand of residue-free agricultural produce, growing organic food market and easier registration than chemical pesticides are some of the key drivers of the biopesticide market. Globally, the use of biopesticides is increasing steadily by 10% every year. About 90% of the microbial biopesticides are derived from just one entomopathogenic bacterium, Bacillus thuringiensis. More than 200 products are being sold in the US market, compared to only 60 comparable products in the EU. More than 225 microbial biopesticides are manufactured in 30 OECD countries [4]. The NAFTA countries (USA, Canada, and Mexico) use about 45% of the biopesticides sold, while Asia lacks behind with the use of only 5% of biopesticides sold world over [5].

Most of the countries have amended their policies to minimize the use of chemical pesticides and promote the use of biopesticides; however biopesticides are still largely regulated by the system originally designed for chemical pesticides. This has created market entry barriers by imposing burdensome costs on the biopesticide industry [6]. Although for effective utilization of biopesticides several technological and policy gaps have been identified, they need to be addressed properly at the country level. Policy measures need to be strengthened in order to reduce excessive use of chemical pesticides and to promote the use of biopesticides.

One of the major obstacles in promoting biopesticides as alternative to chemical pesticides is the lack of profile of biopesticide, which reflects weakness of the supporting policy network. Relative immaturity of the policy network, limited resources and capabilities, and lack of trust between regulators and producers are some of the serious problems. Better understanding of the mode of action of biopesticides, their effects and regulatory issues that arise in their adoption may help further to raise their profile among the public, policy-makers and hence enable them to realize their contributions to sustainability. Since the environmental safety is a global concern, we need to create awareness among the farmers, manufacturers, government agencies, policy makers and the common men to switch-over to biopesticides for the pest management requirements.

RECENT ADVANCES

The science of biopesticide is still considered to be young and evolving. In-depth research is needed in many areas such as production, formulation, delivery and commercialization of the products. Some of the biopesticides, currently under development, may prove to be excellent alternatives to the chemical pesticides. Many of them are based on the locally available plants like beshram, neem, garlic, triphala, pinus kesia etc. which can be easily processed and made available to the farmers to improve biopesticide consumption. In addition to the continuous search for new biomolecules and improving efficiency of the known biopesticides, recombinant DNA technology is also being deployed for enhancing efficacy of biopesticides. Novel fusion proteins are being designed to develop next-generation biopesticides. The technology allows a toxin (not toxic to higher animals) to be combined with a carrier protein which makes it toxic to insect pests when consumed orally, while it was toxic only when injected into a target prey by a predator [7]. The fusion protein may be produced as a recombinant protein in microbial system, which can be scaled up for industrial production and commercial formulations. Several other innovative approaches are also being applied to develop biopesticides as effective, efficient and acceptable pest control measures.

FUTURE PROSPECTS

Biopesticides are attracting global attention as safer strategy to manage pest populations such as weeds, plant pathogens and insects while posing less risk to human being and the environment. In the US, biopesticides are monitored by Environmental Protection Agency which supports their registration based on the findings of "no unreasonable adverse effects" to human and the environment to permit their sale and distribution under the Federal Insecticide, Fungicide, and Rodenticide Act (FIFRA), as well as ensures a "reasonable certainty of no harm" under the Federal Food, Drug, and Cosmetic Act (FFDCA) to provide pesticide residue-free food and feed [8]. Most of the times, it is the farmers who are affected by the problems of pesticide resistance and withdrawal of plant protection products, and yet they are 'policy takers' rather than 'policy makers'. Hence, a public-private sector approach to the development, manufacturing and sale of environment friendly alternatives to chemical pesticides for developing countries is the need of the day.

Research in production, formulation and delivery may greatly assist in commercialization of biopesticides. More research is needed towards integrating biological agents into production system, improving capability of developing countries to manufacture and use biopesticides. At the same time, it is also required to encourage public funded programmes, commercial investors and pesticide companies to take up biopesticide enterprises. Equally important is the development of strict regulatory mechanisms to maintain the quality and availability of the biopesticides at affordable cost in the developing countries. Thus, various aspects of biopesticides covering the current status, constraints, prospects and regulatory network towards their effective utilization for the benefit of human kind need to be reviewed regularly.

CONCLUDING REMARKS

The world production and utilization of biopesticides are increasing at a rapid pace. The interest in organic farming and pesticide residue free agricultural produce would certainly warrant increased adoption of biopesticides by the farmers. Training on production and quality control to manufacturers, and organizational training to extension workers and farmers to popularize biopesticides may be essential for better adoption of this technology. As environmental safety is a global concern, we need to create awareness among the farmers, manufacturers, government agencies, policy makers and the common men to switch-over to biopesticides for pest management requirements. It is also believed that biological pesticides may be less vulnerable to genetic variations in plant populations that cause problems related to pesticide resistance. If deployed appropriately, biopesticides have potential to bring sustainability to global agriculture for food and feed security.

The views expressed here are those of the authors only. These may not necessarily be the views of the institution/organization the authors are associated with.

REFERENCES

1. Kumar S (2012) Biopesticides: a need for food and environmental safety. J Biofertil Biopestici 3:e107.
2. Nicholson GM (2007) Fighting the global pest problem: preface to the special toxicon issue on insecticidal toxins and their potential for insect pest control. Toxicon 49:413-422.
3. Al-Zaidi AA, Elhag EA, Al-Otaibi SH, Baig MB (2011) Negative effects of pesticides on the environment and the farmers awareness in Saudi Arabia: a case study. J Anim Plant Sci 21:605-611.
4. Hubbard M, Hynes RK, Erlandson M, Bailey KL (2014) The biochemistry behind biopesticide efficacy. Sustainable Chemical Processes 2:18.
5. Bailey KL, Boyetchko SM, Längle T (2010) Social and economic drivers shaping the future of biological control: a Canadian perspective on the factors affecting the development and use of microbial biopesticides. Biol Control 52:221–229.
6. Kumar S, Singh A (2014) Biopesticides for integrated crop management: environmental and regulatory aspects. J Biofertil Biopestici 5: e121.
7. Fitches E, Edwards MG, Mee C, Grishin E, Gatehouse AMR, Edwards JP, Gatehouse JA (2004) Fusion proteins containing insect-specific toxins as pest control agents: snowdrop lectin delivers fused insecticidal spider venom toxin to insect haemolymph following oral ingestion. J Insect Physiol 50: 61–71.
8. Leahy J, Mendelsohn M, Kough J, Jones R, Berckes N (2014) Biopesticide oversight and registration at the U.S. Environmental Protection Agency. In Biopesticides: state of the art and future opportunities. Eds Coats et al. ACS Symposium Series, American Chemical Society: Washington, DC.

CHAPTER 4

PLANT BASED BIOPESTICIDES: SAFER ALTERNATIVE FOR ORGANIC FOOD PRODUCTION

Nagappan Raja and Getinet Masresha

Organic food production and consumer demand is increasing recent times in developed and developing countries. The increased demand in organic food and beverages is due to awareness among the consumer and producer about the negative consequences associated with synthetic chemical pesticides. The expected global organic food and beverage market in 2015 to be $104.50 billon. Among the European countries, Germany is the biggest consumer for organic food and beverages with a share of 32%. The estimated organic food consumption in Japan is 54% in 2010 which is one of the leading countries in Asia. The expected growth rate of organic food market in Asia is 20.6% of CAGR from 2010 to 2015. Among the various organic produces, fresh fruits and vegetables are most dominated food categories with a share of 37%. The estimated CAGR of 22.3% from 2010 to 2015 in organic industries are associated with organic supplements. By realizing health benefits and eco-safety several government and non-governmental organizations are also supporting conventional farmers to switch over organic farming practices.

Sustainable organic farming practices needs proper eco-friendly pest and disease management practices in addition to balanced nutritional supplement to improve the quality and quantity of the agricultural outputs. The discovery of synthetic pesticides contributed much for the achievement of sustainable crop protection and production after green revolution. However, indiscriminate application of their utilization in crop protection leads several disadvantages to target and non-target organism in addition to environmental pollution. Due to residual problem and toxicity to the living environment synthetic chemical pesticides are not suitable for organic food production. In this scenario, green pesticides from plant origin are given enormous importance in recent times to develop better alternatives to chemical pesticides by considering eco-friendliness, multiple mode of action against insect pests. Prehistorically many plants and their parts are used extensively for the protection of crops against pests in the field as well as in storage.

In general, botanical pesticides are eco-chemicals isolated from parts of the plants such as leaves, roots, barks, fruits, seeds or seed kernels. By nature, several higher plants have the ability to synthesis and produce numerous secondary metabolites which will be unpalatable to insect pests. Some of the secondary metabolites alter the behaviour and life cycle of insect's pests which are called as semiochemicals. In Asia,

Citation: Raja N, Masresha G (2015) Plant Based Biopesticides: Safer Alternative for Organic Food Production. J Fertil Pestic 6: e128. doi:10.4172/jbfbp.1000e128

insecticidal property of several Chrysanthimum species is known for centuries. Many insecticidal compounds have been isolated from dried flower buds of Chrysanthimum species including six terpenoid esters which are successfully patented and marketed. Azadirachta indica is commonly called as neem which is another most promising plant used effectively and extensively for insect pest management program. The compound azadirachtin isolated from the seed kernel is contributed much for the development of several commercial bio-pesticide formulations. More than 100 commercial products are developed with azadirachtin including Margosan-O, Bio-neem, Azatin, Neemies, Safer's ENI, Wellgro, RD-Repelin, Neemguard, Neemark, Neemazal, Nimbin, Nimbicidine etc., which are used successfully in many parts of the world. The devotion and dedication of scientific community, chemical structure of azadirachtin have been successfully synthesized and developed as synthetic azadirachtin in 2007 which will be useful to develop bio-pesticides in the future. Several research reports highlights that neem products may not leave any toxic residue even though plants absorbed and transported to all tissue. According to Environmental Protection Agency, azadirachtin is classified as class IV due to low mammalian toxicity. Till today several farmers in Indian villages collect the seeds to prepare crude seed kernel extract for pest control program.

In addition, many plants contain essential oil which is a complex mixture of volatile compounds accumulated in seeds, flowers and leaves. These essential oils are includes various alcohols (eg. linalool, geraniol, citronellol), cyclic alcohol (eg. menthol, isopulegol, terpeniol), bicyclic alcohol (eg. borneol, verbenol), phenols (eg. thymol, carvacrol), ketones (eg. carvone, menthonen thujone), aldehydes (eg. citronellal, citral), acids (eg., chrysanthemic acid) etc., which will be released by the plants to protect against herbivores and pathogens. The essential oils of Matricaria recutita contain precocenes a compound which stimulate the production of juvenile hormone from the endocrine gland of insects which will suppress the insect growth during the time of molting. The juvabione from balsam fir wood suppress the insect development. Ocimum basilicum contain juvocimenes, an analogue of insect juvenile hormones. Aromatic plants like French marigold and coriander produce strong smells, which will be useful repellent to protect crops nearby. In general, anti-insect compounds are accumulated in several species of Myrtaceae, Lauraceae, Rutaceae, Lamiaceae, Asteraceae, Apiaceae, Cupressaceae, Poaceae, Zingiberaceae and Piperaceae families. The bioactive compounds isolated so far is countless and some of the compounds may also contribute in future to develop novel plant based biopesticides for organic food production. The appropriate selection of biomolecules to prepare biopesticides with multiple mode of action against target pests is unquestionably safer alternative for organic food production. Recent development in this field of research is disseminated to the scientific world through journal of bio-pesticides and bio-fertilizers are greatly appreciated.

CHAPTER 5

IMPACT OF PESTICIDES ON THE BASIS OF THEIR PHYSICO-CHEMICAL PROPERTIES

Anupama Pradhan, S. K. Markande And Rakesh Kumar Kurre

Keywords: Solubility, Vapour pressure, Adsorption coefficient, Hydrolysis, BCF Octanol/water partition coefficient

INTRODUCTION

The Food and Agriculture Organization of the United Nations defines pesticide as any substance or mixture of substances intended for preventing, destroying or controlling any pest, including vectors of human or animal disease, unwanted species of plants or animals causing harm during or otherwise interfering with the production, processing, storage or marketing of food, agricultural commodities, wood and wood products or animal stuffs or which may be administered to animals for the control of insects, arachnid or other pest in or on their bodies (Food and Agricultural Organization of the United Nations. 1986). Pesticides include herbicides for destroying weeds and other unwanted vegetation, insecticides for controlling a wide variety of insects, fungicides used to prevent the growth of moulds and mildew, disinfectants for preventing the spread of bacteria and compounds used to control mice and rats (Pesticides, 2011).

Naturally occurring compounds or natural extracts have been used as pesticides since ancient times. The earliest pesticides were most likely salt, sulphurous rock, and extracts of tobacco, red pepper, and the like. A pesticide class is a group of pesticidal compounds that share a common chemistry. For example, all pesticides in the class organophosphate (OP) are derivatives of phosphoric acid, and all pesticides in the class organochlorine are composed of carbon, hydrogen, and chlorine. Depending on their chemical properties they may leach to groundwater and surface water, persist in soil or enter the organism bioaccumulating in food chain and consequently influence human health too. Now the rapidly using pesticide use is a source of poisoning and health hazards among exposed population (Das et al. 2006).

This article aims to understand interrelation between physical and chemical properties of pesticides and their distribution in the environment which would be beneficial for manufacturing pesticides with low persistence.

Physico-chemical properties of pesticides

Pesticides are distributed in the environment by physical processes such as sedimentation, adsorption and volatilisation depending on the pesticidal compound itself or the pesticide product or formulation. In pesticides the compound itself is also known as the active ingredient the chemical responsible for killing the target pest. The formulation is the manner in which

Citation: Anupama Pradhan, S. K. Markande and Rakesh Kumar Kurre, Impact of Pesticides on the Basis of Their Physico-Chemical Properties, ISSN: 0970-2083.

the active ingredient is delivered. Typical formulations include liquids, dusts, wettable powders and emulsifiable concentrates. The pesticide formulation includes the active ingredient as well as other ingredients. The process of degradation will largely be governed by the compartment in which the pesticide is distributed and this distribution is governed by the physical processes.

Solubility

Solubility is a measure of the ability of a pesticide to dissolve in a solvent, usually water. Pesticides highly soluble in water dissolve easily and tend to not be adsorbed on soil and living organisms. Such pesticides are more likely to move with water in surface runoff or to move through the soil in water than are less-soluble pesticides. Solubility of a pesticide depends on dipole moment, hydrogen bonding, molecular size, pH and temperature.

Octanol/water partition coefficient (Kow)

Kow is defined as the ratio of a chemicals concentration in Octanol divided by its concentration in water Higher values (greater than 1000) indicate a pesticide that is very strongly attached to soil and is less likely to move unless soil erosion occurs. Lower values (less than 300-500) indicate pesticides that tend to move with water and have the potential to leach or move with surface runoff. Large Kow means low water solubility. Adsorption occurs because of an attraction between the chemical and soil particles. Adsorption increases with decreasing soil pH for ionizable pesticides (e.g. 2,4-D,2,4,5-T, picloram, and atrazine) (Andreu and Pico, 2004.). Kow values are important in that they can be used to estimate many chemical properties such as solubility and bio concentration factor since they are proportional to Kow. Thus Kow gives an overall estimate as to where a chemical will be distributed in the environment.

Vapour pressure

Vapour pressure and volatility are interrelated in that how chemicals are transported from a surface into the atmosphere. Vapour pressure is defined as the pressure that a chemical in the gas phase exerts over a surface. Pesticide volatilization depends on temperatures, wind, solubility, chemical properties and soil. Volatility is also more likely under conditions of low relative humidity. The potential for a pesticide to volatilize is measured by its vapor pressure. This measurement may be described in units of Pa (Pascals) or mmHg (millimetres of mercury). Pesticides that have high vapour-pressure values are more volatile. Vapours from such pesticides can move off-site and cause injury to susceptible plants. Vapours derived from volatilization of residue from previous spraying events combined with rainfall can also contribute to non-target exposure (Marrs, et al. 1989; Marrs, et al. 1991; Marrs, 1993 and Obrigawitch, et al. 1998).

Soil adsorption coefficient (Koc)

Soil adsorption coefficient measures the tendency of pesticides to be attached to soil particles. Kd is called the sorption coefficient and it measures the amount of chemical adsorbed onto soil per amount of water but organic content of soil is not considered. Soils vary in the amount of organic carbon content, which is mainly what determines the amount of pesticide adsorbed. Therefore the preferred value for determining soil's ability to adsorb is Koc, since it considers the organic content of soil.

$$K_{oc} = K_d \times 100 \ / \ \% \text{ organic carbon}$$

Koc depends on polarity, salinity, pH and organic content.

Hydrolysis

Hydrolysis is the reaction of pesticides with water to give new product. This reactivity is largely determined by the substituents bound to the pesticide. Hydrolysis depends on temperature and pH. Hydrolysis half life values helps to estimate how long a chemical will persist in an aqueous environment. If the pesticide resists hydrolysis then it may degrade via some other pathway such as microbial metabolism.

Persistence

Persistence is the ability of a pesticide to remain present and active in its original form for an extended period before degrading. A chemical's persistence is described in terms of its half-life, a comparative measure of the time needed for the chemical to degrade. The longer a pesticide's half-life, the more persistent the pesticide. Persistent pesticide residues are sometimes desirable because they provide longterm pest control and reduce the need for repeated applications. However, some persistent pesticides applied to soil, plants, lumber, and other surfaces or spilled into water or on soil can later harm sensitive plants or animals, including humans. It is especially important to prevent persistent pesticides from moving off-site through improper handling, application, drift, leaching, or runoff. The rate of pesticide degradation relates to the persistence of the pesticide.

Degradation processes break down pesticide compounds into simpler and often less-toxic chemicals. Some pesticides break down rapidly in a matter of days or even hours. Other pesticides can be detected in the environment for a year or more.

Bioconcentration factor

It is an indicator of how much a chemical will accumulate in living organisms such as fish. Once absorbed into an organism chemical can move through food chain. It depends on polarity, solubility and lipid content in organism. BCF can be an indicator of a pesticide's tendency to accumulate in the food chain.

Photolysis, microbial reduction

In atmosphere pesticides are degraded by photochemical reactions and microbial reduction. In photochemical reactions pesticides are broken down in the presence of sunlight. Microbial reduction is the process of degradation of pesticides by microorganisms present in soil. Pesticides not degraded by these processes are likely to accumulate in soil and contaminate ground water.

Following table provides summarised information of physico-chemical properties of some pesticides and gives an idea how they will be distributed in the environment. It is clear from the above table that pesticide having high water solubility will remain in water and tend not to be adsorbed on soil and living organisms. As the size increases, the water solubility decreases. Vapour pressure indicates volatilization which provides information about method of transportation by which the pesticide will be dispersed in the environment (air, water and soil). Koc means increase in persistence as pesticide is protected from degradation. Pesticide movement rating is derived from relation between half life and sorption in soil. Half life of a pesticide in soil measures persistence. Thus by considering the overall physico-chemical properties of a pesticide we can evaluate their impact whether it will leach, persist in soil or accumulate in organism.

RESULTS AND DISCUSSION

The worldwide use of pesticides in agriculture results in the residues commonly found in environment from cropping fields and orchards to rivers, estuaries and oceans and even urban environment (Sanchez-Bayo, et al. 2011). The extreme toxicity of most of these manmade chemicals affect not only the target pests but also many other species of animals, although in different degrees (Sanchez-Bayo, et al. 2011). Pesticides are often considered a quick, easy and inexpensive solution for controlling weeds and insect pests in urban landscapes. However, pesticide use comes at a significant cost. Pesticide drift can account for a loss of 2 to 25% of the chemical being applied, which can spread over a distance of a few yards to several hundred miles. As much as 80–90% of an applied pesticide can be volatilized within a few days of application Majewski, 1995). Some pesticide drift occurs during every application, even from ground equipment (Glotfelty and Schomburg, 1989). Pesticide contamination poses significant risks to the environment and non-target organisms ranging from beneficial soil microorganisms, to insects, plants, fish and birds. The health effects of pesticide exposure vary from one pesticide to another. While considering the potential environmental and health effects of pesticides, it is important to consider the toxicity of the active ingredient as well as the other ingredients in the formulation. These physico-chemical properties can be used to understand the underlying basis of distribution in non target life. Understanding the chemical and physical characteristics of a pesticide allows the applicator to make better decisions about which pesticide active ingredient to use for a particular situation. We need to understand the physicochemical properties so that precautionary measures may be taken to mitigate their negative effects in human health and environment.

REFERENCES

1. Andreu V, Pico' Y. 2004. Determination of pesticides and their degradation products in soil: critical review and comparison of methods. Trends Anal Chemistry. 23 (10Ã¢ÂÂ11) : 772Ã¢ÂÂ789.
2. Das, G.P., Shaik, A.P. and Jamil, K. 2006 Estimation of apoptosis and necrosis caused by pesticides in vitro on human lymphocytes using DNA diffusion assay. Drug ChemToxicol. 29 (2) : 147-156.
3. Food and Agricultural Organization of the United Nations, 1986. International code of conduct on the distribution and use of pesticides, Rome.
4. Glotfelty, J. and Schomburg, J. 1989. Volatilization of pesticides from soil in reactions and movements of organic chemicals in soil. In: Sawhney, B.L., Brown, N. editors. Madison, WI: Soil Science Society of America Special Pubmed.
5. Pesticides, 2011. National Institute of Environmental Health Sciences. National Institutes of Health. 2011. http://www.niehs.nih.gov/health/topics/agents/pesticides/index.cfm
6. Marrs, R.H., Williams, C.T., Frost, A.J. and Plant, R.A. 1989. Assessment of the effects of herbicide spray drifts on a range of plant species of conservation interest. Environmental Pollution. 59 : 71-86.
7. Marrs, R.H., Frost, A.J. and Plant, R.A. 1991. Effects of herbicide spray drift on selected species of nature conservation interest: the effects of plant age and the surrounding vegetation structure. Environmental Pollution. 69 : 223-235.
8. Marrs, R.H., Frost, A.J., Plant, R.A. and Lunnis, P. 1993. Determination of buffer zones to protect seedlings of non-target plants from the effects of glyphosate spray drift. Agriculture, Ecosystems and Environment, 45 : 283-293.
9. Obrigawitch, T.T., Cook, G. and Wetherington, J. 1998. Assessment of effects on non-target plants from sulfonylurea herbicides using field approaches. Pesticide Science. 52 : 199-217.
10. Sanchez-BayoF.,Van den Brink, P.J. and Mann, R.M. edsm. 2011. Ecological Impacts of Toxic Chemicals. Bentham Science Ltd. Online. pp. 281; 63-87.
11. Majewski, M. 1995. Pesticides in the atmosphere: distribution, trends, and governing factors. In: Capel, P. editor. Volume one, Pesticides in the Hydrologic System. Ann Arbor Press Inc; p. 118.

CHAPTER 6

TOXICOLOGY OF PESTICIDES

Francisco Sánchez-Bayo and Richard Ortega

Since the mid-1960s, environmental toxicology focussed on the effects of bioaccumulation of organochlorine insecticides in organisms, and their consequences for populations of species in the wild. Prompted by the release of Silent Spring [1], scientists sifted focus to the ecological effects of pesticides, thus expanding the narrow field of pesticide toxicology that had been restricted to its effects on pests, weeds and pathogenic fungi since its beginnings. The ensuing decades will witness a tremendous gathering of data related to the toxic impacts that insecticides, herbicides and fungicides have on organisms and ecosystems [2].

Despite these efforts, our understanding of the mechanisms of toxicity at different levels of biological organisation has not kept abreast with the overwhelming progress experienced in the development of new pesticides. While chemical companies introduced new plant protection products in the market at a staggering pace, environmental toxicology has trailed behind. Part of the reason is that the impacts of those new chemicals in the environment are not apparent immediately after their release, but usually it takes years for the negative consequences of their activity to be noticed. Let's not forget that it took 25 years from the introduction of DDT in agriculture until the decline in population of raptors was observed [3], and another 10 years to prove that this and other organochlorine insecticides were responsible for such declines [4].

Chemical companies have moved away from producing substances that accumulate in the body of organisms (typically lipophilic substances), and are now developing hydrophilic compounds that can be easily disposed of by the animal's metabolism. The new pesticides are systemic, meaning they can be taken up by the plants and animals and distributed through their tissues without accumulating in any particular organ or structure (e.g. fatty tissues). This applies to herbicides as much as to fungicides and insecticides. In addition, hormone-mimicking chemicals and growth regulators specific to arthropods are replacing the traditional neurotoxic insecticides, because most of the latter products are broad-spectrum insecticides that cause numerous fatalities among applicators and wildlife alike [5-7]. And yet, the environmental toxicology of most of these new compounds remains largely unexplored.

What have we learned from the recent history of ecotoxicology? Are we in a better position to assess the ecological impact of new pesticides? Do we understand the

Citation: Sánchez-Bayo F, Ortega R (2012) Toxicology of Pesticides. J Environ Anal Toxicol S4:e001. doi: 10.4172/2161-0525.S4-e001

pathways that lead to sub-lethal effects in organisms? Have we developed more effective ways of evaluating the toxicity of chemicals? It is regrettable that we are still using methods that consider only fixed times at short periods to evaluate the acute toxicity of chemicals while ignoring the toxic dynamics with time. When would the regulatory authorities establish the much needed time-to-event toxicity protocols as the standard test for ecotoxicity? How can we predict indirect effects on pesticides on communities and ecosystems? These and many other questions pose serious doubts to our ability to interpret and analyse all the toxicological information available to scientists and regulators. We must admit that our current methods for risk assessment of chemicals are deficient and inadequate, so many are the gaps in knowledge that need to be covered. Unless we improve our ways of doing environmental toxicology, human health and environmental protection will be compromised in the future.

This special issue provides a glimpse of the questions that remain to be answered as well as the new directions undertaken to provide answers in this field of research. For a start, Tennekes and Sanchez- Bayo [8] address the toxicology of Neonicotinoids, carcinogens and other compounds with time-dependent toxicity from a toxic dynamic perspective. Based on sound toxicological principles and models, they show empirical evidence that confirm the long-term effects of the novel insecticides on aquatic arthropods and ecosystems. This contrasts with the more familiar toxicology of metals and other compounds that do not have cumulative effects over time. In any case, the toxic dynamic model used to predict the effects of either type of chemical is the same. Its implication for a new approach to risk assessment is sketched.

Sanchez-Bayo [9] reviews the current knowledge status about the toxicity of insecticides to non-target organisms, focusing on the mode of action as the key to understand why some insecticides are more toxic than others to particular groups of organisms. This is a comparative study based on acute toxicity values obtained from several sources. But effects are not restricted to acute toxicity, and there are many other endpoints that need to be considered in ecotoxicology. In this regard, for many years the properties and mode of action of neurotoxic insecticides have been studied on insects (e.g. cockroach, flies). However, the review by McVey et al. [10] on the astounding features of a humble organism, the nematode Caenorhabditis elegans, opens up a new field in neurotoxicological research. The simple structure of this organism will enable the study of toxicological endpoints, their gene expression and the location of the site of action of insecticides with a detail never seen before. The similarities of its nervous system with that of vertebrates make C. elegans an ideal model organism for neurotoxicity research.

The identification of the specific receptors targeted by the pesticides has taken also a new dimension with the introduction of imaging techniques that reveal the site of action in biological samples. Ortega and Carmona [11] review the recent applications in pesticide toxicology of analytical methods with high detection sensitivity and high spatial resolution such as the ion beam, synchrotron, or mass spectrometry based imaging methods. Such methods enable the determination in situ of the distribution of a toxic chemical in the tissues, as well as the speciation of inorganic and organometallic pesticides.

Several clinical disorders in humans have been associated with pesticide usage in agricultural communities, and clinical evidence obtained in recent decades indicates that neurotoxic insecticides are among the substances to blame [12]. Indeed, the variety of sublethal effects that these highly toxic substances cause is only starting to unravel, as Esquivel-Senties and Vega explain [13]. Apart from the obvious neurotoxic effects of the insecticides, some metabolites of organophosphorus compounds produce also immunological disturbances by reducing the viability of Tc lymphocytes, which are essential to kill pathogen-infested cells. Thus, the ability of exposed individuals to deal with viral infections and cancerous cells is hampered, not only in humans but in animals as well.

Immunological sublethal effects of the neonicotinoid imidacloprid, one of the most common insecticides used worldwide, in chickens are demonstrated by Kammon and Brar [14]. These authors show the decline in immunoglobulins and lymphocytic depletion in the medulla and cortex in animals treated with this insecticide. This finding is key to understand the recent observations involving infectious diseases and neonicotinoid usage. This weakening effect in chickens, however, can be ameliorated by supplementation of vitamin E and selenium, which appear to restore the function of the spleen. Further epidemiological studies on neonicotinoids and the honey bee Colony Collapse Disorder should take into account these findings.

In a final contribution to this issue, the controversial teratogenic effects of high doses of glyphosate in frog and chicken embryos are discussed by Fagan and Robinson [15] in relation to other industrybased studies on this matter. The authors question the assessment reports of some government authorities and call for a more transparent risk evaluation to be carried out by independent scientists with no links to industry or government bodies. The underlying hurdle, however, is not so much the biased approached of some industry studies, but rather the misinterpretation of the factual data due to inappropriate knowledge about the sublethal effects that pesticides exert on organisms.

While this selection of articles is small, we hope the topics covered may prompt further research on the toxicology of pesticides from new perspectives. Only thus we will be able to tackle the above questions in a more appropriate way.

REFERENCES

1. Carson R (1962) Silent Spring, Houghton-Mifflin, Boston, MA
2. Sánchez-Bayo F, van den Brink PJ, Mann RM (2011) Ecological Impacts of Toxic Chemicals. Bentham Science Publishers Ltd. Online, 281.
3. Lockie JD, Ratcliffe DA (1964) Insecticides and Scottish golden eagles. British Birds 57: 89-101.
4. Dunlap TR (1981) DDT, Scientists, Citizens and Public Policy, Princeton University Press, Princeton, NJ.
5. Garry VF, Harkins ME, Erickson LL, Long-Simpson LK, Holland SE, et al. (2002) Birth defects, season of conception, and sex of children born to pesticide applicators living in the Red River Valley of Minnesota, USA. Environ Health Perspect 110: 441–449.
6. Mineau P, Whiteside M (2006) Lethal risk to birds

from insecticide use in the United States - A spatial and temporal analysis. Environ Toxicol Chem 25: 1214-1222.

7. Konradsen F, van der Hoek W, Cole DC, Hutchinson G, Daisley H, et al. (2003) Reducing acute poisoning in developing countries--options for restricting the availability of pesticides. Toxicology 192: 249-261.

8. Tennekes HA, Sánchez-Bayo F (2012) Time-dependent toxicity of neonicotinoids and other toxicants: implications for a new approach to risk assessment. J Environ Anal Toxicol S4-001.

9. Sánchez-Bayo F (2012) Insecticides mode of action in relation to their toxicity to non-target organisms. J Environ Anal Toxicol S4: S4-002.

10. McVey KA, Mink JA, Snapp IB, Timberlake WS, Todt CE, et al. (2012) Caenorhabditis elegans: An emerging model system for pesticide neurotoxicity. J Environ Anal Toxicol S4: S4-003.

11. Ortega R, Carmona A (2012) High spatial resolution chemical imaging of inorganic and organometallic pesticides. J Environ Anal Toxicol S4: S4-005.

12. Parrón T, Requena M, Hernández AF, Alarcón R (2011) Association between environmental exposure to pesticides and neurodegenerative diseases. Toxicol Appl Pharmacol 256: 379-385.

13. Esquivel-Senties MS, Vega L (2012) Organophosphorous pesticides metabolite reduces human T CD8 homeostasis and proliferation by inducing cellular death. J Environ Anal Toxicol S4: S4-004.

14. Kammon AM, Brar RS (2012) Ameliorating effects of vitamin E and selenium on immunological alterations induced by imidacloprid chronic toxicity in chickens. J Environ Anal Toxicol S4: S4-007

15. Fagan JB, Robinson CJ (2012) Teratogenic effects of glyphosate-based herbicides and political and scientific controversy. J Environ Anal Toxicol S4: S4-006

CHAPTER 7

DISTRIBUTION BEHAVIOUR OF DIMETHOATE IN TEA LEAF

Shivani Jaggi, Bikram Singh, Adarsh Shanker

Keywords: Tea, Cuticle, Dimethoate, Dissipation

INTRODUCTION

Tea, Camellia sinensis (L) O. Kurtze, is the most important plantation crop in India occupying 420,000 ha of land. All over the world it is a popular invigorating and refreshing drink having excellent medicinal properties. Considering that an estimated amount of 18 - 20 billion cups are consumed daily in the world its economic and social interest is clear [1]. Like any other crop tea plantations are also subjected to ravages of insects, mites, plant pathogens, nematodes etc. The perennial nature of the crop and the more equitable weather pattern prevailing in tea areas are favorable for insect pests resulting in 250-500 million kg of annual loss of crop. In terms of monetary loss it could be approximately 500 million-1 billion US $ [2]. The insects target almost all plant parts such as roots, stem, leaves and buds. Thus every part of the tea plant is a potential target for a wide spectrum of pests and disease causing organisms.

Tea is an unusual crop where leaves are sprayed directly with pesticides, harvested and processed even without washing. The shoots of the tea plant are thin and tender (233 - 291 μm) with cuticle thickness 4 - 10 μm and surface area per unit weight of leaf (tender leaf 41.7 cm2 /gm and mature leaf 15.9 cm^2 / gm respectively).Tea leaf, with thin cuticle, relatively larger surface area and short interval between pesticide application and harvest, is expected to be permeable to various groups of chemicals. Pesticide thus could have negative impact both on ecology and quality of tea when applied [3]. Consequently tea represents a significant potential of human exposure to pesticide residues by virtue of high application of pesticides to tea crop coupled with the average intake of 6 gms of dried (made) tea per day per individual [4,5]. Some basic studies on plant cuticles as barriers against the diffusion of chemicals have been reported [6,7]. Pesticide penetration into the leaf surface plays important practical implications as it allows the residues to stick/persist thus maintaining its efficacy even if it rains after the treatment [8]. Moreover once the pesticide has penetrated the epicuticular wax solar radiations acting on the pesticide molecule have to cross the cuticle thus reducing the photodegradative activity [9]. Furthermore, cuticular wax can hold on the pesticide residues resulting in low volatility from the leaf surface. The information available on the fate of pesticides on tea leaf and role leaf cuticle, plays in the dissipation under different environmental conditions is scanty in literature. Hence a study was initiated to understand the

Citation: S. Jaggi, B. singh and A. Shanker, "Distribution Behaviour of Dimethoate in Tea Leaf," Journal of Environmental Protection, Vol. 2 No. 4, 2011, pp. 482-488. doi: 10.4236/jep.2011.24056.

penetrating and dissipation behavior of dimethoate on tea leaf surface. Fate of dimethoate in tea and its brew have been reported but still its exact behaviour on the tea leaf surface is not known thoroughly [10,11].

EXPERIMENTAL DETAILS

Field Trials

Field trials were carried out in dry and wet seasons at Institute of Himalayan Bioresource Technology (IHBT) tea experimental farm at Banuri, Palampur (1300 msl, 32°6′20″N × 76°33′29″E), India. The maximum and minimum temperature during dry and wet seasons as recorded from the experimental farm was 32°C, 23°C and 30°C, 18°C respectively. Relative humidity was 64% and 82% respectively and the total rainfall was 97 mm during wet season where as dry season was without any rainfall. The commercial formulation of dimethoate was sprayed (spray volume 400 l/ha) on tea bushes considering each plot of 100 bushes per replicate at recommended dose (200 gm a.i./ha) and double of the recommended dose (400 gm a.i./ha). In control treatment (T0), water was sprayed. Treatments were carried out in dry and wet seasons. Spray was done with a calibrated Knapsack sprayer. The weather parameters were continuously recorded in the experimental period to monitor the effect of environmental conditions.Green tea leaves (two leaves and a bud) were plucked from each replicate of both the treatment and control plots and brought to the laboratory each time at 0 (immediately and 4 hours after spraying), 1,3,5,7,10,14 and 21days after the treatment. To see the effect of leaky cuticle damaged leaves were also collected from the same plots. Further to analyze the effect of cuticle on the photodegradation of Dimethoate a laboratory experiment was carried out in parallel by spraying dimethoate on glass plate (i.e. without leaf) and other with leaf under same environmental conditions to provide estimated behavioral information. The weather parameters during the experimental time are graphically represented in figure below (see Figure 1).

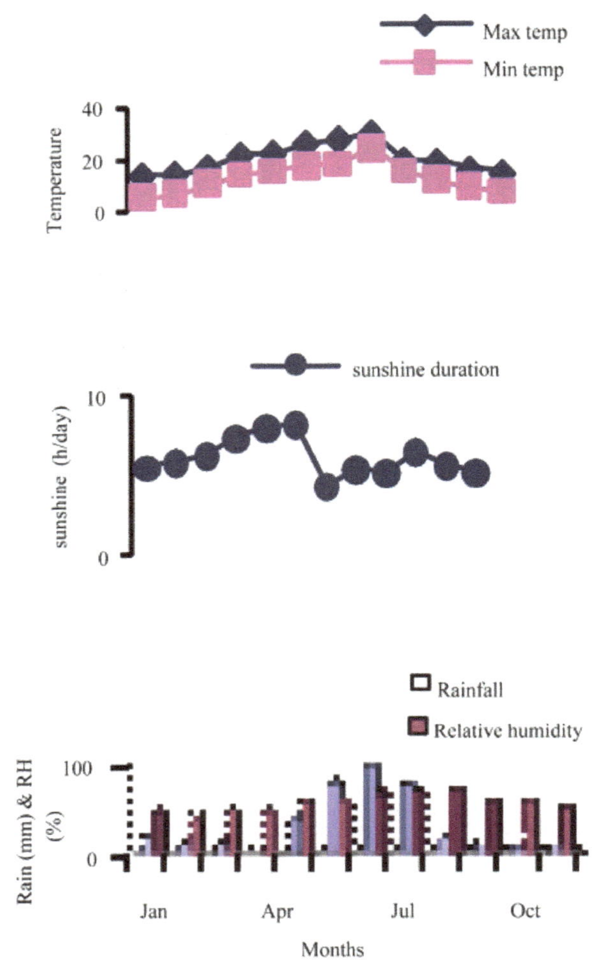

Figure 1: Weather parameters.

Analytical Standards and Working Solutions

An analytical grade of dimethoate was obtained from Dr.Ehrenstorfer Laboratories, Augsburg, Germany (reported purity > 98%). For the field studies, formulation grade of dimethoate (Rogor® 30 Emulcifiable Concentrate EC, Isagro Agrochemicals Pvt. Ltd., Mumbai) was procured from the local market. Standard solution (1000 mg/l) was prepared in acetone and the spiking solution (50mg/l) was diluted from the stock solution and the solutions required for preparing a standard curve (0.2, 0.5, 1.0, 1.5, 5.0 and 10.0 mg/l) were prepared from the stock solution by serial dilutions. All chemicals used for extraction and analysis of the residues and activated carbon were products of Merck India Limited, Mumbai India. Anhydrous sodium sulphate AR (Analytical Reagent) used was supplied by S.d. fine-chemicals, Mumbai.

Apparatus

Gas Chromatograph

A Hewlett-Packard 5890 series II gas chromatograph (Avondale, PA-USA) supported by a nitrogen phosphorus detector (NPD), a HP-7673 autosampler and integrator (Hewlett-packard) using split-splitless injector, connected to HP 3365 Chemstation system software (Hewlett-packard) was used. The detection was done using Nitrogen Phosphorus Detector (NPD). Peak resolution was done on a HP-17 medium polar capillary column (25 m length × 0.2 mm id) containing 50% phenyl and 50% methyl polysiloxane coated fused silica (0.25 μm film thickness) (Hewlett-Packard, Co., Wilmington, DE). Detailed analytical conditions were as follows. The injection was made using a split mode (50:1), injector temperature held at 260°C. The temperature of the NPD was held at 280°C. The oven temperature was programmed at 150°C for the initial 2 minutes and then ramped 10°C /min to 300°C and finally maintained for 5 minutes. Carrier gas was nitrogen (purity 99.99%) at column flow rate of 1 ml/min. The samples were filtered through Millipore membrane teflon filters (0.45 μm particle size) before injection into the chromatographic column.

STANDARD CALIBRATION CURVE

Standard curve was prepared by diluting the stock solution to five different concentrations in acetone. The column was conditioned by repeated injections (3 times) of the standard under constant operating conditions until the peaks obtained were reproducible. Dimethoate was injected at 0.2, 0.5, 1.0, 5.0 and 10.0 mg/l to validate the method.

Recovery Assay

Before laying the experiments in the field, recovery studies were performed at 50.0 mg/l fortification level of active ingredient (three replicates) of each matrix (green leaves, dried leaves and soil). These samples were prepared by adding known amount of standard in matrix before extraction. The extraction was carried out as described below in section The duplicate injections of each extract were made in Gas Chromatograph (GC-NPD).

EXTRACTION OF PESTICIDE FROM LEAF SURFACE

Extraction of dimethoate was done with Chloroform (recovery > 90%) The extract was agitated mechanically with acetonitrile for 3 hours on a horizontal shaker. The mixture was filtered through Whatman no.1 filter paper and the cake was washed twice with 20 ml solvent each time. The combined water extract was partitioned with 150ml of acetonitrile twice in a 500 ml separating funnel. Discarding the aqueous layer, the organic layer was concentrated to near dryness on a water bath and reconstituted with 1 ml of acetone for final analysis. The effect of washing was thus confirmed by laboratory washing and in case of samples collected from the treated fields in dry and wet seasons, the residue was extracted in dichloromethane. The final eluate was evaporated to near dryness and the residue was reconstituted with 1ml acetone for quantification.

Extraction of Pesticide from Epicuticular Wax

Epicuticular wax extraction was done using the method described by Mc. Donald et al. [12]. After thorough washing to remove the surface pesticides, the tea leaves were soaked in 100 ml of chloroform and shaken on an automatic horizontal shaker for 1 minute. Extract was filtered through Whatman No.1 filter paper and concentrated to 5 ml followed by passing through an adsorbent column containing florisil topped with 1 cm of anhydrous sodium sulphate prewashed with chloroform. The extract was eluted with 200 ml of chloroform, concentrated on a vacuum rotatory evaporator using a water bath at 35°C - 40°C. The residue was finally reconstituted with 1ml of acetone and quantified by GC (NPD).

Extraction of Pesticide from Cell Wall

Extraction of dimethoate was done by soaking the tea leaves in 100 ml of chloroform and shaken on an automatic horizontal shaker for 1 minute. Extract was filtered through Whatman No.1 filter paper and concentrated to 5 ml followed by passing through an adsorbent column containing florisil topped with 1 cm of anhydrous sodium sulphate prewashed with chloroform. The extract was eluted with 200 ml of chloroform, concentrated on a vacuum rotatory evaporator using a water bath at 35°C - 40°C. The extract was finally eluted with dichloromethane (200 ml) from the florisil column. The eluate was evaporated to dryness and reconstituted to 1 ml in acetone and 2 μl of it was analysed by GC (NPD).

DETECTION AND QUANTIFICATION

Detection Limit Test

To determine the limit of detection made tea samples were spiked with different concentration levels of dimethoate standard and analysed by GC (NPD). The detection limit was evaluated by the peak signal/noise (S/N) ratio. An S/N ratio greater than 3 was considered as a detectable peak.

RESULTS AND DISCUSSION

Quantification

The GC analytical conditions were optimized in terms of temperature program that allowed an improvement of the time and the chromatographic run resolution. Moreover to avoid the cross contamination between high and low spiked samples, the sequence of injections was in the following order: solvent, blank sample, sprayed samples and finally standard solution. No interfering peaks were present during the analysis of any samples as before each run the solvent was injected.

Moreover, the adopted oven programming allowed a good chromatographic separation of dimethoate. The total run time was 14 minutes and the retention time of the dimethoate in the given chromatographic conditions was 8.68 minutes and constant for each series of samples. Chromatographic separation by HP-17 column provided good results for the quantification of the samples.

Linearity

The calibration curve of the analysed dimethoate gave a good regression line ($R^2 = 0.8827$) in the range of explored concentrations, 0.1 - 10.0 mg/l. The detection limit of dimethoate was taken to be 0.01 mg/kg, which were much lower than the maximum residue limits fixed by European Commision for dimethoate in tea (0.2 mg/kg). Residues below 0.01 mg/kg were detected but not quantified. This low detection limit was achieved because of the efficient cleanup step that allowed the elimination of all the possible interfering peaks, giving a low noise value.

Method Validation

The recovery of the fortified (50 mg/kg) samples of dimethoate in made tea (in triplicate) ranged from 92.9% - 94.6%. The results showed good recovery and reproducibility. The compounds of interest were well resolved from other co-extractives. These results indicated that the method used in this study provided a good cleanup.

Field Studies

The shoots of the tea plant are thin and tender (233 - 291 μm) with cuticle thickness 4 - 10 μm and relatively larger surface area per unit weight of leaf (tender leaf 41.7 and mature leaf 15.9 cm2 /gm respectively). It is an unusual crop where leaves are sprayed directly with pesticides, harvested and processed even without washing. In the preliminary experiments with tea leaf cuticle penetration of dimethoate was measured immediately after application as evaporation of water also affected the rate of penetration [13].As indicated by data presented in Tables 2-5, the residues of dimethoate on leaf surface at 0 day (immediately after spray) was found to be 9.07 ± 0.14 mg/kg and 18.31 ± 0.34 mg/kg whereas its concentration was 9.01 ± 0.10 mg/kg and 18.19 ± 0.34 mg/kg respectively at two different treatments when the samples were collected 4 hours after spray. No penetration effect observed in the epicuticular wax and cell wall when the leaves were collected immediately after spray. This indicated that during the evaporation of water the penetration rate was negligible. In dry season the residue concentration in the epicuticular wax was 0.14 ± 0.05 and 0.11 ± 0.10 mg/kg and in the cell wall was 2.97 ± 0.02 and 4.41 ± 0.08 mg/kg in normal leaf when the samples were collected 4 hours after spray at 200 and 400 gm a.i/ha respectively. While the concentration in injured leaf was 0.17 ± 0.02 and 0.68 ± 0.06 mg/kg in epicuticular wax and 3.04 ± 0.06 and 6.12 ± 0.12 mg/kg in cell wall. Further, the concentration in leaf surface was found to be 0.02 ± 0.00 mg/kg and 0.04 ± 0.00 mg/kg at two different treatments on 7th day after spray.

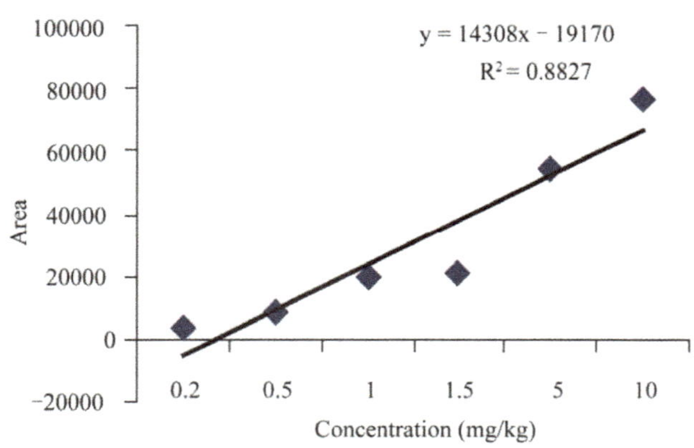

Figure 2: Standard curve.

No residues were detected on leaf surface after 10th day of treatment. In wet season, the residue concentration in the cell wall was 3.24 ± 0.06 mg/kg and 6.25 ± 0.19 mg/kg respectively at two different treatments in normal leaf and 3.32 ± 0.11 mg/kg and 7.20 ± 0.17 mg/kg in injured leaves whereas in wax the residue concentration was 0.03 ± 0.00 mg/kg, 0.08 ± 0.01 mg/kg and 0.08 ± 0.00 mg/kg, 0.08 ± 0.00 mg/kg in normal and injured leaves respectively. Further, this concentration in wax was negligible in normal leaf and injured leaf on 3rd day after spray, which declined to no detectable limit in 7th day after spray. As observed from the data, the residues found on the epicuticular wax and cell wall was comparatively more in the damaged cuticle. Residues observed in the cell wall and tissues confirm its good penetrating ability inspite of its hydrophilic nature. Higher penetration in wet season as observed from the tables indicated the route could be through the stomatal pores also. Little variation in the results as observed from Tables 2-5 for normal and damaged cuticle confirmed that cuticle was also acting as a barrier during penetration of dimethoate residue. The tea leaf having thin cuticle is expected to be permeable to various groups of pesticides and dimethoate residue in the wax and cell wall confirmed it but cuticle thickness alone may not be responsible for the dimethoate penetration in the leaf. Data in Table 1 proved that physical properties of the

Table 1: Physico chemical properties of Dimethoate.

COMMON NAME	DIMETHOATE
CHEMICAL NAME	O,O-DIMETHYLS-METHYL-CARBAMOYL-METHYL PHOSPHORODITHIOATE
EMPIRICAL FORMULA	$C_5H_{12}NO_3PS_2$
MOLECULAR WEIGHT	229.3
VAPOUR PRESSURE	2.5×10^{-4} Pa at 25°C
PHYSICAL STATE	COLOURLESS CRYSTALLINE SOLID.
MELTING POINT	45 - 52.5°C
BOILING POINT	107°C at 0.05 mmHg
VOLATILITY	1.107 mg/m^3
SOLUBILITY IN WATER	39 g/l
SOLUBILITY IN ORGANIC SOLVENTS	HIGHLY SOLUBLE IN CHLOROFORM, METHYLENE CHLORIDE, BENZENE, TOULENE, ALCOHOLS, ESTERS AND KETONES.
SPECIFIC GRAVITY AT 25°C	1.281

Table 2: Dimethoate distribution in tea leaf in dry season (200 gm a.i/ha).

DAS	Residue in mg/kg ± standard deviation					
	Distribution in normal leaf surface			Distribution in injured leaf		
	Leaf surface	Wax	Cell wall	Leaf surface	Wax	Cell wall
0(1)	9.07 ± 0.14	ND	ND	8.96 ± 0.17	0.02 ± 0.00	ND
0(2)	9.01 ± 0.10	0.14 ± 0.05	2.97 ± 0.02	8.65 ± 0.13	0.17 ± 0.02	3.04 ± 0.06
1	6.17 ± 0.15	0.11 ± 0.09	2.03 ± 0.00	5.92 ± 0.12	0.21 ± 0.02	2.79 ± 0.06
3	1.46 ± 0.07	0.02 ± 0.00	0.03 ± 0.00	1.30 ± 0.01	0.02 ± 0.00	0.02 ± 0.00
5	0.05 ± 0.00	ND	ND	0.04 ± 0.00	ND	ND
7	0.02 ± 0.00	ND	ND	ND	ND	ND
10	ND	ND	ND	ND	ND	ND
14	ND	ND	ND	ND	ND	ND
21	ND	ND	ND	ND	ND	ND

Table 3: Dimethoate distribution in tea leaf in dry season (400 gm a.i/ha).

DAS	Residue in mg/ kg ± standard deviation					
	Distribution in normal leaf			Distribution in injured leaf		
	Leaf surface	Wax	Cell wall	Leaf surface	Wax	Cell wall
0(1)	18.31 ± 0.34	ND	ND	17.60 ± 0.30	0.03 ± 0.00	0.02 ± 0.00
0(2)	18.19 ± 0.31	0.11 ± 0.10	4.41 ± 0.08	17.36 ± 0.25	0.68 ± 0.06	6.12 ± 0.12
1	11.39 ± 0.23	0.90 ± 0.07	4.10 ± 0.10	11.18 ± 0.16	0.33 ± 0.07	5.93 ± 0.06
3	3.13 ± 0.13	0.06 ± 0.00	0.04 ± 0.00	2.95 ± 0.07	0.03 ± 0.00	0.03 ± 0.00
5	0.10 ± 0.01	ND	ND	0.06 ± 0.00	ND	ND
7	0.04 ± 0.00	ND	ND	ND	ND	ND
10	ND	ND	ND	ND	ND	ND
14	ND	ND	ND	ND	ND	ND
21	ND	ND	ND	ND	ND	ND

Table 4: Dimethoate distribution in tea leaf in wet season (200 gm a.i/ha).

DAS	Residue in mg/ kg ± standard deviation					
	Distribution in normal leaf surface			Distribution in injured leaf		
	Leaf surface	Wax	Cell wall	Leaf surface	Wax	Cell wall
0 (1)	4.15 ± 0.13	ND	ND	3.86 ± 0.10	ND	ND
0 (2)	4.00 ± 0.01	0.03 ± 0.00	3.24 ± 0.06	3.65 ± 0.08	0.02 ± 0.10	3.32 ± 0.11
1	0.08 ± 0.00	0.05 ± 0.05	4.14 ± 0.09	0.06 ± 0.00	0.08 ± 0.13	4.25 ± 0.03
3	0.02 ± 0.00	0.02 ± 0.00	0.82 ± 0.03	0.03 ± 0.00	0.01 ± 0.00	0.94 ± 0.02
5	ND	0.03 ± 0.00	0.02 ± 0.00	ND	0.02 ± 0.00	0.02 ± 0.00
7	ND	ND	ND	ND	ND	ND
10	ND	ND	ND	ND	ND	ND
14	ND	ND	ND	ND	ND	ND
21	ND	ND	ND	ND	ND	ND

Table 5: Dimethoate distribution in tea leaf in wet season (400 gm a.i/ha).

DAS	Residue in mg/ kg± standard deviation					
	Distribution in normal leaf			Distribution in injured leaf		
	Leaf surface	Wax	Cell wall	Leaf surface	Wax	Cell wall
0(1)	8.03 ± 0.07	ND	ND	7.90 ± 0.05	ND	ND
0 (2)	7.83 ± 0.05	0.08 ± 0.01	6.25 ± 0.14	7.44 ± 0.08	0.05 ± 0.00	7.20 ± 0.17
1	0.14 ± 0.02	0.08 ± 0.01	5.24 ± 0.91	0.10 ± 0.01	0.05 ± 0.00	6.64 ± 0.08
3	0.04 ± 0.00	0.05 ± 0.01	1.34 ± 0.09	0.04 ± 0.00	0.04 ± 0.00	1.42 ± 0.07
5	ND	0.05 ± 0.00	0.05 ± 0.00	ND	0.04 ± 0.00	0.03 ± 0.00
7	ND	ND	ND	ND	ND	ND
10	ND	ND	ND	ND	ND	ND
14	ND	ND	ND	ND	ND	ND
21	ND	ND	ND	ND	ND	ND

Residue and environmental conditions might be equally involved. Low partition coefficient K_{ow} (0.7) and high water solubility of 39 g/l might have enabled it to penetrate inside the inner region of the cuticle. They are rapidly absorbed under high humid conditions, supporting the view that there was an aqueous route traversing the cuticle and maximum penetration might be due to stomatal pores. Thus the permeation of active ingredients was influenced by their solubility characteristics as evident by their partition coefficients. The K_{ow} reflected the lipophilicity of the compound and was related to the degree and rate at which it would be absorbed by leaf [14]. Furthermore, penetration as observed in the leaf surface could be attributed to the emulsifiable concentrate formulation used as they allow better deposits and different adjuvants keep the deposit in binded form and minimize the early loss of pesticide by increasing the rate of penetration. The adhension, retention and distribution of agrochemicals sprayed on plant surfaces also depends on target wettability [15]. However it could be envisaged that temperature and humidity could have roles to play.

CONCLUSIONS

Above studies confirmed that the dimethoate distribution on the tea leaf surface and decrease in surface residue is due to the collective behaviour of cuticle, its solubility, penetration, partition coefficient, vapour pressure and the formulation along with the environmental conditions at the time of experiments.

ACKNOWLEDGEMENTS

We are especially grateful to Director, IHBT for providing necessary facilities and CSIR, India for financial assistance. The authors wish to thanks Guru Nanak Dev University, Amritsar, India for the guidance.

REFERENCES

1. T. C. Choudhuri, "Pesticide Residues in Tea," Global advances in Tea Science, 1999, pp. 369-378.
2. Anonymous, "Tea," The Planters Chronicle, Vol. 90, No. 7-9, 1990, p. 319.
3. N. Muraleedharan, "Pesticide Residues in Tea: Problems and Perspectives." The Planters Chronicle, Vol. 9, 1994, pp. 371-375.
4. Q. Chen, "Tea—the Best Drinking for Health," China Tea, Vol. 3, No. 28, 1985.
5. Z. Deng, B. Tao and X. Li, "Effect of Tea on the Living Time of Musca Domesticas and the Anti-Stress of KM Rats." Journal of Nanchang University, Vol. 19, No. 2, 1997, pp. 69-72.
6. G. S. Hartley and I. J. Graham-Bryce, "Physical Principles of Pesticide Behaviour," Vol. 1-2, Academic Press, London, 1980.
7. J. Schonherr, and P. Baur, "Cuticle Permeability Studies: a Model for Estimating Leaching of Plant Metabolites to Leaf Surface." Journal of Aerial Plant Surface Microbiology, 1989, pp. 1-23.
8. P. Cabras, A. Angioni, P. Caboni, V. L. Garau, M. Melis, F. M. Pirsi and F. Cabitza, "Distribution of Folpet on the Grape Surface after Treatment," Journal of Agriculture and Food Chemistry, Vol. 48, No. 3, 2000, pp. 915-916. doi:10.1021/jf990069u
9. P. Cabras, A. Angioni, V. Garau, M. Melis, F. M. Pirsi and E. V. Minelli, "The Effect of Epicuticular Waxes on Fruits of Fenthion," Journal of Agriculture and Food Chemistry, Vol. 45, No. 9, 1997, pp. 3681-3683. doi:10.1021/jf970102h
10. S. Jaggi, C. Sood, V. Kumar, S. D. Ravindranath and A. Shanker, "Leaching of Pesticide in Tea Brew," Journal of Agricultural and Food Chemistry, 2001, Vol. 49, No. 11, pp. 5479-5483. doi:10.1021/jf010436d
11. C. Sood, S, Jaggi, V. Kumar, S. D. Ravindranath and A. Shanker, "Effect of Various Manufacturing Stages on Pesticide Residues in Tea." Journal of the Science of Food and Agriculture. Vol. 84, No. 15, 2004, pp 2123-2127. doi:10.1002/jsfa.1774
12. R. E. McDonald, H. E. Nordby and T. G. Mccollum, "Epicuticular wax morphology and composition related to grape fruit injury," Horticulture Science, Vol. 28, 1993, pp. 311-312.
13. P. Baur, "Effects on Cuticular Penetration of Neutral Polar Compounds: Dependence on Humidity and Temperature," Journal of Agriculture and Food

Chemistry, Vol. 47, No. 2, 1999, pp. 753-761. doi:10.1021/jf980507h

14. G. G. Briggs, R. H. Bromilow and A. A. Evans, "Relationship between Lipophilicity and Root uptake and Translocation of Non-Ionised Chemicals in Barley." Pesticide Science, Vol. 13, No. 5, 1982, pp. 294-504. doi:10.1002/ps.2780130506

15. R. E. Gaskin, K. D. Steele and W. A. Forster, "Characterizing Plant Surfaces for Spray Adhesion and Retention." New Zealand Plant Protection, Vol. 58, 2005, pp. 179-183.

CHAPTER 8

TOXICITY AND FEEDING RESPONSE OF ADULT CORN EARWORM (LEPIDOPTERA: NOCTUIDAE) TO AN ORGANIC SPINOSAD FORMULATION IN SUCROSE SOLUTION

Juan D. López Jr., Mohamed A. Latheef, Wesley C. Hoffmann

Keywords: Entrust; Attract-and-Kill; Helicoverpa zea; Adult Control; Bioinsecticide

INTRODUCTION

Entrust™ is a natural insect control product formulated from the spinosyn family of insecticides for the organic growers. The spinosyns are fermentation by-products of the soil borne actinomycete bacterium, Saccharopolyspora spinosa Mertz and Yao [1]. Spinosad consists of two principal fermentation factors, Spinosyns, A and D and is a fast acting broad spectrum chemical that acts on the insect primarily through ingestion or contact with the sprayed surface [2]. It affects the nervous system of the insect and activates the nicotinic acetylcholine receptors and causes loss of muscle control, exhaustion and culminates in the death of the insect. In the tobacco budworm larvae, Helithis virescens (F), Spinosyn A causes diuresis and widespread tremors of the extremities and the larvae curl up and lay on their sides [3]. Public awareness of the hazards associated with pesticides has burgeoned consumer interest in organically produced farm products in the United States [4]. This has resulted in the organic farming sector to continuously increase its market share each year and has now become a $30 billion industry [5]. Organic farms have increased from 11 million ha in 1999 to 37.2 million ha in 2011 worldwide [6]. Concomitant with these developments in organic farming, there has been a renewed interest in the reformulation of pesticides that are compatible for usage in organic farms. For instance, the inert ingredient, propylene glycol, contained in SpinTor® 2SC was replaced with more ecologically compatible kaolinite clay in Entrust™ (SpinTor® 2SC; MSDS 2012; Entrust™ 80 W; MSDS 2013, Dow AgroSciences, Indianapolis, Indiana). With the approval from the Organic Materials Review Institute (OMRI) for use in organic farming and gardening, Entrust is also classified as an organic substance by the USDA National Organic Standards Board, and is in conformity with the FAO/WHO "Codex Alimentarius" and IFOAM (International Federation of Organic Agriculture Movements) standards.

Pesticide control of heliothine insect pests is traditionally conducted targeting larval instars which feed on fruiting structures of host plants. However, several researchers contend that adult control of highly mobile heliothine insects would be more beneficial compared to traditional method of control of larvae with broadcast application of synthetic pesticides. For instance, heliothine adults were 10 to 100 times more susceptible to insecticides compared to larvae, and that adults were much less likely to develop resistance to insecticides compared to larvae [7]. Also, higher detoxification associated

Citation: López, J. , Latheef, M. and Hoffmann, W. (2014) Toxicity and feeding response of adult corn earworm (Lepidoptera: Noctuidae) to an organic spinosad formulation in sucrose solution. Advances in Entomology, 2, 33-41. doi: 10.4236/ae.2014.21006.

with cuticular penetration, internal accumulation, excretion of applied toxicants and their metabolites occurred more rapidly in larvae compared to that in adults [8].

Adult females upon emergence from pupal cells in their natural habitat disperse in quest of carbohydrate-rich food source, usually obtained from plant exudates, before resuming their reproductive activity [9-11]. This nocturnal behavior of H. zea has the potential for exploitation in developing pest management strategy for organic farming systems. Researchers have developed attractants for several noctuid species of Lepidoptera and that when the attractant composition is mixed with a toxicant, it could serve as a lethal food source [12]. However, despite the worldwide growth of organic agriculture, there has been a lack of research-based information on arthropod pest management strategies suitable for such farming systems [13].

Objectives of this study were to determine rate of ingestion, toxicity and proboscis extension response of adult corn earworm, Helicoverpa zea (Boddie) relative to an organic formulation of spinosad, Entrust when mixed with sucrose solution as a feeding stimulant. The intent of this study was to determine whether Entrust, when mixed with a sugar solution as a feeding stimulant, could serve as a cynosure of attraction, delivering a lethal food source for foraging moths.

MATERIALS AND METHODS

Test Solutions

We weighed 1.25 g of Entrust™ 80 W (EPA Reg.# 62719-282; 80% spinosad and D, 3.4% kaolin, 2% silica gel and the balance 14.6%; MSDS 2013; Dow AgroSciences, Indianapolis, Indiana) in a Sartorius balance (Model No. LA 120S). Using 10% sugar (Sigma Chemical Co., St Louis, Missouri) solution as a feeding stimulant, we prepared a stock solution of the pesticide at 10,000 mg·L^{-1}. The sugar solution was prepared by weighing 100 g of sugar and made up to a volume of 1 L. Various concentrations of test solutions were then prepared by appropriate dilution with the sugar solution.

Laboratory-Reared Test Insects

Corn earworm eggs were obtained from Department of Biochemistry, Molecular Biology, Entomology and Plant Pathology, Mississippi State University, Mississippi. Eggs were held for hatching in the laboratory maintained at 23.9°C ± 0.38°C, RH 64.5% ± 4.6% with a photoperiod of 14:10 L:D. Larvae were reared on a soybean-wheat germ diet [(Stonefly Heliothis Diet, Ward's Natural Science (www.wardsci.com)]; using similar techniques described earlier [14]. During the rearing procedure, approximately 4 g of the diet was dispensed into a 22.2 ml plastic soufflé cup using a caulking gun and an individual larva was placed on the diet and sealed with a lid. About 250 cups were prepared each time and were stored in a 1/6- 57# paper bag in the laboratory. About 3 wks thereafter, pupae were harvested, sorted by gender, and male and female pupae were placed separately in 4 L jars for moth emergence.

Field-Collected Test Insects

The natural populations of corn earworm comprised of those captured in pheromone-baited wire cone traps baited with Zealure®, the synthetic male sex attractant (Hercon Environmental, Emigsville, Pennsylvania). Traps were established in an agricultural production area in the Brazos Bottom Region in Burleson County, southwest of College Station, Texas (30.6278°N, 96.3342°W). Males captured during the previous night were collected early in the morning and were placed in a BugDorm-1 (www.megaview.com.tw) insect rearing cage, and kept in the laboratory for testing.

Feeding Mechanism

The feeding apparatus used in this study was described earlier [15,16]. Amount of Entrust ingested by each corn earworm was determined by providing test solutions of the chemical in a 0.5 ml disposable centrifuge tube. Test solutions were weighed on an electronic balance before and after feeding. To account for the evaporation loss during the feeding period, extra tubes containing the test solutions on which the moths did not feed were used to obtain the amount loss between before and after feeding. Each moth was placed in an apparatus equipped with alligator clips to hold the wings in a vertical position. Test solutions in centrifuge tubes were placed in a hole drilled in a Plexiglass® block. Immediately, thereafter, the moths extended their proboscides to feed on the test solutions. Moths that did not extend the proboscides were teased with an insect pin to initiate feeding and to ensure adequate feeding, insects were teased multiple times.

Determination of Lethal Concentration (LC) Values

Both male and female laboratory-reared corn earworms that emerged overnight in the laboratory and feral males captured overnight in pheromone-baited traps were used in this study. Each test consisted of moths fed various sub-lethal concentrations of Entrust at 0.1875, 0.375, 0.25, 0.50, 1.0 mg·L^{-1}. Control moths were fed 10% sucrose solutions alone. These sub-lethal concentrations were determined after conducting preliminary tests to assess the range of concentrations that would provide appropriate mortality data. In each test, six moths were fed Entrust at each concentration, and the test was replicated 22 times. Immediately after cessation of feeding, moths were sorted by treatment and were placed in a 946 ml jar where 10% sugar solution was provided in a 22.2 ml soufflé cup closed with a lid through which a cotton wick in contact with the sugar solution was inserted. Two strips of paper towel were left hanging inside the jar to enable the moths to rest and move around within the jar. Mortality was determined 24, 48 and 72 h after feeding.

The assessment of mortality is usually based upon the criterion that the moths could not right themselves when placed upside down [16]. In this study, we observed variant symptoms of poisoning between individual moths after the ingestion of Entrust by the corn earworm. Often the moths which fed to satiation had bloated abdomen, the proboscides were extended with the terminal end being rolled in and the wings were lifted up. Some moths had their genitalia extruded, and lay on their sides inside the cup with the wings lifted up and the body twitching. We considered moths showing such symptoms of poisoning dead because they were incapacitated and were moribund.

Determination of Mean Lethal Time

In order to determine mean lethal time, we chose the 50 mg·L^{-1} concentration of Entrust, the minimum spray application rate at 46.8 L·ha^{-1} for control of corn earworm larvae in sweet corn (Specimen Label, Dow AgroSciences, Indianapolis, IN). We conducted two tests relative to the determination of mean lethal time. In test 1, we determined ingestion of Entrust at 50 mg·L^{-1} by feeding feral males captured overnight in pheromone-baited traps using the feeding apparatus described earlier. A total of 156 moths were fed Entrust in groups of 6 and were compared to control moths fed 10% sucrose solution alone. In test 2, moths fed at 50 mg·L^{-1} were placed individually in a 22.2 ml soufflé cup after feeding, and were examined every 15 min. for mortality. A total of 66 moths were fed in groups of 6 and were compared to control moths relative to mortality.

Feeding Response at Lethal Concentrations

Moths were fed Entrust at concentrations of 0.1, 1.0, 10, 100 and 1000 mg·L^{-1} in order to determine the effect of lethal concentrations of the pesticide relative to ingestion. Control moths were provided only 10% sucrose solutions. Test moths comprised of both laboratory-reared and field-collected corn earworm. These moths were grouped into two categories. Group 1 comprised of corn earworm that emerged overnight in the laboratory as well as those captured overnight in pheromone-baited traps. Similarly, group 2 comprised of both laboratory-reared and field-collected corn earworm held for 24 h without feeding. A total of 30 to 36 replications were conducted in each group.

Proboscis Extension Bioassay

The proboscis extension response assay measures the taste behavior of H. zea and is a useful technique to measure the sense of taste. Stimulation of gustatory receptor neurons on the antennae, the tarsi and the mouthparts elicits the proboscis extension response in tobacco budworm, H. virescens [17]. The methods used to determine the proboscis extension response were similar to those described earlier [18]. Briefly, they comprised of holding a moth with the index finger and the thumb and touching the front tarsi to the test solutions in a porcelain multiwall plate by raking the front legs across it while avoiding contact of other body parts with the test solution. The proboscis extension response comprised of three phases. If the proboscis was completely extended (a positive response), a rating of 2 was assigned, and if the proboscis was partially uncoiled but was retracted without fully extending (a partial response), a rating of 1 was recorded and if there was no extension of the proboscis (a negative response), a rating of zero was recorded.

The proboscis extension response was evaluated in the laboratory in the afternoon using H. zea captured overnight in pheromone-baited traps and those held for 24 h without feeding. Moths comprising of the two age groups were exposed to concentrations of the chemical at 0.1, 1, 10, 100 and 1000 mg·L^{-1}. Five replications comprising of 20 males per concentration were conducted for each age group of the insect. A total of 100 males per concentration were used in each test.

Data Analysis

All statistical analyses of the data were conducted using SAS 9.3 version [19]. Lethal concentration data were analyzed using the Proc Probit log10 procedure with LACKFIT and INVERSECL options. The failure of 95% fiducial limits to overlap was used as a criterion to separate LC_{50} values between 24-, 48- and 72 h responses in the dose-response models [20]. Statistical validity of this criterion to separate LC values for data with large sample size and approximately equal standard errors was demonstrated by Payton et al. using a computer simulation model [21]. Data reported here include tests with large sample size (N = 204 to 372 moths) and nearly equal standard errors (See Tables 1-3) between the slopes of probit regressions. Traditionally, we assume a dose response relationship between the levels of a factor representing increasing amounts x of Entrust and the response y (mean % proboscis extension or the feeding response), and execute the regression of y on x. In this study, neither the feeding response nor the proboscis extension response exhibited a normally expected functional relationship between y and x. Instead, we found that variations between individual moths predominated in each of these test variables without any apparent dose response relationship. For instance, some moths fed to satiation at higher concentrations of Entrust to the extent that they succumbed soon after ingestion of the toxicant. This behavior demonstrated that regression analysis is not appropriate for this study and that a variance analysis instead will adequately describe the relationship between the variables. Therefore, data on proboscis extension response and feeding studies were analyzed using PROC GLIMMIX model. When means were significant ($p < 0.05$), least square means were separated using PDMIX800 letter grouping procedure with adjust = Tukey ($p < 0.05$) [22]. Variability in the amount of Entrust ingested and the concentrations of pesticide offered to the insect was equalized by transforming the data into natural log before conducting ANOVA procedure. The corn earworm lethal time data relative to the rate of ingestion of Entrust was conducted using the PROC REG procedure.

Table 1. Probit statistics relative to toxicity of Entrust 80 W mixed with 10% sucrose solution fed to male corn earworm, H. zea captured overnight in pheromone-baited trap.

Probit statistics	Number of hours feeding		
	24	48	72
Slope (±SEM)	3.55 ± 0.38	2.68 ± 0.34	2.55 ± 0.38
$p > \chi^2$	0.75 ns	0.96 ns	0.24 ns
LC_{10}[a]	0.21a	0.10b	0.08b
95% CL	(0.16 - 0.24)	(0.06 - 0.14)	(0.05 - 0.11)
LC_{50}	0.48a	0.31b	0.26b
95% CL	(0.43 - 0.53)	(0.26 - 0.35)	(0.23 - 0.30)
LC_{90}	1.09a	0.92b	0.84b
95% CL	(0.91 - 1.44)	(0.75 - 1.27)	(0.64 - 1.34)
LC_{99}	2.16a	2.27a	2.16a
95% CL	(1.61 - 3.38)	(1.57 - 4.12)	(1.35 - 4.98)

[a]LC values (mg·L^{-1}) within each row followed by the same lower case letter are not significantly different based upon lack of overlap in 95% confidence limits (N = 372 moths).

Table 2. Probit statistics relative to toxicity of Entrust 80 W mixed with 10% sucrose solution fed to laboratory-reared male corn earworm, H. zea which emerged overnight.

Probit statistics	Number of hours feeding		
	24	48	72
Slope (±SEM)	2.95 ± 0.44	2.86 ± 0.41	3.19 ± 0.46
$P > \chi^2$	0.18 ns	0.88 ns	0.88 ns
LC_{10}[a]	0.31a	0.17ab	0.15b
95% CL	0.22 - 0.38	0.11 - 0.23	0.09 - 0.20
LC_{50}	0.83a	0.49b	0.37b
95% CL	0.72 - 1.02	0.42 - 0.57	0.31 - 0.43
LC_{90}	2.27a	1.38ab	0.95b
95% CL	1.66 - 3.90	1.08 - 2.07	0.78 - 1.29
LC_{99}	5.12a	3.20a	2.02a
95% CL	3.16 - 12.13	2.12 - 6.57	1.44 - 3.60

[a]LC values ($mg{\cdot}L^{-1}$) within each row followed by the same lower case letter are not significantly different based upon lack of overlap in 95% confidence limits (N = 204 moths).

Table 3. Probit statistics relative to toxicity of Entrust 80 W mixed with 10% sucrose solution fed to laboratory-reared female corn earworm, H. zea which emerged overnight.

Probit statistics	Number of hours feeding		
	24	48	72
Slope (±SEM)	3.25 ± 0.46	3.32 ± 0.44	3.43 ± 0.44
$P > \chi^2$	0.14 ns	0.51 ns	0.64 ns
LC_{10}[a]	0.31a	0.19ab	0.17b
95% CL	0.23 - 0.38	0.13 - 0.24	0.12 - 0.22
LC_{50}	0.77a	0.47b	0.41b
95% CL	0.68 - 0.92	0.41 - 0.54	0.35 - 0.46
LC_{90}	1.92a	1.14ab	0.97b
95% CL	1.46 - 3.05	0.94 - 1.57	0.81 - 1.27
LC_{99}	4.02a	2.36a	1.95a
95% CL	2.63 - 8.39	1.69 - 4.10	1.44 - 3.20

[a]LC values ($mg{\cdot}L^{-1}$) within each row followed by the same lower case letter are not significantly different based upon lack of overlap in 95% confidence limits (N = 220 moths).

RESULTS AND DISCUSSION

Toxicity

Table 1 shows that for natural populations of male corn earworm captured overnight in pheromone-baited traps, the dosage mortality equations were in agreement with the probit model for 24-, 48- and 72-h responses (Table 1). The LC_{50} (95% CL) was 0.48 (0.43 - 0.53) $mg{\cdot}L^{-1}$ for 24 h response and was significantly different from those for 48 and 72-h responses with 0.31 (0.26 - 0.35) and 0.26 (0.23 - 0.30) $mg{\cdot}L^{-1}$, respectively. There was, however, no significant difference between 48 and 72 h responses for both LC_{50} and LC_{90} values. In an earlier study with spinosad (Tracer®44.2% spinosyn A and D; inert ingredients including propylene glycol ≈ 55.8%;

MSDS 2001) mixed with 2.5 M sucrose solution, we reported that LC_{50} and LC_{90} values for feral male corn earworm were 4.96 (4.29 - 5.67) and 21.83 (17.35 - 29.84) $mg{\cdot}L^{-1}$ for 24 h responses, respectively [23]. Compared to spinosad, Entrust is 10- and 20-fold more toxic to feral male corn earworm, respectively, as indicated by LC_{50} and LC_{90} values. The increased toxicity of Entrust to H. zea is more likely due to a 2-fold increase in concentration of the spinosad A and D in Entrust compared to that in spinosad.

Table 2 shows that the LC_{50} and LC_{90} values of Entrust for laboratory-reared male corn earworm which emerged overnight were 0.83 (0.72 - 1.02) and 2.27 (1.66 - 3.90) $mg{\cdot}L^{-1}$, respectively. These values were significantly greater than those for the pheromone trap-captured males. It is likely that the feral corn earworm might have been leaner compared to the laboratory-reared moth, and that the corn earworm probably responded to the toxicant in direct proportion to body weight. This is in agreement with Australian researchers who reported that pyrethroid susceptible old world bollworm, H. armigera (Hübner) pupae were lighter than those of the resistant pupae, although differences in resistance frequencies were not significantly related to body weight of pupae collected from maize, pigeon pea and cotton [24]. However, researchers have cautioned against unquestioned use of proportional adjustment of dose to body weight without testing the hypothesis that the response is proportional to body weight. This may result in erroneous conclusions about relative toxicities [25].

Table 3 shows LC_{50} and LC_{90} values of Entrust for laboratory-reared female corn earworm which emerged overnight were 0.77 (0.68 - 0.92) and 1.92 (1.46 - 3.05) $mg{\cdot}L^{-1}$, respectively. These values were not significantly different from those reported for laboratory-reared males (Table 2).

Proboscis Extension Response

Entrust concentrations tested in this study did not significantly influence the proboscis extension response for the moths captured overnight in pheromone-baited traps for any of the three phases of the response: positive, negative and partial ($F = 0.76$, $p > 0.59$ for positive; $F = 0.47$; $p > 0.79$ for negative and $F = 0.55$; $p > 0.74$ for partial, each with 5, 20 df), respectively. However, the frequency of extending their proboscides positively upon contact with Entrust solutions for moths captured overnight was significantly different from that for moths held for 24 h ($F = 171.51$; df = 1, 24; $p < 0.0001$; Table 4). Similarly, the negative response of the moths not responding to Entrust solutions upon contact varied significantly between 24 h old moths and those captured overnight ($F = 140.61$; df = 1, 24; $p < 0.0001$); however, the response was conversely related. Entrust did not significantly in-fluence partial extension of the proboscis for feral corn earworm captured overnight in pheromone-baited traps when compared to those held for 24 h thereafter in the laboratory ($F = 0.89$; df = 1, 24; $p > 0.36$). There was no significant interaction between moths captured overnight and those starved for 24 h relative to any of the components of proboscis extension response ($F = 0.49$, $p > 0.78$ for positive; $F = 0.76$, $p > 0.59$ for negative; $F = 0.56$, $p > 0.73$ for partial, each with 5, 24 df).

The ability of the moth to extend its proboscis upon contact with a toxicant solution is indispensable for feeding initiation. Regardless of concentrations, 24 h old h old corn earworm positively responded to Entrust solutions by extending their proboscides completely more frequently compared to moths captured overnight in pheromone-baited traps. This suggests that 24 h old moths were more appetitive compared to moths captured overnight in pheromone-baited traps. Also, the 24 h starvation time appears to have brought the corn earworm to a proper responsive state. The frequency of deterrence of the corn earworm to feed on Entrust solutions was significantly more common for corn earworm captured overnight in pheromone-baited traps than for those held for 24 h without feeding. The percentage of moths that exhibited partial response to Entrust solutions was minimal with less than 10% of the moths extended their proboscides, but retracted soon thereafter.

Table 4. Proboscis extension response (±SEM) of H. zea males captured in pheromone-baited traps to various concentrations of Entrust 80 W mixed with 10% sucrose solution.

Concentration ($mg{\cdot}L^{-1}$)	Time (h)	Mean Percentage Response[a] ± SEM		
		Positive	Negative	Partial
0	Overnight	38.0 ± 5.4b	55.0 ± 6.5a	7.0 ± 2.0a
	24	77.0 ± 7.3a	20.0 ± 6.5b	4.0 ± 1.9a
0.1	Overnight	31.0 ± 9.4b	67.0 ± 9.8a	2.0 ± 1.2a
	24	77.0 ± 7.3a	20.0 ± 3.2b	5.0 ± 5.0a
1	Overnight	42.0 ± 7.2b	53.0 ± 8.0a	5.0 ± 1.6a
	24	73.0 ± 7.7a	24.0 ± 5.8b	3.0 ± 3.0a
10	Overnight	42.0 ± 4.3b	55.0 ± 5.0a	3.0 ± 1.2a
	24	79.0 ± 4.0a	18.0 ± 4.9b	3.0 ± 1.2a
100	Overnight	37.0 ± 4.4b	58.0 ± 7.2a	5.0 ± 3.2a
	24	80.0 ± 8.2a	22.0 ± 7.2b	2.0 ± 1.2a
1000	Overnight	33.0 ± 4.6b	60.0 ± 4.5a	7.0 ± 1.2a
	24	66.0 ± 6.2a	30.0 ± 6.9b	5.0 ± 1.6a

[a]Means followed by lower case letter within each response category between moths captured overnight in pheromone-baited traps and those held for 24 h thereafter were not significantly different according to Concentration*Time Least square means computed by *t* statistic of Proc Glimmix procedure ($p < 0.01$). Original means and standard errors are presented here (N = 100 moths).

The proboscis of the tobacco budworm, H. virescens exhibited 100% positive response to 1.0 M sucrose, but showed a weak or no response to an insect deterrent, 1.0 M sinigrin monohydrate [17]. Stimulation of gustatory receptor neurons located in the antennae and the proboscis of the moth elicits the proboscis extension response in H. virescens [26]. Data reported here demonstrate that the lethal concentrations of Entrust did not inhibit neural transmission of information from the gustatory receptor neurons in the corn earworm to elicit proboscis extension response.

Feeding Response at Lethal Concentrations

Figures 1 and 2 show that the feeding response of laboratory-reared female corn earworm to concentrations of Entrust did not significantly differ for moths that emerged overnight ($F = 2.25$; df = 5, 165; $p > 0.05$) as well as for moths held for 24 h without feeding ($F = 1.10$; df = 5, 187; $p > 0.36$) when compared to female fed 10% sucrose solutions alone. Similarly, the feeding response of 24 h old laboratory-reared male corn earworm to Entrust did not vary significantly between concentrations ($F = 1.23$; df = 5 and 191; $p > 0.29$) when compared to control male fed 10% sucrose solution alone (Figure 3). Nevertheless, the feeding response for male moths captured overnight in pheromone-baited traps did vary significantly between concentrations of Entrust ($F = 2.28$; df = 5, 183; $p > 0.049$) when compared to control moths fed 10% sucrose solution alone (Figure 4).

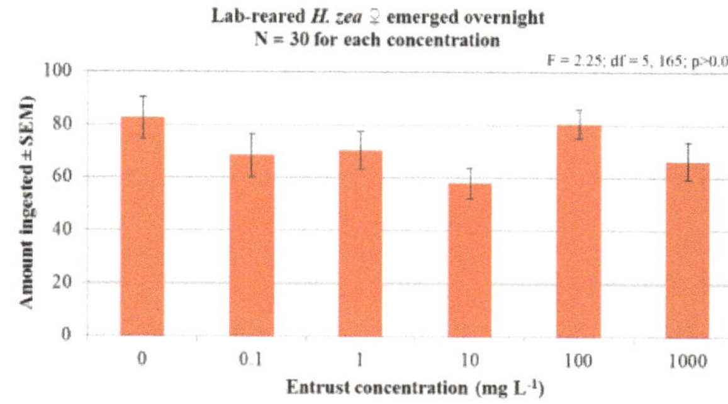

Figure 1. Mean (±SEM) amount of Entrust ingested by labreared H. zea female emerged overnight when fed various concentrations of the chemical mixed with 10% sucrose solution.

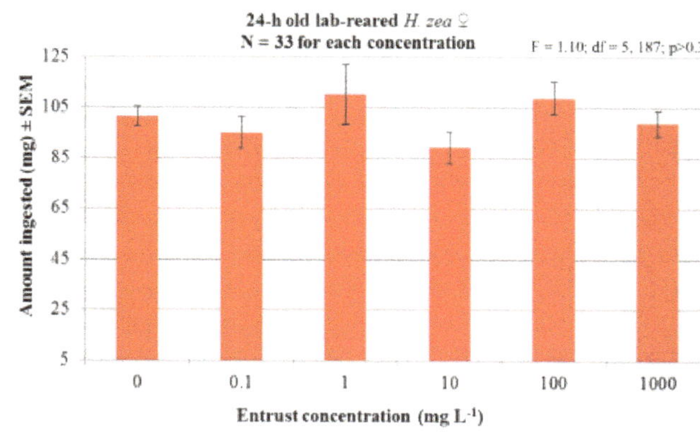

Figure 2. Mean (±SEM) amount of Entrust ingested by 24-h old lab-reared H. zea female when fed various concentrations of the chemical mixed with 10% sucrose solution.

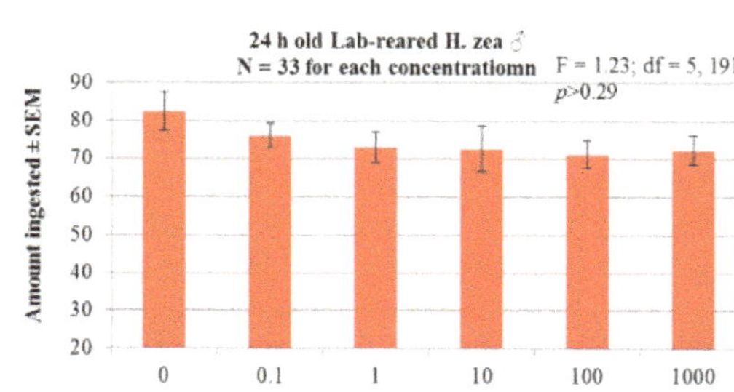

Figure 3. Mean (±SEM) amount Entrust ingested by 24-h old lab-reared male H. zea when fed various concentrations of the chemical mixed with 10% sucrose solution.

Corn earworm male moths fed significantly less Entrust at 1000 $mg{\cdot}L^{-1}$ compared to those fed Entrust at 0.1 $mg{\cdot}L^{-1}$. There was no significant difference in ingestion between moths fed Entrust at 0.1 $mg{\cdot}L^{-1}$ and those fed 10% sucrose solution alone. Ingestion of Entrust at 1, 10 and 100 $mg{\cdot}L^{-1}$ was comparable to one another, and did not vary significantly from control moths as well. However, there was no significant difference in feeding response between moths captured in pheromone-baited traps and held in the laboratory for 24 h without feeding and control moths fed 10% sucrose solutions alone (Figure 5; $F = 1.63$; df = 5, 210; $p > 0.15$). Data show that the inhibition of ingestion of Entrust at the lethal dose of 1000 mg·L^{-1} occurred only with H. zea male captured overnight in pheromone-baited traps and that inhibition was not evident in any of the other more exhaustive tests conducted in this study. This suggests that the inhibition of feeding of Entrust at the lethal dose may not be a genuine phenomenon but that it is likely to be an artifact.

Mean Lethal Time

Figure 6 shows that in test 1, corn earworm consumed significantly less Entrust at 50 mg·L^{-1}compared to control moths fed 10% sucrose solution only ($F = 4.96$; $df = 1, 232$; $p > 0.027$). In test 2, the analysis of the data relative to ingestion of Entrust at 50 mg·L^{-1} and lethal time revealed a significant curvilinear relationship which leveled off asymptotically (Figure 7). There is a decided tendency, as shown in Figure 7, for the corn earworm to succumb to the ingestion of the pesticide within 5 h. With the X variate converted to natural log, the regression of lethal time on ingestion of Entrust showed that lethal time decreased as the amount of Entrust ingested by the corn earworm increased (Figure 8). The regression model was $Y = -0.857\ln(X) - 0.2303$ with $R^2 = 0.3587$. The regression model indicated that only 36% of

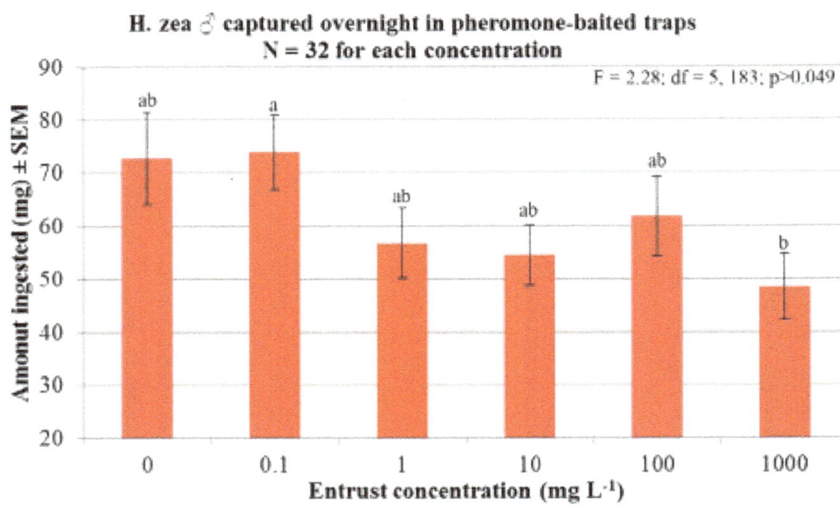

Figure 4. Mean (±SEM) amount of Entrust ingested by male H. zea captured overnight in pheromone-baited traps when fed various concentrations of the chemical mixed with 10% sucrose solution. Least square means were separated using PDMIX800 letter grouping procedure with adjust = Tukey ($p < 0.05$). Bar with the same lower case letter is not significantly different from each other.

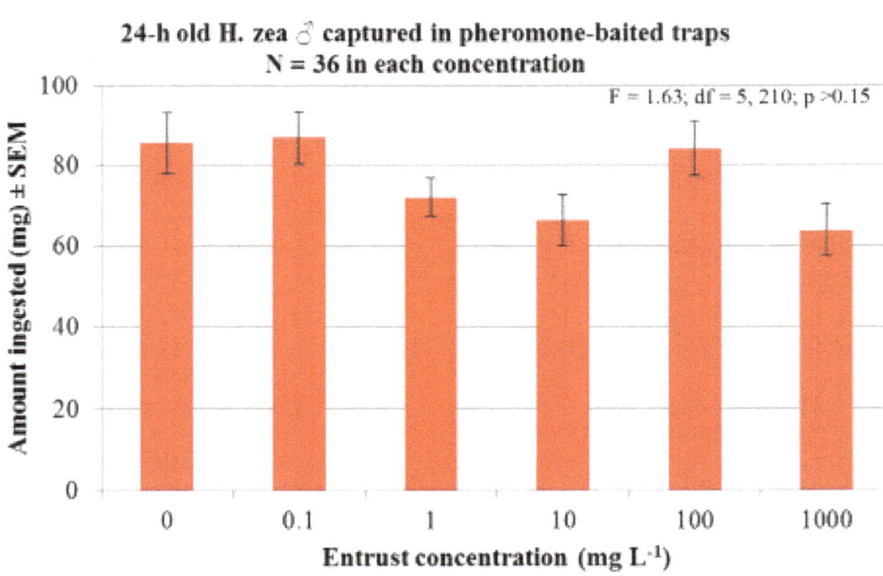

Figure 5. Mean (±SEM) amount of Entrust ingested by 24-h old male H. zea captured in pheromone-baited traps when fed various concentrations of the chemical mixed with 10% sucrose solution.

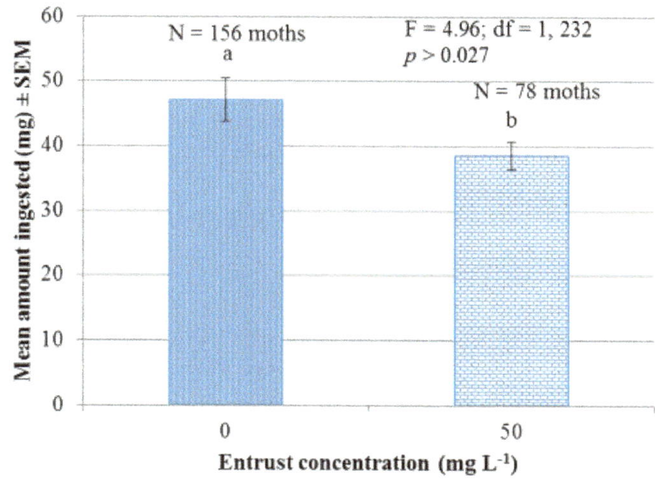

Figure 6. Mean (±SEM) amount of Entrust at 50 mg·L^{-1} ingested by corn earworm compared to 10% sucrose solution.

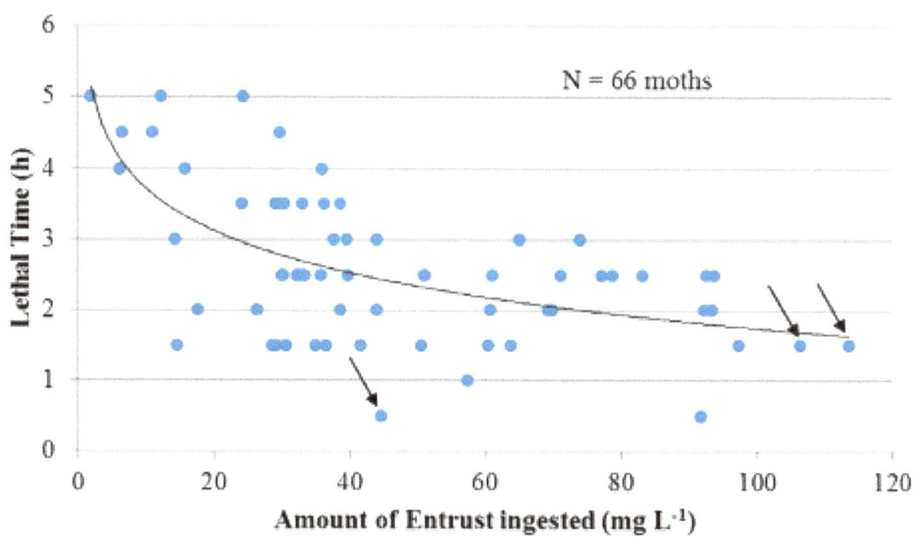

Figure 7. Relationship between amount of Entrust at 50 mg·L^{-1} ingested and lethal time for H. zea male captured overnight in pheromone-baited traps. Arrows show two moths which each ingested 106.4 and 113.5 mg·L^{-1} of Entrust had a lethal time of 1.5 h, and another moth which ingested only 44.7 mg·L^{-1} of Entrust died within 0.5 h.

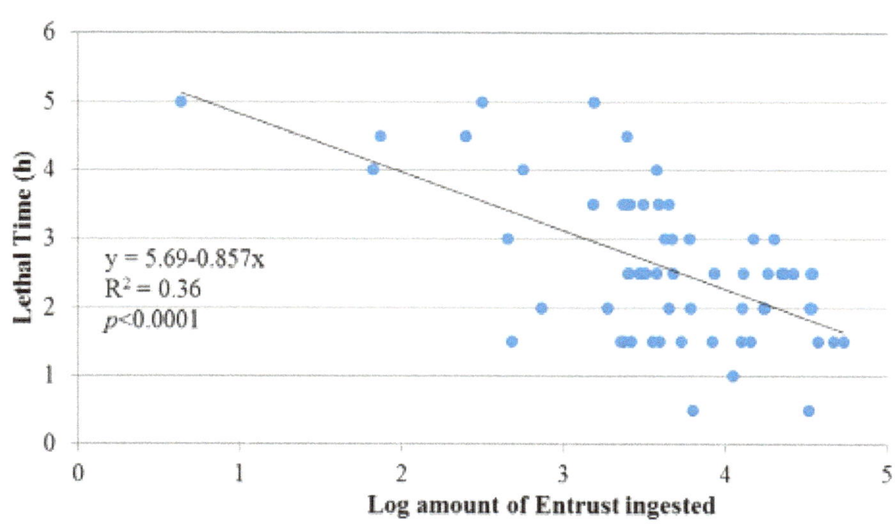

Figure 8. Relationship between log amount of Entrust at 50 mg·L^{-1}ingested and lethal time for H. zea male captured overnight in pheromone-baited traps.

The variation in the ingestion of the chemical was explained by the variations in lethal time. The low R^2 value appears to be due to considerable variability in lethal time between individual corn earworm relative to ingestion of Entrust. For instance, Figure 7 shows that two moths which ingested 106.4 and 113.5 $mg \cdot L^{-1}$ of the chemical took 1.5 h each to die, while one of moths which consumed 44.7 $mg \cdot L^{-1}$ of the pesticide died within 0.5 h. Fourteen percent of the moths, which died at 2 h, exhibited 5.3-fold difference in the ingestion of the pesticide between individual insect. Overall, mean lethal time for the corn earworm was 2.56 ± 0.13 h with ingestion of Entrust at 50 $mg \cdot L^{-1}$. We reported earlier that a similarly negatively linear relationship existed between lethal time and ingestion of spinosad for feral corn earworm captured in pheromone-baited traps in the Brazos Bottom region in Texas [23]. Mean lethal time was 5.3 h with the ingestion of spinosad at 73 $mg \cdot L^{-1}$. Our data are in agreement with researchers in Australia who found that spinosad produced very high mortality of the old world cotton bollworm, H. armigera and H. punctigera, but that moths took much longer to die [27]. Rapid incapacitation or mortality of test moths is important for sampling dead moths near treated rows while evaluating the efficacy of insecticidal baits in an attract-and-kill management strategy [27]. They, Del Socorro et al. [27] found significantly more dead moths near rows treated with methomyl compared to those treated with spinosad. This suggests that quick acting Entrust would be preferable over spinosad in field trials during development of a behavioral-based pest management strategy for heliothine insects.

CONCLUSION

Recent trend in increased awareness of organically produced fruits and vegetables concomitant with the public willingness to pay premium prices for these products has attracted many growers to organic farming. Organic food market grew at 12% per year from 2000 to 2010 with sales of natural and organic foods exceeding $40 billion in 2010, and is expected to grow at 8% from 2010 through 2013 [28]. Nevertheless, the organic farms are not growing fast enough to meet the surging demand for organic meat and dairy products in the United States. For instance, in order to meet the domestic needs of this industry, the value of organic soybean imports from China and India to the United States doubled last year and is expected to surpass $100 million in value in 2013 [29]. Data reported here indicate that Entrust will be a useful tool as applicable to attract-and-kill technology to control heliothine insects in organic farming systems. This technology is not gender specific and targeting virgin females before they mate and reproduce will be an effective management program. Furthermore, organic farms are usually small scale operations and treating small acreage of vegetation with syrup-based feeding stimulant/toxicant mixture using a backpack sprayer will annihilate large populations of reproducing of H. zea on host crops. It was estimated that in the Coastal Plains area of Texas that nearly a million moths could be killed by treating one ha of row of corn using only 20 g of toxicant and 190 L of a sugar-syrup-based feeding stimulant [30]. Soon after the emergence of H. zea from pupae in corn fields, moths climb up corn stalks and feed on exudates from the stalks [10]. Furthermore, the corn earworm moths do not oviposit until 2 d after emergence [10,31]. This behavior provides some windows for conducting spray applications, and can be exploited for the development of an attracticide-based insecticidal bait formulation for controlling corn earworm on its host crop. Even though our results show encouraging trends in the control of heliothine species, additional studies are needed to ascertain the efficacy of attract-and-kill technology in field plots.

ACKNOWLEDGEMENTS

We appreciate the assistance of Curtis Hubbard who serviced and maintained the pheromone traps. Parker Knutson helped in conducting the tests on ingestion, toxicity and proboscis extension response reported in this study.

DISCLAIMER

Mention of a commercial or proprietary product does not constitute an endorsement for its use by the US Department of Agriculture. USDA is an equal opportunity employer.

REFERENCES

1. Crouse, G.D. and Sparks, T.C. (1998) Naturally derived materials as products and leads for insect control: The spinosyns. Reviews in Toxicology, 2, 133-146.
2. Thompson, G.D., Dutton, R. and Sparks, T.C. (2000) Spinosad—A case study: An example from a natural products discovery programme. Pest Management Science, 56, 696-702. http://dx.doi.org/10.1002/1526-4998(200008)56:8<696::AID-PS182>3.0.CO;2-5
3. Salgado, V.L. and Sparks, T.C. (2005) The spinosyns: Chemistry, biochemistry, mode of action, and resistance. In: Gilbert. L.I., Latrou, K. and Gill, S.S., Eds., Comprehensive Molecular Insect Science, Elsevier, Oxford, 137- 173.
4. Dimitri, C. and Greene, C. (2000) Recent growth patterns in the U. S. organic foods market, 1-21. www.ers.usda.gov/aib777
5. USDA News Release (2013) Release No. 0096. www.usda.gov/wps/portal/usda/usdamediafb?contentid=2013/05/0096
6. Willer, H. and Lernoud, J. (2013) The world of organic agriculture. The results of latest survey on organic agriculture worldwide. BioFach Congress 2013, Nürnberg Session, The World of Organic Agriculture, FiBL and IFOAM Publications.http://orgprints.org/22324/1/willer-lernoud-2013-world-of-organic.pdf
7. Joyce, R.J.V. (1981) A critical review of the role of chemical pesticides in Heliothis management. In: Reed, W., Ed., Proceedings of International Workshop, Heliothis Management, ICRISAT, Patancheru, 173-188.
8. Leonova, I.N. and Slynko, N.M. (1996) Comparative study of insecticide susceptibility and activities of detoxifying enzymes in larvae and adults of cotton bollworm. Insect Biochemistry and Physiology, 32, 157-172. http://dx.doi.org/10.1002/(SICI)1520-6327(1996)32:2<157::AID-ARCH1>3.0.CO;2-W
9. Lingren, P.D., Raulston, J.R. and Wann, E.V. (1988) Emergence and dispersal of adult corn earworms. In: Motes, J. Ed., Proceedings of 6th Annual Horticulture Industry Show, Oklahoma Co-operative Extension

Service, Oklahoma State University, Stillwater, 73-77.

10. Lingren, P.D., Warner, W.B., Raulston, J.R., Kehat, M., Henneberry, T.J., Pair, S.D., Zvirgzdins, A. and Gillespie, J.M. (1988) Observations on the emergence of adults from nocturnal populations of the corn earworm, Heliothis zea (Boddie). Environmental Entomology, 17, 254- 258.
11. Beerwinkle, K.R., Shaver, T.N. and Lopez Jr., J.D. (1993) Field observations of adult emergence and feeding behavior of Helicoverpa zea (Lepidoptera: Noctuidae) on dallisgrass ergot honeydew. Environmental Entomology, 22, 554-558.
12. Lopez Jr., J.D., Shaver, T.N., Beerwinkle, K.R. and Lingren, P.D. (2000) Feeding attractant and stimulant for adult control of noctuid and/or other lepidopteran species. US patent No. 6 074634.
13. Zehnder, G., Gurr, G.M., Kühne, S., Wade, M.R., Wratten, S.D. and Wade, M.R. (2007) Arthropod pest management in organic crops. Annual Review of Entomology, 52, 57- 80.http://dx.doi.org/10.1146/annurev.ento.52.110405.091337
14. López Jr., J.D. and Lingren, P.D. (1994) Feeding response of adult Helicoverpa zea (Lepidoptera: Noctuidae) to commercial phagostimulants. Journal of Economic Entomology, 87, 1653-1658.
15. Clemens, C.G. (1996) Effects of feeding stimulant and insecticide mixtures on feeding response and mortality of adult male corn earworm, Helicoverpa zea (Boddie) (Lepidoptera: Noctuidae). MS Thesis, Texas A&M University, College Station, Texas.
16. Lopez Jr., J.D., Latheef, M.A. and Hoffmann, W.C. (2010) Effect of emamectin benzoate on mortality, proboscis extension, gustation and reproduction of the corn earworm. Journal of Insect Science, 10, 1-16. http://dx.doi.org/10.1673/031.010.8901
17. Jørgensen, K., Kavello, P., Almaas, T. J. and Mustaparta, H. (2006) Two closely located areas in the suboesophageal ganglion and the tritocerebrum receive projections of the gustatory receptor neurons located on the antennae and the proboscis in the moth Heliothis virescens. Journal of Comparative Neurology, 496, 121-134.http://dx.doi.org/10.1002/cne.20908
18. López Jr., J.D., Lingren, P.D. and Bull, D.L. (1995) Proboscis extension response of adult Helicoverpa zea (Lepidoptera: Noctuidae) to dry sugars. Journal of Economic Entomology, 88, 1271-1278.
19. User's Guide Version 9.3 (2008) SAS Institute, Cary, North Carolina.
20. Robertson, J.L. and Priesler, H.K. (1992) Pesticide bioassays with arthropods. CRC Press, Boca Raton.
21. Payton, M.E., Greenstone, M.H. and Schenker, N. (2003) Overlapping confidence intervals or standard error intervals: What do they mean in terms of statistical significance? Journal of Insect Science, 3, 34. http://insectscience.org/3.34/
22. Saxton, A. (2012) User's guide for design and analysis SAS macro collection DandA.SAS. Department of Animal Science, University of Tennessee, Tennessee.
23. López Jr., J.D., Latheef, M.A. and Hoffmann, W.C. (2011) Mortality and reproductive effects of ingested spinosad on adult bollworms. Pest Management Science, 67, 220- 225.http://dx.doi.org/10.1002/ps.2055
24. Daly, J.G. and Fitt, G.P. (1990) Monitoring for pyrethroid resistance in relation to body weight in adult Helicoverpa armigera (Hübner) (Lepidoptera: Noctuidae). Journal of Economic Entomology, 83, 705-709.
25. Robertson, J.L., Russell, R.M., Preisler, H.K. and Savin, N.E. (2007) Bioassays with arthropods. 2nd Edition, CRC Press, Taylor & Francis, Boca Raton.
26. Jørgensen, K., Almaas, T.J., Marion-Poll, F. and Mustaparta, H. (2007) Electrophysiological characterization of responses from gustatory receptor neurons of sensilla chaetica in the moth Heliothis virescens. Chemical Senses, 32, 863-879.http://dx.doi.org/10.1093/chemse/bjm057
27. Del Socorro, A.P., Gregg, P.C. and Howes, A.J. (2010) Development of a synthetic plant volatile-based attracticide for female noctuid moths. III. Insecticides for adult Helicoverpa armigera (Hübner) (Lepidoptera: Noctuidae). Australian Journal of Entomology, 49, 31-39.http://dx.doi.org/10.1111/j.1440-6055.2009.00735.x
28. Annie's Prospectus (2011) http://www.annies.com
29. Peters, M. (2013) A gap in organic food chain. The Wall Street Journal, Dow Jones & Co., New York.
30. Cole, Y. (2000) Mortality of adult Helicoverpa zea (Lepidoptera: Noctuidae) in corn and cotton treated with a feeding-based attracticide. MS Thesis, Texas A&M University, College Station, Texas.
31. Callahan, P.S. and Casio, T. (1963) Histology of the reproductive traits and transmission of sperm in the corn earworm, Heliothis zea. Annals of Entomological Society of America, 56, 535-556.

CHAPTER 9

PRODUCTION OF LOW COST BACILLUS THURINGIENSIS BASED-BIOPESTICIDE FOR MANAGEMENT OF CHICKPEA POD-BORER HELICOVERPA ARMIGERA (HUEBN)

Abida Bibi, Khalique Ahmed, Najma Ayub, Sadia Alam

Keywords: Beef Blood; Molasses; Indigenous B.t. Isolate PA-Sb-46.3; Sporulation; Entomotoxicity; Biopesticide

INTRODUCTION

Among the insect pests, chickpea pod-borer, Helicoverpaarmigera occupies a prominent position and has attained a status of topmost agricultural pest in Pakistan, China and India [1]. The most destructive pest H. armigera is polyphagous in nature and has been recorded by Iqbal, and Mohyuddin, 1990 [2] on 62 host plants, and on more than 100 plant hosts by different researchers [3-6]. Synthetic chemical insecticides for the control of insect pests are commonly used in Pakistan which are not only expensive but also have created a number of problems like water pollution, biological and environmental hazards, and development of resistant in pests [6]. H. armigera has also shown resistance to various groups of chemicals in Pakistan. These problems have increased the importance for the development and the use of safe and target specific bio-insecticides, e.g., Bacillus thuringiensis (B.t.). The entomopathogenic bacterium (Bacillus thuringiensis (B.t.)) during sporulation produces crystalline proteins which are associated with the insecticidal activity of B.t. against different insects larvae of Lepidopteran, Dipteran, Coleopteran and some other pests. These crystalline proteins are harmless to humans, vertebrates and plants, are completely biodegradable and cause no toxic residual products to accumulate in the environment. That is why this bacterium is widely used as microbial insecticide in agriculture and forestry for the control of pests, and in human health sector for the elimination of disease vectors [7]. Hence due to the safety associated with B.t., tremendous interest has been developed towards the production of a new commercial B.t. products. B.t. products are being used successfully on large scales in India, China, US, Australia and many other countries of the world whereas in Pakistan no attention has been given towards their production and use. The main objective of this diligent effort is the production of low cost and effective B.t. biopesticide by a simple and effective process (shake flask/ fermentation technology) to manage H. armigera infesting chickpea in Pakistan.

MATERIALS AND METHODS

Laboratory Scale Production of B.t.-Biopesticide against Helicoverpa armigera

Biopesticide was prepared in liquid form with spore counts ×109 /ml by using shake flask/fermentation technology [8].

Citation: Bibi, A. , Ahmed, K. , Ayub, N. and Alam, S. (2013) Production of low cost Bacillus thuringiensis based-biopesticide for management of chickpea pod-borer Helicoverpa armigera (Huebn). Natural Science, 5, 1139-1144. doi: 10.4236/ns.2013.511140.

Indigenous B.t. isolate, PA-Sb-46.3 that had bipyramidal and cuboidal crystals and was 73.6 times toxic against H. armigera than reference standard strain B.t. var. kurstaki (HD-I-S-1980) used in this study Toxicity was evaluated against 1st instar larvae of the test insect chickpea pod-borer, H. armigera mass reared on artificial diet according to the method reported by scientists [9,10].

Composition of Medium

Local available inexpensive raw material was selected as culture medium for the laboratory scale production of B.t. biopesticide which comprised, dried beef blood 30.0 g, molasses 15.0 ml, CaCl2 0.03 g and salt solution 1.0 ml ($ZnCl_2$, $MgCl_2$, $MnCl_2$, $CaCl_2$, $FeCl_3$ and 5 drops of HCl) in1000 ml distilled water

Preparation of Medium

Beef blood obtained from slaughterhouse was dried in an oven at 90°C for 24 hour. Dried blood crystals were ground and sieved through muslin cloth in order to obtain a very fine powder. Thirty gram of dried beef blood powder was added into flask containing 350 ml of distilled water. Flask was tightly plugged with cotton wool covered with polythene paper to avoid absorbance of suspension in the cotton plug during shaking. This flask was placed in a shaking water bath for proper mixing of blood in distilled water at 160 rpm for 03 h at 30°C ± 2°C.

The blood-water mixture was transferred into flask of one litre capacity and other contents of medium i.e., molasses 15 ml and CaCl2 0.03 g were added and volume was made up to one litre with distilled water. Flask was placed into water bath for an hour at 80°C with continuous stirring for proper mixing of medium ingredients. This mixture was then sieved through six-fold of muslin cloth in order to remove the traces of solid beef blood. This process was repeated twice to obtain suspension free of solid blood traces. The volume was again made up to one litre by adding some distilled water, which was evaporated during heating. The medium was then equally distributed into ten flasks (500 ml capacity) in such a way that each flask contained 100 ml of the medium. All the flasks were tightly plugged and autoclaved at 121°C for 20 minutes at 15 lbs/inc^2 .

Inoculation of Medium

When medium was cool down approximately to 60°C then each flask was inoculated with 100 μl of inoculum which was prepared by adding loop full from 72 h old, pure 95% - 98%. sporulated B.t. culture (examined in a phase contrast microscope (PCM) at 100×) into 5.0 ml of sterile salt solution and vortexed. Smear was prepared from this suspension and examined in PCM to check the purity of B.t. culture.

Fermentation of Medium

Inoculated flasks were placed in a shaking water bath for 72 hours at 30°C ± 2°C and 160 rpm. After 72 h flasks were removed from shaking water bath, smear was prepared from each flask and examined in a PCM in order to check the purity and growth stage of fermented culture. Flasks that contained pure and 95% - 98% sporulated culture was pooled into flask of 2-litre capacity.

Suitability of Medium for the Growth of B.t.

Medium giving high yield of spore and crystal were considered suitable for the production of biopesticide and was further subjected for toxicity evaluation through bioassay. Bioassay of fermented culture Diet reported by scientists was used for all bioassays experiments performed during this study [10]. Six different concentrations i.e., 0.5%, 1%, 2%, 4%, 8% and 16% of fermented culture of biopesticide were prepared in total volume of 400 ml artificial diet (Table 1). Four hundred milliliter diet of each concentration was prepared by mixing fermented culture with diet as given in Table 1 and poured with the help of pouring bottles in glass vials and allowed to cool and solidify. Separate pouring bottles were used for each concentration and control. Four replicates were maintained for each concentration and each replicate comprise 25 vials. Similarly four replicates of control without fermented cultures were also carried out in parallel. Each vial containing intoxicated diet and that of control was aseptically infested with the single 1st in star larvae with sterilized soft camel hair brush. Vials were tightly plugged with sterilized cotton wool and incubated in an inverted position at 26°C ± 2°C for 7 days. At the end of incubation period, experiment was terminated and mortality was recorded by counting dead and alive larvae in each vial The LC_{50} values of the toxins were worked out through probit analysis computer programme [11].

Table 1: Concentration of fermented culture used in diet for bioassay.

S. Nos	Concentration	Fermented culture "A"	Diet "B"	Total volume "A" & "B"
1	0.5%	2.0 ml	398 ml	400 ml
2	1%	4.0 ml	396 ml	400 ml
3	2%	8.0 ml	392 ml	400 ml
4	4%	16.0 ml	384 ml	400 ml
5	8%	32.0 ml	368 ml	400 ml
6	16%	64.0 ml	336 ml	400 ml

Preparation of Biopesticide Formulation

Storage of biopesticide for a long period at room temperature diluents and preservatives i.e., Glycerol 10.0 ml, Boric acid 10.0 g, Corn starch 35 g, Methyl-Para-hydroxybenzoate 10.0 g were added into one litre fresh fermented B.t. culture and mixed well by shaking. The pH was noted and placed in a dark room.

Bioassay of Biopesticide Formulation

Toxicity of biopesticide formulation was evaluated against larvae of the H. armigera using the same method and concentrations in 400 ml of diet as used for fermented culture.

Influence of Diluents and Preservatives

Influence of preservatives and diluents on toxicity of biopesticide was also noted by comparing values: pH, CFU × 10^9 /ml and LC_{50} μg/ml diet of the fermented culture and biopesticide formulation formed after adding diluents and preservatives. Diluents and preservatives showing no effect on toxicity was considered suitable for biopesticide preservation and shelf life.

Storage and Shelf Life Evaluation of Biopesticide

Five more batches (each batch of one litre) of biopesticide were prepared by the same procedure as used for the production of first batch. The six batches were combined and toxicity was evaluated; pH was checked and stored at room temperature in a dark room. Bioassay experiments were also conducted against H. armigera at three month's time interval over a period of 30 months in order to measure the stability period of toxin and effectiveness period of preservatives and diluents in the biopesticide placed at room temperature.

Concentrations 4%, 8% and 16% of pooled batch of biopesticide showed 100% mortality (Figure 1). Therefore shelf-life was evaluated with reduced concentrations i.e., 0.125%, 0.25%, 0.5%, 1.0%, 2.0%, and 4.0%, (same for all experiment i.e., 1st to 10th) of the biopesticide prepared in total volume of 400 ml of artificial diet (Table 2).

All bioassay steps and method of determination of LC_{50} values were same as used for the toxicity evaluation of fermented culture.

Viable spore counts colony forming units (CFU) in 1.0 ml of biopesticide was calculated for each batch of

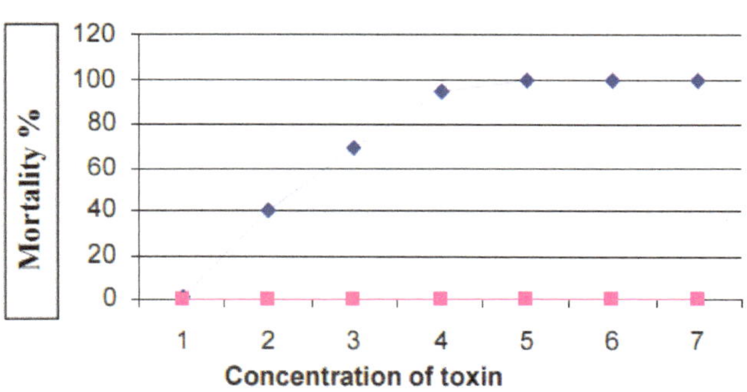

Figure 1: Pooled batch of biopesticide

Table 2: Preparation of different concentrations of biopesticide in artificial diet.

S.Nos	Concentration (biopesticide)	Biopesticide "A"	Diet "B"	Total volume "A" & "B"
1	0.125%	0.5 ml	399.5 ml	400 ml
2	0.25%	1.0 ml	399 ml	400 ml
3	0.5%	2.0 ml	398 ml	400 ml
4	1.0%	4.0 ml	396 ml	400 ml
5	2.0%	8.0 ml	392 ml	400 ml
6	4.0%	16 ml	384 ml	400 ml

One litre, pooled batch of six litres and after every three months during shelf-life evaluation (Table 3). For this purpose 1.0 ml of biopesticide was added into 9.0 ml of sterile distilled water in sterilized test tube and vortexed. Ten fold dilutions of this sample was prepared and 100 µl of dilution 10^{-7} was spread-plated (four replicates) on the surface of solid BGM after heat shock at 80°C for 10.0 min and incubated at 30°C for 24 h. After 24 h, colonies showing B.t. like morphology were counted under magnifying lens and confirmed as B.t. by randomly selecting 5 - 6 colonies per plate and observing in phase contrast microscope. Mathematical average of four replicates was calculated. Number of CFU/mg was calculated by the following formula:

$$\text{Colony Forming Units/mg} = \frac{\text{Number of colony forming units}}{\text{ml} \times \text{Dilution factor}}$$

RESULTS

Suitability of Medium Selected for the Preparation of Biopesticide

Results of fermented media as indicated in Table 4 revealed that the selected media was suitable for the growth of B.t. and the production of biopesticide as B.t. showed 95% - 99% sporulation and produced high yield of crystal after 72 h at adjusted conditions i.e., rpm, temperature time and size of flask. It also showed high toxicity i.e. LC_{50} value against 1st instar larvae of H. armigera 0.53 µg/ml diet.

Table 3: Effect of preservatives and diluents on the toxicity of biopesticide

Culture	pH	spores × 10^9/ml	LC50 µg/ml diet
Fermented culture	7	3.97	0.53
Biopesticide formulation	7	4.25	0.50

Table 4: Toxicity of different batches and combined batch of biopesticide against H. armigera

Batches of biopesticide	Biopesticide pH	No. of spores/ml (×10^9)	LC50 µg/ml Diet
1	7	4.25	0.50
2	7	4.54	0.39
3	7	3.61	0.91
4	7	3.89	0.69
5	7	4.37	0.93
6	7	3.81	0.65
Pooled batch	7	4.01	0.59

Influence of Preservatives and Diluents on the Toxicity of Biopesticide

Toxicity results of fermented culture and biopesticide formulation against 1st instar larvae of H. armigera as shown in Table 5 indicated no effect of preservatives and diluents on pH, number of spores ×10^9 /ml and toxicity as they did not reduce or enhance toxicity because there is no difference between the LC_{50} value of fermented culture and LC_{50} value of biopesticide formulation prepared from the same fermented culture.

Toxicity Evaluation of Biopesticide

The LC_{50} value of six batches and pooled batch of biopesticide as in Table 6 showed that biopesticide was effective against H. armigera. Their pH value and spores $\times 10^9$ /ml were also given. These values also indicated that no correlation exists between number of spores and toxicity of biopesticides as the toxicity value did not increase or decrease with increase or decrease of number of spores.

Mortality Increase with the Increase of Toxin Concentration

Mortality % observed in six batches and pooled batch of biopesticides given in Figures 1 and 2 indicated that with the increase of toxin concentration in diet, mortality of larvae also increased.

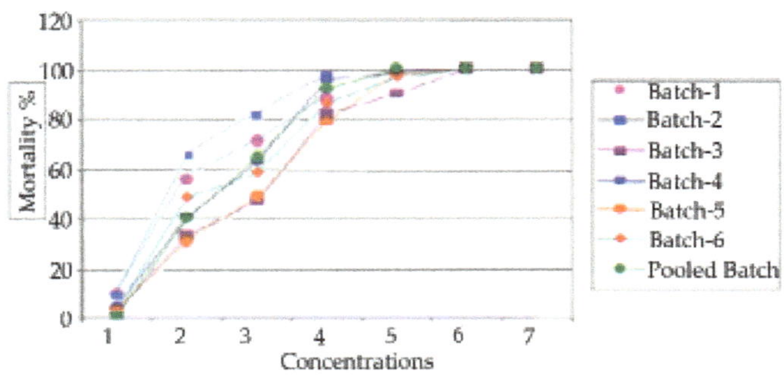

Figure 2: Mortality % of different concentrations of H. armigera.

Shelf Life Evaluation of Biopesticide

Bioassay experiments performed as results indicated in Table 3 at three months' time interval over a period of 30 months showed that there was gradual decrease in the toxicity of biopesticide after nine months but no change in the number of spores and no contamination was observed during this time period. Biopesticide was still considered effective because its LC_{50} µg/ml diet is 4.95 which is slightly higher than LC_{50} value that is 4.54 µg/ml diet 4.54 of the same isolate PA-Sb-46.3.

Effectiveness of Preservatives and Diluents in Biopesticide

Results of shelf-life evaluation of biopesticide (Table 3) indicated that preservatives and diluents used were effective because no: 1) change in pH value 2) significant change in number of spores 3) growth of other microorganism (bacteria and fungi) was observed during spore counting over a period of thirty months

DISCUSSION

Due to the safety associated with B.t. production scientists all over the world are trying to produce effective B.t. biopesticide by using inexpensive and locally available raw material as medium in order to lower the production cost and compete with the commercial B.t. products. Obeta and Okafor (1984) formulated five different media from the seeds of legumes dried beef blood and mineral salts and assessed growth and production of insecticidal toxins of B.t. which were effective against A. aegypti, C. quinquefasciatus, A. gambiae [12]. Bioorganic wastes (chicken feathers) as medium for the production B.t. biopesticide were also used. A similar attempt has been made here for the production of effective B.t. biopesticide against H. armigera by selecting local, cheap and easily available medium ingredients consisting of e.g., molasses as a carbohydrate source, beef blood as protein source and salt solution as inorganic ions for the enhancement of sporulation. Similar requirements are reported by Prasertphon (1996) that the sporulation and crystal production depends upon a source of carbon, nitrogen, minor elements and growth factor [8]. Bernhard and Utz (1993) stated that sporulation was stimulated by the inorganic ions particularly Ca^{+2} and Mg^{+2} [13].

Table 5: Characteristics of fermented medium of biopesticide.

Fermented medium		Time	pH	Sporulation	CFU/mL ($\times 10^9$)	LC50 mg/mL diet
B.t. isolate	Medium Composition					
PA-Sb-46.3	Blood, Molases, CaCl, Distilled water	72 h	7	95% - 99%	3.97	0.53

Table 6: Shelf life evaluation of biopesticide.

S.Nos	Interval (in months)	Time period (in months)	pH	No. of spores/ml ($\times 10^9$)	LC50 µg/ml diet
1	00 (Fresh)	00	7	3.89	0.59
2	3	03	7	3.71	0.23
3	3	06	7	4.40	0.30
4	3	09	7	3.55	1.22
5	3	12	7	4.27	1.83
6	3	15	7	3.21	2.08
7	3	18	7	3.70	2.34
8	3	21	7	3.45	3.23
9	3	24	7	4.30	3.80
10	3	27	7	3.65	4.14
11	3	30	7	3.93	4.95

Medium contained entire nutrient in proper ratio necessary for the optimal growth of B.t. and for the production of crystal in good quality and quantity. During process of bacterial growth no smell of ammonia was observed indicating an appropriate amount of protein in the medium These results were also in agreement with the result reported by Prasertphon (1996) who stated that good quality and quantity of crystal production can be achieved by carefully balancing the nutrition ratio i.e., carbohydrate and protein in the medium [8]. If the nutrition ratio is not properly balanced it will prevent the B.t. to sporulate. Insufficient protein in the medium results poor quantity of crystal and too rich of protein results in bacterial lysis giving odor of ammonia. The neutral pH of fermented culture and biopesticide formulations was observed that indicated appropriate amount of carbohydrates and protein in the media. Similar pH was also reported by Morris et al., 1998 [14]. Conditions for shake flask technique such as temperature, rpm, time size of flask was suitable for the growth of B.t. Temperature, rpm and time were in close agreement with the values reported by Yusoff et al., 2003 [15]. Insect bioassay is the best way of finding the toxicity of B.t. preparation. All bioassays results showed that the fermented culture and biopesticide formulation were toxic against the H. armigera and was suitable to control them different concentrations used showed that with the increase of toxin, mortality also increased. Ahmed et al., (1996) have also reported similar results of B.t. var kurstaki against H. armigera. They found with the increase of toxin concentration mortality was also increased [16]. All bioassay results also indicated that there was no correlation between the number of spores and toxicity value of biopesticide which are in agreement with the results that there is no relationship between the number of spores in preparation and its insect killing power which is true for lepidopterous active isolate [17]. Toxicity test of biopesticide stored at room temperature against H. armigera at three month's time interval over a period of 30 months indicated that B.t. biopesticide can be stored at room temperature for more than 30 months without losing its effectiveness by using preservatives and diluents. These results were in agreement with Prasertphon (1996) results who stated that fresh liquid B.t. culture could be stored at room temperature fore more than 24 months without losing its effectiveness by using preservatives and diluents [8]. Some characteristic s such as no change in pH value, number of spores and no growth of other microorganism (bacteria and fungi) also supported these results.

CONCLUSION

Cost analysis of raw material used as culture medium indicated that it is highly economical (7 US Dollars for the production of 10 litre biopesticide formulation), and bioassay result indicated that production of indigenous B.t. biopesticide on commercial scale can serve as a substitute of chemical pesticides which will be a remarkable achievement in the field of pest management in Pakistan. It will reduce the use of highly toxic chemical insecticides, save foreign exchange used in their import, help to control insects that have developed resistance to chemical insecticides and will save our environment from pollution problems which are the major concerns at present.

REFERENCES

1. Regupathy, A., Kranthi, K., Singh, J., Iqbal, A., Wu, Y. and Russell, D. (2003) Patterns and magnitude of insecticide resistance levels in India, Pakistan and China. Proceeding of World Cotton Research Conference, Cape Town, 9-13 March 2003, 30.9.
2. Iqbal, N. and Mohyuddin, A.I. (1990) Eco. Biology of Heliothis spp in Pakistan. Pakistan Journal of Agricultural Research, 2, 257-266
3. Baloch, A.A. (1989) Insect pests of cotton, their identification, mode of damage and control strategy. Proceedings of workshop organized by CWM Project of Sindh in Collaboration with USAID, Sakrand, 20-25 May 1989, 20.
4. Baloch, A.A., Kalroo, A.M. and Sanjrani, M.W. (2000) A perspective review on eco-biological aspect of Helicoverpa (Heliothis) armigera Hubn (Lepidoptera: Noctuidae) as a pest of cotton in Pakistan. I. Taxonomy, biology, ecology and population dynamics. Balochistan Journal of Agricultural Science, 1, 36-43.
5. Hazara, A.H., Khan, J., Shakeel, M., Iqbal, M. and Bajoi, A.H. (2000) Population dynamics and control of Helicovepa (Heliothis) armigera, Hubner (Lepidoptera; Noctuidae) on different crops in Balochistan. Balochistan Journal of Agricultural Science, 1, 52-62.
6. Malik, M.F., Hussainy, S.W., Rahman, D.U., Munir, A. and Ali, L. (2002) Efficacy of synthetic pheromone for the control of Helicoverpa armigera in tomato. Asian Journal of Plant Sciences, in press.
7. Schnepf, E., Crickmore, N., Van Rie, J., Lereclus, D., Baum, J., Feitelson, J., Zeigler, D.R. and Dean, D.H. (1998) Bacillus thuringiensis and its pesticidal crystal proteins. Microbiology and Molecular Biology Reviews, 62, 775-806.
8. Prasertphon, S. (1996) Historical background on use of Bacillus thuringiensisin Thailand. Proceeding of 2nd Rim Conference on Biotechnology of B.t. and Its Impact on the Environment, 1-14.
9. Ahmed, K., Kongming, Wu, Liang, G. and Guo, Y. (2006) Cross resistance of Cry1Ac resistant cotton bollworm Helicovera armigerato various spore-delta endotoxin of Bacillus thuringiensis Berliner. Pakistan Journal of Biological Sciences, 9, 1639-1649. http://dx.doi.org/10.3923/pjbs.2006.1639.1649
10. Ahmed, K., Khalique, F. and Malik, B.A. (1998) Evaluation of synergistic interactions between Bacillus thuringiensis and malic acid against Chickpea Pod-Borer, Helicoverpa armigera (Huebn) (Lepidoptera: Noctuidae). Pakistan Journal of Biological Sciences, 1, 105-108. http://dx.doi.org/10.3923/pjbs.1998.105.108
11. LeOra Software (1987) POLO-PC-a user's guide to probit or logit analysis. LeOra Software, Berkeley.
12. Obeta, J.A.N. and Okafor, N. (1984) Medium for the production of primary powder of Bacillus thuringiensissubsp, israelensis. Applied and Environmental Microbiology, 47, 863-867
13. Bernhard, K. and Utz, R. (1993) Production of Bacillus thuringiensisinsecticide for experimental and commercial uses. In: Entwistle, P. F., Cory, J.S., Baily, M.J. and Higgs, S., Eds., Bacillus thuringiensis, an Environmental Biopesticide: Theory and Practice. Wiley & Sons, Chichester, New York, Toronto, 255-267.
14. Morris, O.N., Converse, V., Kanagaratnam, P. and Cote, J.C. (1998) Isolation, Characterization and Culture of Bacillus thuringiensis from soil and dust from grain storage bins and their toxicity for Mamestraconfigurata (Lepidoptera: Noctuidae). The Canadian Entomologist, 130, 515-537. http://dx.doi.org/10.4039/Ent130515-4
15. Yusoff, W.M.W., Masri, M.M.M. and Mei, C.C. (2003) Effect of ammonium sulphate on the sporulation of Bacillus thuringiensis subsp. AizawaiSN2 (A local isolate) during batch fermentation. Journal Teknology, 39, 53-60.
16. Ahmed, K., Khalique, F., Malik, B.A. and Ferro, D.N. (1996) Susceptibility of larval instars of Helicoverpa (Heliothis) armigera to HD-1-δ-1980 and relative toxicities of commercial Bacillus thuringiensis. The 2nd Pacific Rim Conference on Biotechnology of B.t., Chiang Mai, 579-594.
17. Dulmage, H.T. and Rhodes, R.A. (1971) Production of pathogens on artificial media. In: Burges, H.D. and Hussay, N.W., Eds., Microbial Control of Insect Pests and Mite, Academic Press, New York, 161.

CHAPTER 10

SYNTHESIS AND BIOACTIVITY OF N-BENZOYL-N'-[5-(2'-SUBSTITUTED PHENYL)-2-FUROYL] SEMICARBAZIDE DERIVATIVES

Zining Cui, Yun Ling, Baoju Li, Yongqiang Li, Changhui Rui, Jingrong Cui, Yanxia Shi and Xinling Yang

Keywords: chitin synthesis inhibitors; benzoylphenylurea; semicarbazide; synthesis; bioactivity

INTRODUCTION

Chitin, the β-(1→4) glycoside polymer of N-acetyl-D-glucosamine, is a major structural component of insect cuticles. In addition to the insect cuticles, chitin is also present in cell walls of fungi and protozoa, but is absent in higher plants and vertebrates. This species-specificity provides the rationale to select chitin as a safe target for pest control agents [1,2]. Chitin synthesis inhibitors (CSIs), which can interfere with chitin formation, will affect the normal growth and development process of insects and fungi but have no effect on plants and vertebrates. The unique mode of action coupled with excellent activity on target and lower toxicity to non-target organisms (including many beneficial arthropods) made these compounds a new tool for integrated pest management (IPM) [3–15]. Benzoylphenylureas (BPUs) have been developed as a typical kind of chitin synthesis inhibitors since Dimilin (diflubenzuron) was introduced into market in the 1970s [3,4]. Their general structures A (Scheme 1) consist of three parts including the benzoyl (X), the urea linkage (Y), and the aniline (Z) [7].

Numerous modifications on the benzoyl (X) and aniline (Z) parts have resulted in the discovery of many commercial insecticides, such as chlorfluazuron, teflubenzuron, bistrifluoron, and noviflumuron [7–11]. However, modification on the urea linkage (Y) has been considered less, although some efforts on this part have been made. For example, Grosscurt found that the compounds had good insecticidal properties when the urea linkages were converted into carbamoyl-2-pyrazolines [12]. Wang's group reported that the compounds resulting from substitution of the hydrogen on the nitrogen atom of the urea linkage with carbamylosulfenyl or carbamate groups could retain the insecticidal activity [13–15].

Citation: Zining Cui , Yun Ling , Baoju Li , Yongqiang Li , Changhui Rui , Jingrong Cui , Yanxia Shi and Xinling Yang, Synthesis and Bioactivity of N-Benzoyl-N'-[5-(2'-substituted phenyl)-2-furoyl] Semicarbazide Derivatives, doi:10.3390/molecules15064267

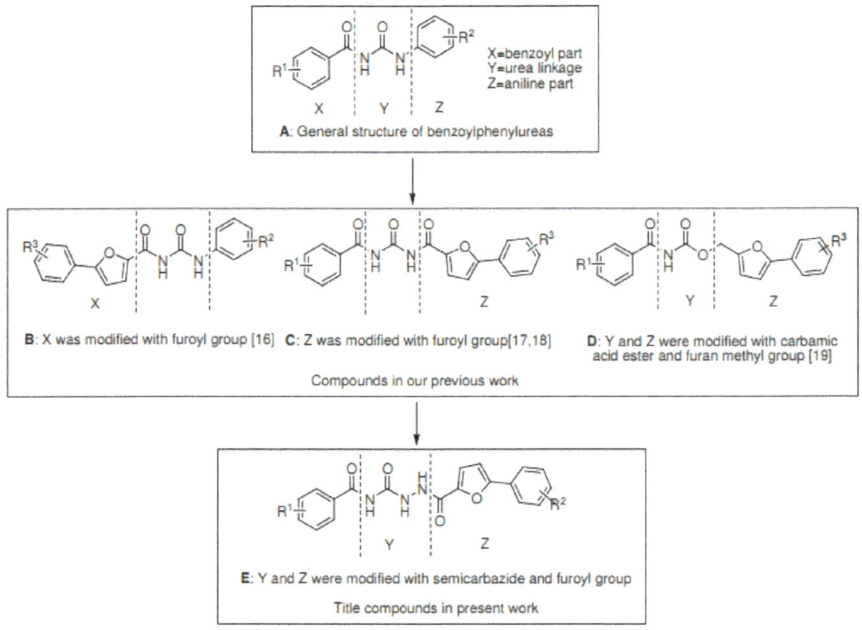

Scheme 1: Design strategy for title compounds E.

In our previous work, the benzoyl (X) part was modified with a furoyl group to get benzoylureas B [16], and the aniline (Z) part was replaced with a furoyl group to obtain dibenzoylureas C [17,18]. The bioassay results indicated that some of the resulting compounds had certain insecticidal activity, whereas when the Y and Z moieties were modified with carbamic acid ester and furan methyl groups, the insecticidal activity disappeared and the compounds exhibited good fungicidal activity [19]. In the present work, an effort of structure optimization was carried out, in which the urea linkage was converted to a semicarbazide, while the aniline part was replaced with a 5-phenyl-2-furoyl group (Scheme 1). Fifteen novel N-benzoyl-N'-[5-(2'-substituted phenyl)-2-furoyl] semicarbazides (E) were designed and synthesized for the purpose of new pesticide and anticancer drug discovery. Their in vivo insecticidal activity and in vitro fungicidal and antitumor activities were preliminarily evaluated.

RESULTS AND DISCUSSION

Chemistry

The synthetic route of compounds E is shown in Scheme 2, where the starting materials were substituted anilines and benzoic acids. All of the title compounds were prepared by the nucleophilic addition reaction of 5-substituted aryl-2-furoyl hydrazine with benzoyl isocyanate under an anhydrous atmosphere.

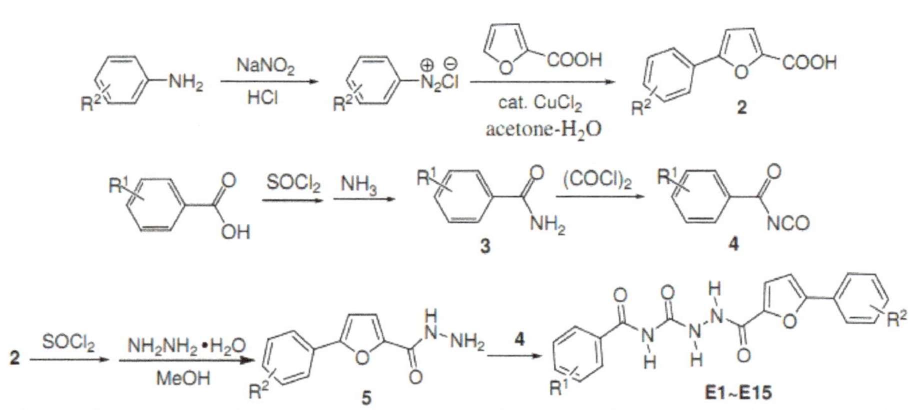

E1: R^1=H, R^2=4-Cl; **E2**: R^1=2,6-di-F, R^2=4-F; **E3**: R^1=3-CH_3, R^2=4-Cl; **E4**: R^1=2,6-di-F, R^2=4-Cl; **E5**: R^1=2-Cl, R^2=4-Cl; **E6**: R^1=2,6-di-Cl, R^2=4-CH_3; **E7**: R^1=2,6-di-F, R^2=4-CH_3; **E8**: R^1=2-Cl, R^2=4-CH_3; **E9**: R^1=2-OCH_3, R^2=2-NO_2; **E10**: R^1=3-CH_3, R^2=2-Cl; **E11**: R^1=2,6-di-F, R^2=2-Cl; **E12**: R^1=2-OCH_3, R^2=2-Cl; **E13**: R^1=2,6-di-Cl, R^2=2,4-di-F; **E14**: R^1=2-Cl, R^2=2,4-di-F; **E15**: R^1=2-OCH_3, R^2=4-Cl.

Scheme 2: General synthetic procedure for title compounds E

All of the structures of the title compounds were confirmed by ^{1}H-NMR, IR, and elemental analyses. In the IR spectra, the compounds showed absorption bands around 3,500 and 3,200 cm^{-1} originating from the N-H stretching vibration. The strong bands around 1,750 cm^{-1} could be assigned to the C=O stretching vibration. The bands between 1,690 and 1,650 cm^{-1} were carbonyl vibration of the secondary amide. Absorption bands around 1,610, 1,520 and 1,480 cm^{-1} were attributed to the frame vibrations of the phenyl and furan rings.

In the ^{1}H-NMR spectrum, one sharp peak in the range from 9.70 to 11.50 ppm was due to the presence of NH. The splits of most compounds were normal, except for the compounds with fluorine substitution because of the coupling and splitting between fluorine and hydrogen. The fluorine atom splits a hydrogen proton into a doublet, which complicated the proton signals. The protons on phenyl rings were mostly split into multiple peaks in the range from 7.20 to 8.10 ppm and the protons on the furan ring were split into a doublet in the range from 6.90 to 7.40 ppm.

The structures were further conformed by single crystal X-ray analysis of a typical example, compound E2. Figure 1 gives a perspective view of the compound sad the crystal data are presented in Table 1. Some important bond lengths, angels, and torsion angles of compound E2 are given in Table 2. It could be seen from the X-ray analysis of E2 that the single bonds distances of C11-N1, C12-N2, C13-N3, and C12-N3 (1.363(3), 1.342(3), 1.369(3), and 1.398(3) Å) are equal to the van der Waals' radii for a C–N double bond (1.35 Å), the single bonds C4-C7, C8-C11, and C13-C14 (1.461(4), 1.470(4), and 1.504(4) Å) are shorter than the standard C–C single bond (1.54 Å), but longer than C–C double bond (1.34 Å), and the N1–N2 (1.387(3) Å) single bond is shorter than the standard N–N single bond (1.45 Å), but longer than a N–N double bond (1.25 Å). All of these clearly indicated that the p orbital of N atoms conjugated with the π molecular orbital and formed the delocalized π-bonds with the conjoint furan and benzene ring. Unexpectedly, the p orbitals of N1, N2, and N3 seemed not to be conjugated with the π molecular orbital of the C11–O2 ,C12–O3, and C13-O4 double bonds, which was explained by the bond length of C11–O2, C12-O3, and C13–O4 (1.228(3), 1.224(3), and 1.219(3) Å) that followed in the normal range of C–O double bonds (1.19-1.23 Å).

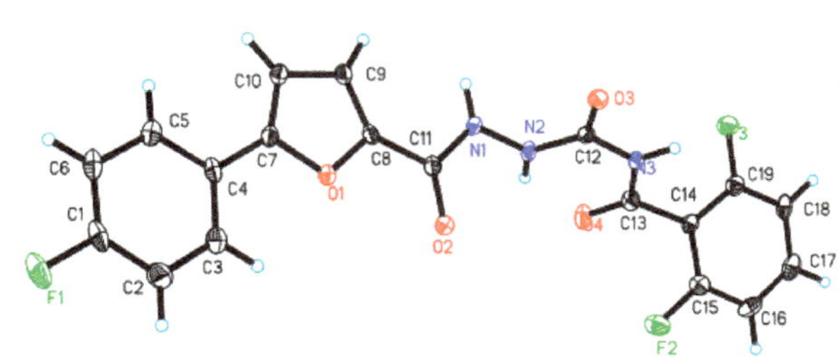

Figure 1: Molecular structure of compound E2, showing 30% probability ellipsoids, H atoms were shown as small spheres of arbitrary radii.

Table 1: Crystal and experimental data of compound E2.

Empirical formula	$C_{19}H_{12}F_3N_3O_4$
Formula weight	403.32
T	173(2) K
Wavelength	1.54178 Å
Crystal system	Triclinic
Space group	$P1$
Unit cell dimensions	a = 6.8462(12) Å, α = 107.173(13)° b = 11.552(2) Å, β = 104.549(12)° c = 11.667(2) Å, γ = 93.363(13)°
Volume	844.4(3) Å^3
Z	2
D_x	1.586 Mg/m^3
Absorption coefficient	1.171 mm^{-1}
F (0 0 0)	412
Crystal dimensions	0.20 x 0.13 x 0.10 mm
θ range for data collection	4.05 to 68.19
Completeness to θ = 68.19	96.7 %
Limiting indices	$-8 \le h \le 8$, $-13 \le k \le 13$, $-13 \le l \le 14$
Reflection collected/unique	8794/2990 [R(int) = 0.0529]
Absorption correction	Numerical
Max. and min. transmission	0.8919 and 0.7995
Data/restraints/parameters	2990 / 0 / 263
Goodness-of-fit on F^2	1.088
Final R indices [$I > 2\sigma(I)$]	R_1 = 0.0555, wR_2 = 0.1218
$2\theta_{max}$	136.38° with Cu K_α
$(\Delta\rho)_{max}$	0.301 eÅ^{-3}
$(\Delta\rho)_{min}$	-0.318 eÅ^{-3}
Program system	SHELXS-97, SHELXL-97
Structure determination	Direct method
Refinement	Full-matrix least-squares on F^2
CCDC No.	769209

Table 2: Selected bond lengths, angels, and torsion angles of compound E2.

Lengths	(Å)	Angles	(°)	Torsion angles	(°)
C(4)-C(7)	1.461(4)	O(2)-C(11)-N(1)	123.0(3)	C(11)-N(1)-N(2)-C(12)	-113.9(3)
C(8)-C(11)	1.470(4)	O(2)-C(11)-C(8)	123.4(3)	C(6)-C(1)-C(2)-C(3)	2.0(5)
C(13)-C(14)	1.504(4)	O(3)-C(12)-N(3)	119.9(3)	F(1)-C(1)-C(2)-C(3)	-177.7(3)
O(2)-C(11)	1.228(3)	O(3)-C(12)-N(2)	124.9(3)	C(5)-C(4)-C(7)-O(1)	176.3(2)
O(3)-C(12)	1.224(3)	O(4)-C(13)-C(14)	120.6(3)	C(7)-O(1)-C(8)-C(9)	0.0(3)
O(4)-C(13)	1.219(3)	O(4)-C(13)-N(3)	124.2(3)	N(2)-N(1)-C(11)-O(2)	4.9(4)
N(1)-C(11)	1.363(3)	N(2)-C(12)-N(3)	115.2(2)	N(1)-N(2)-C(12)-O(3)	4.1(4)
N(2)-C(12)	1.342(3)	N(3)-C(13)-C(14)	115.2(3)	N(1)-N(2)-C(12)-N(3)	-176.2(2)
N(3)-C(13)	1.369(3)	C(13)-N(3)-C(12)	127.7(2)	C(12)-N(3)-C(13)-O(4)	6.4(4)
N(3)-C(12)	1.398(3)	C(12)-N(2)-N(1)	119.9(2)	O(4)-C(13)-C(14)-C(19)	122.7(3)
N(1)-N(2)	1.387(3)	C(11)-N(1)-N(2)	118.4(2)	C(17)-C(18)-C(19)-F(3)	179.9(3)

In the crystal of the structure, C(1), C(2), C(3), C(4), C(5), and C(6) formed a plane with a mean deviation of 0.0099 Å, defined as plane I; C(7), C(8), C(9), C(10), and O(1) formed a plane with the a mean deviation of 0.0009 Å, defined as plane II; O(2), C(11), N(1), and N(2) were nearly coplanar with a mean deviation of 0.0144 Å, defined as plane III; O(3), C(12), N(3), C(31) and O(4) were nearly coplanar with a mean deviation of0.0163 Å, defined as plane IV; C(14), C(15), C(16), C(17), C(18), and C(9) formed a plane with a mean deviation of 0.0075 Å, defined as plane V (Figure 1). Plane II, plane III, plane IV and plane V form a dihedral angle with plane I of 4.2, 3.3, 73.3, and 17.5°. Plane III, plane IV and plane V form a dihedral angle with plane II of 7.2, 75.8, and 19.9°. Plane IV and plane V form a dihedral angle with plane III of 70.1 and 14.5. And the dihedral angle between plane IV and plane V is 55.9°. The related data are summarized in Table 3.

Table 3: The dihedral angles and the mean deviation of the planes in compound E2.

Dihedral angles (°)	
Plane I and plane II	4.2
Plane I and plane III	3.3
Plane I and plane IV	73.3
Plane I and plane V	17.5
Plane II and plane III	7.2
Plane II and plane IV	75.8
Plane II and plane V	19.9
Plane III and plane IV	70.1
Plane III and plane V	14.5
plane IV and plane V	55.9
The mean deviation of the plane (Å)	
Plane I	0.0099
Plane II	0.0009
Plane III	0.0144
Plane IV	0.0163
Plane V	0.0075

Biological Activity

Considering that the lead compounds B and C had good insecticidal activity against dipterous and lepidopterous insects, and D had good fungicidal activity, we chose five strains of fungi and three kinds of insects to evaluate whether the designed compounds retained the insecticidal and fungicidal activity.

The bioassay showed that the title compounds exhibited lower fungicidal activity in vivo against the five strains of fungi at the concentration of 50 μg mL^{-1} (Table 4). In the insecticidal activity shown in Table 5, some title compounds possessed good activity to the Plutella xylostella L. at the concentration of 500 μg mL^{-1}, such as E10 and E15 were 95.0% and 85.0%, respectively.

Table 4: Fungicidal activity of compounds E against five fungus species at 50 μg mL^{-1} .

Compd.	Inhibitory rate (%)				
	Phytophthora Capsici	*Botrytis Cinerea*	*Fusarium Oxysporum*	*Rhizoctonia Solanii*	*Corynespora Cassiicola*
E1	1.94	13.61	7.50	0.00	2.22
E2	9.72	9.17	37.50	3.61	14.44
E3	22.50	6.11	29.17	1.39	8.33
E4	37.50	23.33	10.28	41.39	6.39
E5	23.61	54.72	32.22	0.00	8.06
E6	49.17	49.17	14.17	0.00	11.39
E7	8.89	29.17	5.83	0.00	5.83
E8	31.94	48.89	14.44	8.33	8.33
E9	10.28	28.61	28.89	0.56	10.28
E10	12.50	0.00	20.83	0.00	8.33
E11	19.44	0.00	9.72	50.00	6.94
E12	20.83	45.28	4.72	0.00	12.22
E13	13.06	4.17	8.61	0.00	19.72
E14	21.67	7.78	8.61	0.00	18.06
E15	4.17	10.56	30.28	0.00	5.00
DMF(control)	4.17	5.56	22.78	13.06	14.72
fungicides[a]	86.39 a	69.72 b	68.33 c	76.67 d	68.61 e

[a]Control fungicides: a. 50% dimethomoph WP; b. 40% dimetachlone WP; c. 70% thiophanate-methyl WP; d. 3% jinggangmycin AS; e. 75%chlorothalonil WP

Table 5: Insecticidal activity of compounds E at 500 μg mL^{-1} .

Compd.	Inhibitory rate (%)		
	Plutella xylostella L.	*Aphis gossypii*	*Tetranchus urticae*
E1	15.0	20.0	0
E2	32.0	20.0	0
E3	33.0	29.4	0
E4	30.0	17.1	0
E5	25.0	23.1	0
E6	20.0	12.9	0
E7	14.0	27.3	0
E8	24.0	32.7	0
E9	0	18.5	0
E10	95.0	15.4	0
E11	45.0	23.2	0
E12	16.0	19.2	0
E13	10.0	38.1	0
E14	0	24.5	0
E15	85.0	14.8	0
CK	0	2.4	0
Hexaflumuron	100	22.6	100
RH-5849	100	22.1	100

NT: not detected.

All the title compounds exhibited lower in vitro insecticidal activity towards Aphis gossypii at the concentration of 500 μg mL^{-1}. The highest mortality was 38.0% of E13. The commercial pesticides RH-5849 and hexaflumuron, which display similar structures as the title compounds also showed lower activity to Aphis gossypii (the results were 22.1% and 22.6%), which indicated that these kinds of structures were not suitable for the control of Aphis gossypii. None of the title compounds had activity towards Tetranchus urticae at the concentration of 500 μg mL^{-1} .

Ren [20] and Nishat [21] reported that compounds containing semicarbazides showed excellent anticancer activity. Enlightened by the results from Ren and Nishat, we also studied the anticancer activity of the title compounds, in which the urea linkage was converted into a semicarbazide. Four kinds of cancer cells lines, human promyelocytic leukemic cell line (HL-60), human hepatocellular carcinoma cell line (Bel-7402), human gastric carcinoma cell line (BGC-823), and human nasopharyngeal carcinoma cell line (KB) were chosen for the bioassay. As shown in Table 6, most of the compounds E showed good activity against HL-60. Moreover, some of them exhibited good activity to the solid tumor cells BGC-823 and Bel-7402. Among them E15 exhibited higher activity and broader spectra than others. It had excellent activity of 0.14, 0.36 and 0.09 mM against HL-60, Bel-7402, and BGC-823, respectively.

Table 6: The IC_{50} values of antitumor activity of compounds E.

Compd.	IC_{50} (mM)			
	HL-60	Bel-7402	BGC-823	KB
E1	1.56	-	-	-
E2	1.26	-	-	-
E3	-	-	-	-
E4	-	-	-	-
E5	0.13	-	-	-
E6	-	-	-	-
E7	11.99	5.39	-	-
E8	-	-	-	-
E9	5.39	-	-	-
E10	-	-	-	-
E11	0.44	11.02	1.42	-
E12	2.93	-	-	-
E13	0.18	-	59.46	-
E14	2.63	-	-	-
E15	0.14	0.36	-	0.09

- means IC_{50} > 100 mM.

Comparing the title compounds E with lead compounds B, C, and D, it can be seen that the linkage (Y) is important for the bioactivity and spectra. When the linkage was urea and semicarbazide, the compounds exhibited insecticidal activity, especially towards lepidopterous insects, but had lower effects on fungi. When the linkage was converted to a carbamic acid ester, the compounds had no insecticidal activity, but possessed good fungicidal activity. Moreover, the title compounds E exhibited anticancer activity.

EXPERIMENTAL

Materials and methods

All the melting points were determined with a Cole-Parmer melting point apparatus and are uncorrected. IR spectra were recorded on a Thermo Nicolet Nexus 470 FT-IR spectrometer as KBr pellets. ^{1}H-NMR spectra were recorded on a Bruker DPX300 instrument (Switzerland), with DMSO-d_6 as solvent and tetramethylsilane as the internal standard. Elemental analysis was performed by the Analytical Center in the Institute of Chemistry, Chinese Academy of Sciences, using a Flash EA 1112 elemental analyzer. The solvents and reagents were mainly purchased from the Beijing Chemical Reagents Co., P. R. China.

General procedure for the preparation of key intermediates 2 and 4

The different substituted benzoyl isocyanates 4 were obtained by the reaction of the corresponding benzamides and oxalyl dichloride according to the literature [22]. The 5-substituted phenyl-2- furancarboxylic acids 2 were prepared according to the method given in reference [23].

General synthetic procedure for compounds E

According to the literature [23], different 5-(substituted phenyl)-2-furoyl hydrazines 5 were prepared. Then 4 (5 mmol) was added to a solution of compound 5 (5 mmol) in purified toluene (25 mL). The reaction mixture was kept at room temperature for 2 h. The solvent were evaporated off under reduced pressure, and the resulting solid was purified by vacuum column chromatography on silica gel using petroleum ether (60–90 °C) and ethyl acetate as the eluent to yield E.

N-benzoyl-N'-[5-(4'-chlorophenyl)-2-furoyl] semicarbazide (E1): White powdery crystals: yield 78.9%, m.p. 238–239 °C. ^{1}H-NMR δ: 7.22 (d, J = 3.57 Hz, 1H, FuH), 7.34 (d, J = 3.63 Hz, 1H, FuH), 7.52–7.72 (m, 5H, 2ArH-Fu + 3ArH), 7.92–8.04 (m, 4H, 2ArH-Fu + 2ArH), 10.13 (s, 1H, NHCO), 10.71 (s, 1H, CONH), 11.11 (s, 1H, CONHCO); IR ν: 3405.9, 3255.7, 1686.8, 1653.8, 1604.8, 1534.9, 1474.4, 1441.7, 1271.5, 1093.0, 1025.6 cm-1; Anal. calcd.(%) for $C_{19}H_{14}ClN_3O_4$: C 59.46, H 3.68, N 10.95; found C 59.73, H 3.58, N 10.89.

N-2,6-difluorobenzoyl-N'-[5-(4'-fluorophenyl)-2-furoyl] semicarbazide (E2): Light yellow powdery crystals: yield 75.8%, m.p. 207–208 °C. ^{1}H-NMR δ: 7.15 (d, J = 3.60 Hz, 1H, FuH), 7.23–7.40 (m, 5H, FuH + 2ArH-Fu + 2ArH), 7.57–7.67 (m, 1H, ArH), 7.99–8.06 (m, 2H, ArH-Fu), 9.72 (s, 1H, NHCO), 10.63 (s, 1H, CONH), 11.48 (s, 1H, CONHCO); IR ν: 3425.0, 3262.8, 3131.9, 2951.2, 1738.0, 1698.2, 1648.5, 1626.0, 1592.9, 1512.0, 1482.2, 1315.9, 1284.2, 1265.3, 1234.1, 1161.2, 1109.4, 1030.2, 1014.6 cm^{-1}; Anal. calcd.(%) for $C_{19}H_{12}F_3N_3O_4$: C 56.58, H 3.00, N 10.42; found C 56.53, H 3.08, N 10.37.

N-3-methylbenzoyl-N'-[5-(4'-chlorophenyl)-2-furoyl] semicarbazide (E3): Light yellow powdery crystals: yield 83.6%, m.p. 221–222 °C. ^{1}H-NMR δ: 2.39 (s, 3H, CH_3), 7.23 (d, J = 3.57 Hz, 1H, FuH), 7.34 (d, J = 3.66 Hz, 1H, FuH), 7.43–7.47 (m, 2H, ArH), 7.58 (dd, J = 6.71, 1.94 Hz, 2H, ArH-Fu), 7.80–7.86 (m, 2H, ArH), 7.99–8.02 (m, 2H, ArH-Fu), 10.13 (s, 1H, NHCO), 10.72 (d, J = 1.08 Hz, 1H, CONH), 11.05 (s, 1H, CONHCO); IR ν: 33401.9, 3245.5, 3131.9, 1712.5, 1669.7, 1586.1, 1538.4, 1510.3, 1473.8, 1410.8, 1318.8, 1278.0, 1234.9, 1095.5, 1034.1 cm^{-1}; Anal. calcd.(%) for $C_{19}H_{14}ClN_3O_4$: C 60.38, H 4.05, N 10.56; found C 60.35, H 4.20, N 10.47.

N-2,6-difluorobenzoyl-N'-[5-(4'-chlororophenyl)-2-furoyl] semicarbazide (E4): Light brown powdery crystals: yield 82.6%, m.p. 220–221 °C. ^{1}H-NMR δ: 7.22–7.28 (m, 3H, FuH + 2ArH), 7.34 (d, J = 3.66 Hz, 1H, FuH), 7.56–7.72 (m, 3H, 2ArH-Fu + ArH), 7.98–8.02 (m, 2H, ArH-Fu), 9.74 (s, 1H, NHCO), 10.67 (s, 1H, CONH), 11.48 (s, 1H, CONHCO); IR ν: 3425.0, 3266.2, 3143.5, 1738.7, 1699.1, 1649.4, 1625.3, 1592.1, 1527.1, 1470.1, 1314.6, 1282.4, 1265.2, 1236.8, 1111.4, 1094.7, 1012.7 cm^{-1} ; Anal. calcd.(%) for $C_{19}H_{12}ClF_2N_3O_4$: C 54.36, H 2.88, N 10.01; found C 54.57, H 3.10, N 10.00.

N-2-chlorobenzoyl-N'-[5-(4'-chlorophenyl)-2-furoyl] semicarbazide (E5): White powdery crystals: yield 85.1%, m.p. 196–197 °C. ^{1}H-NMR δ: 7.22 (d, J = 3.60 Hz, 1H, FuH), 7.34 (d, J = 3.63 Hz, 1H, FuH), 7.43–7.62 (m, 6H, 2ArH-Fu + 4ArH), 7.99–8.02 (m, 2H, ArH-Fu), 9.84 (s, 1H, NHCO), 10.68 (s, 1H, CONH), 11.26 (s, 1H, CONHCO); IR ν: 3733.6, 3419.6, 3239.0, 1727.9, 1689.1, 1650.9, 1523.6, 1488.8, 1471.0, 1433.8, 1313.9, 1281.7, 1246.6, 1112.3, 1093.7, 1056.4, 1028.9 cm^{-1}; Anal. calcd.(%) for $C_{19}H_{13}Cl_2N_3O_4$: C 54.56, H 3.13, N 10.05; found C 54.23, H 3.30, N 9.86.

N-2,6-dichlorobenzoyl-N'-[5-(4'-methylphenyl)-2-furoyl] semicarbazide (E6): White powdery crystals: yield 78.6%, m.p. 210–211 °C. ^{1}H-NMR δ: 2.35 (s, 3H, CH3), 7.10 (d, J = 3.30 Hz, 1H, FuH), 7.29–7.32 (m, 3H, 2ArH-Fu + FuH), 7.46–7.60 (m, 3H, ArH), 7.86 (d, J = 7.83 Hz, 2H, ArH-Fu), 9.83 (s, 1H, NHCO), 10.63 (s, 1H, CONH), 11.54 (s, 1H, CONHCO); IR ν: 3247.1, 3135.7, 2973.3, 1716.4, 1700.4, 1677.6, 1596.8, 1535.3, 1486.2, 1433.1, 1307.0, 1260.4, 1211.8, 1144.4, 1019.7 cm^{-1}; Anal. calcd.(%) for $C_{20}H_{15}Cl_2N_3O_4$: C 55.57, H 3.50, N 9.72; found C 55.61, H 3.76, N 9.67.

N-2,6-difluorobenzoyl-N'-[5-(4'-methylphenyl)-2-furoyl] semicarbazide (E7): Light yellow powdery crystals: yield 78.2%, m.p. 211–212 °C. ^{1}H-NMR δ: 2.35 (s, 3H, CH3), 7.09 (d, J = 3.60 Hz, 1H, FuH), 7.23–7.32 (m, 5H, FuH + 2ArH-Fu + 2ArH), 7.57–7.65 (m, 1H, ArH), 7.86 (d, J = 8.16 Hz, 2H, ArHFu), 9.72 (s, 1H, NHCO), 10.59 (s, 1H, CONH), 11.47 (s, 1H, CONHCO); IR ν: 3276.1, 3124.8, 3023.9, 2950.5, 1739.5, 1697.2, 1650.4, 1625.5, 1593.2, 1535.1, 1468.1, 1368.1, 1316.2, 1282.0, 1233.4, 1112.2, 1058.7, 1029.8, 1012.4 cm^{-1}; Anal. calcd.(%) for $C_{20}H_{15}F_2N_3O_4$: C 60.15, H 3.79, N 10.52; found C 60.20, H 4.00, N 10.31. N-2-chlorobenzoyl-N'-[5-(4'-methylphenyl)-2-furoyl] semicarbazide (E8): Light yellow powdery crystals: yield 79.5%, m.p. 206–207 °C. ^{1}H-NMR δ: 2.35 (s, 3H, CH3), 7.09 (d, J = 3.60 Hz, 1H, FuH), 7.29–7.32 (m, 3H, 2ArH-Fu + FuH), 7.43–7.61 (m, 4H, ArH), 7.86 (d, J = 8.16 Hz, 2H, ArH-Fu), 9.81 (s, 1H, NHCO), 10.59 (s, 1H, CONH), 11.23 (s, 1H, CONHCO); IR v: 3262.8, 3128.0, 1725.3, 1685.5, 1657.5, 1544.0, 1484.7, 1318.4, 1286.8, 1246.9, 1224.8, 1101.2, 1055.8, 1031.2 cm^{-1}; Anal. calcd.(%) for $C_{19}H_{14}ClN_3O_4$: C 60.38, H 4.05, N 10.56; found C 60.17, H 4.09, N 10.44.

N-2-methoxybenzoyl-N'-[5-(2'-nitrophenyl)-2-furoyl] semicarbazide (E9): Brown powdery crystals: yield 73.4%, m.p. 191–192 °C. ^{1}H-NMR δ: 3.93 (s, 3H, OCH3), 6.95 (d, J = 3.66 Hz, 1H, FuH), 7.10 (td, J = 7.50, 0.73 Hz, 1H, ArH),7.20–7.23 (m, 1H, ArH), 7.39 (d, J = 3.63 Hz, 1H, FuH), 7.55–7.58 (m, 1H, ArH), 7.68–7.73 (m, 2H, ArH + ArH-Fu), 7.81–7.86 (m, 1H, ArH-Fu), 8.00–8.03 (m, 2H, ArH-Fu), 10.00 (s, 1H, NHCO), 10.50 (s, 1H, CONH), 10.63 (s, 1H, CONHCO); IR v: 3358.1, 3227.9, 3124.2, 1715.7, 1672.0, 1598.8, 1528.0, 1478.3, 1364.7, 1292.9, 1248.9, 1225.1, 1175.6, 1107.8, 1038.0, 1015.9 cm^{-1}; Anal. calcd.(%) for $C_{20}H_{16}N_4O_7$: C 56.61, H 3.80, N 13.20; found C 56.76, H 4.03, N 13.07.

N-3-methylbenzoyl-N'-[5-(2'-chlorophenyl)-2-furoyl] semicarbazide (E10): Light yellow powdery crystals: yield 81.2%, m.p. 209–210 °C. ^{1}H-NMR δ: 2.39 (s, 3H, CH3), 7.33 (d, J = 3.69 Hz, 1H, FuH), 7.39 (d, J = 3.69 Hz, 1H, FuH), 7.41–7.55 (m, 4H, 3ArH-Fu + ArH), 7.62 (dd, J = 7.91,0.83 Hz, 1H, ArH),7.80–7.86 (m, 2H, ArH), 8.23 (dd, J = 7.88, 1.70 Hz, 1H, ArH-Fu), 10.14 (s, 1H, NHCO), 10.75 (d, J = 1.08 Hz, 1H, CONH), 11.05 (s, 1H, CONHCO); IR v: 3413.4, 3243.4, 1711.8, 1667.3, 1516.9, 1469.5, 1316.6, 1281.4, 1231.0, 1085.0, 1029.4 cm-1; Anal. calcd.(%) for $C_{19}H_{14}ClN_3O_4$: C 60.38, H 4.05, N 10.56; found C 60.56, H 4.11, N 10.55.

N-2,6-difluorobenzoyl-N'-[5-(2'-chlorophenyl)-2-furoyl] semicarbazide (E11): Light yellow powdery crystals: yield 84.3%, m.p. 192–193 °C. ^{1}H-NMR δ: 7.22–7.28 (m, 2H, ArH), 7.33 (d, J = 3.69 Hz, 1H, FuH), 7.38 (d, J = 3.69 Hz, 1H, FuH), 7.41–7.55 (m, 2H, 2ArH-Fu), 7.60–7.63 (m, 2H, ArH-Fu + ArH), 8.23 (dd, J = 7.85, 1.70 Hz, 1H, ArH-Fu), 9.73 (s, 1H, NHCO), 10.69 (s, 1H, CONH), 11.47 (s, 1H, CONHCO); IR v: 3406.3, 3271.5, 3163.4, 1728.0, 1700.1, 1673.5, 1627.1, 1593.0, 1549.9, 1490.9, 1468.0, 1317.4, 1283.9, 1236.7, 1029.5, 1011.8 cm^{-1}; Anal. calcd.(%) for $C_{19}H_{12}ClF_2N_3O_4$: C 54.36, H 2.88, N 10.01; found C 54.23, H 3.08, N 10.06.

N-2-methoxybenzoyl-N'-[5-(2'-chlorophenyl)-2-furoyl] semicarbazide (E12): White powdery crystals: yield 84.3%, m.p. 190–191 °C. ^{1}H-NMR δ: 3.88 (s, 3H, OCH3), 7.10 (td, J = 7.51, 0.81 Hz, 1H, ArH), 7.20–7.23 (m, 1H, ArH), 7.33–7.63 (m, 6H, 2FuH + 3ArH-Fu + ArH), 7.69–7.71 (m, 1H, ArH), 8.23 (dd, J = 7.82, 1.58 Hz, 1H, ArH-Fu), 10.02 (s, 1H, NHCO), 10.52 (d, J = 1.08 Hz, 1H, CONH), 10.72 (s, 1H, CONHCO); IR v: 3362.4, 3226.6, 1715.6, 1669.5, 1649.9, 1598.6, 1521.2, 1479.2, 1317.9, 1292.0, 1248.7, 1225.8, 1175.3, 1016.6 cm^{-1}; Anal. calcd.(%) for $C_{20}H_{16}ClN_3O_5$: C 58.05, H 3.90, N 10.15; found C 57.70, H 3.67, N 10.59.

N-2,6-dichlorobenzoyl-N'-[5-(2',4'-difluorophenyl)-2-furoyl] semicarbazide (E13): Light yellow powdery crystals: yield 78.6%, m.p. 224–225 °C. ^{1}H-NMR δ: 6.98 (brs, 1H, FuH), 7.30–7.35 (m, 2H, FuH + ArH-Fu), 7.44–7.61 (m, 4H, ArH-Fu + 3ArH), 8.26–8.31 (m, 1H, ArH-Fu), 9.85 (s, 1H, NHCO), 10.73 (s, 1H, CONH), 11.54(s, 1H, CONHCO); IR v: 3421.2, 3265.8, 3158.9, 2962.2, 1739.3, 1691.4, 1665.6, 1597.3, 1535.3, 1513.6, 1483.3, 1432.0, 1314.6, 1272.2, 1225.5, 1147.4, 1103.9, 1033.7 cm^{-1}; Anal. calcd.(%) for $C_{19}H_{11}Cl_2F_2N_3O_4$: C 54.36, H 2.88, N 10.01; found C 54.26, H 2.87, N 10.18.

N-2-chlorobenzoyl-N'-[5-(2',4'-difluorophenyl)-2-furoyl] semicarbazide (E14): Light yellow powdery crystals: yield 86.2%, m.p. 216–217 °C. ^{1}H-NMR δ: 6.98 (t, J = 3.72 Hz, 1H, FuH), 7.30–7.37 (m, 2H, FuH + ArH-Fu), 7.43–7.62 (m, 5H, ArH-Fu + 4ArH), 8.23–8.31 (m, 1H, ArH-Fu), 9.86 (s, 1H, NHCO), 10.73 (s, 1H, CONH), 11.27 (s, 1H, CONHCO); IR v: 3411.1, 3237.3, 1729.7, 1685.3, 1658.7, 1573.2, 1526.8, 1508.7, 1482.5, 1431.9, 1312.6, 1272.0, 1241.9, 1148.5, 1104.0, 1033.9 cm^{-1}; Anal. calcd.(%) for $C_{19}H_{12}ClF_2N_3O_4$: C 50.24, H 2.44, N 9.25; found C 50.09, H 2.51, N 9.54.

N-2-methoxybenzoyl-N'-[5-(4'-chlorophenyl)-2-furoyl] semicarbazide (E15): White powdery crystals: yield 84.6%, m.p. 192–193 °C. ^{1}H-NMR δ: 3.93(s, 3H, OCH3), 7.10(td, J = 7.51,0.79 Hz,1H, ArH),7 .20–7.24(m,2H, FuH+ ArH), 7.34(d, J = 3.57 Hz, 1H, FuH), 7.56–7.62 (m, 4H, 2ArHFu+2ArH), 7.99–8.02(m, 2H, ArH-Fu), 10.01 (s, 1H, NHCO), 10.52 (s, 1H, CONH), 10.70 (s, 1H, CONHCO); IR v: 394.2, 3331.0, 2969.1, 1742.1, 1721.9, 1660.1, 1597.9, 1478.0, 1408.6, 1295.7, 1253.2, 1228.8, 1091.0, 1049.3, 1018.4 cm^{-1}; Anal. calcd.(%) for $C_{20}H_{16}ClN_3O_5$: C 58.05, H 3.90, N 10.15; found C 57.76, H 3.66, N 10.42.

X-ray structure determination of E2

Compound E2 was recrystallized from methanol to obtain colorless crystal suitable for X-ray single crystal diffraction. Cell constants at 173(2) K were determined by a least-square fit to the setting parameters of E2 independent reflections measured on a Rigaku raxis Rapid IP Area Detector diffractometer with a graphite-monochromated Cu Kα radiation (λ = 0.154178 nm) and operating in the phi and scan modes. The structure was solved by direct method with SHELXS-97 [24,25] and refined by the full-matrix least squares method on F2 data using SHELXL-97 [25,26]. The empirical absorption corrections were applied to all intensity data. H atom of N—H was initially located in a difference Fourier map and was refined with the restraint Uiso(H) = 1.2 Ueq(N). Other H atoms were positioned geometrically and refined using a riding model, with d(C...H) = 0.093—0.097 nm and Uiso(H) = 1.2 Ueq(C) or 1.5 Ueq(C-methyl). Crystallographic data for the structure have been deposited with the Cambridge Crystallographic Data Center as supplementary publication No. CCDC 769209. These data can be obtained free of charge from the CCDC via www.ccdc.cam.ac.uk/data_request/cif.

Biological Assays

(a) The preliminary fungicidal activity in vitro was tested against five kinds of strains: Phytophthora Capsici, Botrytis Cinerea, Fusarium Oxysporum, Rhizoctonia Solanii and Corynespora Cassiicola. All the strains were conserved in the Institute of Vegetable and Flowers, Chinese Academy of Agricultural Science. Commercialized fungicides: 50% dimethomoph WP, 40% dimetachlone WP, 70% thiophanate-methyl WP, 3% jinggangmycin AS and 75% chlorothalonil WP were used as controls for the above five strains, respectively.

The fungicidal activity of the title compounds E against above five strains in vitro was evaluated using the mycelium growth rate test [27]. Both control fungicides and the title compounds were dissolved in DMF at the concentration of 50 μg mL-1. The culture media was obtained by mixing the solution of compounds E in DMF with potato dextrose agar (PDA), on which fungus cakes were placed. The blank test was made using DMF. The culture had been stored in an incubator at 24 ± 0.5 °C for 2 days. Three replicates were performed. After the mycelia grew completely, the diameters of the mycelia were measured and the inhibitory rates were calculated according to the formula: in which I stands for the inhibition (%), C for the diameter of mycelia in the blank control test (in mm), and T for the diameter of mycelia in the presence of compounds E (in mm). The results are shown in Table 4.

(b) Insecticidal activity against Plutella xylostella L., Aphis gossypii and Tetranchus urticae was evaluated using the immersion method [28]. Test solutions were made by dissolving the title compounds E in DMSO, adding a little 0.1% Tween-80 as the emulsifier, and then diluting to 500 μg mL^{-1} with water. The insects were raised at 27 ± 1 °C, with 12:12 h (light/dark) photoperiod and 80% relative humidity. The results were observed after 72 h and expressed by percentage death. The solvent of DMSO was set as blank control. Hexaflumuron and RH-5849 were used as insecticidal controls. Three replicates were performed. The results are shown in Table 5.

(c) Anticancer activity was screened against four different cell lines: a human promyelocytic leukemic cell line (HL-60), a human hepatocellular carcinoma cell line (Bel-7402), a human gastric carcinoma cell line (BGC-823), and a human nasopharyngeal carcinoma cell line (KB). All the title compounds were dissolved in DMSO. The four types of cell line were grown and maintained in RPMI- 1640 medium supplemented with 10% fetal bovine serum (FBS), penicillin (100 U mL^{-1}), and streptomycin (100 μg $mL^{-1)}$ at 37 °C in humidified incubators in an atmosphere of 5% CO_2.

All the experiments were performed on exponentially growing cancer cells. Numbers of viable cancer cells were determined by MTT [3-(4,5-dimethylthiazol-2-yl)-2, 5-diphenyl tetrazolium bromide] [29] and SRB [30] assays. The cancer cells (1~2.5 × 104 cells mL-1) were inoculated in 96-well culture plates (180 μL/well). After 24 h, 20 μL of culture medium containing compounds of various concentrations were added to the wells and, the cells were incubated for 48 h. 20 μL of RPMI-1640 medium was added to the control cells. HL-60 cells were assayed by MTT, and the Bel-7402, BGC- 823 and KB cells were assayed by SRB. The absorbance of each well was measured using a microculture plate reader at 570 nm (MTT) and 540 nm (SRB). The inhibition rate was calculated according to the following formula:

Inhibition rate = (ODcontrol - ODtreated)/ODcontrol × 100%

Three replicates were performed. The IC_{50} values of some active target compounds were evaluated using logit analysis [31]. The results are shown in Table 6.

CONCLUSIONS

In summary, a series of novel semicarbazide derivatives were synthesized by the nucleophilic addition reaction of 5-substituted aryl-2-furoyl hydrazines with benzoyl isocyanates. Compared with the lead compounds, the title compounds showed good insecticidal activity, especially towards lepidopterous insects, but exhibited lower activity against the five kinds of common plant pathogens tested. Inspiringly, the title compounds possessed obvious anticancer activity against human promyelocytic leukemic cell line (HL-60), and some of the title compounds also had activity against solid human tumor cells. The results indicated that the linkage (Y) of the lead compounds was important for the bioactivity and spectra and that modification on the urea linkage was an effective strategy to discover new pesticide and drug candidates.

ACKNOWLEDGEMENTS

We are grateful to the National High Technology Research and Development Program of China (2006AA10A201), the National Key Project for Basic Research (2010CB126104), the National Natural Science Foundation of China (20972185) and the Scientific Research Foundation of the Graduate School of China Agricultural University.

REFERENCES

1. Cohen, E. Chitin synthesis and inhibition: A revisit. Pest Manag. Sci. 2001, 57, 946–950.
2. Ruiz-Herrera, J.; San-Blas, G. Chitin synthesis as a target for antifungal drugs. Curr. Drug Targets Infect. Disord. 2003, 3, 77–91.
3. Wellinga, K.; Mulder, R.; Dallen, J.V. Synthesis and laboratory evaluation of 1-(2,6-disubtituted benzoyl)-3-phenylureas, a new class of insecticides. I. 1-(2,5-Dichlorobenzoyl)-3- phenylureas. J. Agric. Food Chem. 1973, 21, 348–354.
4. Oberlander, H.; Silhacek, D.L. New Perspectives on the Mode of Action of Benzoylphenyl Urea Insecticides. In Insecticides with Novel Modes of Action: Mechanism and Application, 1st ed.; Ishaaya, I., Degheele, D., Eds.; Springer-Verlag: Berlin, Germany, 1998; pp. 92–105.
5. Oberlander, H.; Silhacek, D.L. Mode of action of insect growth regulators in Lepidopteran tissue culture. Pestic. Sci. 1998, 54, 300–302.
6. Qian, X.H. Quantitative studies on structure-activity relationship of sulfonylurea and benzoylphenylurea type pesticides and their substituents' bioisosterism using synthons' activity contribution. J. Agric. Food Chem. 1999, 47, 4415–4418.
7. Nakagawa, Y.; Kitahara, K.; Nishioka, T.; Iwamura, H.; Fujita, T. Quantitative structure- activity studies of benzoylphenylurea larvicides: I. Effect of substituents at aniline moiety against Chilo suppressalis walker. Pestic. Biochem. Physiol. 1984, 21, 309–325.
8. Tecle, B.; Ruzo, L.O.; Casida, J.E. Radiosynthesis of [benzoyl-3,4,5-3H]diflubenzuron by a route applicable to other high-potency Insect Growth Regulators. J. Agric. Food Chem. 1988, 36, 178–180.
9. Hashizume, B. Atabron 5E, a new IGR insecticide (chlorfluazuron). Jpn. Pestic. Inf. 1988, 58, 32–34.
10. Sbragia, R.J.; Johnson, G.W.; Karr, L.L.; Edwards, J.M.; Schneider, B.M. Preparation of benzoylphenylurea

insecticides to control cockroaches, ants, fleas, and termites. WO 9819542, 1998; [Chem. Abstr. 1998, 129, 13497].

11. Yoon, C.; Yang, J.O.; Kang, S.H.; Kim, G.H. Insecticidal properties of bistrifluron against sycamore lace bug, Corythucha ciliata (Hemiptera:Tingidae). J. Pestic. Sci. 2008, 33, 44–50.

12. Grosscurt, A.C.; Van, H.R.; Wellinga, K. 1-Phenylcarbamoyl-2-pyrazolines, a new class of insecticides. 3. Synthesis and insecticidal properties of 3,4-diphenyl-1-phenylcarbamoyl-2- pyrazolines. J. Agric. Food Chem. 1979, 27, 406–409.

13. Chen, L.; Wang, Q.M.; Huang, R.Q.; Mao, C.H.; Shang, J.; Bi, F.C. Synthesis and insecticidal evaluation of propesticides of benzoylphenylureas. J. Agric. Food Chem. 2005, 53, 38–41.

14. Chen, L.; Huang, Z.Q.; Wang, Q.M.; Shang, J.; Huang, R.Q.; Bi, F.C. Insecticidal benzoylphenylurea-S-carbamate: A new propesticide with two effects of both benzoylphenylureas and carbamates. J. Agric. Food Chem. 2007, 55, 2659–2663.

15. Sun, R.F.; Zheng, Y.L.; Chen, L.; Li, Y.Q.; Li, Q.S.; Song, H.B.; Huang, R.Q.; Bi, F.C.; Wang, Q.M. Design, synthesis and insecticidal activities of new N-benzoyl-N-phenyl-N- sulfenylureas. J. Agric. Food Chem. 2009, 57, 3661–3668.

16. Yang, X.L.; Ling, Y.; Wang, D.Q.; Chen, F.H. The synthesis and biological activity of N-phenylN-(5-phenyl-2-furoyl) ureas. Chin. J. Synth. Chem. 2002, 10, 510–512.

17. Yang, X.L.; Wang, D.Q.; Chen, F.H.; Ling, Y.; Zhang, Z.N.; Shang, Z.Z. Studies on the design, synthesis and biological activity of a novel type of acylurea compound. Chem. J. Chin. Univ. 1997, 18, 395–398.

18. Yang, X.L.; Wang, D.Q.; Chen, F.H.; Ling, Y.; Zhang, Z.N. The synthesis and larvicidal activity of N-aroyl-N-(5-aryl-2-furoyl) ureas. Pestic. Sci. 1998, 52, 282–286.

19. Li, Y.; Li, B.J.; Ling, Y.; Miao, H.J.; Shi, Y.X.; Yang, X.L. Synthesis and Fungicidal Activity of Aryl Carbamic Acid-5-aryl-2-furanmethyl Ester. J. Agric. Food Chem. 2010, 58, 3037–3042.

20. Ren, S.J.; Wang, R.B.; Komatsu, K.; Bonaz-Krause, P.; Zyrianov, Y.; McKenna, C.E.; Csipke, C.; Tokes, Z.A.; Lien, E.J. Synthesis, biological evaluation, and quantitative structure-activity relationship analysis of new Schiff bases of hydroxysemicarbazide as potential antitumor agents. J. Med. Chem. 2002, 45, 410–419.

21. Nishat, N.; Ahamad, T.; Alshehri, S.M.; Parveen, S. Synthesis, characterization, and biocide properties of semicarbazide-formaldehyde resin and its polymer metal complexes. Eur. J. Med. Chem. 2010, 45, 1287–1294.

22. Speziale, A.J.; Smith, L.R. New and convenient synthesis of acyl isocyanates. J. Org. Chem. 1962, 27, 3742–3743.

23. Cui, Z.N.; Huang, J.; Li, Y.; Ling, Y.; Yang, X.L.; Chen, F.H. Synthesis and bioactivity of novel N,N'-diacylhydrazine derivatives containing furan(I). Chin. J. Chem. 2008, 26, 916–922

24. Bruker (1998) SMART. Bruker AXS Inc.: Madsion, WI, USA, 1998.

25. Sheldrick, G. M. (1997) SHELXS97 and SHELXL 97. University of Göttingen: Germany, 1997.

26. Bruker (1999) SAINT and SHELXTL. Bruker AXS Inc.: Madison, WI, USA, 1999.

27. Chen, N.C. Bioassay of Pesticides; Beijing Agricultural University Press: Beijing, China, 1991; pp. 161–162.

28. Chen, N.C. Bioassay of Pesticides; Beijing Agricultural University Press: Beijing, China, 1991; p. 54.

29. Denizot, F.; Lang, R. Rapid colorimetric assay for cell growth and survival. Modifications to the tetrazolium dye procedure giving improved sensitivity and reliability. J. Immunol. Methods 1986, 89, 271–277.

30. Monks, A.; Scudiero, D.; Skehan, P.; Shoemaker, R.; Paull, K.; Vistica, D.; Hose, C.; Langley, J.; Cronise, P. Vaigro-Wolff, A.; Gray-Goodrich, M.; Campbell, H.; Mayo, J.; Boyd, M. Feasibility of a high-flux anticancer drug screen using a diverse panel of cultured human tumor cell lines. J. Natl. Cancer Inst. 1991, 83, 757–766.

31. Berkson, J. Application of the logistic function to bio-assay. J. Am. Statistical Assoc. 1944, 39, 357–365.

CHAPTER 11

HEALTH ASPECTS OF ORGANOPHOSPHOROUS PESTICIDES

M Balali-Mood, K Balali-Mood, M Moodi, and B Balali-Mood

INTRODUCTION

Background

Over the past decades, organophosphorous (OP) pesticides were commonly used in agriculture, especially in Asian countries. Organophosphorous pesticides poisoning, either in its acute or chronic forms is a serious health threat. Although OP pesticides residues in fruits and vegetables may not induce early clinical features, nonetheless they could still affect the human health (1, 2). Hence, raising awareness among medical and health professionals is imperative. This awareness should not only cover the toxicology behind poisoning, but it should also include methods of prevention and appropriate management of OP poisoning.

How this review article was prepared

This review was prepared based on the experience of the fist author and the available literature between 1980 and 2011. Pub Med was searched with different names of organophosphorous, organophosphate, pesticides, insecticides and search terms including human exposure, organophosphorous pesticides poisoning and its complications. The first author's collections of literature on OP including the books, monographs and historically relevant articles were also used for this review. It was aimed to describe the brief basic chemistry and toxicology of OP as well as its clinical effects and long term complications. Special attention was given to the studies and reports from Asian countries. Therefore, relevant references were selected and the headings and subheadings were chosen based on the above objectives. This is neither a Meta-analysis nor a critical review on OP. Herein we present a descriptive text on health aspects of OP for health professionals with special reference to the Asian countries.

History and size of the problem

Aside from the large scale use of OP pesticides in agriculture, OP compounds have also been used as chemical warfare agents (tabun and sarin) by the Iraqi army against the Iranian troops (Majnoon Island) and civilians in Halabjah (1). A few OP compounds (glyphosate, merphos) are used as herbicides, but they are structurally different from the OP pesticides (2).

Von Hofmann synthesized an OP compound called methyl phosphor chloride in 1837. Michaels introduced a compound with P-CN bond, which led to the synthesis of a number of

Citation: M Balali-Mood , K Balali-Mood , M Moodi , B Balali-Mood, Health Aspects of Organophosphorous Pesticides, http://www.ncbi.nlm.nih.gov/pmc/articles/PMC3494223/

insecticides and the nerve agent tabun before the World War II (3, 4).

Over the past decades, numerous structurally different OP compounds have been synthesized and used as pesticides, which poisoned even the children of agricultural workers in India (2, 5). Currently, over 100 different OP compounds are used worldwide as insecticides (6). Low level exposures either as occupational or via the consumption of OP contaminated fruits and vegetables have been reported (7–10). OP compounds are not ideal pesticides because of the lack of target vector selectivity, and severe toxicity in human beings and domestic animals. On the other hand, OP pesticides are readily available and are widely used which explains the high number of reported intoxications (11, 12).

In some parts of the developing world particularly in Asian countries, pesticide poisoning causes more deaths than infectious diseases (11). Use of pesticides is poorly regulated and controlled in the Asian countries and thus, their easy availability may induce self-poisoning. In 1985, Food and Agriculture Organization (FAO) of the United Nation produced a voluntary code of conduct for the pesticide industry to limit the harmful effects of pesticides. Unfortunately, inadequate governmental attention in some developing countries has made this code ineffective (1, 11). The World Health Organization (WHO) has recommended restricting highly toxic pesticides, but this was not applied in a number of developing countries. As a result, OP pesticides exposure has remained common in these countries and continues to induce health problems as well as environmental hazards (8–16).

It was estimated that in 2002–2005, around 3,000,000 human beings were intoxicated by OP pesticides worldwide (6, 14, 15).

It was later indicated that OP poisoned 3 million and kills at least 250,000 people every year, mostly in Asian countries (17, 18). In 25 villages of three townships of Jiangsu and Shandong provinces in China, more than 5000 cases of OP exposure as sprayers were reported (19). From July 1985 through December 2006, 4799 OP exposures were recorded in Taiwan (20). An outbreak of food poisoning in Singapore of an imported green leafy vegetable (Brossica alboglabra) contaminated by two OP (metamidophos and profenfos) poisoned 105 people (21).

The above information clearly shows that OP pesticides are the cause of high number of human morbidities and mortalities particularly in the Asian region. Therefore, health authorities should act on the regulation, control and prevention of this common serious poisoning.

Chemical structures and classification

OP compounds including organophosphates are derived from phosphoric, phosphonic, phosphinic and thiophosphoric acids (2, 22). Organophosphates are usually esters, amides or thiol derivatives of phosphoric, phosphonic or phosphinic acids. The general structure of an OPcompound is shown in Fig. 1 (22, 23).

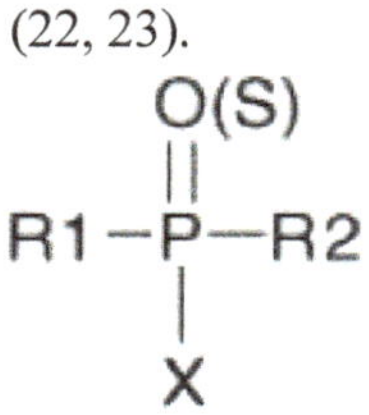

Figure 1: General chemical structure of an organophosphorous compound. R1 and R2 are alkyl-, alkoxy-, alkylthio- or amido groups. X is the acyl residue (cyano-, substituted or branched aliphatic, aromatic or heterocyclic groups)

OP compounds are divided into two main groups; pesticides and chemical warfare nerve agents. OP pesticides have varied chemical structures. Variations in the chemical structure of main groups of OP pesticides are summarized in Table 1.

Table 1: Chemical structures of main groups of OP pesticides and examples in each group

Type of groups	Outline of structure	Examples
Phosphate	O ‖ $(R\text{-}O)_2$-P-O-X	chlorfenvinphos, dicrotophos, crotoxyphos, dichlorvos, heptenphos, mevinphos
Phosphorothioate	S ‖ $(R\text{-}O)_2$-P-S-X	bromophos-ethyl, bromophos-methyl chlorpyriphos-methyl, coumaphos, dichlofenthion, fenchlorphos, parathion
O-alkyl Phosphorothioate	S ‖ $(R\text{-}O)_2$-P-O-X	demeton-S-methyl, omethoate vamidothion, phoxim,
Phosphorodithioate	S ‖ $(R\text{-}O)_2$-P-S-X	azinophos-ethyl, azinophos-methyl, malathion, mecarbam, menazon, morphothion, phenthoate

OP compounds exhibit markedly different actions depending on the specific substituents at R1, R2, and X. For example, parathion is 1000 times more toxic than malathion (22).

Mechanism of action

The well known mechanism of action of OP is the inhibition of cholinesterases. Two types of cholinesterase are involved:

Acetyl cholinesterase (AChE), which is a specific enzyme for the diagnosis of OP poisoning and is referred to as true cholinesterase. It is usually estimated in red blood cells (RBC) and as such it is also called RBC AChE or erythrocyte acetyl cholinesterase.

Butyryl cholinesterase (BChE); which is less specific but more sensitive than AChE is also called pseudo cholinesterase. BChE is usually estimated in Plasma and is thus known as plasma cholinesterase.

Some proteolytic enzymes (e.g. trypsin, chymotrypsin) may also be inhibited by OP. OP pesticides like parathion are detoxified in part through a two-step pathway involving bioactivation of the parent compound by the cytochrome P450 system, followed by hydrolysis of the resulting oxygenating metabolite (Oxon) by serum and liver paraoxygeanse 1 (PON1). Serum PON1 has been shown to be polymorphic in human populations (24).

Although all OP compounds have a common mechanism of action, their effectiveness as inhibitors of AChE, can be significantly different. OP compounds are classified as direct or indirect inhibitors of AChE. Direct inhibitors are effective without undergoing any further metabolic modifications in the body, whereas, indirect inhibitors need to be transformed in the body to become active (22). People with BChE genetic variations may be at risk for taking succinylcholine. The clinically most important variant is atypical (D70G) BChE. The people with this variation may have apnea after receiving a dose of succinylcholine which is intended to paralyze muscles for 3–5 minutes in anaesthesia (23, 25).

Furthermore, OP covalently binds to other serine esterase, such as carboxyl esterase (CaE), neuropathy target esterase (NTE), trypsin and chymotrypsin (26). In OP binding to a tyrosine, residue of human serum albumin has also been reported (27).

The persistence of unbound OP in the body depends on the physico-chemical properties and the activity of endogenous OP hydrolyzing enzymes, such as paraoxonases (25). Lipophilic OP, like parathion and its active form paraoxon may penetrate into deep compartments resulting in long-term toxicity (27).

Toxicokinetics

Absorption

Absorption varies by route of exposure.

Dermal exposure

Absorption by the skin tends to be slow, however as the OP pesticides are hard to remove from the skin. The presence of aqueous dispersing agents or organic solvents in a spray or other formulations may enhance absorption.

On the basis of radio autographic studies, it appears that skin absorption of parathion is trans-epidermal. The rate of dermal absorption of parathion in rabbit is reported 0.059 mg/min/cm^2 (16).

Following administration of ^{14}C-malathion to the ventral forearm of 12 volunteers, 8.2% of the total dose was recovered from their urine during the course of 5 days. After IV injection of ^{14}C-malathion, 90.2% of the radioactivity was recovered in the urine (16, 22).

Inhalation exposure

In a study, OP exposure by respiratory and dermal routes was compared in workers spraying parathion. They either breathed a pure air supply but did not wear protective clothing, or wore protective clothing but did not have any respiratory protection. Total urinary output of 4-nitrophenyl as derived from the respiratory source, compared with that derived from the dermal source, was 1.2% and 12%, respectively (16).

Oral exposure

After ^{32}P-dimethoate was given orally to volunteers, 76 to 100% of the radioactivity appeared in the urine over 24 hours (16).

Distribution

The absorbed OP compounds are going under bio-transformations and reactions with tissue constituents. In view of the inherent instability of the OP pesticides, retention in human tissue is not prolonged.

Metabolism

OP compounds are mainly metabolized via oxidation and hydrolysis by esterases and by reaction with glutathione. Demethylation and glucuronidation may also occur. Oxidation of OP pesticides may result in potentially toxic products. In general, phosphorothioates are not directly toxic and require oxidative metabolism to produce toxic metabolite. In reverse, glutathione transferase reactions induce products that are usually less toxic (28).

The half-life of most OP pesticides and their inhibitory metabolites in vivo is relatively short. For instance, the serum half-life of malathion was 2.89 hours in a 24-year-old white male who, in a suicidal attempt, injected approximately 3 ml of 50% malathion intravenously into his right forearm (22).

Excretion

The elimination of the OP and metabolites is mostly by the urine and lesser amounts in the feces and expired air. In summary, the rates of OP excretion usually reach a peak within two days and decline quite rapidly (2,16).

Clinical Effects

The lipophilic diethyl phosphoryl pesticides such as azinophos-ethyl, bromophos-ethyl, chlorpyriphos, coumaphos, diazinon, parathion, phosalone and sulfotep may remain in the body for many days in severe cases. This may promote a recurrence of clinical effects after an initial period of apparent recovery (2, 28,29).

Clinical effects of OP exposure are categorized into acute and chronic poisonings.

Acute Poisoning

Initial clinical manifestations following acute exposure vary according to the route of exposure.

Inhalation

Inhalation of OP pesticides depends on volatility of the compound, formulation and the technique of application. However, clinical effects appear immediately or shortly after OP inhalation (22).

Exposure to low vapor concentrations may affect only the eyes, nose and airways. Miosis, copious secretion, visual disturbances, rhinorrhoea and or some degree of dyspnea develop within seconds to several minutes. The extent of severity of dyspnea is dose dependent. Usually, these effects do not progress significantly once the patient is removed from the contamination area. After inhalation of high vapor concentrations, victims lose consciousness within one or two minutes and then have seizures, flaccid paralysis and apnea. Involuntary micturation/defecation may also occur in severe cases (2, 22).

Skin

Symptoms and signs usually appear about 2–3 hours following dermal absorption. A small concentration of OP may retain in fat tissues which can delay the clinical manifestation of symptoms for up to 24 h (2). Dermal absorption of OP varies depending on the body site exposed and the ambient temperature. Droplets containing near-lethal or lethal dose, may cause loss of consciousness, seizures, flaccid paralysis and apnea. The onset of these effects is sudden, after an asymptomatic interval of 10 to 30 minutes (23, 30).

Eyes

Following splash exposure or eye contact with OP vapor and later if at all after systemic poisoning, miosis may occur. Unilateral miosis can occur, if only one eye has been exposed. Miosis may be accompanied by deep, aching eye pain, conjunctival irritation, and visual disturbances following direct OP exposure (4).

Gastrointestinal

Accidental ingestion may occur in children and even in adults due to improper storage of OP pesticides at home. Following oral ingestion, nausea and vomiting may occur. Abdominal pain and diarrhoea together with a cholinergic syndrome, CNS and cardiovascular effects may be observed in moderate to severe OP poisoning (16). Clinical features of cholinergic syndromes, CNS and cardiovascular effects are described in the following relevant sections.

Parenteral

Intradermal injection of paraoxon or surface application of maloxon or dichlorvos to human skin produced a long-lasting local sweating over a few minutes. Intramuscular administration of an OP pesticide (diisopropylfluorophosphonate or DFP) to people with psychosis, and to normal controls at a rate of 2 mg/man per day (about 0.028 mg/kg per day) for seven days caused anorexia, vomiting, and diarrhea more severe in normal than in psychotic patients (31).

Cholinergic syndromes

These syndromes are due to the acetylcholine accumulation at the nerve endings, stimulating both muscarinic and nicotinic receptors. Muscarinic syndrome include increased bronchial secretion, excessive sweating, salivation, and lachrymation, pinpoint pupils, bronchoconstriction, vomiting, diarrhoea, abdominal cramps urinary frequency, bradycardia and hypotension and in severe intoxicated patients; pulmonary edema may occur. Nicotinic syndrome include tachycardia, hypertension, mydriasis, twitching and fasciculation of muscles, and in more severe cases; paralysis of diaphragm and respiratory muscles (2, 16, 22).

Central nervous system effects

Central nervous system effects include headache, dizziness, restlessness, anxiety, mental confusion, convulsions and coma. Depression of the respiratory and vasomotor centers in brain may occur and further complicate the clinical picture of OP poisoning (3, 16, 32).

Cardiovascular effects

Cholinesterase inhibition increases the vagal nerve and thereby slows the heart rate. In accidentally poisoned patients, however, other factors, such as fear, hypoxia, and ganglionic stimulation, may accelerate the heart rate (16).

ECG abnormalities other than bradycardia have been described in human OP pesticides poisoning. These include atrial fibrillation, idioventricular dysrhythmias, multiform ventricular extrasystoles, torsade de pointes, ventricular fibrillation, and complete heart block (33). Sudden death occurring after a patient has appeared to recover from the respiratory and neurologic effects of acute OP insecticide exposure has been reported (34).

Intermediate Syndrome

The intermediate syndrome consists of marked weakness of the proximal skeletal musculature (including the muscles of respiration-intercostal muscles) and cranial nerve palsies, which may occur within 1–4 days of certain acute OP poisoning. This syndrome is probably a consequence of cholinergic over activity at the neuromuscular junction. It appears that there is a correlation between the acute phase and OP-induced myopathy (32, 35, 36).

Severity Grading of intoxication

Severity grading of OP poisoning can be categorized based on clinical manifestations, cholinesterase activity and initial atropine dose required for atropinisation.

Clinical

The severity of OP poisoning can be divided into four groups of mild, moderate, severe and fatal according to the symptoms and signs of poisoning (Table 2) (2, 22):

Table 2:: Severity grading of OP poisoned patients based on symptoms and signs of poisoning

Grade	Symptoms	Signs
Mild	Dizziness, anxiety, headache, nausea, weakness, tightness of breath.	failure of eye accommodation, rhinorrhoea, sweating, salivation, coughing, lachrymation
Moderate	(Worsening of the above features plus the followings): Restlessness, confusion, dyspnea, disorientation, abdominal pain, diarrheal	Pallor, miosis, lack of concentration, tachycardia, hypertension, muscle twitching, fasciculation, respiratory depression, bronchorrhea, loss of consciousness, bronchospasm.
Severe	(Worsening of the above features plus the followings) Loss of conscious, seizure.	Convulsions, respiratory failure, pulmonary edema, flaccid paralysis, involuntary micturation/defecation, Cyanosis, deep coma.
Fatal	(Worsening of the above features plus the followings) Respiratory arrest, cardiac arrest.	Coma, convulsions, miosis hypersecretions and apnea, within a few minute after exposure.

Inhibition of Cholinesterases

The severity of OP poisoning may be divided into three groups according to their cholinesterase activities as shown in Table 3 (2, 16, 22).

Table 3: Severity grading of poisoned patients based on their cholinesterase activities

Grade	BChE activity (%)	AChE activity (%)
1. Mild	40-50	50-90
2.Moderate	10-40	10-50
3. Severe	<10	<10

As it can be observed in Table 3, BChE concentration has less quantitative value than AChE activity.

Atropine dose

Acute OP poisoning can also be divided into three groups according to the initial dose required for atropinisation:

1. Mild <2mg
2. Moderate <2–10mg
3. Severe >10mg

The patients with OP pesticides poisoning require much more atropine doses and thus the above atropine dosing for the severity grading of OP pesticides should be five to ten times higher (13).

Mixed Poisoning

Concomitant poisoning of OP with other compounds such as organochlorine, fungicide, copper sulphate and kerosene may occur. The organic solvents used for dissolution of OP may also potentiate the intoxication. A report of three patients with mixed poisoning who were successfully treated with greater focus on OP poisoning was reported (37).

Chronic Poisoning

Chronic and/or sub-acute OP poisonings are usually occupational and may occur in workers who have daily exposure. Chronic poisoning is most common among agricultural workers involved in spraying of OP pesticide or in sheep divers. Since chronic OP poisoning is much less common than acute poisoning, unless the physician pays attention to the occupation of the patient, the diagnosis will be missed out (2, 22).

The great majority of OP compounds are rapidly metabolized and excreted and thus sub-acute or chronic poisoning may not occur. However, since several OP compounds cause slowly reversible inhibition of cholinesterase, accumulation of this effect can occur (22).

The farmers who exposed to OP revealed lower AChE activity and higher urinary dialkylphosphate and 8-hydrox-29-deoxyguanosine than the controls, indicating that they had chronic OP poisoning. They also had higher DNA damage than the controls (38).

Delayed neuropathy

OP induced delayed neuropathy (OPIND) is a symmetrical sensorimotor axonopathy, tending to be more severe in long axons and occurring 7–14 days after exposure. In severe cases, it is an extremely disabling condition, but is very rare. Inhibition of neuropathy target esterase (NTE) claimed to be necessary for OPIND to develop. However, other mechanisms may be involved e.g. trophic factor (ornithine decarboxylase), a growth related enzyme, which decreased in spinal cord following diisopropylfluorophosphate (DFP) poisoning (2, 22).

Electrodiagnostic procedures including electromyography of the extremities and nerve conduction velocity of the upper and lower nerves of the limbs revealed that sensory nerve dysfunction of the lower extremities was more common than motor nerves, which was predominantly a distal sensory deficit (39).

Diagnosis

Initial diagnosis of OP poisoning can be made based on the history of exposure and clinical manifestations. In low-level exposure, the route of absorption may affect the clinical features, but in high-level exposure, the occurrence time is faster through inhalation than by skin absorption (16).

Estimation of AChE in erythrocytes is required to confirm diagnosis and to estimate severity of OP intoxication. BChE is more sensitive and declined earlier, but it is not specific and may be low naturally in some people due to genetic variations (40).

Reasonable relationships exist between red blood cells or plasma cholinesterase inhibition and the clinical signs of acute intoxication. Monitoring of neuromuscular transmission during the course of severe OP poisoning revealed that disturbances occur when AChE activity reached below 30 % (41).

TOXICOLOGICAL ANALYSES

Cholinesterases determination

Determinations of AChE and BChE activities are well known screening methods to establish exposure to OP pesticides. Modifications of the original colorimetric Elman assay (40) allowed determination of AChE activity in whole blood and of BChE activity in the plasma more accurately (42).

Standard determination of AChE and BChE activity may indicate inhibition of the enzyme which may be due to OP or other cholinesterase inhibitors like carbamates. Thus, reduced activity of AChE and or BChE activity indicate an exposure to a cholinesterase inhibitor without specifying the agent. However, determination of cholinesterase activities is a valuable tool for confirming the clinical diagnosis of OP poisoning. Clinical symptoms are expected at inhibition of more than 50% of brain AChE and 70% of diaphragm AChE, respectively (27). Inhibition levels greater than 90% are associated with severe toxicity.

Erythrocyte AChE showed to be a more specific parameter than BChE for the diagnosis of OP poisoning and the assessment of antidotal efficacy (16, 40, 42, 43).

Detection of OP compounds and their metabolites

Identification and quantitative analysis of trace concentrations of OP compounds in plasma after human exposure requires sophisticated instruments such as gas chromatography-mass spectrometry (GC–MS) or liquid chromatography-mass spectrometry (LC–MS) and well trained operators (44). It is not really required for the clinical management of OP poisoning.

MANAGEMENT

First aid advice for medical and para-medical personnel

The first rule is that the emergency responders must protect themselves to avoid contamination resulting from contact with casualties and the polluted environment. This can be done by appropriate personal protective equipments. At minimum, rescuers should wear a protective mask (mask containing a charcoal filter, not a surgical or similar mask) and heavy rubber gloves and avoid skin contact with victims until decontamination has been carried out (2, 22).

The victims should be removed from the contaminated area as soon as possible, and decontamination must be initiated. Antidotes (e.g. auto injector containing atropine, obidoxime and diazepam) should be used at the onset of clinical symptom/sign. For unconscious or severely intoxicated patients, priorities must follow the ABCs of resuscitation. Oxygen administration and assisted ventilation should be undertaken as soon as possible in those with respiratory insufficiency (2).

It is important to improve tissue oxygenation before atropine administration to minimize the risk of ventricular fibrillation. Advanced life support, including IV line placement, should be provided to all victims with signs of severe OP toxicity (12).

Decontamination

If the eyes have been exposed, they should be irrigated as with running water or normal saline. Skin decontamination should be done by pouring on large amounts of a light chlorine-liberated solution such as 5.0% hypochlorite solution (household bleach) followed by several water rinsing. If bleach is not available, the skin should be washed up by an alkaline soap and water followed by a water rinse. Water alone can be used if nothing else is available as it will dilute and physically wash away the agent, but it will not hydrolyze it. Contaminated clothing and jewellery should be removed before decontamination. Care should be taken to clean under the nails, intertriginous areas, auxilla, groin, and hair (22).

Recombinant DNA-derived AChEs revealed a great improvement as bioscavengers (45). Immobilized Escherichia coli with surface-expressed organophosphorous hydrolase were made to detoxify OP poisoning (46). By protein engineering techniques one butyryl cholinesterase mutant G117H was made to hydrolyze OP but reacts much too slowly (47).

Antidotes

The well known antidotes (atropine, oxime) do not effect in all severe OP pesticides poisoning and may not prevent respiratory insufficiency. However, appropriate administration of these antidotes and intensive care management are the main treatment for acute OP poisoning. Cinical investigations revealed that blood alkalinisation by sodium bicarbonate is effective and should be added to the treatment regime of OP poisoning (48). Although oximes have been designed to reactivate the inhibited acetylcholinesterase, clinical experience has revealed that they are not always effective and none of them can be regarded as a broad-spectrum antidote (49). Liver function tests should be checked regularly during obidoxime therapy to avoid hepatotoxicity (13,49–52).

Blood alkalinisation by sodium bicarbonate

Effects of sodium bicarbonate in OP pesticide poisoning were studied in patients with moderate to severe intoxication. It was aimed to make a mild alkalinisation to obtain the arterial blood pH of 7.45 to 7.55. The preliminary results were promising (53) and the final results were satisfactory (48).

Roberts and co-workers (54) were concern about the safety of alkalinisation regime but the investigators replied with the evidence of safety data (55).

Intravenous lipid emulsions combined with extracorporeal purification particularly charcoal hemoperfusion has been recommended for adjunct treatment of severe OP poisoning (56). However, this should be investigated by a carefully designed study in severe human different OP poisonings.

Advances in the treatment of acute organophosphorous poisonings were reported in 2006 and 2012 (57, 58).

Pesticides Residues

OP pesticide abuse in growing fruit and vegetable was found in 65% in Tianjin area. Around 32% of the fruits and vegetable samples collected in summer from this city were positive for high toxic OP pesticides. Significant decrease of pesticide residue (up to 80%) in fruits and vegetables was achieved by scaling, immersion in 0.15% and 0.30% detergent solution, as well as peeling and cutting root. The authors concluded that it is necessary to strengthen pesticide abuse control and market surveillance and inspection to reduce the harmful effects of pesticide residue in fruit and vegetables to human health (59).

Over 27,000 tons of pesticides were used in the Islamic Republic of Iran during 2000 and 2001, of which 16,000 tons are formulated in the country. Of the 241 pesticides used in this country, the group order was insecticides 33%, herbicides 30%, fungicides 20%, acaricides 6.2%, rodenticides 3.8%, nematicides 1.5 % and others for 5.5%. The country spent US$125 million on pesticide imports in 2002. Although this huge volume of pesticides is distributed all over the country, 60 % of all pesticides were applied in the three northern provinces, close to the Caspian Sea, while rice production alone accounts for a quarter of the national pesticide usage (60). Unregistered and illegal imports of pesticides, which have not been formally reported, should be added to the size of this health problem.

Contamination of crop samples by organic chemicals, mainly OP pesticides has become a pressing problem in many Arab countries. Safety status was assessed by comparing the current contamination level with that of WHO maximum residue limits (MRL). Low contamination levels were detected in cucumber and tomato in Palestine, Jordan and Egypt. Elevated levels of contamination were detected in vegetables from Pakistan, Egypt and in grapes from Jordan. Several poisonous cases and plant food contamination were reported in Morocco, Egypt, Iraq, Saudi Arabia, Sudan, Syria, Jordan, UAE, Pakistan and Yemen in the past years. Further detailed studies of these problems showed accumulation of these organic contaminants in food consumer bodies and farm workers who deal directly with agricultural products. This problem occurred probably due to misuse and/or overuse of pesticides in the environment. The author concluded that these countries should implement control measures to reduce pesticide use and awareness programs to enhance food safety (61).

Ethion and diazinon concentrations in Iranian pistachio nuts have been analyzed by use of matrix solid-phase dispersion (MSPD) followed by gas chromatography with nitrogen–phosphorus detection (GC–NPD). The limits of detection were 0.02 mg kg^{-1} for ethion and 0.035 mg kg^{-1} for diazinon; these were lower than the maximum residue limits (MRL) established by WHO/FAO (62). However, regular pesticides monitoring on this product is recommended.

Preventive measures

The persons are going to use OP pesticides should be provided with safety information and equipments before application. Protective devices for low toxic OP pesticides may include a long-sleeved shirt, long trousers or overall suit with appropriate hat, but for the highly toxic OP pesticides, waterproof suit, thick gloves and rubber boots are needed. The protective devices should be washed out every day after use. The contaminated items must be washed up separately. To protect possible splashing on the eyes, goggles or a face shield should be worn.

Contact lenses are advised to be removed before using an OP pesticide, because it may seep in behind the lenses. For spraying the highly toxic OP pesticides, a respirator may be required. The label of OP pesticides may specify when this is necessary.

More precautions are needed when mixing the highly toxic OP pesticides and thus physical protection must be applied. Mixing the OP pesticides should be carefully done by a stick or paddle. The risk of pesticide spraying, increases on windy days due to possible inhaling spray drift or contaminating the skin and thus appropriate protections are required. After spraying OP pesticides, taking shower and changing the clothes are necessary. Hands should be washed out carefully before eating, drinking or smoking.

All chemicals including OP pesticides should be stored preferably in a locked shed, out of the reach of children and animals. OP pesticides should also be kept away from work areas for other purposes. They also must be stored separated from other materials such as animal food Stuff. OP pesticides as any other chemicals should be kept in their original containers and must have never been transferred to the containers which are normally used for food or drink. The new container must be labelled properly.

Decontamination and clean-up procedures of OP pesticides should be performed by a mild alkaline solution such as 10% sodium carbonate (washing soda solution) to the contaminated area. After bushing well, it should be left for at least 8 hours.

For workers who are employing to use OP pesticides on a regular basis, determination of their baseline cholinesterase levels is advisable. These tests should also be repeated on a regular basis to determine whether exposure is occurring with sub-clinical exposure. If the red blood cell or plasma cholinesterase falls below 25% of baseline levels, workers must be taken off the job and should not return to work until their cholinesterase levels return to normal range (63). Bacterial enzymes including OP hydrolases have demonstrated prophylactic and antidotal efficacy against a few different OP classes in animal models (18).

CONCLUSIONS AND RECOMMENDATIONS

OP pesticides have induced a lot of human morbidities and mortalities, particularly in the Asian countries. OP pesticides are still used in most parts of the world and unfortunately are easily available in some developing countries and thus occupational and accidental exposure and even intentional ingestion are common and induced health problems.

WHO has recommended that access to highly toxic pesticides be restricted and where this has been done, suicide rates have fallen. Proper legislations and pesticides control particularly on OP compounds which are the most commonly used pesticides are recommended. Biological pest control that has recently been applied in some countries should be extended and advanced to replace the use of OP pesticides.

ETHICAL CONSIDERATIONS

Ethical issues (Including plagiarism, Informed Consent, misconduct, data fabrication and/or falsification, double publication and/or submission, redundancy, etc) have been completely observed by the authors.

ACKNOWLEDGMENTS

Partial financial support of the Medical Toxicology Research Center of Mashhad University of Medical Sciences is acknowledged. The authors declare that there is no conflict of interests.

REFERENCES

1. Balali-Mood M, Balali-Mood K. Neurotoxic disorders of organophosphorous compounds and their managements. Arch Iranian Med. 2008;11(1):65–89. [PubMed]
2. Jeyaratnam J, Maroni M. Organophosphorous compounds. Toxicology. 1994;91(1):15–27.
3. Sungurtekin H, Gürses E, Balci C. Evaluation of several clinical scoring tools in organophosphate poisoned patients. Clin Toxicol. 2006;44(2):121–26.
4. Holmsted B. The third symposium on the prophylaxis and treatment of chemical poisons. Fund Appl Toxicol. 1985;5:S1–S9.
5. Rastogi SK, Tripathi S, Ravishanker D. A study of neurologic symptoms on exposure to organophosphate pesticides in the children of agricultural workers. Indian J Occup Environ Med. 2010;14(2):54–57.
6. Kwong T. Organophosphate pesticides: biochemistry and clinical toxicology. Therc Drug Monit.2002;24(1):144–49.
7. Lotti M. Low level exposures to organophosphorus esters and peripheral nerve function. Muscle & Nerve.2002;25(4):492–504.
8. Amr M. Pesticide monitoring and its health problems in Egypt, a Third World country. Toxicol Lett.1999;107(1–3):1–13.

9. Cocker J, Mason H, Garfitt S, Jones K. Biological monitoring of exposure to organophosphate pesticides. Toxicol Lett. 2002;134(1–3):97–103.

10. Brown M, Brix K. Review of health consequences from high-, intermediate-and low-level exposure to organophosphorus nerve agents. J Appl Toxicol. 1998;18(6):393–408. [PubMed]

11. Eddleston M, Karalliedde L, Buckley N, Fernando R, Hutchinson G, Isbister G, Konradsen F, Murray D, Piola J, Senanayake N. Pesticide poisoning in the developing world; a minimum pesticides list. The Lancet. 2002;360(9340):1163–67.

12. Thiermann H, Szinicz L, Eyer F, Worek F, Eyer P, Felgenhauer N, Zilker T. Modern strategies in therapy of organophosphate poisoning. Toxicol Lett. 1999;107(1–3):233–39.

13. Balali-Mood M, Shariat M. Treatment of organophosphate poisoning. Experience of nerve agents and acute pesticide poisoning on the effects of oximes. J of Physiol-Paris. 1998;92(5–6):375–78.

14. Forget G. Pesticides and the third world. J ToxicolEnviron Health, Part A. 1991;32(1):11–31.

15. Eddleston M, Gunnell D, Karunaratne A, De Silva D, Sheriff M, Buckley N. Epidemiology of intentional self-poisoning in rural Sri Lanka. Brit J Psychiat. 2005;187(6):583–584.

16. Worek F, Koller M, Thiermann H, Szinicz L. Diagnostic aspects of organophosphate poisoning.Toxicology. 2005;214(3):182–89.

17. Mohamed F, Gawarammana I, Robertson T, Roberts M, Palangasinghe C, Zawahir S, Jayamanne S, Kandasamy J, Eddleston M, Buckley N. Acute human self-poisoning with imidacloprid compound: A neonicotinoid insecticide. PLoS One. 2009;4(4) e5127(1–5).

18. Bird S, Dawson A, Ollis D. Enzymes and bioscavengers for prophylaxis and treatment of organophosphate poisoning. Front Biosci (Scholar edition) 2010;2(1):209–220.

19. Gan W, Chen S, Tao B. An epidemiological study on pesticide poisoning with mixed preparation. Chin J Prev Med. 2001;35(1):13–15.

20. Lin T, Walter F, Hung D, Tsai J, Hu S, Chang J, Deng J, Chase P, Denninghoff K, Chan H. Epidemiology of organophosphate pesticide poisoning in Taiwan. Clin Toxicol. 2008;46(9):794–801.

21. Goh K, Yew F, Ong K, Tan I. Acute organophosphorus food poisoning caused by contaminated green leafy vegetables. Arch Environ Health. 1990;45(3):180–184.

22. Bradbery SM, Vale JA. Organophosphorous insecticides. In: Brent, Wallace, Bukhart, Philips, Donovan, editors. Critical Care Toxicology. 1st ed. Elsevier Mosby; Philadelphia, USA: pp. 937–942.

23. Ooms A, Van Dijk C. The reaction of organophosphorus compounds with hydrolytic enzymes-III: The inhibition of chymotrypsin and trypsin. Biochem Pharmacol. 1966;15(9):1361–1377.

24. Josse D, Lockridge O, Xie W, Bartels C, Schopfer L, Masson P. The active site of human paraoxonase (PON1) J Appl Toxicoly. 2001;21(S1):S7–S11.

25. Boter H, Ooms A. Stereospecificity of hydrolytic enzymes in their reaction with optically active organophosphorus compounds--II:: The inhibition of aliesterase, acetylesterase, chymotrypsin and trypsin by S-alkyl p-nitrophenyl met-hylphosphonothiolates. Biochem Pharmacol. 1967;16(8):1563–69.

26. Sogorb M, Vilanova E. Enzymes involved in the detoxification of organophosphorus, carbamate and pyrethroid insecticides through hydrolysis. Toxicol Lett. 2002;128(1–3):215–28.

27. Eyer P, Worek F, Kiderlen D, Sinko G, Stuglin A, Simeon-Rudolf V, Reiner E. Molar absorption coefficients for the reduced Ellman reagent: reassessment. Anal Biochem. 2003;312(2):224–27

28. Young G, Koplovitz I. Acute toxicity of cyclohexylmethylphosphonofluoridate (CMPF) in rhesus monkeys: serum biochemical and hematologic changes. Arch Toxicol. 1995;69(6):379–83.

29. Ecobichon D, Comeau A. Pseudocholinesterases of mammalian plasma: Physicochemical properties and organophosphate inhibition in eleven species. Toxicol Appl Pharmacol. 1973;24(1):92–100.

30. Gordon R, Feaster S, Russell A, LeJeune K, Maxwell D, Lenz D, Ross M, Doctor B. Organophosphate skin decontamination using immobilized enzymes. Chem-Biol Interact. 1999;119–120:463–70.

31. Rowntree DW, Nevin S, Wilson A. The effects of diisopropylfluorophosphonate in schizophrenia and manic depressive psychosis. J Neurol Neurosurg Psychiat. 1950;13(1):47–62.

32. Senanayake N, Karalliede L. Neurotoxic effects of organophosphorous insecticides. An intermediate syndrome. N Engl J Med. 1987;316:761–63.

33. Vijayakumar S, Fareedullah M, Ashok Kumar E, Mohan Rao K. A prospective study on electrocardiographic findings of patients with organophosphorus poisoning. Cardiovasc Toxicol.2011;11(2):113–17.

34. De Candole C, Douglas W, Evans C, Holmes R, Spencer K, Torrance R, Wilson K. The failure of respiration in death by anticholinesterase poisoning. Br J Pharmacol Chemother. 1953;8(4):466–475.

35. Furlong C, Li W, Richter R, Shih D, Lusis A, Alleva E, Costa L. Genetic and temporal determinants of pesticide sensitivity: role of paraoxonase (PON1) Neurotoxicology. 21(1–2):91.

36. De Bleecker J, Van Den Neucker K, Willems J. The intermediate syndrome in organophosphate poisoning: Presentation of a case and review of the literature. Clin Toxicol. 1992;30(3):321–29.

37. Thunga G, Sam K, Khera K, Xavier V, Verma M. Profile of acute mixed organophosphorus poisoning.Am J Emerg Med. 2009;27(5) 628 (e1–3)

38. Atherton K, Williams F, Egea González F, Glass R, Rushton S, Blain P, Mutch E. DNA damage in horticultural farmers: a pilot study showing an association with organophosphate pesticide exposure. Biomarkers. 2009;14(7):443–51.

39. Jalali N, Balali Mood M, Jalali I, Shakeri M. Electrophysiological Changes in Patients with Acute Organophosphorous Pesticide Poisoning. Basic Clin Pharmacol Toxicol. 2010;108(4):251–255.
40. Ellman G, Courtney K. A new and rapid colorimetric determination of acetylcholinesterase activity.Biochem Pharmacol. 1961;7(2):88–90.
41. Thiermann H, Zilker T, Eyer F, Felgenhauer N, Eyer P, Worek F. Monitoring of neuromuscular transmission in organophosphate pesticide-poisoned patients. Toxicol Lett. 2009;191(2–3):297–304.
42. Worek F, Mast U, Kiderlen D, Diepold C, Eyer P. Improved determination of acetylcholinesterase activity in human whole blood. Clin Chim Acta. 1999;288(1–2):73–90.
43. Mortensen S, Brimijoin S, Hooper M, Padilla S. Comparison of thein VitroSensitivity of Rat Acetylcholinesterase to Chlorpyrifosoxon: What Do Tissue IC50 Values Represent? Toxicol Appl Pharmacol. 1998;148(1):46–49.
44. Katagi M, Nishikawa M, Tatsuno M, Tsuchihashi H. Determination of the main hydrolysis product of O-ethylS-2-diisopropylaminoethyl methylphosphonothiolate, ethyl methylphosphonic acid, in human serum. J Chromatograph B: Biomed Sci Appl. 1997;689(2):327–33.
45. Wolfe A, Rush R, Doctor B, Koplovitz I, Jones D. Acetylcholinesterase prophylaxis against organophosphate toxicity. Fundam Appl Toxicol. 1987;9(2):266–70.
46. Caranto G, Waibel K, Asher J, Larrison R, Brecht K, Schutz M, Raveh L, Ashani Y, Wolfe A, Maxwell D. Amplification of the effectiveness of acetylcholinesterase for detoxification of organophosphorus compounds by bis-quaternary oximes. Biochem Pharmacol. 1994;47(2):347–57.
47. Caranto GR, Waibel KH, Asher JM, Larrison RW, Brecht KM, Schutz MB, Raveh L, Ashani Y, Wolfe AD, Maxwell DM, Bhupedra P. Amplification of the effectiveness of acetylcholinesterase for detoxification of organophosphorus compounds by bis-quaternary oximes. Biochem Pharmacol. 1994;47(2):347–57.
48. Balali-Mood M, Ayati M, Ali-Akbarian H. Effect of high doses of sodium bicarbonate in acute organophosphorous pesticide poisoning. Clin Toxicol. 2005;43(6):571–74.
49. Van Helden H, Busker R, Melchers B, Bruijnzeel P. Pharmacological effects of oximes: how relevant are they? Archiv Toxicol. 1996;70(12):779–86.
50. Corvino T, Nahata M, Angelos M, Tschampel M, Morosco R, Zerkle J, Nelson R. Availability, Stability, and Sterility of Pralidoxime for Mass Casualty Use. Annals Emerg Med. 2006;47(3):272–77.
51. Worek F, Widmann R, Knopff O, Szinicz L. Reactivating potency of obidoxime, pralidoxime, HI 6 and HLö 7 in human erythrocyte acetylcholinesterase inhibited by highly toxic organophosphorus compounds.Arch Toxicol. 1998;72(4):237–43.
52. Dawson R. Review of oximes available for treatment of nerve agent poisoning. J Appl Toxicol. 1994;14(5):317–31.
53. Balali-Mood M, Salimifar H, Shariate M. Effects of sodium bicarbonate in human organophosphate poisoning. "Proceedings of the third international Chemical and Biological Medical treatment symposium; Spiez, Switzerland. May 7–12; 2000. pp. 18–27.
54. Roberts DM, Dawson AH, Hittarage A, Jeganathan K, Sheriff MH, Buckley NA. Plasma alkalinization for acute organophosphorus poisoning--is it a reality in the developing world? Clin Toxicol (Phila)2007;45(1):90–91.
55. Balali-Mood M, Afshari R, Kahrom M, Ayati M, Ali-Akbarian H, Zare G. Letter to the Editor: Use of high doses of sodium bicarbonate in acute organophosphorous pesticide poisoning is advancing" Clin Toxicol. 2007;45(1):92–93.
56. Zhou Y, Zhan C, Li Y, Zhong Q, Pan H, Yang G. Intravenous lipid emulsions combine extracorporeal blood purification: a novel therapeutic strategy for severe organophosphate poisoning. Med Hypotheses.2010;74(2):309.
57. Balali-Mood M, Balali-Mood K, Hosseini Shirazi F. Recent advances in treatment of acute organophosphorous nerve agents poisoning. Iran J Pharm Res. 2006;2:82–88.
58. Balali-Mood M, Saber MR. Recent advances in the treatment of acute organophosphorous poisonings.Iran J Med Sci. 2012;37(2):74–91.
59. Jiang G, Huo F, Li J, Wang Y, Cao H. Studies on use and residue levels of pesticides in fruit and vegetable in Tianjin Area and its control measures. Chin J Prev Med. 2003;37(5):351–54.
60. Heidari H. Farmer field schools (FFS) slash pesticide use and exposure in Islamic republic of Iran. Agro-Chemicals Report. 2003;3(1):23–26.
61. El Nahhal Y. Contamination and safety status of plant and food in Arab countries. J Appl Sci.2004;4(3):411–7.
62. Husain S, Kiarostami V, Morrovati M, Tagebakhsh M. Multiresidue determination of diazinon and ethion in pistachio nuts by use of matrix solid phase dispersion with a lanthanum silicate co-column and gas chromatography. Acta Chromatographica. 2003;13:208–14.
63. Temple WA, Smith NA. 1989. last updated by Szinicz L, Karalliedde L, Ostapenko Y, Jonitz W, Balali-Mood M, Wong A, Socrates J (1999). Organophosphorous pesticides PIM, IPCS/WHO.http://www.inchem.org/documents/pims/chemical/pimg001.htm.

CHAPTER 12

LIVER δ--AMINOLEVULINATE DEHYDRATASE ACTIVITY IS INHIBITED BY NEONICOTINOIDS AND RESTORED BY ANTIOXIDANT AGENTS

Elisa Sauer, Angela M. Moro, Natália Brucker, Sabrina Nascimento, Bruna Gauer, Rafael Fracasso, Adriana Gioda 6, Ruy Beck, José C. F. Moreira, Vera Lucia Eifler-Lima and Solange Cristina Garcia,

Keywords: neonicotinoids; δ-ALA-D activity; toxicity; antioxidants

INTRODUCTION

The widespread use of pesticides in agriculture has resulted in an increase of environmental pollution and health risks for non-target organisms, culminating in cases of acute and chronic poisoning [1]. Neonicoitinoids are currently the most important chemical class of insecticides marketed worldwide since the synthesis of the pyrethroids. The neonicotinoids have similar structures to nicotine and act on its site of action at the nicotinic acetylcholine receptor (nAChR) [2]. These compounds are classified as N-nitroguanidines (imidacloprid, thiamethoxam, dinotefuran, and clothianidin) and N-cyanoaminides (acetamiprid and thiacloprid) [3]. In 1991, this new class of pesticides was introduced into the market in the form of its precursor imidacloprid (IMI, 1-(6-chloro-3-pyridylmethyl)-N-nitroimidazolidin-2-ylideneamine) [4]. Since then, the widespread development of additional neonicotinoids for protection of modern crops reflects the importance of this chemical class, which is used for crop protection against piercing–sucking insects of cereals, vegetables, tea and cotton, and for flea control in cats and dogs [5]. Neonicotinoid pesticides represent 17% of all processed insecticides on the global market, with the class precursor imidacloprid being the most commercialized, representing 41.5% of sales [3,4].

Recent studies have shown that pesticides induce toxicity by several mechanisms. Some research has demonstrated that the biotransformation of pesticides generates reactive oxygen (ROS) and nitrogen (NOS) species, and that these free radicals are associated with the toxicity induced by these pesticides culminating in development of oxidative stress [2]. Oxidative stress is characterized by an imbalance between the production of free radicals and antioxidant defenses of the organism. Increased production of ROS may result from pathological conditions and by action of xenobiotics such as pesticides inducing tissue damage in several organs such as the heart, brain, kidney and liver [2,6,7].

Taking into account that δ-aminolevulinate dehydratase (δ-ALA-D) or porphobilinogen synthase is a metalloenzyme with thiol groups (-SH) that requires zinc ions for its activity [8], this enzyme can be inhibited by substances that compete with zinc, or by substances that oxidize-SH groups. Therefore, the δ-ALA-D activity can be inhibited by oxidation by different soft electrophiles or chemical elements that compete with Zn(II) in its active site. Recent studies have shown that this enzyme is a marker protein of oxidative stress situations. Indeed, numerous researches have shown a negative correlation

Citation: Elisa Sauer, Angela M. Moro, Natália Brucker, Sabrina Nascimento, Bruna Gauer, Rafael Fracasso , Adriana Gioda , Ruy Beck , José C. F. Moreira , Vera Lucia Eifler-Lima and Solange Cristina Garcia, Liver δ-Aminolevulinate Dehydratase Activity is Inhibited by Neonicotinoids and Restored by Antioxidant Agents, doi:10.3390/ijerph111111676

between enzyme activity and the occurrence of oxidative stress [9].

In vertebrates, the liver, with its high metabolic rates and high concentrations of enzymes from the endogenous antioxidant system is the main organ involved in detoxification of xenobiotics [10]. The aim of this study was to evaluate how the presence of imidacloprid affects the activity of hepatic δ-ALA-D *in vitro*. Furthermore, we evaluated the protective effect of antioxidant agents such as resveratrol, curcumin, ascorbic acid and GSH against the potential toxic effects caused by this pesticide. Additionally, the presence of chemical elements which could interfere with the enzymatic activity of δ-ALA-D or increase its toxicityand not declared in the composition of imidacloprid was determined.

MATERIALS AND METHODS

Chemicals

Imidacloprid (IMI, 1-(6-chloro-3-pyridin-3-methyl)-N-nitroimidazolidin-2-ylidenamine, Evidence®, 70% technical grade was obtained from Bayer CropScience (Morrisville, NC, USA). δ-Aminolevulinic acid (δ-ALA), dithiotreitol (DTT), ascorbic acid (L-3-ketothreohexuronic acid lactone), L-glutatione reduced (GSH), resveratrol, curcumin, Bradford reagent and bovine serum albumin were purchased from Sigma (St. Louis, MO, USA). Zinc chloride ($ZnCl_2$) was purchased from Proquimios (Bangu, RJ, Brazil). All chemicals and solvents used were of analytical reagent grade quality and were used as received. Twice-deionized water was used.

Animals

The study was conducted using male adult Wistar rats weighing 270 ± 60 g, aged 6–8 weeks obtained from the Fundação Estadual de Produção e Pesquisa em Saúde (FEPPS, Porto Alegre, Brazil), maintained at 22 ± 28 °C under a 12/12 h light/dark cycle, receiving standard food and water *ad libitum*. The animals treatment was conducted in accordance with the "Guiding Principles in the Care and uses of Animals" [11]. This study was approved by the local Ethics Committee of Universidade Federal do Rio Grande do Sul, No. 18427.

Tissue Preparation

Rats (*n* = 4) were sacrificed with an overdose of ketamine and xylazine anesthesia. Each liver sample was divided into equal parts of 1 g and stored at −80 °C until homogenization. Liver samples were homogenized with 50 mM Tris-Cl, pH 7.4 (1/10, *w/v*) and kept on ice. Homogenates were centrifuged at 581 g for 10 min to yield a low-speed supernatant (S1) fraction. Freshly prepared S1 was used for δ-ALA-D assays to obtain IC_{50} values and for enzyme activity reversibility tests.

Protein

Protein levels from supernatants were determined according to Bradford [12], using bovine serum albumin as standard.

δ-ALA-D Activity

δ-ALA-D activity was assayed by the method of Sassa (1981) [13], with some modifications. After a pre-incubation period, enzymatic reaction was initiated by adding the substrate (δ-ALA) in the medium and incubating for 1 h at 37 °C. The incubation was stopped by adding trichloroacetic acid solution (10% TCA) with 10 mM $HgCl_2$. Porphobilinogen (PBG) was mixed with modified Ehrlich's reagent, and the color developed was measured photometrically (555 nm) against a blank. Results were reported as nmol PBG/mg protein/h. All experiments were performed four times, and 1 g of liver from each rat as used.

Inhibitory Effect of Imidacloprid to *δ-ALA-D* Activity and IC_{50} Determination

The effect of imidacloprid on the liver δ-ALA-D activity was determined in the presence of different concentrations of pesticide (2–40 mM). The freshly prepared S1 was pre-incubated at 37 °C for 10 min with imidacloprid and after this time, the substrate (δ-ALA) was mixed to start the reaction. After data evaluation the IC_{50} value was determined and utilized to study the protective effect of resveratrol, curcumin, ascorbic acid and GSH.

Effect of Dithiothreitol (DTT) and Zinc Chloride ($ZnCl_2$)

We verified the effect of DTT (3 mM) and zinc chloride ($ZnCl_2$) (100 mM) in restore δ-ALA-D inhibition caused by imidacloprid (IC_{50}). For that, imidacloprid (at IC_{50} concentration) was pre-incubated with freshly prepared S1 of liver tissue containing DTT or $ZnCl_2$ for 10 min at 37 °C. After this time the reaction was started by the addition of substrate (δ-ALA).

Effect of Resveratrol, Curcumin, Ascorbic Acid and Reduced Glutathione on Liver *δ-ALA-D* Activity in the Presence of Imidacloprid

The protective effects of curcumin, resveratrol, ascorbic acid and GSH were studied in the presence of imidacloprid (IC_{50}concentration). The freshly prepared (S1) hepatic tissue was pre-incubated at 37 °C for 10 min with imidacloprid plus resveratrol or curcumin (0.001, 0.1, 1, 5, 10, 100 and 1000 μM), and imidacloprid plus ascorbic acid or GSH (10, 100 and 1000 μM).

Quantification of Chemical Elements in Imidacloprid

The chemical elements ^{75}As, ^{27}Al, ^{114}Cd, ^{59}Co, ^{53}Cr, ^{65}Cu, ^{208}Pb, ^{60}Ni, ^{55}Mn, ^{202}Hg and ^{88}Sr were quantified in samples of commercial imidacloprid by inductively coupled plasma mass spectrometry (ICP-MS: NexION 300X, PerkinElmer, Norwalk, CT, USA). For the measurement of chemical elements, 1.0 mL of 65% nitric acid PA (redistilled) was added to 100 mg of pesticide in a sterile polypropylene tube. The mixture was digested by heating at 95 °C for 8 h. The extracts were cooled at room temperature and the volume was made up to 10.0 mL with ultrapure water. Calibration was performed using standard solutions of 10 $\mu g \cdot L^{-1}$ (Perkin Elmer 29 and Merck Titrisol) and acidified with bidistilled nitric acid. Calibration curve concentrations ranged from 5 $\mu g \cdot L^{-1}$ to 80 $\mu g \cdot L^{-1}$, and the internal standard used was rhodium at a concentration of 400

$\mu g \cdot L^{-1}$ for calibration. Precision and accuracy of the analytical method were monitored through the use of reference standards that were analyzed in intervals of 15 samples. For differences greater than 10%, a new calibration was applied. The limit of detection (LOD) was calculated using the formula LOD = 3 × (SD/S) and the limit of quantification (LOQ) was determined by the formula LOQ = 10 × (SD/S), where SD represents the standard deviations of the readings of 10 blanks and S is the sensitivity of the analytical curve (slope).

Statistical Analysis

Data were expressed as mean ± S.D. Statistical analysis was performed by one-way ANOVA followed by Bonferroni's post-hoc tests. Values of $p < 0.05$ were considered statistically significant. The IC_{50} value was determined by linear regression from individual experiments using GraphPad software (GraphPad software, San Diego, CA, USA).

RESULTS

Inhibitory Effect of Imidacloprid on *δ-ALA-D* Activity and Determination of IC_{50}

Hepatic δ-ALA-D activity was significantly inhibited by imidacloprid at the concentrations 2, 5, 10, 20 and 40 mM (Figure 1), in a dose-dependent manner. The IC_{50} value was 20.06 ± 0.17 mM. Next, the potential protective effect of the antioxidants curcumin, resveratrol, acid ascorbic and GSH was tested utilizing the IC_{50} value of imidacloprid.

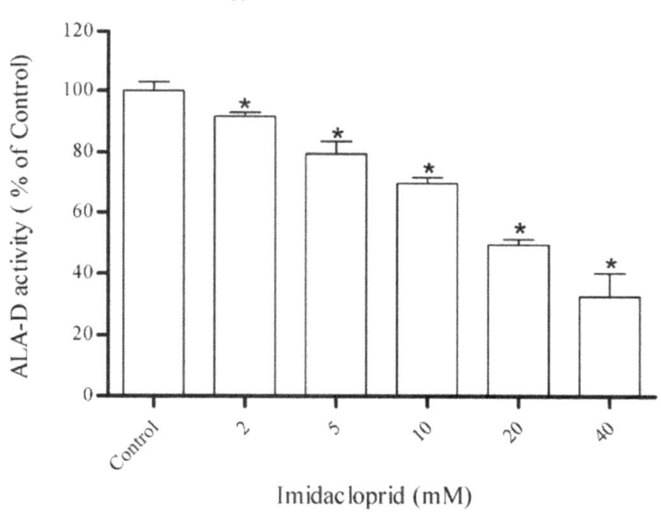

Figure 1; Effect of imidacloprid on δ-ALA-D activity from rat liver. Data are expressed as mean ± SD, (n = 4). δ-ALA-D activity of control (100%) was of 13.57 ± 0.17 (mean ± SD) nmol of porphobilinogen per mg protein per hour.

Effect of Dithiothreitol (DTT) and Zinc Chloride ($ZnCl_2$)

The inhibitory effect of imidacloprid (20 mM) on hepatic δ-ALA-D activity was completely (100%) restored by the addition of DTT (3 mM) and partially restored (75%) by $ZnCl_2$ (100 mM) when compared to the initial enzyme activity (Figure 2).

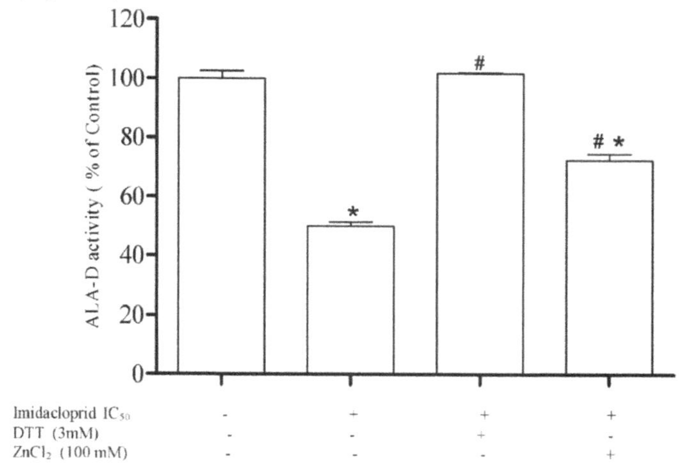

Figure 2: Effect of DTT and $ZnCl_2$ as restoring agents δ-ALA-D inhibition caused by imidacloprid (IC_{50} = 20 mM). Data are expressed as mean ± SD, (n = 4).

Effect of Resveratrol, Curcumin, Ascorbic Acid and Reduced Glutathione on Liver *δ*-AlA-D Activity in the Presence of Imidacloprid

Results showed that resveratrol at 0.1, 1, 5, and 10 μM restored the δ-ALA-D activity inhibited by imidacloprid (20 mM) at 59%, 61%, 61% and 58%, respectively, when compared to the initial enzymatic activity. However, resveratrol at 100 μM did not restore the inhibitory effect of imidacloprid (20 mM) on δ-ALA-D activity, and at 1000 μM had an inhibitory effect on enzymatic activity, which decreased to 29% when compared to the baseline activity (Figure 3).

Curcumin at 0.001, 0.1, 1, 5 and 10 μM restored the enzyme activity inhibited by imidacloprid (20 mM) at 55%, 55%, 63%, 65% and 58%, respectively, when compared to the initial enzyme activity, while at 100 and 1000 μM was not able to restore enzyme activity (Figure 4).

We verified that ascorbic acid treatment at 10, 100 and 1000 μM was not able to restore the enzymatic inhibition (Figure 5), and that reduced glutathione at 100 and 1000 μM partially restored the inhibition to 53% and 67% (Figure 6).

Determination of Chemical Elements in Imidacloprid

The concentrations of chemical elements analyzed in commercial imidacloprid are shown in Table 1.

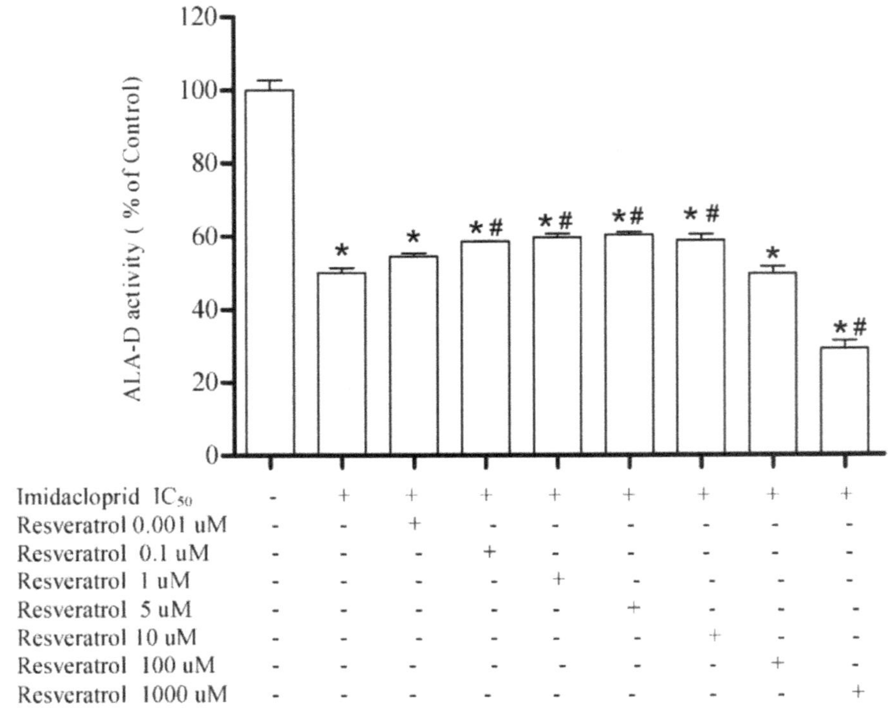

Figure 3: Effect of resveratrol (0.001, 0.1, 1, 5, 10, 100 and 1000 μM) as restoring agent for δ-ALA-D inhibition caused by imidacloprid (IC_{50} = 20 mM).Data are expressed as mean ± SD, (n = 4).

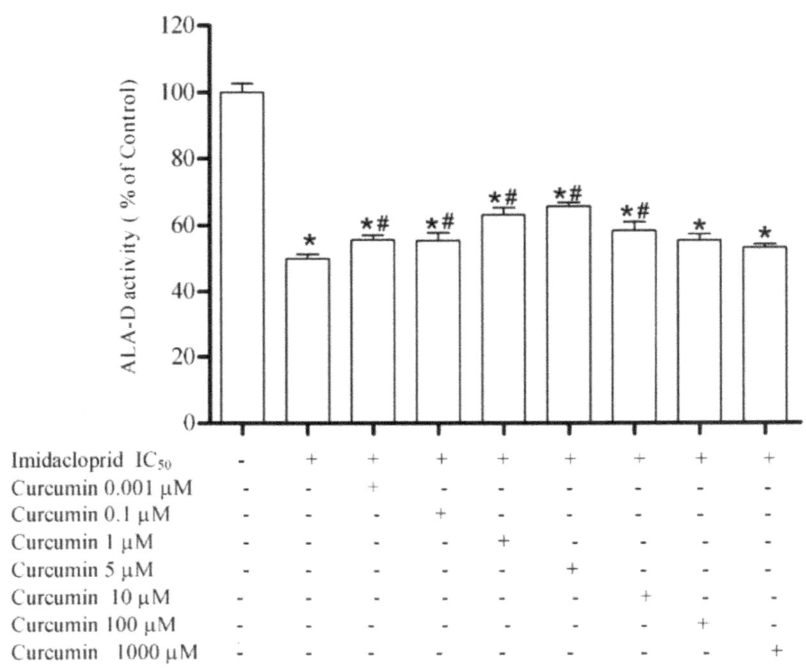

Figure 4: Effect of curcumin (0.001, 0.1, 1, 5, 10, 100 and 1000 μM) as restoring agent for δ-ALA-D inhibition caused by imidacloprid (IC_{50} = 20 mM). Data are expressed as mean ± SD, (n = 4).

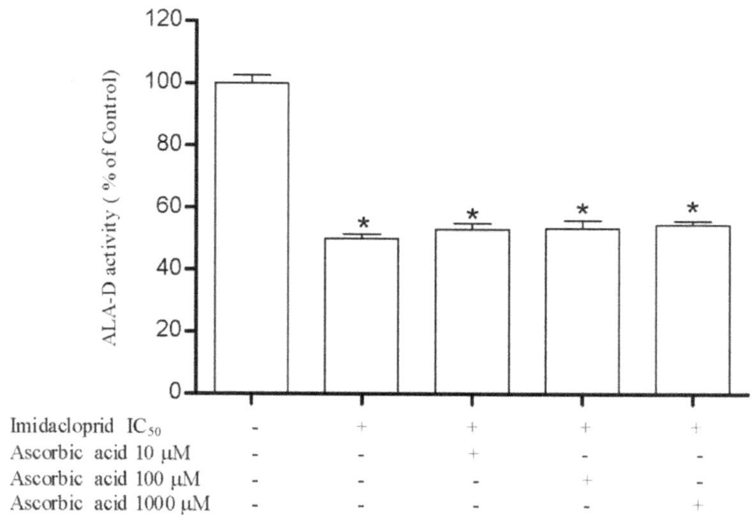

Figure 5: Effect of ascorbic acid (10, 100 and 1000 μM) as restoring agent for δ-ALA-D inhibition caused by imidacloprid (IC_{50} = 20 mM). Data are expressed as mean ± SD, (*n*= 4).

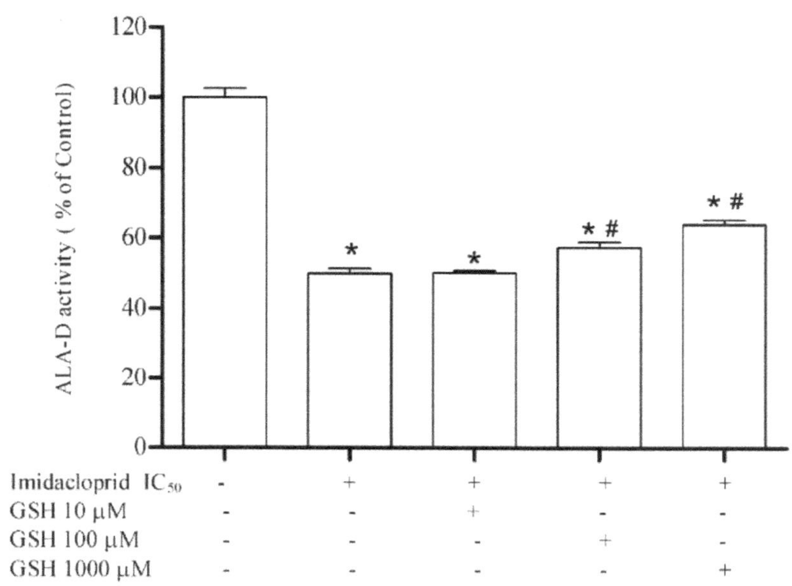

Figure 6: Effect of reduced glutathione (10, 100 and 1000 μM) as restoring agent for δ-ALA-D inhibition caused by imidacloprid (IC_{50} = 20 mM). Data are expressed as mean ± SD, (*n* = 4).

Table 1: Concentration of chemical elements present in imidacloprid quantified by ICP-MS.

Chemical elements	Concentration ($mg \cdot L^{-1}$)
Aluminum	8.43
Arsenic	0.28
Cadmium	0.02
Cobalt	0.05
Copper	2.98
Chromium	2.81
Lead	0.11
Manganese	77.62
Mercury	0.11
Nickel	0.51
Strontium	3.27

DISCUSSION AND CONCLUSIONS

Currently, neonicotinoids are classified by the Environmental Protection Agency (EPA) system as toxicity class II and/or class III agents [14], because they block a specific neuron pathway that is more abundant in insects than warm blooded animals, so the toxicity of these insecticides is more selective to insects than mammals [2]. However, these insecticides affect insects by interfering with nAChRs, suggesting that these receptors may also be a target in mammals. Moreover, there are reports of neonicotinoid intoxications, with clinical manifestations including nausea, vomiting, drowsiness, disorientation, dizziness, oral and gastroesophageal erosions, hemorrhagic gastritis, productive cough, fever, leukocytosis, muscle weakness, hypothermia and convulsions [15,16,17]. Calderón-Segura *et al.* [3] demonstrated that commercial neonicotinoid formulations induced DNA damage, reduced the viability of human lymphocytes and caused cell death. Birsen [18] demonstrated that treatment with the neonicotinoid thiacloprid results in increased oxide nitric (NO) levels in rat polymorphonuclear leukocytes and plasma. El-Gendy*et al.* [2] showed that imidacloprid treatment of rats induced a marked increase in the hepatic lipid peroxidation. Moreover another study found changes in liver enzymes, oxidative stress markers, induction of pro-inflammatory cytokines and NO levels in the brain and liver of imidacloprid-exposed rats [5].

In the present study, we demonstrated for the first time that the neonicotinoid imidacloprid is able to inhibit the activity of δ-ALA-D in liver tissue. This enzyme has thiol groups (-SH) in its active site, which are essentially involved in the coordination of Zn(II) ions, and the proximity between these groups renders the enzyme easily oxidizable [19,20]. The δ-ALA-D inhibition by toxic agents, such as imidacloprid, contributes to the increase of circulating levels of the substrate aminolevulinic acid (ALA). ALA is a pro-oxidant compound and a weak γ-aminobutyric acid (GABA) agonist, which is responsible for decreasing GABA release by presynaptic inhibition and may cause neurotoxicity [21]. Additionally, other experimental studies have shown that ALA possibly presents other central nervous system effects such as induction of free radical formation, effects on the uptake and release of glutamate, inhibition of Na^+, K^+, -ATPase activity and seizures induced by glutamatergic mechanisms [22]. Patients affected by disorders characterized by increased levels of aminolevulinic acid, such as occurs in porphyrias, present acute attacks characterized by neurological manifestations, including seizures and psychiatric manifestations such as hysteria, anxiety and depression [22].

Furthermore, δ-ALA-D is directly involved in the synthesis of grouping tetrapyrroles, such as heme. The enzymatic inhibition caused by the addition of imidacloprid may interrupt or interfere with the synthesis of heme groups resulting in damage to the cell metabolism and injury to the health of non-target organisms exposed to pesticides. These alterations may occur both by induction of neurotoxicity or producing an increase in oxidative effects due to the pro-oxidant activity of the accumulated enzyme substrate ALA [9].

Recent studies have shown that the enzymatic activity of δ-ALA-D can be used as a biomarker of pro-oxidant situations because it is extremely susceptible to oxidizing agents and must be in the reduced state to catalyze the substrate formation [9]. Several studies have shown a negative correlation between the activity of δ-ALA-D and the occurrence of oxidative stress. Previous studies have shown that δ-ALA-D activity was inhibited in hemodialysis patients [23,24], in patients after bone marrow transplantation [25] and in patients with diabetes [26]. Furthermore, the activity of δ-ALA-D was inhibited after exposure to other pro-oxidant situations such as hyperoxygenation [27] and after exposure to paints, which contain a broad mixture of solvents [28]. Therefore, based on previous studies that demonstrate that the enzyme is a good marker for pro-oxidant conditions and oxidative stress, we can infer that imidacloprid is a compound capable of causing oxidative stress since it was able to significantly inhibit the enzymatic activity of δ-ALA-D.

Since δ-ALA-D activity may be inhibited by compounds that oxidize the –SH groups or which remove Zn(II) from the enzyme structure, we studied the possible mechanism(s) of imidacloprid toxicity. In this line, it was observed that the enzymatic inhibition caused by imidacloprid was restored by the addition of dithiothreitol (DTT), which is a dithiol that possesses the ability of protecting δ- ALA-D against inhibition by sulfhydryl oxidizing agents [29]. On the other hand, we verified that $ZnCl_2$was partially able to restore δ-ALA-D activity, thus we propose that the mechanism involved in the inhibitory effect of imidacloprid on δ-ALA-D activity is also by zinc displacement of the enzyme structure. Chemical elements found in the composition of the pesticide may be contributing to the direct oxidation of thiol groups –SH or interacting by facilitating the displacement of Zn(II). Thus, the toxic effects caused by pesticide on the enzyme activity are not only resulting from the active principle imidacloprid, but also of chemical elements presents in the formulation, which are not declared on the product label. A study has shown strong reactivity *in vitro* of some chemical elements such as Pb, Hg, Cd, As and Al, which are chemical elements found in the imidacloprid formulation, with–SH, causing inhibition of enzyme activity [9]. Besides that, high concentrations of Mn were found in the imidacloprid formulation. Mn is an essential metal necessary for normal functioning of many biological processes such as energy metabolism and the immune system [30]. Additionally, Mn can be found in the brain as an important co-factor of enzymes involved in the antioxidant system [31]. However, despite its essentiality, several psychomotor and psychiatric disorders are associated with exposure to high levels of Mn, such as Parkinson's disease symptoms, cognitive deficits, memory loss, impaired learning demonstrating its neurotoxic potential [32]. Therefore, the presence of this metal in high concentrations in the imidacloprid formulations could potentiate the neurotoxic effects resulting from the inhibition of the enzymatic activity of ALA-D caused by this pesticide.

We used resveratrol and curcumin as potential antioxidants to reverse the inhibition of δ-ALA-D caused by imidacloprid and other chemical agents found in the pesticide. Resveratrol (3,5,4›-tri- hydroxystilbene) is a phytoalexin found in grapes and in foods such as peanuts, blueberries, and red wines, and along with curcumin is a polyphenolic compound. Curcumin (diferuoylmethane) is the most active component of turmeric, an agent derived from dried rhizomes of the plant turmeric (*Curcuma longa* L.), and is one of the most recently studied chemopreventive compounds [33,34,35]. As shown in the results, both curcumin and resveratrol at low concentrations were effective at partially restoring enzyme activity, in other words, they are able to restore enzyme activity due to their antioxidant activity, protecting the enzyme from the oxidative effects of the pesticide. On the other hand, the highest concentrations of resveratrol tested (100 and 1000 μM) were unable to restore enzyme activity. Indeed Stooco *et al.* [36] have shown that at high concentrations these antioxidants may present pro–oxidant effects. In addition, the concentration 1000 μM caused an increase in enzymatic inhibition induced by the pesticide, demonstrating a pro-oxidant effect of resveratrol, which was not observed with curcumin. Our findings corroborate some reports in the literature, where both were recognized as potential antioxidants at low concentrations, because they present the ability to eliminate free radicals and increase antioxidant effects [33,34,35].

Moreover, we also used GSH and ascorbic acid to test their influence on enzyme activity inhibited by the pesticide. Ascorbic acid is widely known due to its antioxidant properties. It is an excellent source of electrons, acting as a donor of electrons and neutralizing free radicals. Due to its solubility in water, ascorbic acid promotes an antioxidant effect both inside and outside the cell and prevents free radical damage [37,38]. Ascorbic acid may scavenge peroxyl radicals and inhibit cytotoxicity induced by oxidants [39]. El-Gendy *et al.* [2] demonstrated that ascorbic acid promotes protective effects against toxicity induced by imidacloprid in rats as observed by some markers of oxidative stress such as MDA, GSH, CAT, SOD and GPx. In our study, ascorbic acid was not able to restore enzyme activity inhibited by the pesticide. However El-Gendy *et al.* [2] also showed that pre-treatment with ascorbic acid is most effective when compared to post-treatment. In our study, both pesticide and ascorbic acid were incubated simultaneously, and probably would a pre-incubation with ascorbic acid is necessary to obtain the protective effects of this antioxidant.

GSH is a non-protein thiol widely distributed in animal tissues, and closely linked to the antioxidant cell response against the toxic effects of reactive oxygen species [40]. In the present study, GSH demonstrated its antioxidant effect when it was able to partially reverse the enzymatic activity inhibited by imidacloprid at the two highest concentrations tested (100 and 1000 μM). Other studies have shown the benefits of GSH treatment, resulting in a reduction in the oxidant burden at the alveolar epithelial surface in the idiopathic pulmonary fibrosis [41], attenuation of reactive oxygen species generation and increased antioxidant defenses [42], attenuation of lipid peroxidation [43] and prevention of neurotoxicity induced by treatment with oxaliplatin without reducing the clinical activity of oxaliplatin [44].

Our study has some limitations. The imidacloprid concentration range used in our study is very high and may not represent environmental relevance. On the other hand, we aimed to investigate the potential toxic effects of this pesticide in order to assess the risks in cases acute occupational exposure, as well as in cases of accidental or intentional poisoning. A study by Kimura-Kuroda *et al.* [45], evaluated the effect of imidacloprid in cerebellar neurons and found that in concentrations more than 1 M the pesticide exerts excitatory effects of nicotinic acetylcholine receptors (nAChRs) and thus may harm human health, especially in the developing brain. The concentration used in this study was much lower than those used in our study, however, Kimura-Kuroda *et al.* used a primary cell culture model that mimics the conditions of the body.

In view of our data, this study supports the evidence that imidacloprid, an insecticide widely used and classified as being of low toxicity, induces oxidative damage since it significantly inhibited the enzymatic activity of δ-ALA-D. Moreover, the enzymatic inhibition of δ-ALA-D could contribute to accumulation of its enzymatic substrate δ-ALA that may rapidly oxidize to generate ROS such as superoxide ions, hydroxyl radicals and hydroxyl peroxides generating a vicious pro-oxidant cycle [9] that could promote neurotoxic effects [21]. The inhibition was reversed completely after treatment with the reducing agent DTT and the partial restoration by the use of $ZnCl_2$ indicates that the enzyme inhibition does not occur only by oxidation of thiol groups, but also by Zn(II) displacement, which is possibly related to the presence of various chemical elements in the pesticide formulations. Therefore, the toxicity demonstrated by the studied pesticide could be associated to the active principle, imidacloprid, but also to the presence of different chemical elements that are not declared in its formulation, which can contribute to potentiate the toxicity caused by imidacloprid. Knowing that some of the chemical elements found in the pesticide formulation have an influence on the enzymatic activity of δ-ALA-D, future studies using these chemicals elements, mainly manganese, found in pesticide formulations are important to evaluate the effect of these elements on the inhibition enzymatic activity of δ-ALA-D, a point that can be a limitation in our study. Considering our results together with previous findings in the literature, it could be stated that this neonicotinoid, despite its low toxicity classification, should be investigated carefully because it may cause serious damages to non-target organisms, especially after chronic exposure. Hepatio-protective effects were observed in imidacloprid-induced liver toxicity after the use GSH at 1000 μM followed by curcumin at 5 μM, which appeared as the second most powerful antioxidant and resveratrol at 5 and 10 μM concentrations. Therefore, it could be suggested that these compounds could contribute to prevention of inhibition caused by this pesticide along with other chemicals present in the formulation on δ-ALA-D activity.

ACKNOWLEDGMENTS

This work was supported by CNPq and FAPERGS (grant to Solange Cristina Garcia). Solange Cristina Garcia is recipient of CNPq research fellowship. Angela Maria Moro is recipient of CNPq Postdoctoral Junior fellowship (150261/2014-4). Elisa Sauer received PIBIC-CNPq-IC/FUC/PIBIC-CNPq—UFRGS fellowship.

CONFLICTS OF INTEREST

The authors declare no conflicts of interest.

REFERENCES

1. Abdollahi, M.; Ranjbar, A.; Shadnia, S.; Nikfar, S.; Rezaie, A. Pesticides and oxidative stress: A review. *Med. Sci. Monit.*2004, *10*, RA141–RA147.
2. El-Gendy, K.S.; Aly, N.M.; Mahmoud, F.H.; Kenawy, A.; El-Sebae, A.K.H. The role of vitamin C as antioxidant in protection of oxidative stress induced by imidacloprid.

Food Chem. Toxicol. 2010, *48*, 215–221.

3. Calderón-Segura, M.E.; Gómez-Arroyo, S.; Villalobos-Pietrini, R.; Martínez-Valenzuela, C.; Carbajal-López, Y.; Calderón-Ezquerro, M.D.C.; Cortés-Eslava, J.; García-Martínez, R.; Flores-Ramírez, D.; Rodríguez-Romero, M.I. Evaluation of genotoxic and cytotoxic effects in human peripheral blood lymphocytes exposed *in vitro* to neonicotinoid insecticides news. *J. Toxicol.* 2012, *2012*.
4. Jeschke, P.; Nauen, R.; Schindler, M.; Elbert, A. Overview of the status and global strategy for neonicotinoids. *J. Agric. Food Chem.* 2010, *59*, 2897–2908.
5. Duzguner, V.; Erdogan, S. Chronic exposure to imidacloprid induces inflammation and oxidative stress in the liver and central nervous system of rats. *Pestic. Biochem. Physiol.* 2012, *104*, 58–64.
6. Dwivedi, P.; Das, M.; Khanna, S. Role of cytochrome P450 in quinalphos toxicity: Effect on hepatic and brain antioxidant enzymes in RatsITRC communication No. 1965. *Food Chem. Toxicol.* 1998, *36*, 437–444.
7. Yu, F.; Wang, Z.; Ju, B.; Wang, Y.; Wang, J.; Bai, D. Apoptotic effect of organophosphorus insecticide chlorpyrifos on mouse retina *in vivo* via oxidative stress and protection of combination of vitamins C and E. *Exp. Toxicol. Pathol.* 2008,*59*, 415–423.
8. Jaffe, E.K. The porphobilinogen synthase family of metalloenzymes. *Acta Crystallogr. Sect. D* 2000, *56*, 115–128.
9. Rocha, J.B.; Saraiva, R.A.; Garcia, S.C.; Gravina, F.S.; Nogueira, C.W. Aminolevulinate dehydratase (δ ALA-D) as marker protein of intoxication with metals and other pro-oxidant situations. *Toxicol. Res.* 2012, *1*, 85–102.
10. Hinderer, R.K.; Menzer, R.E. Comparative enzyme activities and cytochrome P-450 levels of some rat tissues with respect to their metabolism of several pesticides. *Pestic. Biochem. Physiol.* 1976, *6*, 148–160.
11. Olfert, E.; Cross, B.; McWilliam, A. *Canadian Council on Animal Care—Guide to the Care and Use of Experimental Animals*; Brada Printing Services: Ottawa, ON, Canada, 1993; Volume 1.
12. Bradford, M.M. A rapid and sensitive method for the quantitation of microgram quantities of protein utilizing the principle of protein-dye binding. *Anal. Biochem.* 1976, *72*, 248–254.
13. Sassa, S. Delta-aminolevulinic acid dehydratase assay. *Enzyme* 1981, *28*, 133–145.
14. Meister, R.T. *Farm Chemicals Handbook*; Meister Publishing Company: Willoughby, OH, USA, 1995.
15. Mohamed, F.; Gawarammana, I.; Robertson, T.A.; Roberts, M.S.; Palangasinghe, C.; Zawahir, S.; Jayamanne, S.; Kandasamy, J.; Eddleston, M.; Buckley, N.A. Acute human self-poisoning with imidacloprid compound: A neonicotinoid insecticide. *PLoS One* 2009, *4*.
16. Imamura, T.; Yanagawa, Y.; Nishikawa, K.; Matsumoto, N.; Sakamoto, T. Two cases of acute poisoning with acetamiprid in humans. *Clin. Toxicol.* 2010, *48*, 851–853.
17. David, D.; George, I.A.; Peter, J.V. Toxicology of the newer neonicotinoid insecticides: Imidacloprid poisoning in a human. *Clin. Toxicol.* 2007, *45*, 485–486.
18. Aydin, B. Effects of thiacloprid, deltamethrin and their combination on oxidative stress in lymphoid organs, polymorphonuclear leukocytes and plasma of rats. *Pestic. Biochem. Physiol.* 2011, *100*, 165–171.
19. Markham, G.D.; Myers, C.B.; Harris, K.A.; Volin, M.; Jaffe, E.K. Spatial proximity and sequence localization of the reactive sulfhydryls of porphobilinogen synthase. *Protein. Sci.* 1993, *2*, 71–79.
20. Farina, M.; Barbosa, N.; Nogueira, C.; Folmer, V.; Zeni, G.; Andrade, L.; Braga, A.; Rocha, J. Reaction of diphenyl diselenide with hydrogen peroxide and inhibition of delta-aminolevulinate dehydratase from rat liver and cucumber leaves. *Braz. J. Med. Biol. Res.* 2002, *35*, 623–631.
21. Needleman, H. Lead poisoning. *Annu. Rev. Med.* 2004, *55*, 209–222.
22. Emanuelli, T.; Pagel, F.W.; Alves, L.C.B.; Regner, A.; Souza, D.O. Inhibition of adenylate cyclase activity by 5-aminolevulinic acid in rat and human brain. *Neurochem. Int.* 2001, *38*, 213–218.
23. Valentini, J.; Grotto, D.; Paniz, C.; Roehrs, M.; Burg, G.; Garcia, S.C. The influence of the hemodialysis treatment time under oxidative stress biomarkers in chronic renal failure patients. *Biomed. Pharmacother.* 2008, *62*, 378–382.
24. Roehrs, M.; Valentini, J.; Bulcão, R.; Moreira, J.C.; Biesalski, H.; Limberger, R.P.; Grune, T.; Garcia, S.C. The plasma retinol levels as pro-oxidant/oxidant agents in haemodialysis patients. *Nephrol. Dial. Transplant.* 2009, *24*, 2212–2218.
25. Gonçalves, T.L.; Benvegnú, D.M.; Bonfanti, G.; Frediani, A.V.; Rocha, J.B. δ-ALA-D activity is a reliable marker for oxidative stress in bone marrow transplant patients. *BMC Cancer* 2009, *9*.
26. Fernandez-Cuartero, B.; Rebollar, J.; Batlle, A.; Enriquez de Salamanca, R. Delta aminolevulinate dehydratase (ALA-D) activity in human and experimental diabetes mellitus. *Int. J. Biochem. Cell Biol.* 1999, *31*, 479–488.
27. Rocha, J.B.; Heinzmann Bulow, N.M.; Correa, E.F.; Scholze, C.; Nogueira, C.W.; Barbosa, N.B. Dexmedetomidine protects blood delta-aminolevulinate dehydratase from inactivation caused by hyperoxygenation in total intravenous anesthesia. *Hum. Exp. Toxicol.* 2011, *30*, 289–295.
28. Moro, A.M.; Charão, M.; Brucker, N.; Bulcão, R.; Freitas, F.; Guerreiro, G.; Baierle, M.; Nascimento, S.; Waechter, F.; Hirakata, V. Effects of low-level exposure to xenobiotics present in paints on oxidative stress in workers. *Sci. Total Environ.* 2010, *408*, 4461–4467.
29. Folmer, V.; Bolzan, R.C.; Farina, M.; Zeni, G.; Nogueira, C.W.; Emanuelli, T.; Rocha, J.B.T. Mechanism of delta-aminolevulinate dehydratase inhibition by phenyl selenoacetylene involves its conversion to diphenyl diselenide.*Toxicology* 2005, *206*, 403–411.
30. Erikson, K.M.; Syversen, T.; Aschner, J.L.; Aschner, M. Interactions between excessive manganese exposures

and dietary iron-deficiency in neurodegeneration. *Environ. Toxicol. Pharmacol.* 2005, *19*, 415–421.

31. Aschner, M.; Guilarte, T.R.; Schneider, J.S.; Zheng, W. Manganese: Recent advances in understanding its transport and neurotoxicity. *Toxicol. Appl. Pharmacol.* 2007, *221*, 131–147.
32. Josephs, K.; Ahlskog, J.; Klos, K.; Kumar, N.; Fealey, R.; Trenerry, M.; Cowl, C. Neurologic manifestations in welders with pallidal MRI T1 hyperintensity. *Neurology* 2005, *64*, 2033–2039.
33. Sebastià, N.; Montoro, A.; Montoro, A.; Almonacid, M.; Villaescusa, J.I.; Cervera, J.; Such, E.; Silla, M.A.; Soriano, J.M. Assessment *in vitro* of radioprotective efficacy of curcumin and resveratrol. *Radiat. Meas.* 2011, *46*, 962–966.
34. El-Azab, M.; Hishe, H.; Moustafa, Y.; El-Awady, E.-S. Anti-angiogenic effect of resveratrol or curcumin in Ehrlich ascites carcinoma-bearing mice. *Eur. J. Pharmacol.* 2011, *652*, 7–14.
35. Eybl, V.; Kotyzova, D.; Koutensky, J. Comparative study of natural antioxidants-curcumin, resveratrol and melatonin—In cadmium-induced oxidative damage in mice. *Toxicology* 2006, *225*, 150–156.
36. Stocco, B.; Toledo, K.; Salvador, M.; Paulo, M.; Koyama, N.; Torqueti Toloi, M.R. Dose-dependent effect of resveratrol on bladder cancer cells: Chemoprevention and oxidative stress. *Maturitas* 2012, *72*, 72–78.
37. Bendich, A. Antioxidant micronutrients and immune responses. *Ann. N.Y. Acad. Sci.* 1990, *587*, 168–180.
38. Bindhumol, V.; Chitra, K.; Mathur, P. Bisphenol A induces reactive oxygen species generation in the liver of male rats.*Toxicology* 2003, *188*, 117–124.
39. Yen, G.-C.; Duh, P.-D.; Tsai, H.-L. Antioxidant and pro-oxidant properties of ascorbic acid and gallic acid. *Food. Chem.*2002, *79*, 307–313.
40. Meister, A. Selective modification of glutathione metabolism. *Science* 1983, *220*, 472–477.
41. Borok, Z.; Buhl, R.; Hubbard, R.; Holroyd, K.; Roum, J.; Czerski, D.; Crystal, R.; Grimes, G.; Bokser, A.; Cantin, A. Effect of glutathione aerosol on oxidant-antioxidant imbalance in idiopathic pulmonary fibrosis. *Lancet* 1991, *338*, 215–216.
42. Liu, J.; Wang, X.; Mori, A. Immobilization stress-induced antioxidant defense changes in rat plasma: Effect of treatment with reduced glutathione. *Int. J. Biochem.* 1994, *26*, 511–517.
43. Brzezińska-Ślebodzińska, E.; Ślebodziński, A.; Pietras, B.; Wieczorek, G. Antioxidant effect of vitamin E and glutathione on lipid peroxidation in boar semen plasma. *Biol. Trace Element.* 1995, *47*, 69–74.
44. Cascinu, S.; Catalano, V.; Cordella, L.; Labianca, R.; Giordani, P.; Baldelli, A.M.; Beretta, G.D.; Ubiali, E.; Catalano, G. Neuroprotective effect of reduced glutathione on oxaliplatin-based chemotherapy in advanced colorectal cancer: A randomized, double-blind, placebo-controlled trial. *J. Clin. Oncol.* 2002, *20*, 3478–3483.
45. Kimura-Kuroda, J.; Komuta, Y.; Kuroda, Y.; Hayashi, M.; Kawano, H. Nicotine-like effects of the neonicotinoid insecticides acetamiprid and imidacloprid on cerebellar neurons from neonatal rats. *PLoS One* 2012, *7*.

CHAPTER 13 REPRODUCTIVE EFFECTS OF TWO NEONICOTINOID INSECTICIDES

Yi-hua Gu, Yan Li, Xue-feng Huang, Ju-fen Zheng, Jun Yang, Hua Diao, Yao Yuan, Yan Xu, Miao Liu, Hui-juan Shi, and Wen-ping Xu

Keywords: neonicotinoids; δ-ALA-D activity; toxicity; antioxidants

INTRODUCTION

Pesticides are widespread chemicals mainly utilized in pest control. Only for agricultural purposes, more than 140, 000 tones of pesticides are used annually in the European Union [1], this kind of extensive application raised concerns about hazards of pesticides to human health, including reproductive safety. Imidacloprid (IMI) and acetamiprid (ACE) are two of main compounds in a relatively new class of pesticides, neonicotinoids, which occupied dominant position in global market due to broad spectrum of activity to pests, low residue in environment and low toxicity to human [2], [3]. Despite that they are synthesized to selectively bind to insect nicotinic acetylcholine receptor (nAChRs) in central nervous systems [4], *in vivo*studies demonstrated that IMI, ACE and other neonicotinoid pesticides could adversely affect mammalian reproductive organs such as retardation of testicular development, damage to spermatogenesis, decrease in sperm quality and change of ovary morphology [5], [6], [7], [8], [9].

Sharing partial structure and similar action with nicotine, deleterious effects of IMI and ACE in animal experiments are similar to those of nicotine [10], [11], [12]. To illustrate *in vitro* effects on reproduction and the underlying mechanism, reproductive toxicity study of nicotine exposure on mammalian spermatozoa or oocytes has been conducted for years [13], [14], [15], [16]. However, studies are rarely reported for the *in vitro* effects of IMI and ACE on mammalian reproduction, especially on their direct actions upon fertilization and preimplantation embryonic development. Referring to previous studies of *in vitro* effects of nicotine, we evaluated and compared the impacts of IMI, ACE and nicotine on mouse reproduction by using an integrated testing strategy for reproductive toxicology. To study their direct action upon sperm, sperm parameters were determined, such as motility and DNA integrity. Fertilization capability of the chemical-treated spermatozoa was also estimated by using *in vitro* fertilization (IVF) procedure, which is regarded as a sensitive screening system for reproductive toxicants [17]. The resultant zygotes were kept in culture until blastocyst formation, which could also help determine the impacts of chemical treatment on sperm functions. To evaluate the sensitivities of fertilization and embryos at different preimplantation stages to these chemicals, normal IVF procedure, zygotes and 2-cell embryos were respectively treated with chemicals, cultured in presence of chemicals, and monitored continuously until blastocyst formation.

Citation: Gu Y-h, Li Y, Huang X-f, Zheng J-f, Yang J, et al. (2013) Reproductive effects of two neonicotinoid insecticides, doi:10.1371/journal.pone.0070112.

MATERIALS AND METHODS

Ethical Statement

This study was carried out in full compliance with Guide for the Care and Use of Laboratory Animals. The protocol was approved by the Committee on the Ethics of Animal Experiments of Shanghai Institute of Planned Parenthood Research.

Chemicals

Nicotine ((−)-nicotine) was purchased from Sigma-Aldrich (St Louis, MO) at purities >99%. The neonicotinoid insecticides 1-(6-chloro-3-pyridylmethyl)-N-nitroimidazolidin-2-ylideneamine (IMI, purity >96%) and (E)-N^1-[(6-chloro-3-pyridyl) methyl]-N^2- cyano-N^1-methylacetamidine (ACE, purity >96%) were acquired from Shanghai Pesticide Research Institute (Shanghai, China). They were dissolved in dimethyl sulfoxide (DMSO, Sigma-Aldrich), and their stock solutions (500 mM) were frozen at −20°C immediately prior to use to minimize their inactivation and degradation.

Animals

6–8 weeks old female B6D2F1 (C57BL/6×DBA/2) strain mice were used as oocyte donors, and 10–15 weeks old male B6D2F1 mice were used as semen donors. All mice were housed under controlled light conditions (12 h light: 12 h dark) in the Laboratory Animal Services Facility and were fed a standard mouse diet and water *ad libitum*.

Experimental Design

To investigate the effect of these three substances on fertilization and embryonic development, concentrated ACE, IMI and nicotine were prepared as medium supplements. DMSO was used at final concentration ≤0.1% and this vehicle was used as control to investigate the potential effect of the solvent.

In a previous report, concentrations of 0.1mM to 10 mM were used to approximately represent different ranges of residual nicotine in the testis of light to habitual smokers, wherein the motility of human spermatozoa does not change after exposure to 500 μM of nicotine for 30 minutes [14]. In our preliminary experiment, we also found that nicotine exposure with a dosage of 500 μM for 30 minutes could not impair both motility and fertilization capability of mouse spermatozoa. We then adopted concentration of 5 mM in the sperm exposure experiment.

In sperm exposure experiment, mouse spermatozoa were placed in ACE, IMI or nicotine-containing (500 μM or 5 mM) HTF medium supplemented with bovine serum albumin (HTF-BSA, Sigma) for 30 min first, then washed by and incubated in fresh HTF-BSA medium for another 60 min until capacitation finished, followed by normal IVF procedure. Control spermatozoa were processed with the same procedure except the exposure of chemicals.

To study their effects on the development of early embryos that skipped the stage of fertilization or the first cleavage, zygotes with 2 pronuclei as well as 2-cell stage embryos by natural insemination were cultured in ACE, IMI or nicotine-added KSOM medium (500 μM) to observe how chemicals worked at subsequent developmental stage. Furthermore, the consecutive exposure process from fertilization to blastocyst formation was monitored with exposure concentration of 500 μM both in HTF medium for fertilization and KSOM medium for embryo culture. Concentrations of pesticides were limited to 500 μM, because our preliminary experiments indicated that oocytes and embryos with higher than 500 μM of nicotine would induce massive fragmentation or death the next day.

Collection of Spermatozoa

Caudal epididymides were isolated, gently squeezed out and placed in a 2.0 ml eppendorf tube with HTF-BSA. "Swim-up" spermatozoa were obtained after incubation at 37°C for 10 min.

Collection of Oocytes and Embryos

Mature female mice were superovulated with 10 IU of pregnant mare serum gonadotropin (PMSG) and 5 IU of human chorionic gonadotropin (HCG) at 48 h intervals. 14–16 h after HCG administration, cumulus oocyte complexes (COCs) were collected from the removed oviducts and then maintained in human tubal fluid (HTF, Sage In-Vitro Fertilization, Trumbull, CT) medium supplemented with 10% human serum albumin (HSA, Vitrolife, Gothenburg, SE) at 37°C in an atmosphere of 5% CO_2 in air until use.

With regard to the recovery of the naturally fertilized zygotes and embryos, several female mice were mated with males and examined 12–18 h after HCG injection for the presence of copulation plugs. Fertilized oocytes and 2-cell embryos were recovered by flushing the oviducts 24 h and 40 h later after the HCG injection, respectively. The cumulus of oocytes were dispersed with 0.1% hyaluronidase (Sigma-Aldrich, St. Louis, MO) and washed in several changes of HCZB medium. Fertilized oocytes (identified by the presence of a second polar body and two pronuclei) and 2-cell embryos were then placed in potassium chloride supplemented simplex optimized medium (KSOM medium, Millipore-Chemicon, Billerica, MA), which was designed for culture of implantation stage embryos and previously equilibrated in a humidified atmosphere of 5% CO_2 in air at 37°C.

Sperm Motility Assay

The control droplet consisted of an equivalent volume of DMSO in treated groups. After incubation, a 15-μl aliquot of the treated and control samples was transferred into each of two compartments on a glass cannula slide for computer-assisted sperm analysis (CASA) using the integrated visual optical system (IVOS) motility analyzer (Hamilton-Thorne Research, Inc.). Thirty frames were acquired at a frame rate of 60 Hz. The operational settings of the IVOS were as follows: minimum contrast (40) and size (four pixels), gate thresholds 0.38/1.65 for intensity and 0.42/2.34 for size, static elongation 0/75, progressive minimum path velocities of sperm (VAP) 50 μm/sec, straightness threshold 50%, and magnification 0.82.

Sperm Chromatin Dispersion (SCD) Assay

Generally, SCD assay was developed as the Halosperm® kit (INDAS Laboratories, Madrid, Spain) instructed. An aliquot of each semen sample was diluted to 5–10 million/ml in PBS. The unfixed suspensions were mixed with 1% low-melting-point aqueous agarose (to obtain a 0.7% final agarose concentration) at 37°C. Aliquots of 20 µl mixture were pipetted onto a glass slide precoated with 0.65% standard agarose, covered with a coverslip (22 × 22 mm), and left to solidify at 4°C for 5 min. Then coverslips were carefully removed and slides immediately incubated with freshly prepared acid denaturation solution for 7 min (RT) in the dark to generate restricted single-stranded DNA (ssDNA) motifs from DNA breaks. The denaturation was then stopped, followed by incubation with lysing solution for 23 min (RT). Slides were thoroughly washed in deionized water for 5 min, dehydrated in sequential 70%, 90%, and 100% ethanol baths (2 min each) and air dried. Afterwards, cells were stained with modified Wright-Giemsa stain (Sigma-Aldrich, St. Louis, MO) for bright-field microscopy and a minimum of 400 spermatozoa per sample were evaluated under the × 40 objective of the light microscope. After staining, four SCD patterns were established: sperm heads with (i) large size halos, whose halo width was similar or larger than the minor diameter of the core, (ii) medium size halos, whose halo size was between those with large and with small halo, (iii) small size halos, whose halo width was similar or smaller than one third of the minor diameter of the core, and (iv) without a halo or degraded sperm cells, the latter ones were weakly or irregularly stained. The spermatozoa without DNA damage showed nucleoids with large- or medium-sized halos of spreading DNA loops whereas those with fragmented DNA appeared with a small or no halo. Finally, the percentage of sperm (iii) and (iv) was considered as DNA fragmentation index (DFI) for each semen sample. In this study, spermatozoa pre-incubated in ACE, IMI or nicotine-added HTF medium (5 mM or 500 µM) for 30 min were analyzed for DNA integrity.

In vitro Fertilization and Preimplantation Embryonic Development Procedure

IVF procedure was performed as previously described [18]. HTF medium was equilibrated in a 37°C, 5% CO_2 incubator one day before experiment. Next day, caudal epididymides were collected from adult male mice. A dense sperm mass was squeezed out and then incubated in HTF-BSA medium for 60–90 min at 37°C to develop their fertilization potential (capacitation). A small volume of capacitated sperm suspension was added to a drop of 200 µl HTF-BSA medium containing freshly ovulated oocytes to achieve a final sperm concentration of 10^6/ml. Four to six hours later, fertilized oocytes at pronuclear stage were washed and cultured in KSOM for *in vitro* development to morula/blastocyst stages in 5% CO_2 in air. Oocytes were observed for male and female pronucleus formation (fertilization) at 6 h after the initiation of culture, and the number of 2-cell embryos, 4-cell embryos, morulae and blastocysts after 24 h, 48 h, 72 h and 96 h in culture were checked and recorded respectively.

Statistical Analysis

SPSS for Windows (Version 15.0; SPSS Inc., Chicago, IL, USA) was used for statistical analysis. *In vitro*developmental outcomes and SCD results were evaluated using ^{2} tests and one-way analysis of variance (ANOVA) for significance, respectively. Results were considered statistically significant at P<0.05.

RESULTS

Influences of Chemical Exposure on Sperm Function

With CASA, we were able to obtain objective and quantitative descriptions of changes in sperm kinematic parameters in response to exogenous toxicant. Treated with 500 µM or 5 mM of chemicals for 30 minutes, motility of spermatozoa showed no obvious difference from that of control (data not shown). We then investigated whether toxicant-induced reproductive hazards was associated with sperm DNA lesion using SCD assay. All chemical-treated groups displayed a minor increase in average percentage of DNA fragmented spermatozoa compared with those of control groups without reaching a significant difference (P>0.05), as shown in Figure 1. With respect to the difference between 500 µM and 5 mM of each chemical, the response toward exogenous compounds at current differential concentration was not obvious, as similar effects on sperm motility and DFI were observed.

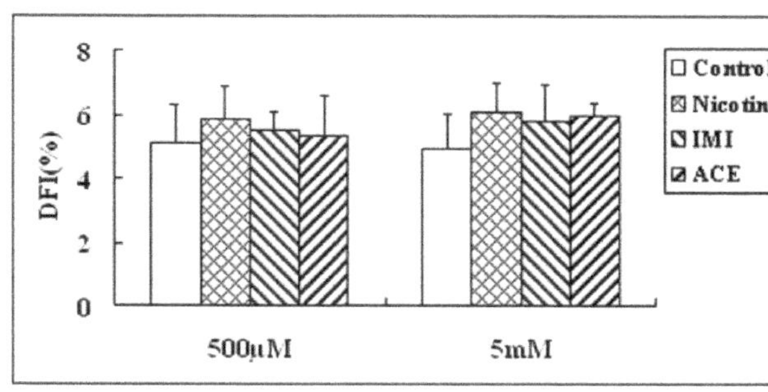

Figure 1: The SCD results of toxicants exposure upon sperm DNA integrity.

When IVF was performed with the spermatozoa pretreated with chemicals adopted herein at the concentration of 500 µM or 5 mM, all fertilized oocytes survived without evident changes in cell morphology. Fertilized oocytes were judged normal by extrusion of second polar body and the presence of 2 pronuclei, which represents success of fertilization. Our preliminary data indicated that treatment with 500 µM of chemicals for 30 min did not induce any significant adverse effect on fertilization potential of the spermatozoa and subsequent embryo development (data not shown). However, during the culture process, embryos originated from spermatozoa pretreated with 5 mM of chemicals were more inclined to encounter failure of the first cleavage, wherein some of them exhibited various degrees of cellular fragmentation and asymmetry (Figure 2A'). Finally, when these embryos were cultured *in vitro* up to 96 h, with fragmentation, loss of cytoplasm or decrease in cytoplasmic clarity, part of them would arrest or degenerate during the developmental progression (Figure 2B'). As shown in Table 1, in the presence of 5 mM toxicant in HTF medium, all treated spermatozoa retained their potential to fertilize oocytes. However, in nicotine and IMI-exposed groups, rates of pronucleus formation (fertilization), the first cleavage and morula/blastocyst formation were remarkably decreased, compared to those of non-treated control (P<0.05). In ACE-exposed group, the first cleavage of zygote and blastocyst formation process were also impaired (91.2% and 58.5%, respectively), compared to those of the control group (98.5% and 74.6%, respectively), whereas the fertilization rate was slightly lower than that of control without reaching a statistical significance. Thus, ACE appeared to pose much weaker adverse effects on mouse spermatozoa, at least in terms of fertilization process*in vitro*. During embryo culture, embryo fragmentation, a process where portions of the embryo's cells have broken off, had attracted our attention. It is preferable to have little or no fragmentation when evaluate a normal embryo, while nicotine and IMI exposure remarkably elevated the fragmented embryo percentage compared with control. Comparisons were also made among treated groups, it was observed that ACE exerted significantly moderate effect, whereas nicotine exposure showed most severe reproductive hazard.

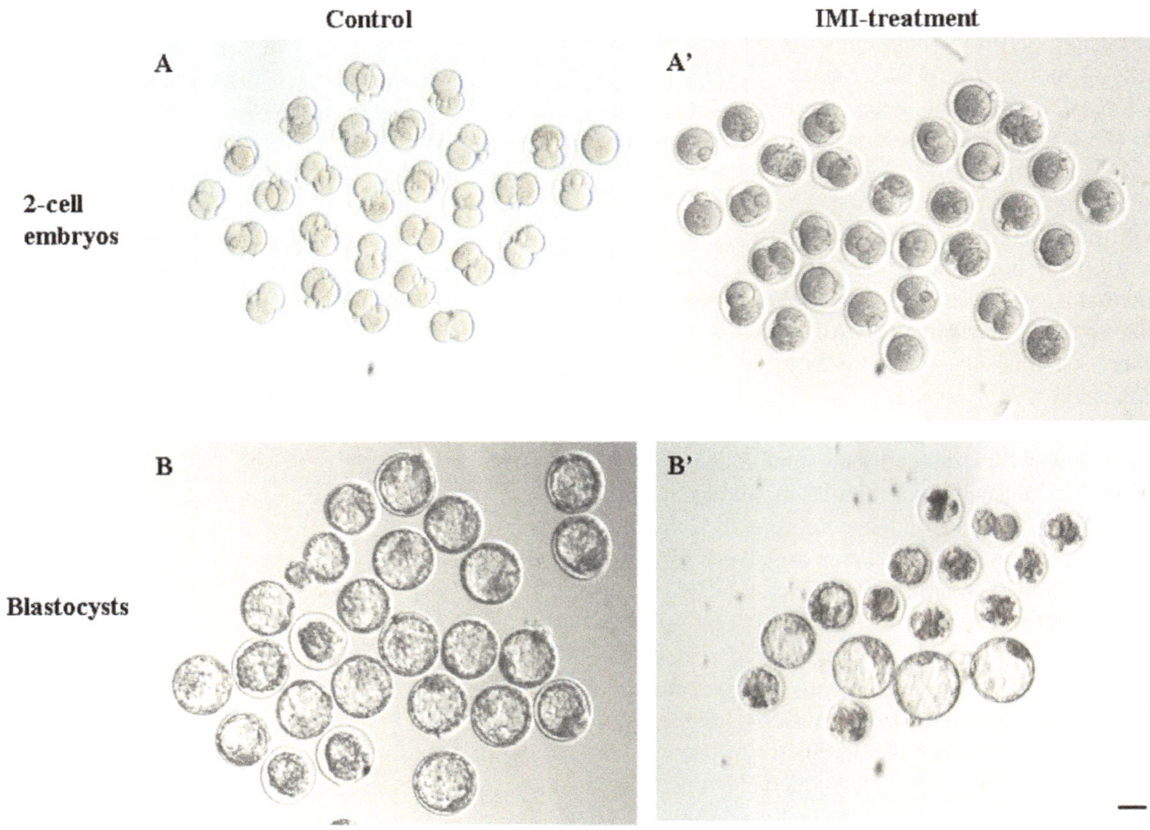

Figure 2: Partial embryos derived from IVF process with control or 5 mM IMI treated spermatozoa.

Table 1: The effects of chemicals upon sperm fertilization capability in IVF procedure and subsequent embryonic development.

Category	No. of oocytes (replicates)	No. with pronuclei formation (%)[a]	No. of 2-cell embryos (%)[b]	No. of fragmented embryos (%)[b]	No. of morulae (%)[b]	No. of blastocysts (%)[b]
Control	283(5)	205(72.4)	202(98.5)	6(2.9)	165(80.5)	153(74.6)
nicotine-exposed	344(5)	186(54.1)*	155(83.3)*	31(16.7)*	93(50.0)*	78(41.9)*
IMI-exposed	301(5)	188(62.5)*, #	160(85.1)*	16(8.5)*, #	112(59.6)*	96(51.1)*
ACE-exposed	225(5)	159(70.7)#,$	145(91.2)*, #	7(4.4)#	122(76.7)#,$	93(58.5)*,#

[a]Based on total oocytes.
[b]Based on total pronuclear embryos.
*, #, $ $P<0.05$, comparisons were made between control group and each treated group, nicotine group and two insecticide groups, and two insecticide groups, respectively.
doi:10.1371/journal.pone.0070112.t001

Influences of Chemical Exposure on Fertilization and Subsequent Embryonic Development *in vitro*

In consecutive exposure experiment with chemical exposure both in HTF and KSOM medium, the concentration of supplementation constricted to 500 μM in both of medium, which allowed the fertilized oocytes proceed to blastocysts without inducing excessive fragmented or dead embryos. It was showed that mixture of oocytes and spermatozoa in chemical-added HTF maintained normal fertilization capacity compared with control (ratio of oocytes with pronuclei formation, $P>0.05$), while the percentages of 2-cell embryo and morula/blastocyst formation decreased significantly ($P<0.05$). Among these three chemicals, ACE appeared most mild in the effect on the first cleavage (ratio of 2-cell embryo formation), with no significance found (Table 2).

Table 2: The effects of chemicals upon the consecutive exposure from fertilization to blastocyst formation.

Category	No. of oocytes (replicates)	No. of oocytes with pronuclei (%)[a]	No. of 2-cell embryos (%)[b]	No. of fragmented embryos (%)[b]	No. of morulae (%)[b]	No. of blastocysts (%)[b]
Control	132(3)	98(74.2)	94(95.9)	4(4.1)	79(80.6)	77(78.6)
Nicotine-exposed	138(3)	99(71.7)	82(82.8)*	10(10.1)	66(66.7)*	63(63.6)*
IMI-exposed	143(3)	102(71.3)	90(88.2)*	7(6.9)	68(66.7)*	67(65.7)*
ACE-exposed	142(3)	104(73.2)	95(91.3)	9(8.7)	70(67.3)*	68(65.4)*

[a]Based on total oocytes.
[b]Based on total pronuclear embryos.
*$P<0.05$, comparisons were made between control group and each treated group.
doi:10.1371/journal.pone.0070112.t002

Influences of Chemical Exposure on Preimplantation Embryonic Development *in vitro*

Considering that exposure of 1 mM chemicals would cause considerable embryo fragmentation or even death in our preliminary experiments (data not shown), we used 500 μM of concentration in culture medium. As shown in Table 3, exposure of these chemicals caused a moderate decline in the percentage of 2-cell embryo formation and a drastic impact on morula/blastocyst formation derived from normal zygotes, compared with control ($P<0.05$). When comparison was made among these three chemicals, exposure of IMI or ACE retarded embryonic development to a more moderate degree than nicotine, but no significant difference existed between IMI and ACE group. Taken together, adverse effects exerted on development of zygotes in the order of nicotine>IMI>ACE.

Table 3: The effects of chemicals upon the development of naturally fertilized zygotes.

Category	No. of oocytes with pronuclei (replicates)	No. of 2-cell embryos (%)[a]	No. of 4-cell embryos (%)[a]	No. of morulae (%)[a]	No. of blastocysts (%)[a]
Control zygotes	86(3)	82(95.3)	82(95.3)	81(94.2)	80(93.0)
Nicotine-exposed zygotes	125(3)	106(84.8)*	93(74.4)*	86(68.8)*	84(67.2)*
IMI-exposed zygotes	141(3)	134(95.0)#	123(87.2)*,#	108(76.6)*	106(75.2)*
ACE-exposed zygotes	128(3)	120(93.8)#	113(88.3)#	105(82.0)*,#	101(78.9)*,#

[a]Based on total oocytes with pronuclei.
*, #$P<0.05$, comparisons were made between control group and each treated group, nicotine group and two insecticide groups, respectively.
doi:10.1371/journal.pone.0070112.t003

Incubated with 500 μM of each chemical, development of naturally fertilized 2-cell embryos was also monitored (Table 4). Under these conditions, treatment with different chemicals did not show significant adverse effects on 2-cell embryos ($P>0.05$), with less extent of effects than those observed in zygotes. These results collectively revealed that the doses up to 500 μM of each chemical used in the study did not exert toxicity at the onset of 2-cell embryo, but fertilization or zygote as well as the subsequent developmental procedure with preceding chemical exposure.

Table 4: **The effects of chemicals upon the development of 2-cell embryos.**

Category	No. of 2-cell embryos (replicates)	No. of 4-cell embryos (%)[a]	No. of morulae (%)[a]	No. of blastocysts (%)[a]
Control 2-cell embryos	72(3)	71(98.6)	70(96.6)	70(97.2)
Nicotine-exposed 2-cell embryos	107(3)	104(97.2)	103(96.3)	100(93.5)
IMI-exposed 2-cell embryos	103(3)	102(99.0)	100(97.1)	98(95.1)
ACE-exposed 2-cell embryos	101(3)	100(99.0)	99(98.0)	95(94.1)

[a]Based on total 2-cell embryos.Haibin Wang.
doi:10.1371/journal.pone.0070112.t004

DISCUSSION

Despite of lower affinity to mammalian nAChRs, neonicotinoid pesticides have been illustrated to impair mammalian reproduction by recent animal studies [5], [6], [7], [8], [9]. In the present study, we used a set of promising *in vitro* models of reproductive toxicology [19], and examined the direct effects of neonicotinoid pesticides, IMI and ACE, on spermatozoa, fertilization procedure and preimplantation embryo development.

Sperm quality, such as motility and DNA integrity, are important in male fertility and in the particular contribution to early embryonic development [20], which is also a sensitive and quick testing strategy for reproductive toxicology [21]. *In vitro* exposure of nicotine to human semen was reported to be able to cause human sperm DNA damage and motility decrease (1 mM for 20 min) [14], [22], [23]. However, we found that motility and DNA integrity were not significantly affected by a high exposure dosage (5 mM for 30 min) of chemicals, even with nicotine, which may result from difference of experimental objects, mouse spermatozoa *versus* human semen. When IVF process was introduced, subtle differences among the spermatozoa caused by pretreatment with different chemicals, nicotine, IMI or ACE, could still be detected through the procedures of fertilization and subsequent embryonic development (Table 1).

Procedure of IVF includes sperm-egg binding, zygote formation and the first cleavage to form 2-cell embryo. After being transferred into KSOM medium, 2-cell embryo could conduct multiple cleavages to form 4-cell embryo, morula then blastocyst successively *in vitro*. In order to determine the specific embryo developmental stages that chemicals could take effect, mixture of spermatozoa and eggs for fertilization, naturally fertilized zygotes and 2-cell embryos were separately prepared, and consecutive chemical exposure with a concentration of 500 μM was conducted until blastocyst formation. We observed that exposure of chemicals during fertilization could adversely affect 2-cell formation and subsequent embryo development (Table 2), normal zygotes with chemical exposure could impair subsequent 4-cell embryo formation and following procedure (Table 3), whereas there was no significant adverse effect on subsequent development when normal 2-cell embryos were treated with these chemicals (Table 4). Compared with the effects on fertilization procedure or zygotes, our results suggested that, 2-cell embryos were most resistant to exposure of 500 μM nicotine, IMI or ACE, which is consistent to the previous study of 2-cell embryos toxicity with nicotine [12].

Although it may cause human reproduction disorder, nicotine could show *in vitro* detriments only with a concentration much higher than the exposure level in an "average" smoker [12], [15], [24], suggesting that nicotine might adversely affect spermatozoa or embryos in an indirect way. Our study supported these previous reports, and implied that IMI and ACE may work with a similar mechanism to nicotine. Studies indicated that acute or chronic exposure of nicotine will cause oxidative stress in animal and human body[24], [25], [26], [27], which could do harm to reproductive organs. Several studies reported that oxidative stress caused by testicular tissue and lymphocyte in semen will impair sperm parameters [24], [27], suggesting that owing to lack of lymphocytes around, "swim-up" mouse spermatozoa in our study are more resist to the exposure of nicotine than human spermatozoa in semen. Human exposure to neonicotinoids is very limited (12.8–350 ng/ml in the urine of farm workers, with or without protection) [28], [29], our study indicated that, at exposure levels, IMI and ACE do not show adverse effects on mouse sperm functions and early embryo development *in vitro* (data not shown). However, recent animal studies showed that IMI and ACE could cause oxidative stress in body [5], [26], and even chronic exposure of IMI with a low concentration could result in oxidative stress in tissues [30], which warned that low level of neonicotinoid exposure in a long period may also exert impacts on reproduction of human, especially for professional populations.

Taken together, in a reproductive toxicity study, we herein integrated several *in vitro* tests reported in our and other previous studies [14], [19], [31], [32], which covered sperm quality, sperm penetration into oocytes, process of oocyte *in vitro* maturation, and preimplantation embryonic development. The results indicated that, at high levels, direct exposure of nicotine, IMI or ACE had harmful effects on sperm function and embryonic development, and stages mainly at fertilization, zygote formation, and first cleavage of zygote, with the extent in an order of nicotine>IMI>ACE. These preliminary but provocative results elucidated the reproductive toxicities of two neonicotinoid insecticides on mammals from a new prospective, which evaluated the direct effects of pesticides on gametes, fertilization and embryonic development. Meanwhile, our study suggested that application of an integrated testing strategy will help developers detect the reproductive toxicity and determine the targets in embryogenesis for a chemical substance sensitively and shortly.

FUNDING STATEMENT

Research support was provided by National Key Technologies R&D Program (2011BAE06B04), The National Natural Science Foundation of China (N0. 30872765), Three National Comprehensive Programs of Reproductive Health & Family Planning (C1–93), and the Basic Research Key Program of Shanghai (10JC1410800). The funders had no role in study design, data collection and analysis, decision to publish, or preparation of the manuscript.

REFERENCES

1. Ramazzini C (2009) Collegium Ramazzini statement on the control of pesticides in the European Union: a call for action to protect human health. Am J Ind Med 52: 176–177
2. Wamhoff H, Schneider V (1999) Photodegradation of imidacloprid. J Agric Food Chem 47: 1730–1734
3. Elbert A, Haas M, Springer B, Thielert W, Nauen R (2008) Applied aspects of neonicotinoid uses in crop protection. Pest Manag Sci 64: 1099–1105
4. Tomizawa M, Casida JE (2005) Neonicotinoid insecticide toxicology: mechanisms of selective action. Annu Rev Pharmacol Toxicol 45: 247–268
5. Kapoor U, Srivastava MK, Bhardwaj S, Srivastava LP (2010) Effect of imidacloprid on antioxidant enzymes and lipid peroxidation in female rats to derive its No Observed Effect Level (NOEL). J Toxicol Sci35: 577–581
6. Kapoor U, Srivastava MK, Srivastava LP (2011) Toxicological impact of technical imidacloprid on ovarian morphology, hormones and antioxidant enzymes in female rats. Food Chem Toxicol 49: 3086–3089
7. Bal R, Naziroglu M, Turk G, Yilmaz O, Kuloglu T, et al. (2012) Insecticide imidacloprid induces morphological and DNA damage through oxidative toxicity on the reproductive organs of developing male rats. Cell Biochem Funct 30: 492–499
8. Bal R, Turk G, Tuzcu M, Yilmaz O, Kuloglu T, et al. (2012) Assessment of imidacloprid toxicity on reproductive organ system of adult male rats. J Environ Sci Health B 47: 434–444
9. Bal R, Turk G, Yilmaz O, Etem E, Kuloglu T, et al. (2012) Effects of clothianidin exposure on sperm quality, testicular apoptosis and fatty acid composition in developing male rats. Cell Biol Toxicol 28: 187–200
10. Jana K, Samanta PK, De DK (2010) Nicotine diminishes

testicular gametogenesis, steroidogenesis, and steroidogenic acute regulatory protein expression in adult albino rats: possible influence on pituitary gonadotropins and alteration of testicular antioxidant status. Toxicol Sci 116: 647–659

11. Ezzatabadipour M, Azizollahi S, Sarvazad A, Mirkahnooj Z, Mahdinia Z, et al. (2012) Effects of concurrent chronic administration of alcohol and nicotine on rat sperm parameters. Andrologia 44: 330–336
12. Baldwin KV, Racowsky C (1987) Nicotine and cotinine effects on development of two-cell mouse embryos in vitro. Reprod Toxicol 1: 173–178
13. Pekarsky A, Rust PF, Varn E, Mathur RS, Mathur S (1995) Effects of nicotine on sperm attachment and penetration of zona-free hamster eggs. Arch Androl 34: 77–82
14. Reddy A, Sood A, Rust PF, Busby JE, Varn E, et al. (1995) The effect of nicotine on in vitro sperm motion characteristics. J Assist Reprod Genet 12: 217–223
15. Gandini L, Lombardo F, Lenzi A, Culasso F, Pacifici R, et al. (1997) The in-vitro effects of nicotine and cotinine on sperm motility. Hum Reprod 12: 727–733
16. Zenzes MT, Bielecki R (2004) Nicotine-induced Disturbances of Meiotic Maturation in Cultured Mouse Oocytes: Alterations of Spindle Integrity and Chromosome Alignment. Tob Induc Dis 2: 151–161
17. Jelks K, Berger T, Horner C, Miller MG (2001) alpha-chlorohydrin induced changes in sperm fertilizing ability in the rat: association with diminished sperm ATP levels and motility. Reprod Toxicol 15: 11–20
18. Wakayama S, Kawahara Y, Li C, Yamagata K, Yuge L, et al. (2009) Detrimental effects of microgravity on mouse preimplantation development in vitro. PLoS One 4: e6753.
19. Lorenzetti S AI, Arabi S, Balduzzi D, Bechi N, Cordelli E, et al. (2011) Innovative non-animal testing strategies for reproductive toxicology: the contribution of Italian partners within the EU project ReProTect.Ann Ist Super Sanita 47: 16
20. D'Occhio MJ, Hengstberger KJ, Johnston SD (2007) Biology of sperm chromatin structure and relationship to male fertility and embryonic survival. Anim Reprod Sci 101: 1–17
21. Claassens OE, Wehr JB, Harrison KL (2000) Optimizing sensitivity of the human sperm motility assay for embryo toxicity testing. Hum Reprod 15: 1586–1591
22. Arabi M (2004) Nicotinic infertility: assessing DNA and plasma membrane integrity of human spermatozoa. Andrologia 36: 305–310
23. Arabi M, Shareghi B (2005) [Anti-fertility effect of nicotine]. Zhonghua Nan Ke Xue 11: 323–330
24. Cope GF (1998) The in-vitro effects of nicotine and cotinine on sperm motility. Hum Reprod 13: 777–778
25. Arrick DM, Mayhan WG (2007) Acute infusion of nicotine impairs nNOS-dependent reactivity of cerebral arterioles via an increase in oxidative stress. J Appl Physiol 103: 2062–2067
26. Jain A, Flora SJ (2012) Dose related effects of nicotine on oxidative injury in young, adult and old rats. J Environ Biol 33: 233–238
27. Vine MF, Tse CK, Hu P, Truong KY (1996) Cigarette smoking and semen quality. Fertil Steril 65: 835–842
28. Marin A, Martinez Vidal JL, Egea Gonzalez FJ, Garrido Frenich A, Glass CR, et al. (2004) Assessment of potential (inhalation and dermal) and actual exposure to acetamiprid by greenhouse applicators using liquid chromatography-tandem mass spectrometry. J Chromatogr B Analyt Technol Biomed Life Sci 804: 269–275
29. Harris SA, Villeneuve PJ, Crawley CD, Mays JE, Yeary RA, et al. (2010) National study of exposure to pesticides among professional applicators: an investigation based on urinary biomarkers. J Agric Food Chem58: 10253–10261
30. Duzgunerb V ES (2012) Chronic exposure to imidacloprid induces inflammation and oxidative stress in the liver & central nervous system of rats. Pesticide Biochemistry and Physiology 104: 7
31. Perreault SD, Cancel AM (2001) Significance of incorporating measures of sperm production and function into rat toxicology studies. Reproduction 121: 207–216
32. Huang XF, Li Y, Gu YH, Liu M, Xu Y, et al. The Effects of Di-(2-ethylhexyl)-phthalate Exposure on Fertilization and Embryonic Development In Vitro and Testicular Genomic Mutation In Vivo. PLoS One 7: e50465.

CHAPTER 14

CLASTOGENIC EFFECTS OF GLYPHOSATE IN BONE MARROW CELLS OF SWISS ALBINO MICE

Sahdeo Prasad, Smita Srivastava, Madhulika Singh, and Yogeshwer Shukla

INTRODUCTION

Pesticides, including herbicides, insecticides, and fungicides are used extensively to improve crop yields and as a result, they accumulate in the environment and humans unavoidably exposed to them [1]. Pesticides tend to be very reactive compounds that can form covalent bonds with various nucleophilic centers of cellular biomolecules, including DNA [2–4]. Because of their biological activity, the indiscriminate use of pesticides may cause undesired effects to human health. For instance, the induction of DNA damage can potentially lead to adverse reproductive outcomes, the induction of cancer, and many other chronic diseases [5–8]. Epidemiological studies demonstrated that occupational exposure to some pesticides may be related to several kinds of cancer, including leukemia [9], bladder [10], and pancreatic cancers [11].

To assess the genetic damage induced by physical and chemical agents including pesticides, various test systems have been described in bacteria, in mammalian cells in vivo and in vitro and in plants [12–14]. Arguably, the most reliable genotoxicity evaluation for human health risk is conducted in mammals by the induction of chromosomal aberrations (CAs) and micronuclei (MN). In this regard, particular attention is focused on CAs because these are considered as early warning signals for neoplastic development [15, 16]. MN are defined as small, round, DNA containing cytoplasmic bodies formed during cell division by loss of acentric chromatin fragments and/or whole chromosomes and are used as a fast and reliable assay for detecting clastogenic or aneugenic action [17]. CAs qualitatively and quantitatively detect clastogenic activity, while the MN assay detects both clastogenic effects and damage to the mitotic apparatus, some of which might have aneugenic consequences[18].

Glyphosate [chemical name: N-(phosphonomethyl) glycine - isopropylamine (IPA) salt; $C_3H_8NO_5P$; Figure 1], commonly sold in the commercial formulation named Roundup, Rodeo, Touchdown, and so forth, has been a frequently used herbicide on both cropland and noncropland areas of the world since its introduction in the 1970s [19]. Roundup (CAS # 1071-83-6) is a liquid water soluble organophosphorus herbicide, containing glyphosate as its active ingredient and surfactant (polyoxyethyleneamine) that enhances the spreading of spray droplets when they contact foliage. As a herbicide Roundup works by being absorbed into the plant not only through its leaves but also through soft stalk tissue and applied at concentrations ranging from 0.26-1.152 % of active ingredient, that is, glyphosate (20). Plants treated

Citation: Sahdeo Prasad, Smita Srivastava, Madhulika Singh, and Yogeshwer Shukla, "Clastogenic Effects of Glyphosate in Bone Marrow Cells of Swiss Albino Mice," Journal of Toxicology, vol. 2009, Article ID 308985, 6 pages, 2009. doi:10.1155/2009/308985

with glyphosate slowly die over a period of days or weeks [20]. Glyphosate is transported throughout the plant where it inhibits the shikimic acid pathway, which participates in the biosynthesis of phenylalanine and tyrosine and is also the major pathway in the biosynthesis of most plant phenolics [21]. Because this specific biologic pathway operates only in plants and microorganisms, the mechanism is not considered to be a risk for humans. Nevertheless, genotoxic, hormonal, and enzymatic effects of glyphosate in mammals have been reported [20, 22–25]. In rats, glyphosate was found to decrease the activity of some detoxifying enzymes, cytochrome P-450, and monooxygenase activities and the intestinal activity of aryl hydrocarbon hydroxylase when injected into the abdomen [26].

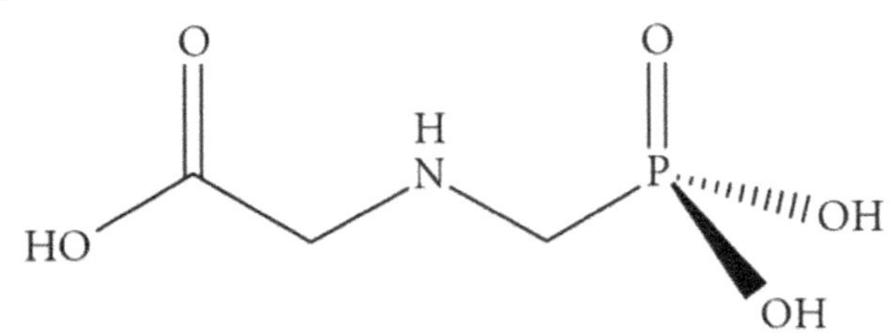

Figure 1: Chemical structure of glyphosate.

Li and Long [27] reported nonmutagenic effects from glyphosate in Salmonella typhimurium, Escherichia coli,Bacillus subtilis, Chinese hamster ovary cells gene mutation assay and chromosomal aberration in rat bone marrow cells. However, some other studies stated that glyphosate treatment on human lymphocytes in vitro resulted in increased sister chromatid exchanges [18, 22], CAs [22, 28], and oxidative stress measured by glucose 6-phosphate dehydrogenase (G6PD, marker of changes in the normal cell redox state) enzyme activity [22]. Roundup was associated with increased DNA adducts in mice [23] and DNA damage in Rana catesbeianatadpolesas assessed by using Comet assay test [29]. Beside these, several assays also have demonstrated genotoxic activities of roundup, such as induction of reverse mutation in S. typhimurium (TA98 and TA100) and sex-linked recessive lethal mutation in Drosophilamelanogaster [12, 28, 30] whereas glyphosate alone did not show these effects. In mammalian cells glyphosate was not also mutagenic [19]. Thus, so far there have been conflicting reports on the genotoxic hazards associated with the use of glyphosate.

On the basis of the information available, U.S. Environmental Protection Agency [31] and the World Health Organization [32] reviewed the toxicology data on glyphosate and concluded that glyphosate is not mutagenic or carcinogenic in humans. On the contrary, few recent studies have demonstrated cytotoxic effects of glyphosate [22, 33, 34]. Considering the widespread and frequent use of glyphosate throughout the world, ongoing risk assessment is of importance. In the present study we reported the genotoxic potential of glyphosate in mouse bone marrow cells.

MATERIALS AND METHODS

Chemicals

Roundup containing active ingredient glyphosate >41% SL (IPA salt) was purchased from, Monsanto India Ltd. (Mumbai, India). Benzo(a)pyrene [B(a)P], colchicine and Giemsa were obtained from Sigma Chemical Company (St. Louis, USA). The rest of the chemicals used in the study were of analytical grade purity and obtained locally.

Animals and Treatment

Swiss albino mice (Male, 18 ± 2 g b.wt.; age: 10–12 weeks) were obtained from the Indian Institute of Toxicology Research (Lucknow, India) animal breeding colony. The ethical approval for the experiment was obtained from Institutional Ethical Committee. Animals were randomly selected and housed in polycarbonate boxes with steel wire tops and rice husk bedding. They were maintained in controlled atmosphere of 12 hours dark/light cycle, 25 ± 2°C temperature, and 57 ± 7% humidity with free access to pelleted feed (M/s. Ashirwad, Chandigarh, India) and fresh tap water.

The animals were divided into four groups of 15 animals each in two sets. The animals of group I were used as a control group and intraperitonialy (i.p.) treatment DMSO (0.2 mL, once only) was given. The animals of group II were served as positive control and only B(a)P was given at the single dose of 100 mg/kg b.wt. i.p. In groups III and IV single dose of glyphosate (diluted appropriately in DMSO) was given i.p. at the dose of 25 and 50 mg/kg b.wt., respectively.

Chromosomal Aberration Assay

After completion of the treatment period 5 animals from each group of set 1 were sacrificed at the sampling time of 24, 48, and 72 hours, respectively, by cervical dislocation (colchicine was given at a dose of 4 mg/kg of the b.wt. at 2 hours prior to sacrificing the animals to arrest cycling cells in metaphase). Cytogenetic analysis was performed as per the protocol of Preston et al. [35]. Briefly, the bone marrow was flushed out from both femurs using Hanks buffered salt solution (pH 7.2). The cells were centrifuged at 1000 rpm for 5 minutes and the pellet was redispersed in a hypotonic solution of 0.56% (w/v) KCl for 30 minutes at 37°C to permit osmotic swelling of cells. Swollen cells were fixed in ice-cold Carnoy's fluid, dropped onto slides, and stained with phosphate-buffered 5% Giemsa solution. A total of 75 well spread metaphase plates per animal in each group was analyzed for chromosomal aberrations at a magnification of 100x and the mitotic index (MI) was calculated from a scan of 2000 cells per animal. The chromosomal aberrations were classified as breaks, fragments, and exchanges. The incidence of aberrant cells was expressed as the percentage of damaged cells (aberrant metaphases).

Mitotic Index (MI) %:

$$\frac{\text{Number of dividing cells} \times 100}{\text{Total number of bone marrow cells counted}}, \quad (1)$$

Incidence of aberrant cells (%):

$$\frac{\text{Total number of aberrant metaphases} \times 100}{\text{Total number of metaphases counted}}. \quad (2)$$

Micronuclei Induction Assay

The rest of 5 animals from each group of set 2 were sacrificed after 24, 48, and 72 hours of treatment and the frequency of micronucleated polychromatic erythrocytes (MNPCEs) was evaluated using a modified protocol of Schmid [36]. The bone marrow was flushed from both femurs using Hanks' buffered salt solution, 1% (w/v) bovine serum albumin, and 0.15% (w/v) EDTA (pH 7.2). Evenly spread bone marrow smears were stained by using the May-Grunwald and Giemsa protocol. A minimum of 2000 erythrocytes was scored for each treated and control group. The stained slides were scored for number of MNPCE's/1000 PCE's.

Statistical Analysis

The data was analyzed for mean values and standard error (mean ± SE) for all groups. Statistical comparisons were made using Students t-test, and P < .05 was considered significant.

RESULTS

In the results of chromosomal aberration assay, the percent incidence of aberrant cells in positive control B(a)P treated groups were found to be 12.76, 14.35, and 15.22 in 24, 48, and 72 hours of sampling time, respectively, in comparison to 1.88, 1.92, and 1.75 of untreated group I (Table 1, Figure 2). The frequency of percentage aberrant cells was also found to be significantly (P < .05) increased in glyphosate treated groups in dose- and time-dependent manner. The frequency of percent aberrant cells in glyphosate (25 mg/kg b.wt.) treated group III was found increased to 5.86, 7.24, and 7.76 in 24, 48, and 72 hours of sampling time, respectively, while in group IV (50 mg/kg b.wt.) it was 7.46, 8.85, and 9.24, respectively (Table 1, Figure 2).

Table 1: Effect of glyphosate treatment on induction of chromosomal aberration in swiss albino mice.

		Groups	Untreated	B(a)P (100 mg/kg b.wt)	Glyphosate (25 mg/kg b.wt)	Glyphosate (50 mg/kg b.wt)
Number of aberrant cells (%) after	24 hours of treatment	Breaks	0.36 ± 0.1	5.65 ± 0.4	2.86 ± 0.2	3.79 ± 0.16
		Fragments	0.17 ± 0.01	1.59 ± 0.03	0.39 ± 0.1	1.94 ± 0.02
		Exchange	0.26 ± 0.02	0.69 ± 0.2	0.47 ± 0.3	0.41 ± 0.01
		Multiple damage	1.02 ± 0.07	4.83 ± 0.3	2.14 ± 0.4	1.32 ± 0.07
		Total no. of aberrant cells	1.81 ± 0.03	12.76 ± 0.17*	5.86 ± 0.12*	7.46 ± 0.14*
	48 hours of treatment	Breaks	0.33 ± 0.2	6.84 ± 0.5	3.37 ± 0.05	4.51 ± 0.07
		Fragments	0.19 ± 0.01	2.63 ± 0.7	0.46 ± 0.03	0.89 ± 0.01
		Exchange	0.23 ± 0.1	0.83 ± 0.03	0.59 ± 0.01	0.54 ± 0.02
		Multiple damage	1.17 ± 0.04	4.05 ± 0.04	2.82 ± 0.06	2.91 ± 0.16
		Total no. of aberrant cells	1.92 ± 0.03	14.35 ± 1.27*	7.24 ± 0.15*	8.85 ± 0.14*
	72 hours of treatment	Breaks	0.34 ± 0.02	6.91 ± 0.10	4.42 ± 0.07	4.49 ± 0.13
		Fragments	0.15 ± 0.01	2.93 ± 0.04	0.53 ± 0.02	0.82 ± 0.02
		Exchange	0.19 ± 0.01	1.65 ± 0.06	0.47 ± 0.03	0.63 ± 0.02
		Multiple damage	1.12 ± 0.04	3.73 ± 0.1	2.34 ± 0.09	3.30 ± 0.15
		Total no. of aberrant cells	1.80 ± .05	15.22* ± 1.19	7.76 ± 0.4*	9.24 ± 0.18*

Mean ± SE of animals $n = 5$.
*$P < .05$.

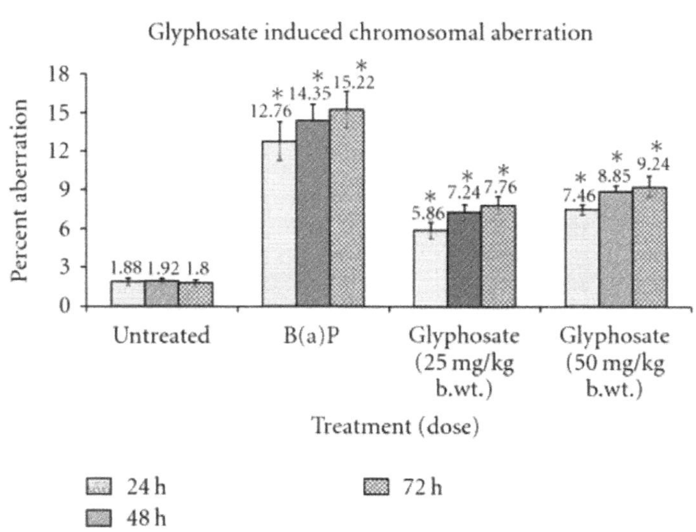

Figure 2: Mutagenic activity of glyphosate in Swiss albino mice showing incidence of aberrant cells at sampling time of 24, 48, and 72 hours. Values are expressed as mean ± SE of 5 animals. *Represent significant increase over untreated control group at their respective sampling time. Data are significant as P < .05.

Significant decrease in MI after B(a)P treatment was noticed and evaluated as percentage of dividing cells which was found to be 2.46, 2.12, and 1.94 in group II in comparison to 4.88, 4.90, and 4.84 of untreated control group I (Table 2, Figure 2). A significant ($P < .05$) decrease in MI was also observed in glyphosate treated groups III and IV in comparison to untreated controls (group I). Low-dose (25 mg/kg b.wt) glyphosate resulted in significant decrease in MI by 4.12, 3.84, and 3.75 in 24, 48, and 72 hours of treatment while high dose (50 mg/kg b.wt.) resulted in 3.54, 3.16, and 3.06, respectively (Table 2, Figure 3).

Table 2: Effects of glyphosate treatment on mitotic index and micronuclei induction in swiss albino mice.

Groups (treatment)	Mitotic index (MI) after treatment			Micronuclei induction (MNPCEs/1000PCEs) after treatment		
	24 hours	48 hours	72 hours	24 hours	48 hours	72 hours
Group I (untreated)	4.88 ± 0.06	4.90 ± 0.02	4.84 ± 0.04	1.24 ± 0.01	1.10 ± 0.01	1.18 ± 0.03
Group II B(a)P (100 mg/kg b.wt)	2.46 ± 0.09[#]	2.12 ± 0.01[#]	1.94 ± 0.02[#]	15.46 ± 0.03[*]	17.50 ± 0.10[*]	18.25 ± 0.12[*]
Group III (glyphosate dose 25 mg/kg b.wt)	4.12 ± .05[#]	3.84 ± 0.04[#]	3.75 ± 0.03[#]	3.87 ± 0.02[*]	5.76 ± 0.08[*]	6.12 ± 0.07[*]
Group IV (glyphosate dose 50 mg/kg b.wt)	3.54 ± 0.01[#]	3.16 ± 0.03[#]	3.06 ± 0.01[#]	6.86 ± 0.04[*]	8.25 ± 0.04[*]	8.48 ± 0.09[*]

Data shows mean ± SE of 5 animals in each group.
[#] $P < .05$ represents significant decrease as compared to untreated control.
[*] $P < .05$ represents significant increase as compared to untreated control.
MNPCEs: Micronucleated polychromatic erythrocytes;
PCEs: Polychromatic erythrocytes.

Figure 3: Cytotoxic effects glyphosate in Swiss albino mice indicated by decrease in mitotic index (MI) at 24, 48, and 72 hours of sampling time. Values are expressed as mean ± SE of 5 animals. *Represent significant decrease over untreated control group at their respective sampling time. Data are significant as $P < .05$.

The frequency of MNPCEs/1000PCEs in the present study was 15.46, 17.50, and 18.25 in 24, 48, and 72 hours of B(a)P treatment (group II) and which was 1.24, 1.10, and 1.18 in control group I (Table 2, Figure 3). Glyphosate (25 mg/kg b.wt.) induced micronuclei induction in group III was 3.87, 5.76, and 6.12 whereas in group IV (50 mg/kg b.wt. glyphosate treated animals) it was 6.86, 8.25, and 8.48, in 24, 48, and 72 hours of sampling period, respectively, (Table 2, Figure 4), suggesting the genotoxic potential of glyphosate.

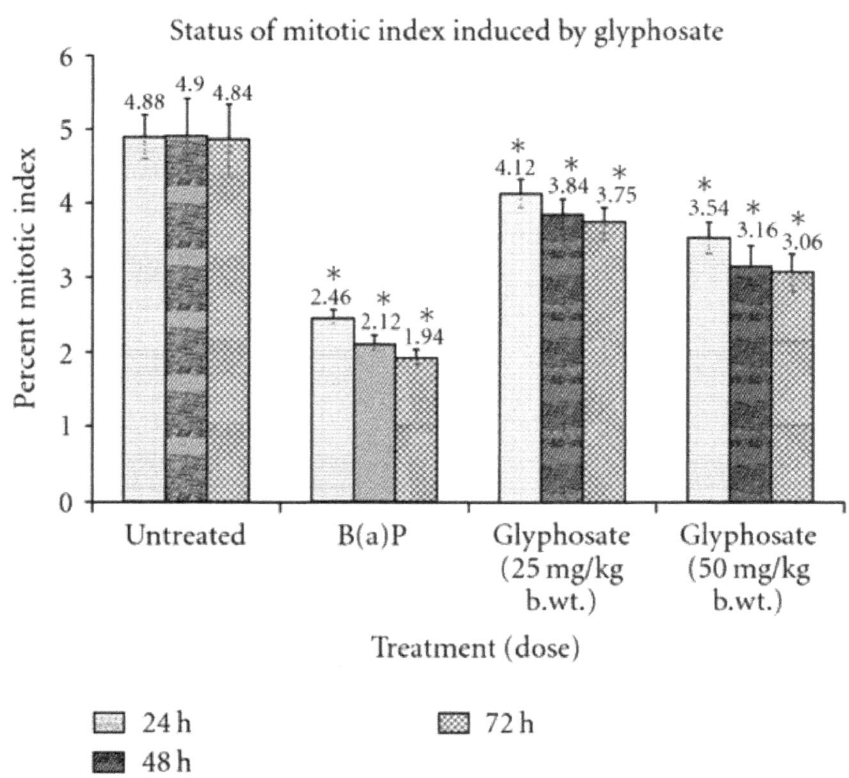

Figure 4: Mutagenic activity of glyphosate in Swiss albino mice showing increased micronuclei (MN) induction at sampling time of 24, 48, and 72 hours. Values are expressed as mean ± SE of five animals. *Represent significant increase over untreated control group at their respective sampling time. Data were significant as $P < .05$. MNPCEs: Micronucleated polychromatic erythrocytes and PCEs: polychromatic erythrocytes.

DISCUSSION

Results of the present study reveals that single dose of glyphosate caused significant incidence of chromosomal aberration and induction of micronuclei in a dose- and time-dependent manner. Various cytogenetic results on commercial glyphosate are problematic. They may depend on purity of the active agent and on the nature of inert components. Surfactants and other inert compounds were previously suggested to increase the toxicity of the herbicide [37]. In a recent study, Caiman latirostris embryos were exposed at early embryonic stage to different sublethal concentrations of Roundup (range from 50–1750 g/egg), results from both the comet assay and the MN test revealed a concentration dependent effect [4].

Glyphosate reported for positive clastogenic and genotoxic effects in vitro [22, 27] which are consistent with our results (Tables 1 and 2). Chromosomal damage is considered to detect early effects of xenobiotic insult and evaluation of the frequency of CAs is a sensitive cytogenetic assay for detecting exposure to mutagens and carcinogens [15]. In the present study, glyphosate induced CAs could be attributed to early changes either an increase in induced DNA lesions or interference with their repair (Table 1, Figure 1). Glyphosate has been reported to cause DNA damage in erythrocytes of bullfrog tadpoles (R. catesbeiana) [29]. However, few studies reported that glyphosate is weak or nonclastogenic in vivo [18, 28, 38].

The MN induction assay was used as an additional sensitive biological indicator of the damage to somatic cell genome of subjects exposed to pesticide mixtures occupationally. It is known that the appearance of MN is related to the loss of chromosome fragments due to chromosome breaks [39]. Our results revealed that there was elevation in the number of micronuclei in the glyphosate exposed animals. Because MN could be the consequence of the mitotic spindle malfunction, it is possible that the glyphosate could also express an aneugenic mode of action as inhibiting cell division and mitotic spindle apparatus.

The molecular mechanisms responsible for the genotoxicity of glyphosate are not yet known clearly. However, the CAs and the micronucleus formation observed in animals clearly indicate that these compounds interact with chromatin DNA and induce damage there. Such interactions/DNA damage may be caused by an increased incidence of alkali labile sites in DNA as observed in kidney and liver with glyphosate treatment in CD-1 mice [23]. Alkali labile sites are generally produced at abasic sites in DNA and may be revealed under conditions that denature DNA secondary structure. Peluso et al. [23] also reported a dramatic increase in the number of oxidized guanine, 8-hydroxylguanine (8-OHdG), residues in DNA of liver cells from mice treated with glyphosate which also may be the reason of chromosomal damage in bone marrow cells of mice as observed in our study. It has also been shown in our study that CAs and MN induction increases in time as well as dose-dependent manner. It could be due to the glyphosate induced toxicity which produces reduced repair of spontaneous 8-OHdG and lead to an accumulation of oxidation products [23].

The sensitivities of two cytogenetic tests, chromosome analysis and the micronucleus test, were compared by using mice exposed to the substances glyphosate and B(a)P (Tables 1 and 2). Both test systems proved equally sensitive for genotoxicity assessment. Glyphosate at the tested doses significantly increased both the CAs rates and the MN induction in comparison to control. Thus, our results indicate that glyphosate is able to induce CAs and MN accompanied by inhibition of cell proliferation in Swiss albino mice following i.p. administration. In view of the earlier reports on mutagenic activity of glyphosate in laboratory experiments and from the present study, further studies are needed to assess the possible health hazard from glyphosate.

ACKNOWLEDGMENTS

Authors express their gratitude toward Dr. Ashwani Kumar, the Director of Indian Institute of Toxicology Research (Council of Scientific & Industrial Research, India), Lucknow for his keen interest and support during the course of the study. Authors are also thankful to Council for Scientific & Industrial Research, New Delhi for funding this work under network Project NWP-17.

REFERENCES

1. H. M. G. van der Werf, "Assessing the impact of pesticides on the environment," Agriculture, Ecosystems and Environment, vol. 60, no. 2-3, pp. 81–96, 1996.
2. D. G. Crosby, "Pesticides as environmental mutagens," in Genetic Toxicology: An Agricultural Perspective, R. A. Fleck and A. Hollander, Eds., pp. 201–218, Plenum Press, New York, NY, USA, 1982.
3. M. F. Simoniello, E. C. Kleinsorge, J. A. Scagnetti, R. A. Grigolato, G. L. Poletta, and M. A. Carballo, "DNA damage in workers occupationally exposed to pesticide mixtures," Journal of Applied Toxicology, vol. 28, no. 8, pp. 957–965, 2008. ·
4. G. L. Poletta, A. Larriera, E. Kleinsorge, and M. D. Mudry, "Genotoxicity of the herbicide formulationRoundup® (glyphosate) in broad-snouted caiman (Caiman latirostris) evidenced by the Comet assay and the Micronucleus test," Mutation Research, vol. 672, no. 2, pp. 95–102, 2009. ·
5. F. Lander, L. E. Knudsen, M. O. Gamborg, H. Jarventaus, and H. Norppa, "Chromosome aberrations in pesticide-exposed greenhouse workers," Scandinavian Journal of Work, Environment and Health, vol. 26, no. 5, pp. 436–442, 2000.
6. R. Meinert, J. Schüz, U. Kaletsch, P. Kaatsch, and J. Michaelis, "Leukemia and non-Hodgkin›s lymphoma in childhood and exposure to pesticides: results of a register-based case-control study in Germany,"American Journal of Epidemiology, vol. 151, no. 7, pp. 639–646, 2000.
7. B.-T. Ji, D. T. Silverman, P. A. Stewart, et al., "Occupational exposure to pesticides and pancreatic cancer,"American Journal of Industrial Medicine, vol. 39, no. 1, pp. 92–99, 2001. ·
8. S. Zhao, A. Narang, J. Gierthy, and G. Eadon, "Detection and characterization of DNA adducts formed from metabolites of the fungicide ortho-phenylphenol," Journal of Agricultural and Food Chemistry, vol. 50, no. 11, pp. 3351–3358, 2002. ·

9. Blair and S. H. Zahm, "Agricultural exposures and cancer," Environmental Health Perspectives, vol. 103, supplement 8, pp. 205–208, 1995. ·

10. L. R. Webster, G. H. McKenzie, and H. T. Moriarty, "Organophosphate-based pesticides and genetic damage implicated in bladder cancer," Cancer Genetics and Cytogenetics, vol. 133, no. 2, pp. 112–117, 2002. ·

11. T. Clary and B. Ritz, "Pancreatic cancer mortality and organochlorine pesticide exposure in California, 1989–1996," American Journal of Industrial Medicine, vol. 43, no. 3, pp. 306–313, 2003. ·

12. M. Moriya, T. Ohta, K. Watanabe, T. Miyazawa, K. Kato, and Y. Shirasu, "Further mutagenicity studies on pesticides in bacterial reversion assay systems," Mutation Research, vol. 116, no. 3-4, pp. 185–216, 1983. ·

13. D. Yüzbaşioğlu, "Cytogenetic effects of fungicide afugan on the meristematic cells of Allium cepa L.,"Cytologia, vol. 68, no. 3, pp. 237–243, 2003. ·

14. M. Çelik, F. Ünal, D. Yüzbaşioğlu, M. A. Ergün, O. Arslan, and R. Kasap, "In vitro effect of karathane LC (dinocap) on human lymphocytes," Mutagenesis, vol. 20, no. 2, pp. 101–104, 2005. ·

15. S. Bonassi, A. Abbondandolo, L. Camurri, et al., "Are chromosome aberrations in circulating lymphocytes predictive of future cancer onset in humans? Preliminary results of an Italian cohort study,"Cancer Genetics and Cytogenetics, vol. 79, no. 2, pp. 133–135, 1995. ·

16. L. Hagmar, S. Bonassi, U. Strömberg, et al., "Chromosomal aberrations in lymphocytes predict human cancer: a report from the European study group on cytogenetic biomarkers and health (ESCH)," Cancer Research, vol. 58, no. 18, pp. 4117–4121, 1998.

17. M. Fenech, "The in vitro micronucleus technique," Mutation Research, vol. 455, no. 1-2, pp. 81–95, 2000. ·

18. B. D. Dimitrov, P. G. Gadeva, D. K. Benova, and M. V. Bineva, "Comparative genotoxicity of the herbicides Roundup, Stomp and Reglone in plant and mammalian test systems," Mutagenesis, vol. 21, no. 6, pp. 375–382, 2006. ·

19. G. M. Williams, R. Kroes, and I. C. Munro, "Safety evaluation and risk assessment of the herbicide Roundup and its active ingredient, glyphosate, for humans," Regulatory Toxicology and Pharmacology, vol. 31, no. 2, pp. 117–165, 2000. ·

20. G. A. Bresnahan, F. A. Manthey, K. A. Howatt, and M. Chakraborty, "Glyphosate applied preharvest induces shikimic acid accumulation in hard red spring wheat (Triticum aestivum)," Journal of Agricultural and Food Chemistry, vol. 51, no. 14, pp. 4004–4007, 2003. ·

21. D. J. Wilson, S. Patton, G. Florova, V. Hale, and K. A. Reynolds, "The shikimic acid pathway and polyketide biosynthesis," Journal of Industrial Microbiology and Biotechnology, vol. 20, no. 5, pp. 299–303, 1998. ·

22. M. B. Lioi, M. R. Scarfi, A. Santoro, et al., "Cytogenetic damage and induction of pro-oxidant state in human lymphocytes exposed in vitro to gliphosate, vinclozolin, atrazine, and DPX-E9636,"Environmental and Molecular Mutagenesis, vol. 32, no. 1, pp. 39–46, 1998. ·

23. M. Peluso, A. Munnia, C. Bolognesi, and S. Parodi, "P32-Postlabeling detection of DNA adducts in mice treated with the herbicide Roundup," Environmental and Molecular Mutagenesis, vol. 31, no. 1, pp. 55–59, 1998. ·

24. L. P. Walsh, C. McCormick, C. Martin, and D. M. Stocco, "Roundup inhibits steroidogenesis by disrupting steroidogenic acute regulatory (StAR) protein expression," Environmental Health Perspectives, vol. 108, no. 8, pp. 769–776, 2000. ·

25. J. Daruich, F. Zirulnik, and M. S. Gimenez, "Effect of the herbicide glyphosate on enzymatic activity in pregnant rats and their fetuses," Environmental Research, vol. 85, no. 3, pp. 226–231, 2001. ·

26. E. Hietanen, K. Linnainmaa, and H. Vainio, "Effects of phenoxyherbicides and glyphosate on the hepatic and intestinal biotransformation activities in the rat," Acta Pharmacologica et Toxicologica, vol. 53, no. 2, pp. 103–112, 1983.

27. P. Li and T. J. Long, "An evaluation of the genotoxic potential of glyphosate," Fundamental and Applied Toxicology, vol. 10, no. 3, pp. 537–546, 1988. ·

28. J. Rank, A.-G. Jensen, B. Skov, L. H. Pedersen, and K. Jensen, "Genotoxicity testing of the herbicide Roundup and its active ingredient glyphosate isopropylamine using the mouse bone marrow micronucleus test, Salmonella mutagenicity test, and Allium anaphase-telophase test," Mutation Research, vol. 300, no. 1, pp. 29–36, 1993.

29. C. Clements, S. Ralph, and M. Petras, "Genotoxicity of select herbicides in Rana catesbeiana tadpoles using the alkaline single-cell gel DNA electrophoresis (Comet) assay," Environmental and Molecular Mutagenesis, vol. 29, no. 3, pp. 277–288, 1997. ·

30. P. G. Kale, B. T. Petty Jr., S. Walker, et al., "Mutagenicity testing of nine herbicides and pesticides currently used in agriculture," Environmental and Molecular Mutagenesis, vol. 25, no. 2, pp. 148–153, 1995. ·

31. U.S. EPA, "U.S. Environmental Protection Agency Reregistration Eligibility Decision (RED) Glyphosate,"EPA-738-R-93-014, U.S. Environmental Protection Agency, Washington, DC, USA, 1993.

32. WHO, "International programme on chemical safety. Glyphosate," Environmental Health Criteria 159, World Health Organization, Geneva, Switzerland, 1994.

33. B. Kaya, A. Yanikoğlu, A. Creus, and R. Marcos, "Genotoxicity testing of five herbicides in the Drosophila wing spot test," Mutation Research, vol. 465, no. 1-2, pp. 77–84, 2000. ·

34. C. M. Monroy, A. C. Cortés, D. M. Sicard, and H. G. de Restrepo, "Cytotoxicity and enotoxicity of human cells exposed in vitro to glyphosate," Biomédica, vol. 25, no. 3, pp. 335–345, 2005.

35. R. J. Preston, B. J. Dean, S. Galloway, H. Holden, A. F. McFee, and M. Shelby, "Mammalian in vivo cytogenetic assays. Analysis of chromosome aberrations in bone marrow cells," Mutation Research, vol. 189, no. 2, pp. 157–165, 1987.

36. W. Schmid, "The micronucleus test," Mutation Research, vol. 31, no. 1, pp. 9–15, 1975.

37. C. Cox, "Glyphosate (Roundup)," in Global Pesticide Campaigner, E. Hickey, Ed., vol. 9, pp. 12–19, Pesticide Action Network (PAN): North America, San Francisco, Calif, USA, 1999.

38. K. Šiviková and J. Dianovský, "Cytogenetic effect of technical glyphosate on cultivated bovine peripheral lymphocytes," International Journal of Hygiene and Environmental Health, vol. 209, no. 1, pp. 15–20, 2006.

39. J. A. Heddle, M. C. Cimino, M. Hayashi, et al., "Micronuclei as an index of cytogenetic damage: past, present, and future," Environmental and Molecular Mutagenesis, vol. 18, no. 4, pp. 277–291, 1991.

CHAPTER 15

IMPACT OF PARATHION EXPOSURE ON SOME BIOCHEMICAL PARAMETERS IN RABBIT AS A NON TARGET ORGANISM

Nagat Aly, Kawther El-Gendy

Keywords: Relative organ weight; Non target organisms; Biomarkers; Parathion; Rabbits; Liver

INTRODUCTION

Pesticides have played a vital role in controlling agricultural, industrial, home and public health pest worldwide.[1] However, their use poses animal and human health concerns because of their toxicity, widespread use and release into the environment.[2] According to the World Health Organization, 3 million cases of pesticide poisoning occur every year, resulting in more than 250,000 deaths.[3] Despite this alarming figure, there is currently no global system to track and stem poisoning or diseases associated with pesticide use.[4]Real world exposure to pesticides normally occurs through lower level single or repeated exposures (for example, as residues in food products). The organophosphorus pesticides (OPs) are a group of highly toxic compounds and they are readily available commercially for domestic, agricultural, and industrial purposes.[5] They account for over 50% of all insecticides applied world-wide.[3] Parathion (*O*, *O*-diethyl-*O*-(4-nitrophenyl) phosphorothioate) is one of the most acutely toxic pesticides registered by the EPA 1986. Because of its highly toxic nature, parathion is classified as a Restricted Use Pesticide (RUP). [6] It is a well-known AChE inhibitor just like other OPs which leads to the accumulation of acetylcholine and results in excessive stimulation of postsynaptic receptors and consequent signs of toxicity. [7 and 8]

The general physiology of rabbits is similar to humans; therefore, the rabbit has been used as a model for human diseases. The rabbit is large enough to provide adequate quantities of tissue for experimental work without pooling of samples but is small enough to be economical for most studies. However, rabbits do have many advantages and serve to bridge the gap between these small animal models, which are perhaps best suited for discovery phases of research, and larger animal models are often required for preclinical, translational research.[9] Changes in body weight have been used as an indicator of adverse effects of drugs and chemicals. Also, organ weight changes have long been accepted as a sensitive indicator of chemically induced changes to organs and in toxicological experiments.[10]

A biomarker may be any measurable biochemical, cellular, physiological or behavioral change in an organism or population that indicates exposure to chemical pollutants.[11] By focusing on the intermediate, sublethal effects of a pollutant, this developing field aims to reveal environmental threats before obvious toxic effects such as death of organisms are observed. An ideal biomarker will also be nondestructive to

Citation: Nagat Aly, Kawther El-Gendy, Impact of parathion exposure on some biochemical parameters in rabbit as a non-target organism, Alexandria Journal of Medicine, Volume 51, Issue 1, March 2015, Pages 11-17, ISSN 2090-5068, http://dx.doi.org/10.1016/j.ajme.2014.07.004.

the indicator organism. Biomarkers and rabbits have been employed as useful tools for risk assessment of chemical compounds that are exposed in the environment.[12]

The aim of the present work was to evaluate the distribution pattern of ChE, ATPase, CE, GST, ACP, ALP, AST, and ALT in different organs of male rabbits. Besides the effect of repeated sublethal doses of parathion on some biological and biochemical parameters, consequently these parameters can be used as potential biomarkers of damage caused by parathion exposure.

MATERIALS AND METHODS

Animals

Male New Zealand white rabbits (six months old, 3–4 kg weight), were purchased from the Abbis Farm, Faculty of Agriculture; Alexandria University. Animals were individually housed in stainless steel cages at 22–26 °C temperature, 40–70% humidity and controlled environment with a 12 h light/dark cycle. Food and water were given *ad libitum*. The animals were accommodated to laboratory conditions for two weeks before being experimented. All maintenance and care were in accordance with the animal welfare guidelines established at the university.

Chemicals

Technical material (99.6%) parathion was obtained from EPA, Research Triangle Park, N.C. All other chemicals used were of the highest purity grade available from Sigma and Merck Chemical Companies.

Experimental Design

The rabbits were divided into two groups (5 animals per each). Animals in the first group were daily given corn oil (1 ml/kg bw) for two weeks and used as control. Rabbits in the second group orally received parathion (0.2 mg/kg/day). Animals were examined during the 6 weeks of study period (2 weeks of treatment + another 4 weeks without treatment). The body weights of control and treated animals were recorded weekly. At the end of the experiment the animals were sacrificed and dissected, then the brain, liver, kidney and heart were removed, rinsed in saline solution (0.9% NaCl), dried on filter paper and weighted individually in all rabbits and the relative organ weight was calculated (organ weight: body weight).

Biochemical Analysis

Each organ was minced and homogenized separately in ice cold saline solution (10% w/v) in a polytron homogenizer (Tekmar tissumizer). The homogenate was centrifuged at 10,000×*g* for 30 min at 4 °C using a cooling centrifuge. The resultant supernatant was used for different enzymes' assay.

ChE activity was measured spectrophotometrically according to Ellman et al.,[13] using acetyl thiocholine iodide as a substrate. ATPase activity was measured by the colorimetric method of Koch.[14] CE activity was assayed using *p*-nitrophenyl butyrate as substrate according to Verschoyle et al. [15] GST activity was assayed using 1-chloro-2,4-dinitrobenzene as substrate by the method of Vessey and Boyer.[16] The assay was conducted by monitoring the appearance of the conjugated complex CDNB and GSH at 340 nm. Data were expressed as u mole/mg protein/minute. The activities of ACP and ALP were determined according to Bessey et al.[17] with sodium *p*-nitrophenyl phosphate as a substrate in the acid and alkaline medium, respectively. AST and ALT activities were measured by the procedure of Reitman and Frrankel [18] using a commercially available kit from Bio-Merieux. The total protein content was determined by the method of Lowry et al.[19] using bovine serum albumin as the standard.

Statistical Analysis

All data were expressed as mean ± standard error (SE). Data were analyzed using one-way analysis of variance (ANOVA) followed by the Student–Newman–Keuls test to determine significance between different groups. The criterion for statistical significance was set at $p < 0.05$.

RESULTS

Body Weight and Relative Organ Weight

The physiological status of control and treated animals was noticed as the change in the body weight gain and relative organ weights. Male rabbits orally administrated with parathion in a dose of 0.2 mg/kg/day for 2 weeks have shown that no mortality occurred during the experimental period. It is clear that the body weight of the control group was gradually increased during the 6 weeks by 106.45, 108.65, 113.09, 116.65, 121.99, and 125.34% after 1, 2, 3, 4, 5 and 6 week, respectively. On the other hand the body weight of treated animals was gradually decreased until the fourth week and then it was increased (Fig. 1). From this result it is noticed that there is a significant difference ($p < 0.05$) of mean body weight gains between control and treated animals. No significant change in the relative weights of all organs except the liver in treated animals when compared with control was observed (Table 1). The percentage relative weights of the liver in control and treated animals were 3.52 ± 0.3 and 4.53 ± 0.31, respectively.

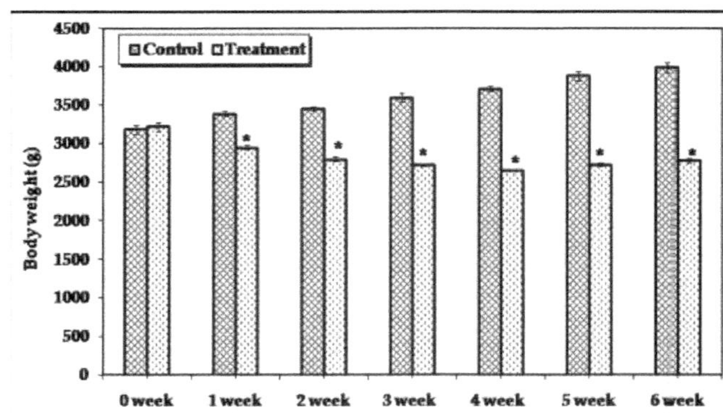

Figure 1: Body weight pattern of rabbits orally administrated to 0.2 mg/kg/day of parathion for two weeks.*Significantly different from the control value at $p < 0.05$.

Table 1: Relative organ weights of rabbits after four weeks of last treatment with parathion.

Organs	Relative organ weight (%)		% Change [a]
	Control	Treatment (0.2 mg/kg/day)	
Brain	0.33 ± 0.02	0.32 ± 0.01	3.03
Liver	3.52 ± 0.3	4.53 ± 0.31*	−27.61
Kidney	0.65 ± 0.06	0.69 ± 0.052	6.153
Heart	0.25 ± 0.03	0.27 ± 0.04	8.0

Data are presented as means of five replicates ± SE.

*Significantly different from control at $p < 0.05$.

[a] Percentage of increase (−) or decrease in treatment weights compared to control.

Biochemical Studies

The distribution pattern of the enzyme activities; ChE, ATPase, CE, GST, ACP, ALP, AST and ALT in the different organs of rabbits was carried out.

ChE activity: The results of this survey detected that the brain contained extremely high activity of ChE, followed by the liver (87.32 and 54.67 u moles acetylthiocholine iodide hydrolyzed/mg protein/min., respectively). Parathion resulted in a significant inhibition of ChE activity in the brain, liver, and kidney by 22.71, 27.02, and 22.42%, respectively (Fig. 2A).

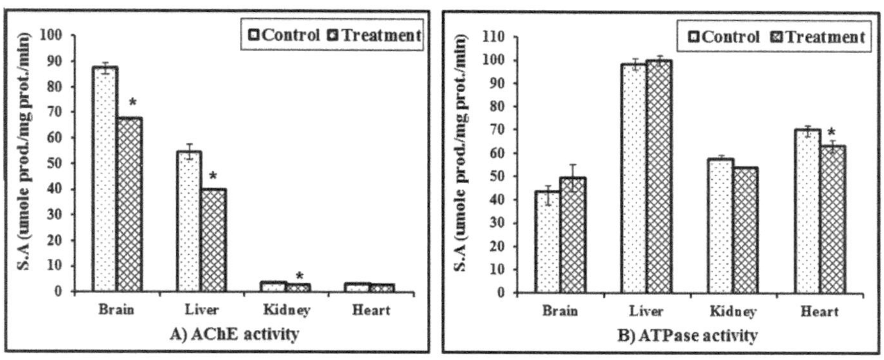

Figure 2: ChE and ATPase activities in different organs of male rabbits treated with 0.2 mg/kg/day for two weeks of parathion after four weeks of last treatment. Values represent the mean ± SE of three replicates from each animal. *Significantly different from the control value at $p < 0.05$.

ATPase activity: The data showed that the liver contained the highest activity of ATPase, which is almost twice as much as the activity in the brain and kidney. It is clear from Fig. 2B that parathion has different effects on ATPase in different organs. Activities oscillating were between activation and inhibition.

CE activity: The CE activities were 27.7 ± 1.3, 18.73 ± 0.75, 13.7 ± 0.9 and 7.2 ± 0.52 m mole/mg protein/min. in the kidney, liver, heart, and brain, respectively (Fig. 3A). The activity in the kidney was about 3.6 times more than that in the brain. CE of treated rabbits in all organs was higher than that of control. The activation power of the tested organs was in the following order: liver > heart > kidney > brain.

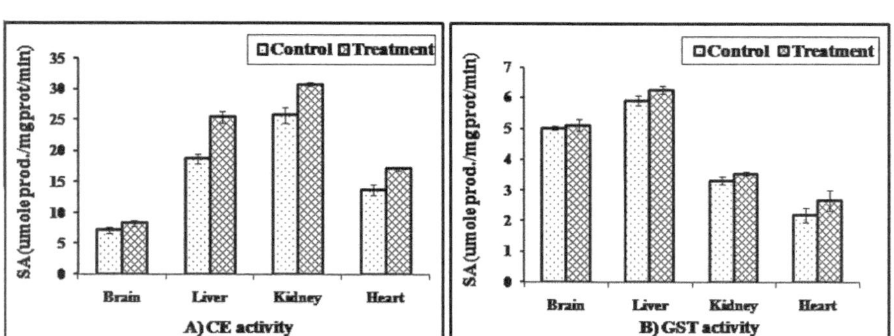

Figure 3: CE and GST activities in different organs of male rabbits treated with 0.2 mg/kg/day for two weeks of parathion after four weeks of last treatment. Values represent the mean ± SE of three replicates from each animal.

GST activity: It was noticed from Fig. 3B that the liver contained the highest GST activity followed by the brain, while the heart contained the least level of enzyme activity. Parathion had slightly stimulatory effects on GST activities in the tested organs.

ACP and ALP activities: Kidney contained the highest activity of ACP and ALP followed by the liver. Parathion reduced ACP activity in the kidney, liver, brain and heart with percentage of control; 29.6, 41.0, 15.1 and 16.6, respectively, while ALP activities in all organs of treated animals were activated except in the heart (Fig. 4A and B).

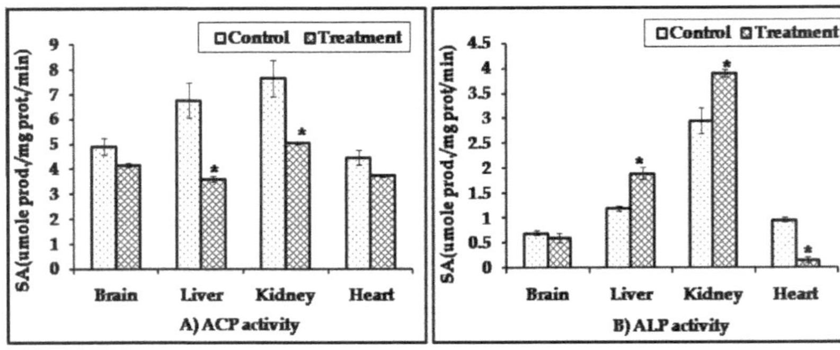

Figure 4: ACP and ALP activities in different organs of male rabbits treated with 0.2 mg/kg/day for two weeks of parathion after four weeks of last treatment. Values represent the mean ± SE of three replicates from each animal. *Significantly different from the control value at $p < 0.05$.

AST and ALT activities: The activity of AST and ALT in the brain was the highest one, while the kidney contained the least activity. AST and ALT levels in all organs were markedly elevated in the treated animals when compared with the control group except in the brain (Fig. 5A and B).

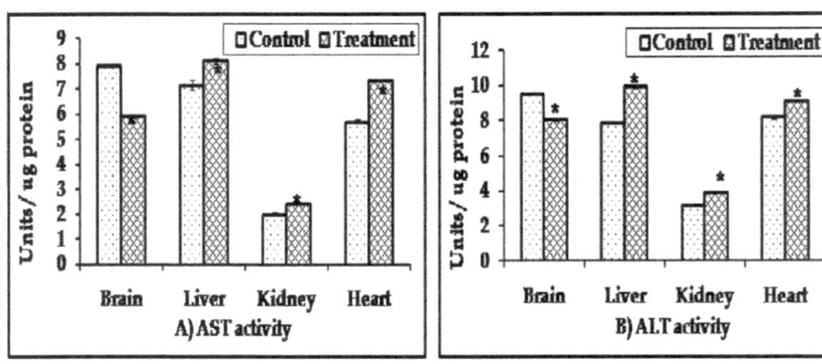

Figure 5: AST and ALT activities in different organs of male rabbits treated with 0.2 mg/kg/day for two weeks of parathion after four weeks of last treatment. Values represent the mean ± SE of three replicates from each animal. *Significantly different from the control value at $p < 0.05$.

DISCUSSION

Pesticides are widely used in order to enhance the food protection by controlling the unwanted insects and disease vectors in agriculture. It is known that the OPs among other pesticides are the most toxic pesticides to the vertebrates. OPs toxicity is an important problem in many countries of the world due to easy accessibility, extensive and unconscious use.[5]

Body Weight and Relative Organ Weight

In toxicological studies body and organ weights are important criteria for the evaluation of toxicity. In the present study, the body weight of parathion treaded rabbits was significantly ($p < 0.05$) lower than that of the control group. This may be attributed to a decreased food intake (anorexia or food avoidance), poor food palatability or increased degradation of lipids and protein due to treatment-related toxicity.[20] Also, weight loss observed in the parathion treatment group may be a result of the combination of oxidative stress and adrenal-mediated stress caused by the inhibition of cholesterol ester hydrolase. Parathion is known to show its toxic effects by inhibiting cholinesterase activity which could be due to the less food consumption and/or fluid and electrolyte loss. Our data are in consonance with those obtained by Ambali et al.[21] and Al-Othman et al.[22]Results showed that there is a significant increase in the relative liver weight in rabbits exposed to parathion compared with control rabbits (Table 1). The increase in relative liver weight in rabbits exposed to parathion seems to be due to toxic potential of pesticide, and it is in agreement with Al-Sarat et al.[23] in rabbits, Institoris et al.[24] in rats.

Biochemical Studies

The classical target of organophosphorus compounds is cholinesterase, which is one of the hydrolytic enzymes for acetylcholine. The inhibition of cholinesterase action is leading to cholinergic hyperactivity resulting in the death of the animal.7 [and] 8 In our study it was found that the brain contained extremely high enzyme activity followed by the liver. Administration of sublethal dose of parathion (0.2 mg/kg/day) for successive two weeks into rabbits elicited highly significant inhibition of ChE in all tested organs. It is well known that there is a good relationship between exposure to OPs and inhibition of ChE activity. Therefore, the level of ChE activity has been considered a good biomarker exposure to this pesticide.[25]

ATPase CE, GST, phosphatases, and transaminases are important indices in the biological processes. They are responsible for detoxification processes, metabolism, and biosynthesis of energetic macromolecules for different essential functions. Any interference with these activities out of the normal range should lead to biochemical impairment and lesions of tissues and cellular function.[26] ATPase plays an important role in the maintenance of cell permeability and energy transformation in the biological system. ATPase activity can be taken as a meaningful index of cellular activity and forms a useful toxicological tool and is considered to be sensitive indicator of toxicity.[27] Data showed that the activity of the liver and brain ATPase was slightly stimulated in rabbit treated with parathion. On the contrary, heart ATPase was significantly inhibited in treated animals than in the control group. It is well known that ATPase is essential for the regulation of ionic content and membrane excitability of myocardial cells, impairment of its function would lead to the coronary artery vasospasm, arrhythmias, ischemic damage, and cardiac failure. This contention is in concert with some findings that certain cardiovascular diseases, such as cardiomyopathy, and hypertension, associate with decreased ATPase activity.[28] On the other hand, Sushma and Rao[27] found that aluminum acetate decreased the total ATPase activity in the brain, liver, kidney, heart, muscle and testis of albino mice. From the results of this study, it is quite clear that ATPase sensitivity toward parathion differs depending on the type of the tissues.[29]

CE is found in almost all organisms, it has been proposed as a possible biomarker for OP and carbamate exposure, but it has not been studied to the extent that AChE has.[30] In this study, it was found that the kidney contained the highest activity of CE followed by the liver. CE level in treated rabbits has been slightly stimulated by parathion. These data are in agreement with the results of El-Gendy et al.[31] who found that hepatic CE was slightly increased in alachlor and butachlor treated mice.

It was noticed that the liver contained the highest activity of GST, while the heart contained the least enzyme (Fig. 3B). We also observed that parathion possesses slightly stimulatory effects on GST in all tested organs. This induction may be due to glutathione and glutathione dependent enzyme systems that provide major protection against the toxic agent.[32] GST is thought to play a physiological role in the detoxification and elimination of toxic and undesirable foreign compounds. This enzyme catalyzes the conjugation of a variety of electrophilic substrates to the thiol group of GSH, producing less toxic forms.[33] Increased GST activity in tissues may indicate the development of a defensive mechanism to counteract the effects of parathion and may reflect the possibility of a more efficient protection against pesticide toxicity.

Regarding ACP and ALP activities in different organs of rabbit, it is clear that the kidney contained the highest activity of ACP and ALP followed by the liver. Treatment with parathion significantly decreased ACP activity, while increased ALP in both the kidney and liver as compared to controls. Also, Igwenyi et al. 2014 reported a significant increase in alkaline phosphatase activity, in serum and liver of experimental animals treated with baygon.[34] ACP is known to be localized in lysosomes and surrounded by a lipoprotein membrane. The decrease in ACP may be related either to leakage of the enzyme into extracellular compartments or to tissue damage.[21] ACP was used as a marker for lysosomal functions in liver cells in order to estimate the interference with catabolic and autophagic processes in the liver. Also, the change in the ACP activity may be related to the biotransformation and elimination of the tested pesticide.[35] The significant elevation in the activity of ALP indicated damage to any or all of the organs producing this enzyme such as the liver and kidney is due to leakage of lysosomal enzymes into the cytoplasm and renal necrosis and pyknotic nuclei. This result is paralleled by the result of Ambali et al.[21] Rahman et al.[36] suggested that the decrease in the activities of ALP and ACP in different tissues might be due to the increased permeability of plasma membrane or cellular necrosis, showing the stress condition of the treated animals.

It is quite clear that the liver contained the highest activity of AST and ALT followed by the brain and heart, while the kidney contained the least activity. AST and ALT are considered to be the liver markers that are used to study varying cell viability and changes in cell membrane permeability.[37] The levels of these enzymes in treated animals were significantly higher than those in the control group in all organs except the brain. The disruption of transaminases from the normal values denotes biochemical impairment and lesions of tissues and cellular function because they are involved in the detoxification process, metabolism and biosynthesis of energetic macromolecules for different essential functions.[21] The liver plays a crucial role in the detoxification process and faces the threat of maximum exposure to xenobiotics and their metabolic by-products, which lead to liver damage and hepatotoxicity.[22] The susceptibility of liver tissues to the stress resulting from exposure to pesticides is a function of overall cellular balance between the degree of oxidative stress and the antioxidant capacity.[38] In the case of liver injury resulting from hepatotoxicity, cellular contents are released, thereby increasing the level of liver enzymes above the normal threshold. In this context, activity levels of liver enzymes (i.e. CE, GST, ALP, ALT, and AST) are primarily employed as biomarkers of hepatic damage and injury. These results are consistent with previous findings indicating that OP exposure correlates with elevation of the enzymatic activity of CE, GST, ALP, ALT, and AST.[33] Our data demonstrated that repeated sublethal doses of parathion caused a significant alteration in the level of tested enzymes especially in the liver, which is the main vital organ of all biochemical processes in the body.[22]

In conclusion: The present study demonstrated that excessive exposure to parathion caused cytotoxic changes in the hepatic biochemical markers. Hence these biomarkers might be used in addition to ChE activity to monitor the non target organisms' exposure to pesticides to take effective measures to avoid serious adverse health effects.

CONFLICT OF INTEREST

None declared.

REFERENCES

1. Bjørling-Poulsen M, Andersen HR, Grandjean P. Potential developmental neurotoxicity of pesticides used in Europe. Environ Health 2008;7(50):1–23.
2. Calvert GM, Karnik J, Mehler L, Beckman J, Morrissey B, Sievert J, et al. Acute pesticide poisoning among agricultural workers in the United States, 1998–2005. Am J Ind Med 2008;51:883–98.
3. Yang C, Deng J. Intermediate syndrome following organophosphate insecticide poisoning. J Chin Med Assoc 2007;70(11):467–72.
4. Ali SM, Chia SE. Interethnic variability of plasma paraoxonase (PON1) activity towards organophosphates and PON1polymorphisms among Asian population. A short review. Indus Health 2008;46:309–17.
5. Aardema H, Meertens JHJM, Ligtenberg JJM, Peters-Polman JE, Tulleken JE, ijlstra G. Organophosphorus pesticide poisoning: cases and developments. Neth J Med 2008;66(4):149–53.
6. Meister RT, editor. Farm Chemicals Handbook. Willoughby, OH: Meister Publishing Company; 1992.

7. Al-Badrany YMA, Mohammad FK. Effects of acute and repeated oral exposure to the organophosphate insecticide chlorpyrifos on open-field activity in chicks. Toxicol Lett 2007;174(1–3):110–6.

8. Hundekari IA, Suryakar AN, Rathi DB. Acute organophosphorus pesticide poisoning in North Karnataka, India: oxidative damage, haemoglobin level and total leukocyte. Afr Health Sci 2013;13(1):129–36.

9. Bosze Z, Houdebine LM. Application of rabbits in biomedical research: a review. World Rabbit Sci 2006;14:1–14.

10. Mukinda JT, Eagles PF. Acute and sub-chronic oral toxicity profiles of the aqueous extract of polygala fruticosa in female mice and rats. J Ethnopharmacol 2010;128:236–40.

11. Depledge MH. The Rational Basis for the Use of Biomarkers as Ecotoxicological Tools. In: Fossi MC, Leonzio C, editors. Nondestructive Biomarkers in Vertebrates. Boca Raton, Florida: Lewis; 1994. p. 271–95.

12. Yousef IM. Aluminium-induced changes in hemato-biochemical parameters, lipid peroxidation and enzyme activities of male rabbits: protective role of ascorbic acid. Toxicology 2004;199:47–57.

13. Ellman GL, Courtney KD, Andreess V, Featherstone RM. A new and rapid colorimetric determination of acetylcholinesterase activity. Biochem Pharmacol 1961;7:88–95.

14. Koch RB. Chlorinated hydrocarbon insecticides: inhibition of rabbit brain ATPase activities. J Biol Chem 1969;193:265–75.

15. Verschoyle RD, Reiner E, Bailey E, Adrige WN. Dimethyl phosphorothioate, reaction with malathion and effects on malathion toxicity. Arch Toxicol 1982;49:293–301.

16. Vessey DA, Boyer TD. Differential activation and inhibition of different forms of rat liver glutathione-S-transferase by the herbicides 2,4-dichloro phenoxy acetate 2,4-D) and 2,4, trichloro phenoxy acetate (2,4, S-T). Toxicol Appl Pharmacol 1984;73:492–9.

17. Bessy DA, Lowry OH, Brock MI. Determination in serum with Pnitrophenylphosphate. J Biol Chem 1946;164:321–9.

18. Reitman S, Frrankel SA. A colorimetric method for the determination of serum glutamic oxaloacetic and glutamic pyruvictransaminases. Am J Clin Pathol 1957;28:56–63.

19. Lowry OH, Rosebrough NJ, Farr AL, Randall RJ. Protein measurement with the Folin phenol reagent. J Biol Chem 1951;193:265–75.

20. Mansour SA, Mossa ATH. Oxidative damage, biochemical and histopathological alterations in rats exposed to chlorpyrifos and the antioxidant role of zinc. Pest Biochem Physiol 2010;96:14–23.

21. Ambali S, Akanbi D, Igbokwe N, Shittu M, Kawu M, Ayo J. Evaluation of sub-chronic chlorpyrifos poisoning on hematological and serum biochemical changes in mice and protective effect of vitamin C. J Toxicol Sci 2007;32(2):111–20.

22. Al-Othman AM, Al-Othman ZA, El-Desoky GB, Yusuf K, Aboul-Soud MAM. Ameliorative effect of a-tocopherol and selenium on effects of malathion on plasmatic biochemical indices and lesions in the liver of rats. Curr Pharm Anal 2012;8:214–8.

23. Al-Sarat AS, Hafiz AM, Bayoumi AE, Hussein HI, AboBaer Y. Impact of fenitrothion thermal fogging on some biological and parameters in New Zealand rabbits as non-target organisms. Int J Agric Biol 2011;13:435–8.

24. Institoris L, siroki O, Undeger U, Basaran N, Desi I. Immunotoxicological investigation in rats dosed repeatedly with combinations of cypermethrin, As(III), and Hg(II). Toxicology 2002;172:59–67.

25. Remor AP, Totti CC, Moreira DA, Dutra GP, Heuser VD, Boeira JM. Occupational exposure of farm workers to pesticides: biochemical parameters and evaluation of genotoxicity. Environ Int 2009;35:273 8.

26. Latner LA. Aminotransferases. In: Saundres WB, editor. Clinical Biochemistry Seventh. London, Toronto: Comp. Philadelphia; 1978. p. 553–68.

27. Sushma NJ, Rao KJ. Total ATPases activity in different tissues of albino mice exposed to aluminium acetate. Environ Biol 2007;28:483–4.

28. Chen CC, Lin-Shiau SY. ATPase activities in the kidney and heart of alloxan induced diabetic mice. Asia Pac J Pharmacol 1988;3:51–5.

29. Fox DA, Rubinstein SD, Hsu P. Development lead exposure inhibits adult rat retinal, but not kidney, Na, K-ATPase. Toxicol Pharmacol 1991;109:482–93.

30. Yoon KJP, Morton CL, Potter PM, Danks MK, Lee RL.Synthesis and evaluation of esters and carbamates to identify critical functional groups for esterase specific metabolism. Bioorg Med Chem 2003;11:3237–44.

31. EL-Gendy KS, Aly NM, Sabra FS. Biochemical effects of a single oral dose of two acetanilide herbicides alachlor and butachlor on female mice. Alex J Pharm Sci 1998;12:87–90.

32. Aly NM, EL-Gendy KS, Mahmoud FH, El-Sebae AH. Protective effect of vitamin C against chlorpyrifos oxidative stress in male mice. Pest Biochem Physiol 2010;97:7–12.

33. Kalender Y, Kaya S, Durak D, Uzun FG, Demir F. Protective effects of catechin and quercetin on antioxidant status, lipid peroxidation and testis-histoarchitecture induced by chlorpyrifos in male rats. Enviorn Toxicol Pharmacol 2012;33:141–8.

34. Igwenyi IO, Aboh N, Nwachukwu N, Ibiam UA, Offor CE, Aja PM, et al. Effect of baygon insecticide on the activities of total, alkaline and acid phosphatases of selected tissues of albino rats. J Pharm Biol Sci 2014;9:41–3.

35. Khan S. Endosulphan concentration alters biomarkers in albino rat. Indian J Pharm Biol Res 2014;2:14–7.

36. Rahman MF, Siddiqui MKJ, Jamil CK. Inhibition of acetylcholinesterase and different ATPases by a novel phosphorothionate (RPR-II) rat brain. Ecotoxicol Environ Saf 2000;47:125–9.

37. Novelli ELB, Vierira EP, Rodrigues NL, Ribas BO. Risk

assessment of cadmium toxicity on hepatic and renal tissues of rats. Environ Res 1998;79 A:102–5.

38. Kalender S, Uzun FG, Durak D, Demir F, Kalender Y. Malathion-induced hepatotoxicity in rats: the effects of vitamins C and E. Food Chem Toxicol 2010;48:633–8.

CHAPTER 16

RELEVANCE OF PLASMA CHOLINESTERASE TO CLINICAL FINDINGS IN ACUTE ORGANOPHOSPHOROUS POISONING

Devanur R.M.M. Prasad; Prasanna S. Jirli; Mahadevaiah Mahesh; Shivanagappa Mamatha

Keywords: Organophosphorous compounds; Acute poisoning; Acetyl Cholinesterase; Pesticide

INTRODUCTION

Pesticide poisoning is a major public health problem in developing world (1). Millions of people are exposed to danger of hazardous occupational practices and unsafe storage of pesticides (2). However, it is deliberate self-poisoning which causes the great majority of deaths and places immense strain on hospital services, particularly in Asia (3,4). According to a World Health Organization report, three million cases of pesticide poisoning occur annually worldwide and most of them are in Asia which at least half of them are due to organophosphorus (OP) poisoning (5).

Poisoning is a common method of suicide, especially in the developing world (6). OP compounds are amongst the most common poisons used for deliberate self-poisoning in India and other parts of the world (7-12). The exact rate of OP poisoning in India is uncertain due to lack of data and proper reporting. In many reports from India, rate of suicidal poisoning with OP compounds ranges from 10.3to 43.8% (8,13,14). Among OP poisoned patients in India, hospital mortality rate is reported to be as high as 20-70% (15,16). However, in United Kingdom, OP compounds are responsible for only about 1% of deaths. This is because in developing countries, facilities are limited for early diagnosis and treatment.

Being predominantly an agricultural country, OP compounds are used abundantly for farming in India. Hence, access to these hazardous chemical substances is easy. OP pesticides inhibit carboxylic esterase enzymes including acetylcholinesterase (AChE) and plasma cholinesterase (PChE). AChE can be found in erythrocytes, nervous tissue and skeletal muscles, while PChE can be found in plasma, liver, heart, pancreas and brain. Most of clinical manifestations associated with exposure to OP compounds have been attributed to inhibition of these enzymes (17).

Although it has not been fully studied, these anti-cholinesterase effects can be associated with the extent of decrease of AChE and PChE. This study was designed to investigate the relevance of PChE to clinical manifestations following OP poisoning and to evaluate usefulness of PChE in predicting clinical outcomes.

METHODS

This was a prospective cross-sectional study which was conducted at Dr. Prabhakar Kore Hospital and Medical Research Centre, Jawaharlal Nehru Medical College, Belgaum, Karnataka from 1st October 2009 to 30th September 2010 after

Citation: Devanur R.M.M. Prasad; Prasanna S. Jirli; Mahadevaiah Mahesh; Shivanagappa Mamatha, Relevance of Plasma Cholinesterase to Clinical Findings in Acute Organophosphorous Poisoning, http://apjmt.mums.ac.ir/article_546.html

taking approval from the ethical committee. 76 patients with definitive diagnosis of OP poisoning were enrolled. Exclusion criteria were liver dysfunction, malnutrition, chronic infections, hypersensitivity reaction, pregnancy, age of more than 60 years and being on some specific medications including succinyl choline, codeine and morphine.

Each patient was assessed according to severity of OP poisoning based on Proudfoot classification (Table 1) (18). Patients who had manifestations suggestive of severe poisoning were assessed and ventilatory support was administered for them if they had any of the following signs: 1) Apnea 2) Obvious hypoventilation 3) Persistent cyanosis in spite of O2 supplementation 4) Persistent tachypnea or respiratory rate >24/ minute 5) Persistent SpO2 <90% with oxygen supplementation 6) Active involvement of accessory muscles of respiration.

Four 5-mL samples of intravenous blood were collected from each patient under strict aseptic precautions on first day. Also, a fifth blood sample was collected and analyzed for PChE level on the fifth day of treatment. This time (day 5th on treatment) was selected as it has been considered to be the average time required for effect of pralidoxime to eliminate respiratory distress and need for mechanical ventilation (19). The PChE level was measured usingDimension Clinical Chemistry System (E.I. Dupont De Nemours & Company Inc., Wilmington, DE, USA). The normal values of PChE range from 5100 to 11700 with mean (SD) of 8440 (1780) IU/L (20,21). Based on Proudfoot classification, mild OP toxicity is defined as less than 10% reduction of PChE, moderate toxicity as 10-50% reduction and severe toxicity as >50% of reduction. In keeping with this definition, 4590-5100 IU/L PChE can be considered as mild, 2550-4590 IU/L as moderate and less than 2550 IU/L as severe toxicity.

Data are shown with frequency and percentage. Mean and standard deviation (SD) were calculated using Statistical Package of Social Sciences (SPSS Inc., Chicago, IL, USA).

RESULTS

Socio-demographic

In this study, 76 patients were enrolled with mean age of 25.5 (range: 21-30) years. Majority of patients were males (n=50, 65.7 %), were from rural areas (n=66, 86.84 %) and were agricultural workers (n=19, 25%) who consumed OP compounds orally with the intension of self-poisoning. Monocrotophos, a highly hazardous OP compound, was the most common used poison among the patients (60%) which could be due to frequent use and easy availability in our state, Karnataka.

Clinical and Laboratory Findings

Main clinical findings at the time of admission were congested conjunctiva (87%), pin point pupil (83%), lacrimation (80%), vomiting (78%), non-reactive pupil (75%), respiratory distress (60%) and abdominal pain (37%). Among 46 patients with respiratory distress, 35 patients required ventilatory support. The average time taken for initiating active weaning was 4.3 days post-admission in the Intensive Care Unit. After an average of 7.4 days, patients were successfully weaned off from ventilator.

Table 1: Assessment of Severity of Acute Organ phosphorous Compound Poisoning

	SEVERITY		
	Mild	Moderate	Severe
Clinical Manifestations	Fatigue, Headache, Paresthesia, Nausea and Vomiting, Diaphoresis, Salivation, Abdominal pain, Diarrhea, Able to ambulate	Symptoms of mild poisoning + Miosis, General weakness, Dysarthria, Fasciculation, Unable to ambulate	Generalized Fasciculation, Marked miosis (Absent pupillary reaction), Flaccid Paralysis, Pulmonary crepitation, Respiratory distress, Cyanosis, Unconsciousness
Plasma Cholinesterase level	< 10 %	10-20 %	< 50 %

Mean (SD) PChE at 6 hours post-exposure was 3672.4 (4200.1) IU/L. PChE level then decreased to 2205.7 (2565.2) at 6 to 12 hours post-exposure and 1739.1 (1583.8) at 12 to 24 hours post-exposure. At 24 to 48 hours post-exposure mean PChE started to rise to 1966.4 (2525.8). After 5 days of treatment, PChE level reached a mean of 8587.7 (4728.3) (Figure 1). At presentation, 62 patients (90%) had PChE values of less than 5000 IU/L. In addition, in over 50% of patients, PChE suppressed to less than 2000 IU/L (severe toxicity).

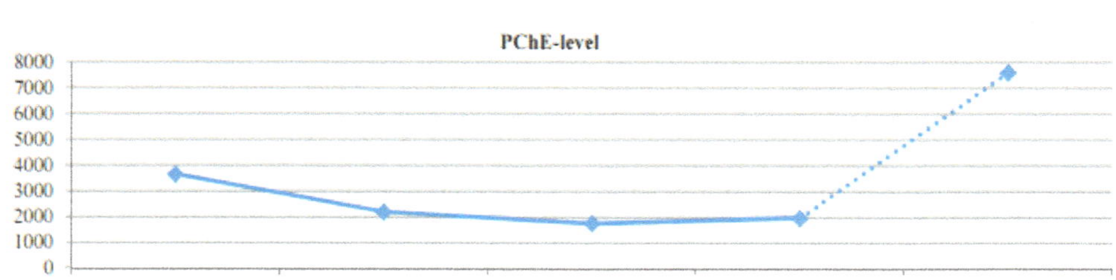

Figure 1. Mean Plasma cholinesterase levels in patients with organ phosphorous poisoning in different times of sampling post-admission.

Relevance of Plasma Cholinesterase to Clinical Manifestations

To assess the relationship of clinical manifestations with levels of PChE, mean PChE level for each manifestation was measured independently at the time of presentation. As it is shown in figure 2, cyanosis, muscle weakness, convulsion, respiratory distress and fasciculation were related to cases with very severe suppression of PChE (>75%). In this respect, cyanosis was noted in 5 cases and was related to the lowest mean PChE level (847.2 IU/L). In association with less than 50% PChE reduction, abdominal pain, dryness of conjunctiva, vomiting and diarrhea were found. For PChE levels of 50 to 75% of normal, pin point and non-reactive pupil, lacrimation and congested conjunctivae were noted.

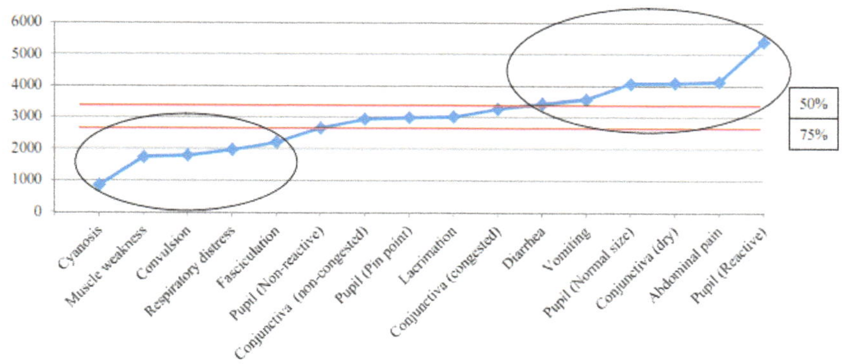

Figure 2. Level of plasma cholinesterase in association with clinical manifestations

Relevance of Plasma Cholinesterase to Morbidity and Mortality

Mean PChE was further measured according to some important complications following OP poisoning (Table 2). Patients who died had the lowest mean PChE level on first day (1270.2). Among survived patients, those who required ventilatory support had the lowest PChE (1383.7) on first day. Subsequently, in the cases presented with muscle weakness, convulsion, respiratory distress and fasciculation, mean PChE on first day was very low as it was reduced to 1739.1, 1899.5, 1966.4 and 2205.7 respectively (severe toxicity). In addition, patients with muscle weakness and fasciculation had the lowest blood oxygen saturation (SpO2<70%) on first day, indicating severe respiratory distress (Table 2). Death was mostly observed among patients who had respiratory distress. Overall mortality was within the first two days.

Table 2: Comparative data of morbidity and mortality

Features	No. of Patients	Oxygen saturation-Day 1 (SpO2), mean (SD)	PChE-Day 1 (IU/L), mean (SD)	PChE-Day 5 (IU/L), mean (SD)
Oxygen therapy with mask	16	80.6 (15.2)	5605.5 (5234.6)	10346.5 (4089.9)
Respiratory distress	46	69.5 (17.9)	1966.4 (2525.8)	7356.6 (4228.3)
Ventilatory support	35	67.7 (17.9)	1383.7 (1232.5)	6636.5 (4277.3)
Fasciculation	17	70.0 (19.3)	2205.7 (2565.2)	6369.4 (5417.6)
Muscle weakness	7	67.8 (22.3)	1739.1 (1583.8)	6164.2 (3500.9)
Convulsion	6	79.5 (14)	1899.5 (1353.8)	7053.4 (2162.2)
Survived	62	80.6 (18.8)	3672.4 (4200.1)	8587.7 (4728.3)
Died	14	70.3 (16.8)	1270.2 (1456.2)	9459.4 (7656.0)*
* 9 patients died within 5 days and 5 others thereafter.				

DISCUSSION

OP poisoning is a major health problem worldwide, especially in developing countries with millions of victims and deaths occurring each year. Determination of AChE and PChE level in blood has remained as a mainstay for the fast initial screening of acute OP exposure which helps health-care professionals to establish early diagnosis and immediate treatment plan (22). However, it has been believed that these tests lack sensitivity and specificity, and additionally they might not be related to severity of poisoning (19,22). In this respect, Aygun et al.

showed that PChE level is useful in diagnosis of OP poisoning in acute phase but it is not correlated to severity of poisoning and also morbidity and mortality (23). Conversely, Goswamy et al. demonstrated that apart from clinical indicators, low PChE levels were of greatest predictive value in OP poisoning (24).

In this study, we found that cyanosis, muscle weakness, convulsion, respiratory distress and fasciculation were linked to very low PChE levels. Moreover, we found that as PChE level falls, the O2 saturation decreases and leads to respiratory distress which was the main cause of death among patients. This can be explained by the fact that mitochondria are the target of OP compounds (25). Therefore, a more severe OP poisoning which shows itself with lower PChE levels is associated with cellular hypoxia and subsequently severer life-threatening manifestations.

Similar to our findings, Kar in 2006 and Tsao et al. in 1990 showed that fatal outcomes following OP poisoning were associated with lower PChE levels (26,27). In addition, they found that all deceased patients had respiratory failure. In this regard, it has been ascertained that the essential cause of death in OP poisoning is respiratory failure which is due to weakness of the respiratory muscles, paralysis of the respiratory centre, bronchospasm and increased bronchial secretion (28). Furthermore, it has been proposed to consider miosis and muscle fasciculation for the control of treatment in OP poisoning (28).

In the present study, we found that deceased patients had the lowest PChE level at presentation. Likewise, Chen et al. showed that low PChE activity with non-rising trend within 48 hours of OP poisoning was associated with higher mortality (29). Moreover, Eddleston et al. revealed that PChE activity can predict death based on the formula of OP compound ingested (30).

LIMITATIONS

Although in this study we tried to identify the relevance of mean PChE level with each clinical manifestation, overlapping of features were present in some cases which can reduce the value of our findings. Therefore, to clarify the controversies, further studies with larger samples are recommended while the amount of OP compound consumed is strictly noted. Furthermore, Eddleston et al. proposed that predicting death with PChE level is possible when the ingested OP compound is known (30). However, in this study, we did not separate the results and outcomes based on the OP poison formula.

CONCLUSION

A relative relationship between PChE level and clinical manifestations and outcomes was found. These findings can assist health professionals to better evaluate patient's prognosis and improve their treatment plan.

ACKNOWLEDGMENT

We would like to thank Dr. Tippe Swamy, Department of Community Dentistry, JSS Dental College and Hospital, Mysore for his timely help in performing statistical analysis.

Conflict of interest: None to be declared.

Funding and Support: None.

REFERENCES

1. Jeyaratnam J. Acute pesticide poisoning: a major global health problem. World Health Stat Q 1990;43(3):139-44.
2. Karalliedde L, Eddleston M, Murray V. The Global Picture of Organophosphate Insecticide Poisoning. In: Karalliedde L, Feldman F, Henry J, Marrs T, editors. Organophosphates and Health. 1st ed. London: Imperial College Press; 2001. p.431-71
3. Van der Hoek W, Konradsen F, Athukorala K, Wanigadewa T. Pesticide poisoning: a major health problem in Sri Lanka. Soc Sci Med 1998 Feb-Mar;46(4-5):495-504.
4. Eddleston M, Sheriff MH, Hawton K. Deliberate self harm in Sri Lanka: an overlooked tragedy in the developing world. BMJ 1998 Jul 11;317(7151):133-5.
5. World Health Organization (WHO), United Nations Environment Programme (UNEP). Public health impact of pesticides used in agriculture. Geneva: WHO press; 1990.
6. Vijayakumar L. Suicide prevention: the urgent need in developing countries. World Psychiatry 2004 Oct;3(3):158-9.
7. Reddy KSN. The Essentials of Forensic Medicine and Toxicology. Hyderabad: Suguna Devi Publication; 2004.
8. Gururaj G, Isaac MK. Epidemiology of suicide in Bangalore. Bangalore: National Institute of Mental Health and Neuro Sciences; 2001.
9. Chugh SN, Aggarwal N, Dabla S, Chhabra B. Comparative Evaluation of "Atropine Alone" and "Atropine with Pralidoxime (PAM)" in the Management of Organophosphorus Poisoning. JIACM 2005;6(1):33-7
10. Srinivas Rao Ch, Venkateswarlu V, Surender T, Eddleston M, Buckley NA. Pesticide poisoning in south India: opportunities for prevention and improved medical management. Trop Med Int Health 2005 Jun;10(6):581-8.
11. Eddleston M, Szinicz L, Eyer P, Buckley N. Oximes in acute organophosphorus pesticide poisoning: a systematic review of clinical trials. QJM 2002 May;95(5):275-83.
12. Latha Ks, Bhat SM. Suicide attempts among youth: Co-relates of medical lethality. Behavioral Med J 1999;2(1):21-9.
13. Ponnudurai R, Jeyakar J. Suicide in madras. Indian J Psychiatry 1980 Apr;22(2):203-5.
14. Nandi DN, Mukherjee SP, Banerjee G, Boral GC, Chowdhury A, Bose J. Is Suicide Preventable By Restricting the Availability of Lethal Agents? A Rural Survey of West Bengal. Indian J Psychiatry 1979;21(3):251-5.
15. Wadia RS. Treatment of Organophosphate Poisoning. Indian J Crit Care Med 2003;7(2):85-7.
16. Pillay VV. Organophosphate/carbamate pesticide poisoning – a primer for physicians. Paper presented at: The 3rd Annual Conference of Indian Society of

Toxicology (Toxocon-3); 2007 April 7-8; Mangalore, India.

17. Karalliedde L. Cholinesterase estimations revisited: the clinical relevance. Eur J Anaesthesiol 2002 May;19(5):313-6.
18. Proudfoot AT. Diagnosis and Management of Acute Poisoning. 1st ed. Oxford: Blackwell Science; 1982.
19. Eddleston M, Buckley NA, Eyer P, Dawson AH. Management of acute organophosphorus pesticide poisoning. Lancet 2008 Feb 16;371(9612):597-607.
20. Vij K. Textbook of Forensic Medicine and Toxicology: Principles and Practice. New Delhi: Elsevier; 2008.
21. Mehta AB, Shah AC, Joshi LG, Kale AK, Vora DD. Clinical features and plasma acetylcholinesterase activity in poisoning with insecticidal organophosphorous compounds. J Assoc Physicians India 1971 Feb;19(2):181-4.
22. Worek F, Koller M, Thiermann H, Szinicz L. Diagnostic aspects of organophosphate poisoning. Toxicology 2005 Oct 30;214(3):182-9.
23. Aygun D, Doganay Z, Altintop L, Guven H, Onar M, Deniz T, et al. Serum acetylcholinesterase and prognosis of acute organophosphate poisoning. J Toxicol Clin Toxicol 2002;40(7):903-10.
24. Goswamy R, Chaudhuri A, Mahashur AA. Study of respiratory failure in organophosphate and carbamate poisoning. Heart Lung 1994 Nov-Dec;23(6):466-72.
25. Kaur P, Radotra B, Minz RW, Gill KD. Impaired mitochondrial energy metabolism and neuronal apoptotic cell death after chronic dichlorvos (OP) exposure in rat brain. Neurotoxicology 2007 Nov;28(6):1208-19.
26. Kar N. Lethality of suicidal organophosphorus poisoning in an Indian population: exploring preventability. Ann Gen Psychiatry 2006 Nov 21;5:17. doi:10.1186/1744-859X-5-17.
27. Tsao TC, Juang YC, Lan RS, Shieh WB, Lee CH. Respiratory failure of acute organophosphate and carbamate poisoning. Chest 1990 Sep;98(3):631-6.
28. Namba T. Cholinesterase inhibition by organophosphorus compounds and its clinical effects. Bull World Health Organ 1971;44(1-3):289-307.
29. Chen HY, Wang WW, Chaou CH, Lin CC. Prognostic value of serial serum cholinesterase activities in organophosphate poisoned patients. Am J Emerg Med 2009 Nov; 27(9):1034-9.
30. Eddleston M, Eyer P, Worek F, Sheriff MH, Buckley NA. Predicting outcome using butyrylcholinesterase activity in organophosphorus pesticide self-poisoning. QJM 2008 Jun;101(6):467-74.

CHAPTER 17

LINKING PESTICIDE EXPOSURE WITH PEDIATRIC LEUKEMIA

Antonio F. Hernández, and Pablo Menéndez

Keywords: infant and childhood leukemia; hematopoietic stem/progenitor cells; chromosomal rearrangements; topoisomerase II;pesticides; DNA double-strand break; oxidative stress

INTRODUCTION

Leukemia is the most common childhood cancer, accounting for 30% of all cancers diagnosed in children under 15 years of age, with an annual incidence of up to 40 cases per million children in developed countries and an incidence peak between three and five years of age [1,2]. Pediatric acute leukemia is a phenotypically- and genetically-heterogeneous disease of immature hematopoietic stem and progenitor cells (HSPCs). Phenotypically, it can target B-cell progenitors (B-cell acute lymphoblastic leukemia (B-ALL)), T-cell progenitors (T-ALL) or myeloid progenitors (acute myeloid leukemia (AML)). Acute leukemia can be further stratified according to the differentiation stage at which HSPCs are blocked; for example, B-ALL can have a pro-B (proB-ALL) or pre-B phenotype (preB-ALL) [3]. Similarly, AML can affect both immature (subtype M0 of the French-American-British classification of AML) and mature lineage-committed types, such as erythroblastic or megakaryoblastic leukemia (subtypes M6 and M7, respectively). Seventy percent of pediatric acute leukemias are ALL and 30% are AML. Genetically, ALL and AML can be further stratified according to molecular cytogenetics [4,5], which represents a prognostic factor.

Fetal hematopoiesis begins in the aorta gonad-mesonephros region to subsequently colonize the fetal liver (FL) and ultimately, just before birth, the bone marrow [6]. FL hematopoiesis entails an active proliferation of progenitors, rendering fetal HSPCs susceptible to oncogenic transformation through DNA damage mediated by chemical exposure during pregnancy [7]. Although the etiology of ALL remains elusive, ionizing radiation, congenital genetic syndromes and *in utero* exposure to specific genotoxic chemicals, including household pesticides, represent prime etiological suspects [8]. Importantly, altered patterns of infection during early childhood might also contribute to acute leukemia in children [9,10,11].

We here review the available experimental and epidemiological evidence linking pesticide exposure with infant and childhood leukemia and provide a mechanistic basis to support the association, focusing on early molecular events. However, the paucity of mechanistic data is a major obstacle to fully understanding the toxicological pathways involved. Causation pathways are likely to be multifactorial, and it is possible that the risk of pediatric leukemia from environmental exposure is influenced by genetic susceptibility.

Citation: Antonio F. Hernández and Pablo Menéndez, Linking Pesticide Exposure with Pediatric Leukemia, doi:10.3390/ijms17040461.

EVIDENCE LINKING PESTICIDE EXPOSURE WITH PEDIATRIC LEUKEMIA

Epidemiological Studies Supporting the Association

There is a growing concern about whether chronic low-level pesticide exposure during pregnancy or childhood increases the risk of childhood leukemia. Epidemiological studies suggest that pesticide exposure may have a greater impact on children than adults [12,13]. Almost all of the available evidence has focused on pediatric leukemia without making a distinction between infant and childhood leukemia, which are etiologically and pathologically different entities. However, most epidemiological studies are limited because no specific pesticides have been directly associated with the risk of leukemia, but rather the broad term "pesticide exposure" [13,14]. Such associations are mainly based on subjects' recall of the pesticide exposure, which hampers the drawing of conclusions because of recall/information bias.

In contrast to childhood leukemia, very few studies have examined the risk of infant leukemia and pesticide exposure. An international collaborative study on transplacental chemical exposure and risk of infant leukemia found an increased risk after *in utero* exposure to household pesticides (propoxur and other methylcarbamate insecticides), the therapeutic analgesic dipyrone and hormonal intake (estrogens). In these cases, infant leukemia was associated with the mixed lineage leukemia (*MLL*) gene fusion, likely as a result of topoisomerase II inhibition [15,16]. Although the aforementioned study was based on a rather small sample size, an increased risk (Odds Ratio—OR: 2.18) of infant leukemia was shown in mothers exposed to domestic insecticides during pregnancy. Since estrogens can be metabolized to catechol estrogen-3,4-quinones [17], the association found for infant leukemia might be due to topoisomerase II inhibition caused by quinone metabolites generated during estrogen metabolism [7]. A further Brazilian study found that over use of pesticides during pregnancy was associated with ALL and AML (OR: 2.10 and 5.01, respectively) in children <1 year of age [18]. Moreover, maternal exposure to the insecticide permethrin (assessed by self-reporting) was associated with a higher risk of leukemia in children <1 year of age, with an OR of 2.47 for ALL and 7.28 for AML. This finding was also supported by a case-control study in China where the use of pyrethroids (assessed by urine levels of major metabolites) was associated with a greater risk of ALL [19].

The presence of the herbicide chlorthal in household dust samples was also associated with an increased risk of ALL in children <8 years, with a significant dose-response trend [20]. The association was greater with the herbicide mixture chlorthal plus alachlor. Other studies, however, report no significant associations. For example, no significant risk of childhood leukemia was found with exposure to some agricultural and residential herbicides, such as metolachlor, bromoxynil, cyanazine and 2,4-dichlorophenoxyacetic acid [20,21]. Furthermore, a case-control study on leukemia in children <1 year old from the American Children's Oncology Group failed to find a significant association between household exposure to insecticides or rodenticides and ALL or AML [22].

Different meta-analyses have consistently shown an increased risk of childhood leukemia associated with pesticide exposure [13,23]. However, this review will focus on the latest quantitative synthesis of evidence from studies. A recent meta-analysis has shown that maternal occupational pesticide exposure during pregnancy and/or paternal occupational pesticide exposure near-to-conception increases the risk of leukemia in offspring [24]. The authors pooled data from 13 case-control studies participating in the Childhood Leukemia International Consortium (CLIC) and found an almost two-fold increased risk of AML in mothers exposed to pesticides during pregnancy, whereas no significant risk was found for paternal exposure around conception. In relation to ALL, the same study observed a 20% increased risk with paternal exposure around conception, which appeared to be more evident for pediatric T-cell ALL. By contrast, no significant association was found between maternal exposure during pregnancy and risk of B or T-cell ALL. In a separate study investigating residential pesticide exposure, Bailey *et al.* [25] pooled data from 12 case-control studies in the CLIC and found a significant increased risk of ALL associated with exposure to any pesticide shortly before conception, during pregnancy and after birth (OR: 1.39, 1.43 and 1.36, respectively). Little variation was observed with the type of pesticide. Regarding AML, an increased risk was found for exposure to any pesticide in the few months prior to conception and during pregnancy (OR: 1.49 and 1.55, respectively); however, exposure after birth failed to demonstrate an increased leukemogenic risk. A recent meta-analysis conducted by Chen *et al.* [12] pooled 16 case-control studies and found that childhood exposure to indoor, but not outdoor, residential insecticides was associated with an increased risk of pediatric leukemia (OR: 1.47). A slightly weaker association was found for herbicide exposure (OR: 1.26). Notwithstanding these positive associations, observational studies on pesticide exposure and pediatric leukemia have a number of weaknesses to claim causal relationships. The consistency of findings across meta-analyses may be due to the considerable overlap in the studies included in the different meta-analyses undertaken. Many epidemiological analyses have not been performed using methodologically-rigorous association studies. Limitations include the lack of an accurate exposure estimate (from both a qualitative and quantitative standpoint), lack of temporal concordance (most studies were case-control in design) and little information on the dose-response relationship. In addition, the available epidemiological evidence may be challenged by endogenous or exogenous factors, such as genetic susceptibility, lifestyle and co-exposure to other environmental agents.

In Vitro Studies

The few *in vitro* studies available so far have shown that captan and captafol (two related chloroalkylthiocarboximide fungicides) decrease the activity of topoisomerase II by 50% and 20%, respectively, at a concentration of 1 μM [26]. Similarly, thiram (a dithiocarbamate fungicide) inhibits topoisomerase II at 10 μM [27]. However, genotoxic potential (*i.e.*, genetic abnormalities, mutations) of these fungicides occurred only at very high doses (10–100 mM) *in vivo* using common fruit flies [26]. More recently, the organophosphate (OP) insecticide chlorpyrifos has been reported to induce DNA double-strand breaks (DSBs) and *MLL* gene rearrangements in human fetal liver CD34+ HSPCs as a consequence of topoisomerase II inhibition [14].

Other OP pesticides have been implicated in leukemogenesis, particularly isofenphos, diazinon and fenitrothion. An *in vitro* study using the human leukemic cell line K562 demonstrated metabolic changes consistent with a leukemogenic potential of isofenphos [28]. In addition, human peripheral blood lymphocytes exposed to isofenphos exhibited dose-dependent damage to chromosomal DNA, as well as disruption of the cholinergic nuclear signaling pathway, which collectively could lead to genomic instability and leukemogenesis [29]. In an *in vitro* study using diazinon, a concentration of 0.1 μM induced hypermethylation of several genes involved in cell cycle arrest, such as cyclin-dependent kinase inhibitor 1A (*CDKN1A*) and 1C (*CDKN1C*), and tumor suppressor genes, such as *p53* and*PTEN* [30]. Fenitrothion at low concentrations (1 μM) also induced chromosomal damage in the B-cell leukemia/lymphoma-2 cell line BCL-2 [31].

GENE-ENVIRONMENT INTERACTIONS

For most pediatric leukemias, multiple genetic polymorphisms of xenobiotic metabolizing enzymes may interact with environmental, dietary and maternal factors to modulate the development of the disease. For example, quinones, which are capable of inhibiting topoisomerase II and can cleave the *MLL* gene at topoisomerase II cleavage sites, may be poorly detoxified depending on the activity of NAD(P)H:quinone oxidoreductase 1 (NQO1), an enzyme that detoxifies chemicals with quinone rings, such as bioflavonoids and benzene metabolites. Thus, genetic polymorphisms of *NQO1* resulting in low-activity variants might be associated with an increased risk of infant leukemia. By contrast, in childhood ALL without *MLL* rearrangements, deficiency of the *NQO1* gene is not associated with the etiology of the disease [32].

Global DNA hypomethylation is associated with activation of oncogenes and neoplastic processes [33], whereas the hypermethylation of 5′ cytosine-phospho-guanine (CpG) islands in promoter regions of some tumor suppressor genes prevents their transcription and promotes the development of tumors [34]. The genetic regulation of folate metabolism may have an influence on the preleukemic clone origin via DNA hypomethylation of key regulatory genes, rendering the genome vulnerable to genomic instability [35]. The presence of some polymorphisms in genes involved in folate metabolism reduces enzyme activity, leading to inadequate folate levels and DNA hypomethylation, ultimately contributing to the neoplastic process [35,36]. The insufficient input of folate increases the plasma concentration of homocysteine and *S*-adenosylhomocysteine, with the latter being a general inhibitor of adenosylmethionine-dependent methyltransferases [37]. Inhibition of these enzymes may alter both DNA methylation and transcriptional regulation [36,38]. The 677C>T gene polymorphism in methylenetetrahydrofolate reductase (*MTHFR*) has been linked to a decreased risk of childhood ALL, likely as a result of higher production of 5,10-MTHF and thymidine, which improve the fidelity of DNA synthesis and repair [39]. On the other hand, inactivating polymorphisms of detoxifying enzymes involved in carcinogen metabolism, such as glutathione *S*-transferases (GST), in parents have been associated with the development of ALL in their children <1 year old. The deletion of both the *GSTT1* and *GSTM1* genes in either parent might affect the risk of infant leukemia [40]. Furthermore, genetic polymorphisms of xenobiotic transport and metabolism pathways are associated with the risk of childhood ALL. In particular, polymorphisms of the *ABCB1* gene, which encodes a membrane transporter of lipophilic compounds, may interact with household insecticide exposures to increase the risk of disease [41]. Genetic variability in DNA repair pathways and cell cycle checkpoints might also interact with environmental, dietary, maternal and other external factors affecting the development of ALL. In summary, the limited data available suggest that dietary and environmental exposure to substances targeting topoisomerases together with the reduced ability of fetuses or their mothers to detoxify such compounds because of polymorphic variants of given genes could contribute to the development of pediatric leukemia [8,42].

The International Childhood Acute Lymphoblastic Leukemia Genetics Consortium revealed limitations in current studies on genetic susceptibility and the risk of ALL because of difficulties in conducting statistically- and methodologically-rigorous investigations [43]. Genome-wide association studies of childhood ALL have provided robust evidence for four low-penetrance susceptibility variants, which confer only a modest increase in risk. Moreover, the well-recognized ethnic differences in the risk of ALL represent a weakness in assessing the interplay between inherited and non-genetic risk factors. Given the small frequency of many ALL subgroups, the identification of differential effects will realistically be possible only through multi-center pooled analyses [43].

EARLY MOLECULAR EVENTS INVOLVED IN PESTICIDE-ASSOCIATED PEDIATRIC LEUKEMOGENESIS

Despite the rather comprehensive epidemiologic evidence linking pesticide exposure during different reproductive stages (pre-conception, pregnancy and early postnatal life) and pediatric leukemia, robust underlying pathological mechanisms remain unknown. The initiating event at the molecular level might be the induction of chromosomal rearrangements as a result of pesticide exposure and subsequent topoisomerase II inhibition or generation of oxidative stress, leading directly or indirectly to DNA damage. A mechanistic explanation follows.

DNA Double-Strand Breaks (DSBs)

Under some circumstances, oxidative lesions can lead to DNA DSBs formation in HSPCs. Environmental exposures to numerous chemicals, including many pesticides, have been shown *in vivo* and *in vitro* to generate oxidative species that can ultimately induce DNA base or sugar oxidative damage, leading to single-strand breaks (SSBs) and DSBs formation in the DNA [44]. For example, OP insecticides (chlorpyrifos, methyl-parathion, malathion), methyl-carbamates (methomyl) and the herbicide paraquat all cause oxidative DNA damage followed by DNA SSBs and DSBs [45,46,47,48]. There is also evidence of pesticide-induced oxidative stress and DNA damage in agricultural workers [47]. Additionally, oxidative species may interact with biological molecules to disrupt normal DNA synthesis and repair, and so, inhibition/inactivation of antioxidant proteins or DNA repair enzymes may also be an underlying molecular mechanism [49]. Along this line, pesticides can disrupt a number of antioxidant enzymes, including superoxide dismutase and catalase [50], rendering oxidative stress [51].

DSBs can arise under different circumstances: (i) when two SSBs form close to each other on opposite strands; (ii) upon enzymatic DNA cleavage next to an SSB on the opposite strand; or (iii) when either DNA replication or transcription takes place at sites of misrepaired DNA. DSBs constitute the first molecular event in the generation of chromosomal aberrations [52]. For instance, chlorpyrifos is reported to cause DNA DSBs and further chromosomal rearrangements (*i.e.*, *MLL*) through oxidative stress in human FL HSPCs [53]. However, chlorpyrifos can also induce DNA DSBs as a result of topoisomerase II inhibition in FL HSPCs in a manner similar to that produced by etoposide [14]. Analogously, blood lymphocytes from pesticide sprayers have greater fragile site breakage than normal individuals following treatment with aphidicolin, an inhibitor of DNA polymerases [54]. Chromosomal fragile sites are regions of the genome prone to breakage following exposure to many chemicals, including environmental and chemotherapeutic agents. During DNA replication, fragile site-inducing conditions can uncouple the helicase complex from the DNA polymerase, resulting in long stretches of single-stranded DNA and further DNA breakage [55]. Aphidicolin can also induce fragile site breakage through a topoisomerase II-mediated mechanism [56].

Topoisomerase II has critical functions in both DNA replication and transcription processes, and the so-called "topoisomerase II poisons" disrupt the DNA-induced topoisomerase II cleavage-religation equilibrium through the stabilization of ternary (drug-DNA-enzyme) complexes, termed cleavage complexes [57]. Chemical-induced breakpoints are strongly associated with predicted topoisomerase II cleavage sites (*i.e.*, *MLL*), thus supporting a role for topoisomerase II-mediated breakage upon exposure to environmental agents. The high frequency of topoisomerase II recognition sites in specific DNA regions and the high expression of this enzyme in human $CD34^+$HSPCs represent favorable conditions for breakage following exposure to agents targeting topoisomerase II activity (*i.e.*, bioflavonoids and quinones). Because $CD34^+$ HSPCs appear to be more sensitive to DNA damage than committed progenitor cells, exposure to low levels of different chemicals may induce DNA breakage at certain sites in HSPCs, increasing the risk of chromosomal rearrangements. If affected cells survive, they continue growing and dividing, thus perpetuating DNA lesions and starting the chain of events that will eventually lead to leukemogenesis [55].

Chromosomal Translocations

Key molecular events leading to pediatric leukemia pathogenesis are chromosomal translocations. These generally result from the exchange of chromosomal arms between heterologous chromosomes, and DNA DSBs are prerequisites for their occurrence. Chromosomal translocations ultimately result in the deregulation of key cellular proteins, especially those encoded by proto-oncogenes and tumor suppressor genes, which are critical functional regulators of the cell [58]. Two functional classes of translocations are known. The first one relocates a proto-oncogene (or genes encoding for non-antigen receptors or transcription factors) into regulatory regions of actively-transcribed genes (such as those encoding for immunoglobulin chains or T-cell receptors), causing dysregulated expression of an intact protein. The second class of translocations juxtaposes two genes to encode a chimeric protein, which is functionally distinct from the wild-type proteins [1].

Although the mechanistic generation of chromosomal translocations is not well understood, they may arise from improper DNA repair or erroneous recombination of variable (V), diversity (D) and joining (J) gene segments (a process known as V(D)J recombination). As for improper DNA repair, reactive oxygen species (ROS)-induced DSBs in human FL $CD34^+$ HSPCs following maternal exposure to chemicals triggers recombination/repair pathways by non-homologous end-joining (NHEJ) [14]. The majority of damaged HSPCs may either successfully repair the DNA DSBs or fail to do so and undergo apoptotic cell death. In a fraction of cells, the repair of the DNA DSBs within particular breakpoint cluster regions (bcr) is not completed correctly, giving rise to chromosomal translocations or deletions [59]. For fusion genes to be leukemogenic, DSBs must occur simultaneously in two chromosomes and must also involve the coding region of the genes to generate an exon-exon in-frame functional chimeric gene product. Importantly, this has to occur in an HSPC that has managed to bypass cell death and displays a sustainable lifespan and clonal potential to propagate the chimeric gene product [60].

Erroneous V(D)J recombination usually occurs in developing lymphocytes during cell maturation, where V(D)J gene segments of immunoglobulin chains or T-cell receptors are rearranged to yield a wide range of immunoglobulins and T-cell receptors. The process entails the cleavage of the V(D)J gene at the flanking recombination signal sequences (RSS) by lymphocyte-specific recombination-activating gene (RAG) endonucleases and subsequent ligation of the segments via the classical NHEJ pathway [61]. In pediatric leukemia, chromosomal translocations and deletions often arise as a result of mistakes in V(D)J rearrangements because RAG enzymes can erroneously recognize and target RSS-like sequences. V(D)J-recombinase-mediated rearrangements may occur at both immune RSS and non-immune cryptic RSS (cRSS), which are widely distributed throughout the genome [62]. There is growing evidence that *in vivo* exposure to DNA-damaging agents, including pesticides, can increase the frequency and alter the recombination site distribution of V(D)J rearrangements at cRSS [63,64]. An increase in V(D)J-recombinase-mediated events at either immune or non-immune RSS following exposure to DNA-damaging agents could play an important role in environmentally-induced genetic alterations associated with leukemia development. Nonetheless, the mechanism by which exposure to DNA-damaging agents could increase the frequency of V(D)J-recombinase-mediated genomic rearrangements remains unclear [64].

PATHOBIOLOGY OF PEDIATRIC LEUKEMIAS

Given the distinct natural history and pathogenesis of infant and childhood leukemia, both entities will be addressed separately, although a chromosomal translocation is frequently the common initiating oncogenic event in both entities.

Infant Leukemia

Infant acute leukemia shows unique clinical and biological features and is commonly associated with rearrangements in the *MLL* gene (*MLL*-r), a master gene located on chromosome 11q23 that regulates normal human hematopoietic development and differentiation [65]. The *MLL* gene encodes a methyltransferase with activity for lysine 4 of histone H3 (H3K4), which mediates changes in chromatin associated with epigenetic transcriptional activation that plays an essential role in regulating gene expression during early development and hematopoiesis [66]. Rearrangements involving the *MLL* gene have been reported to occur only in mice with defects in DNA damage response and not in wild-type animals [67]. *MLL*-r functions as the initiating, and perhaps the sole driving, oncogenic event by dysregulating epigenetic and/or transcriptional programs [33] (Figure 1). Epidemiological and genetic studies have suggested that *MLL*-r may result from transplacental exposure to DNA topoisomerase-II inhibitors during gestation, such as chemotherapeutic agents, benzene metabolites (*i.e.*, benzoquinone), quinolone antibiotics, bioflavonoids present in some fruits and vegetables and some pesticides [7,33,68]. However, exposure to topoisomerase-II inhibitors is not sufficient *per se* for rearrangement of *MLL*, and the genetic background, such as mutations in the DNA damage response pathway, may influence the likelihood of *MLL*-r [67].

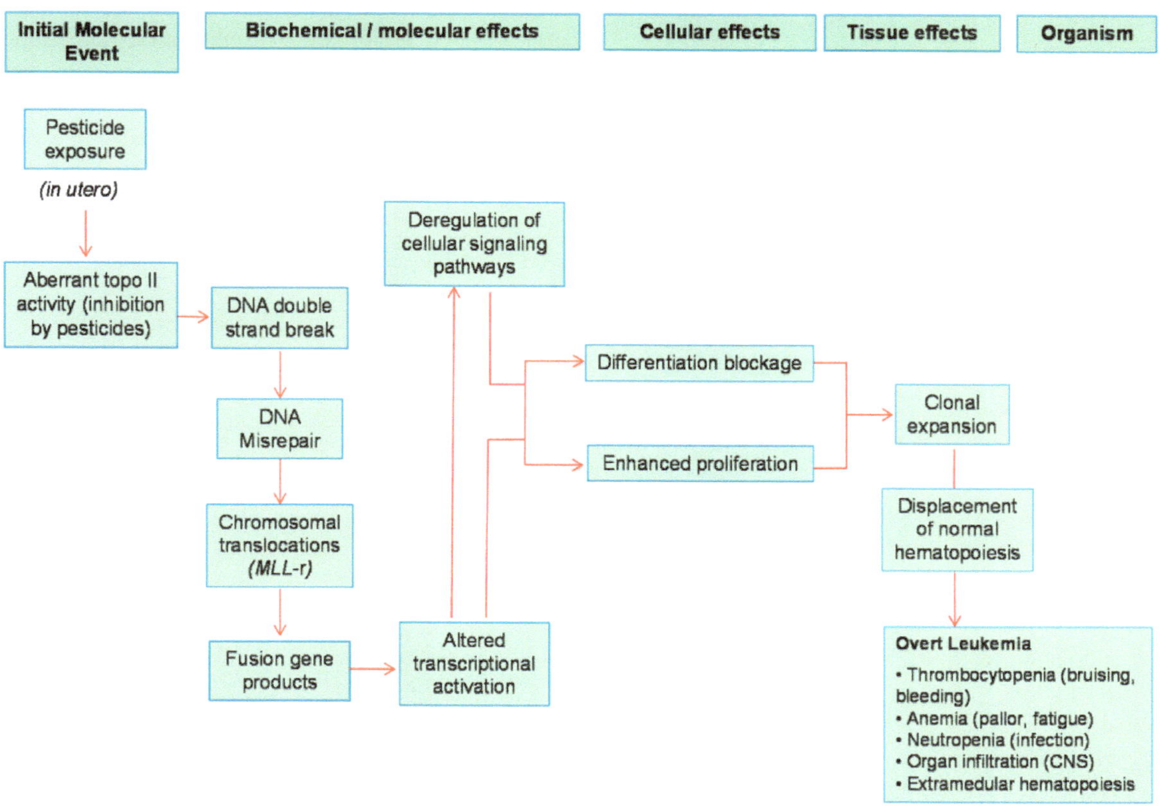

Figure 1: Chain of pathogenic events linking pesticide exposure to the development of infant *MLL*-rearranged acute leukemia.

The existence of recombination-prone sequences in the *MLL* bcr region supports the contention that *MLL*-r results from DNA breakage and recombination events. The genomic instability within *MLL* bcr may be the consequence of increased ROS generation [69]. The *MLL* fusion gene renders HSPCs more vulnerable to DNA repair and cell-cycle deregulation, facilitating the rapid acquisition of additional, secondary genetic changes, particularly upon continued exposure to genotoxic chemicals *in utero* [7,70]. These chemicals target early mesodermal precursors or HSPCs residing mainly in the FL where they inhibit topoisomerase-II activity and produce DNA DSBs within the *MLL* bcr, which are not properly repaired by homologous recombination or NHEJ. Because those mesodermal precursors or HSPCs are rapidly dividing and have high topoisomerase II content, they may be particularly sensitive to damage by topoisomerase II-targeting chemicals during a critical developmental window of vulnerability [33,71,72,73,74,75]. However, because of the very short latency of infant leukemia, it remains obscure whether the fusion gene generated from chromosomal translocations requires additional cooperating oncogenic hits for leukemogenesis. Although recurrent activating mutations of genes associated with cellular proliferation, such as components of the RAS signaling pathway, have been reported [76,77,78,79], functional studies revealed that these mutations are important for tumor maintenance rather than initiation in human HSPCs [80]. *MLL* breakage itself is not sufficient for the development of full-blown infant leukemia, even if the DNA damage response is defective. Activation of cellular proliferation by mutation of other genes might be necessary for overt leukemia [67]. The transformation mediated by the aberrant proteins encoded by fusion genes might depend on alternative (epi)-genetic cooperating lesions at a critical developmentally-earlier window of stem cell vulnerability to develop overt leukemia [33]. Intriguingly, and in contrast to the global dogma of cancer biology, *MLL*-r infant leukemia has been shown to have abnormal hypermethylation in non-enhancer, non-promoter regions, perhaps contributing to genomic stability and a silenced mutational landscape [76,81,82]. Extensive hypermethylation of tumor suppressor genes resulting in gene silencing has been observed in some cases of *MLL*-r infant leukemia [83].

Childhood Leukemia

Childhood leukemia has a prevalence peak at ~3–5 years of age, suggesting that environmental exposures *in utero*or during early childhood might be risk factors [25]. Under the current paradigm, the first initiating oncogenic mutation usually involves structural or numerical chromosomal alterations, impairing normal cell differentiation, while secondary hits more commonly comprise mutations affecting developmentally-regulated master transcription factors or membrane-proximal signaling pathways conferring proliferation and survival advantages to the differentiation-blocked clone [1,7,8,84,85]. The development of leukemia requires the activation of cell proliferation in addition to differentiation blockage [67]. Numerical aberrations (*i.e.*, hyperdiploidy) are also common hallmarks in childhood B-cell ALL.

The most common chromosomal aberrations are *E2A-PBX1*, *TEL-AML1* and *MLL*-r for B-ALL and *AML1-ETO* and*MLL*-r for AML. Similar to *MLL* rearrangements, the resulting aberrant chimeric proteins alter the normal transcriptional program and block normal B-cell and/or myeloid differentiation [8,86,87,88] (Figure 2). Although the*AML1* gene has been linked to anti-topoisomerase II agents, similar to the *MLL* gene, *TEL-AML1* is not sufficient to cause the disease by itself. As this fusion gene is observed in cord blood from about 1% of normal newborns, a significant proportion of the population carries self-limiting preleukemic clones, and the majority of them do not result in disease [3]. The longer latency observed in childhood leukemia unequivocally indicates that the initiating chromosomal translocation itself is unlikely to convert a preleukemic clone into an overt disease, thus suggesting the need for secondary cooperating (epi)-genetic events.

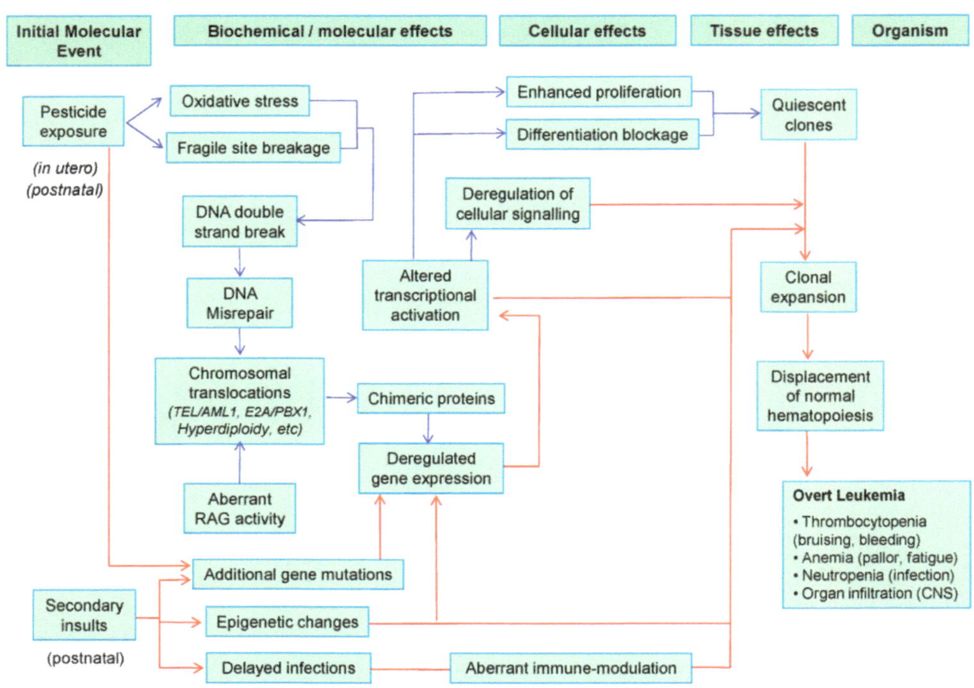

Figure 2: Chain of pathogenic events linking pesticide exposure to the development of childhood leukemia. Blue arrows indicate events related to the "first hit" and red arrows events related to the "second hit" (for more details, see Section 5.2).

Dysfunction of the immune system and delayed infections have been linked to childhood leukemia [9,89]. Two distinct underlying mechanisms might explain this association: (i) a lower repertoire of infections during early immune development; and (ii) an altered congenital responder status to infection resulting in functionally-aberrant clinical presentation of occasional infections. Thus, an untimely and excessive inflammatory response abolishes normal hematopoiesis, promoting selective expansion of a preleukemic clone (Figure 2) because of proliferative advantage and increased likelihood for a second mutation required for the development of the disease to occur [33]. In turn, early childhood infections or vaccination may reduce the likelihood of leukemia [90]. Importantly, the major histocompatibility genes might play a role in the linkage between patterns of infection and leukemia risk, as several HLA haplotypes have been associated with childhood leukemia [3]. However, other studies have suggested that major histocompatibility complex-defined variation in immune-mediated response is unlikely to be a major risk factor [91].

Aberrant RAG activity resulting in genomic rearrangements may be a crucial secondary mechanism leading to B-cell ALL. Aberrant RAG activities can result in various oligoclonal V(D)J recombination events and the inactivation of genes required for B-lineage differentiation [87]. A clear link between RAG and childhood leukemia through inflammatory mechanisms has been recently reported [89], further connecting immune system-RAG-childhood leukemia.

ROLE OF ACETYLCHOLINESTERASE IN LEUKEMOGENESIS

Moderate acetylcholine (ACh) levels are crucial for controlling immune and inflammatory functions in peripheral tissues. An increase in ACh above a certain threshold can suppress the production of pro-inflammatory cytokines. Acetylcholinesterase (AChE) contributes to regulating ACh levels and, thus, modulates inflammation [92]. In particular, ACh produced by the vagus nerve and/or by peripheral leukocytes [93] can potently modulate several classical immune reactions by activating the α7-nicotinic ACh receptor on the leukocyte membrane, which in turn blocks the nuclear factor kappa B (NF-κB)-mediated production of pro-inflammatory cytokines, such as IL1β and tumor necrosis factor alpha [92]. Because mesenchymal stromal/stem cells carry both nicotinic and muscarinic ACh receptors [94], niche-derived cholinergic signals may play a role in hematopoiesis by regulating proliferation and apoptosis of HSPCs undergoing erythroid and myeloid differentiation [95].

The *ACHE* gene includes multiple putative binding sites for hematopoietic transcription factors. Alternative splicing gives rise to "synaptic" (AChE-S) multimers, which control ACh levels in the brain and muscles, "erythrocyte" (AChE-E) dimers and stress-induced "read-through" (AChE-R) monomers [96]. AChE-R is involved in cell proliferation, whereas AChE-S can be induced during apoptosis [97]. Under stress responses, blood AChE-R undergoes C-terminal cleavage rendering a C-terminal peptide (ARP) of 55 kDa, which promotes the myeloproliferation and thrombopoiesis characteristics of cellular stress [98]. Because ARP functions as a hemopoietic growth factor promoting proliferation of $CD34^+$ HSPCs, circulating AChE-R and/or ARP might be involved in directing $CD34^+$ HSPCs towards prolonged granulocytosis [96]. Furthermore, *ACHE* has been reported to play a role in hematopoiesis by regulating proliferation, differentiation and apoptosis of erythroid and myeloid progenitors. This might explain, at least in part, the association of perturbations in *ACHE* gene expression with myeloid leukemia [99], particularly after exposure to anticholinesterase insecticides, such as OPs.

ACHE is located on chromosome 7q22 within a critical region subject to non-random chromosomal abnormalities. The remarkable abundance of SINEs (short interspersed elements), in particular Alu repeats, in the *ACHE* locus implies exceptional susceptibility to retrotransposition events, which are assisted by the existence of chromosomal breakages. Alu repeats also facilitate unequal crossing-over, altogether contributing to the instability of this region. Chromosomal rearrangements could result in the loss of upstream transcription factor binding sites and, thus, may affect *ACHE* gene expression under stress or exposure to anti-AChE agents. This explains the reported chromosomal aberrations involving 7q22 in leukemic patients [100]. The proximal promoter of the *ACHE* gene contains consensus motifs for the leukemia-associated factor AML1/Runx1 and c-fos, a transcription factor known to regulate *ACHE* gene expression under stress [101]. Hence, the loss of DNA on chromosome 7 may play a significant role in AML [95,96,97,98,99,100,101,102]. Furthermore, a study of 1880 children with ALL reported that 4% of them had DNA losses involving chromosome 7 [103].

A pivotal role of AChE has been suggested in apoptosis. While the 55-kDa AChE protein is selectively induced during apoptosis, its suppression inhibits apoptosome formation and rescues cells from apoptosis [104]. The 55-kDa AChE protein is negatively regulated by the activation of the phosphatidylinositol-3 kinase (PI3K)/protein kinase B (Akt) pathway [104,105]. This signaling cascade is crucial to cell cycle progression, transcription, translation, differentiation, apoptosis, motility and metabolism [106]. The decrease in AChE activity and the consequent increased level of ACh could cause cholinergic overstimulation and enhance cell proliferation in lung cancer [97]; however, whether a similar effect can occur in leukemogenesis is unknown. On the other hand, AChE can hydrolyze lipid peroxides, raising the possibility that a reduction in enzyme activity increases oxidative stress and cellular damage [97].

CONCLUSIONS

Overall, there is sustained epidemiological evidence to suggest a risk of pediatric leukemia upon exposure (*in utero*and/or after birth) to some classes of pesticides, but scientific/mechanistic studies to definitively support this association are lacking. Pesticides may induce topoisomerase II inhibition or generation of oxidative stress, consistently leading to misrepaired DNA cleavage and further chromosomal aberrations in HSPCs. This early molecular event might be sufficient for triggering infant leukemia, but not childhood leukemia, which requires further postnatal events for overt disease. The combination of epidemiological and case-based genomic studies together with cell biology analyses would be useful to elucidate the etiology of pediatric leukemia. In particular, this approach would help to better understand the biological and genetic evidence that is pertinent to the mechanisms by which pesticides might impact on the risk of pediatric leukemia.

ACKNOWLEDGMENTS

Antonio F. Hernández research was partially supported by grants from the Council of Health (PI-0682-2013) and the Council of Innovation (P09-CVI-5062) of the Andalusian Government. Work in Pablo Mendéndez's laboratory is supported by the European Research Council (ERC-2014-CoG-646903), the Spanish Ministry of Economy and Competitiveness (MINECO and Instituto de Salud Carlos III (ISCIII)/Fondo Europeo de Desarrollo regional (FEDER), the Foundation Inocente Inocente, the Spanish Association of Cancer Research, the Catalunya Government (SGR330) and Celgene. Pablo Menéndez also acknowledges financial support from The Obra Social La Caixa-Fundaciò Josep Carreras. Pablo Menéndez is an investigator of the Spanish Cell Therapy cooperative network (Red de Terapia Celular, TERCEL).

CONFLICTS OF INTEREST

The authors declare no conflict of interest.

REFERENCES

1. Hunger, S.P.; Mullighan, C.G. Acute lymphoblastic leukemia in children. *N. Engl. J. Med.* 2015, *373*, 1541–

1552

2. World Health Organization. Incidence of Childhood Leukemia, an ENHIS Fact Sheet, 2009. Available online: http://www.euro.who.int/__data./pdf_file/0005/97016/4.1.-Incidence-of-childhood-leukaemia-EDITED_layouted.pdf?ua=1 (accessed on 10 February 2016).
3. Wiemels, J. Perspectives on the causes of childhood leukemia. *Chem. Biol. Interact.* 2012, *196*, 59–67.
4. Pandita, A.; Harish, R.; Digra, S.K.; Raina, A.; Sharma, A.A.; Koul, A. Molecular cytogenetics in childhood acute lymphoblastic leukemia: A hospital-based observational study. *Clin. Med. Insights Oncol.* 2015, *9*, 39–42.
5. Yohe, S. Molecular genetic markers in acute myeloid leukemia. *J. Clin. Med.* 2015, *4*, 460–478.
6. Wang, L.D.; Wagers, A.J. Dynamic niches in the origination and differentiation of haematopoietic stem cells.*Nat. Rev. Mol. Cell Biol.* 2011, *12*, 643–655.
7. Emerenciano, M.; Koifman, S.; Pombo-de-Oliveira, M.S. Acute leukemia in early childhood. *Braz. J. Med. Biol. Res.* 2007, *40*, 749–760.
8. Pui, C.H.; Robison, L.L.; Look, A.T. Acute lymphoblastic leukemia. *Lancet* 2008, *371*, 1030–1043.
9. Greaves, M. Infection, immune responses and the etiology of childhood leukemia. *Nat. Rev. Cancer* 2006, *6*, 193–203.
10. Greaves, M.; Müschen, M. Infection and the perils of B-cell activation. *Cancer Discov.* 2015, *5*, 1244–1246.
11. Martín-Lorenzo, A.; Hauer, J.; Vicente-Dueñas, C.; Auer, F.; González-Herrero, I.; García-Ramírez, I.; Ginzel, S.; Thiele, R.; Constantinescu, S.N.; Bartenhagen, C.; *et al.* Infection exposure is a causal factor in B-cell precursor acute lymphoblastic leukemia as a result of Pax5-inherited susceptibility. *Cancer Discov.* 2015, *5*, 1328–1343.
12. Chen, M.; Chang, C.H.; Tao, L.; Lu, C. Residential exposure to pesticide during childhood and childhood cancers: A meta-analysis. *Pediatrics* 2015, *136*, 719–729.
13. Ntzani, E.E.; Chondrogiorgi, M.; Ntritsos, G.; Evangelou, E.; Tzoulaki, I. Literature Review on Epidemiological Studies Linking Exposure to Pesticides and Health Effects. Available online: http://www.efsa.europa.eu/sites/default/files/scientific_output/files/main_documents/497e.pdf (accessed on 25 March 2016).
14. Lu, C.; Liu, X.; Liu, C.; Wang, J.; Li, C.; Liu, Q.; Li, Y.; Li, S.; Sun, S.; Yan, J.; *et al.* Chlorpyrifos induces MLL translocations through caspase 3-dependent genomic instability and topoisomerase II inhibition in human fetal liver hematopoietic stem cells. *Toxicol. Sci.* 2015, *147*, 588–606.
15. Alexander, F.E.; Patheal, S.L.; Biondi, A.; Brandalise, S.; Cabrera, M.E.; Chan, L.C.; Chen, Z.; Cimino, G.; Cordoba, J.C.; Gu, L.J.; *et al.* Transplacental chemical exposure and risk of infant leukemia with *MLL* gene fusion. *Cancer Res.* 2001, *61*, 2542–2546.
16. Pombo-de-Oliveira, M.S.; Koifman, S.; Brazilian Collaborative Study Group of Infant Acute Leukemia. Infant acute leukemia and maternal exposures during pregnancy. *Cancer Epidemiol. Biomark. Prev.* 2006, *15*, 2336–2341.
17. Cavalieri, E.L.; Stack, D.E.; Devanesan, P.D.; Todorovic, R.; Dwivedy, I.; Higginbotham, S.; Johansson, S.L.; Patil, K.D.; Gross, M.L.; Gooden, J.K.; *et al.* Molecular origin of cancer: Catechol estrogen-3,4-quinones as endogenous tumor initiators. *Proc. Natl. Acad. Sci. USA* 1997, *94*, 10937–10942.
18. Ferreira, J.D.; Couto, A.C.; Pombo-de-Oliveira, M.S.; Koifman, S.; Brazilian Collaborative Study Group of Infant Acute Leukemia. *In utero* pesticide exposure and leukemia in Brazilian children <2 years of age. *Environ. Health Perspect.* 2013, *121*, 269–275.
19. Ding, G.; Shi, R.; Gao, Y.; Zhang, Y.; Kamijima, M.; Sakai, K.; Wang, G.; Feng, C.; Tian, Y. Pyrethroid pesticide exposure and risk of childhood acute lymphocytic leukemia in Shanghai. *Environ. Sci. Technol.* 2012, *46*, 13480–13487.
20. Metayer, C.; Colt, J.S.; Buffler, P.A.; Reed, H.D.; Selvin, S.; Crouse, V.; Ward, M.H. Exposure to herbicides in house dust and risk of childhood acute lymphoblastic leukemia. *J. Expo. Sci. Environ. Epidemiol.* 2013, *23*, 363–370.
21. Ma, X.M.; Buffler, P.A.; Gunier, R.B.; Dahl, G.; Smith, M.T.; Reinier, K.; Reynolds, P. Critical windows of exposure to household pesticides and risk of childhood leukemia. *Environ. Health Perspect.* 2002, *110*, 955–960.
22. Slater, M.E.; Linabery, A.M.; Spector, L.G.; Johnson, K.J.; Hilden, J.M.; Heerema, N.A.; Robison, L.L.; Ross, J.A. Maternal exposure to household chemicals and risk of infant leukemia: A report from the Children's Oncology Group. *Cancer Causes Control* 2011, *22*, 1197–1204.
23. Turner, M.C.; Wigle, D.T.; Krewski, D. Residential pesticides and childhood leukemia: A systematic review and meta-analysis. *Environ. Health Perspect.* 2010, *118*, 33–41.
24. Bailey, H.D.; Fritschi, L.; Infante-Rivard, C.; Glass, D.C.; Miligi, L.; Dockerty, J.D.; Lightfoot, T.; Clavel, J.; Roman, E.; Spector, L.G.; *et al.* Parental occupational pesticide exposure and the risk of childhood leukemia in the offspring: Findings from the childhood leukemia international consortium. *Int. J. Cancer* 2014, *135*, 2157–2172.
25. Bailey, H.D.; Infante-Rivard, C.; Metayer, C.; Clavel, J.; Lightfoot, T.; Kaatsch, P.; Roman, E.; Magnani, C.; Spector, L.G.; Th Petridou, E.; *et al.* Home pesticide exposures and risk of childhood leukemia: Findings from the childhood leukemia international consortium. *Int. J. Cancer* 2015, *137*, 2644–2663.
26. Rahden-Staron, I. The inhibitory effect of the fungicides captan and captafol on eukaryotic topoisomerases *in vitro* and lack of recombinagenic activity in the wing spot test of *Drosophila melanogaster*. *Mutat. Res.* 2002, *518*, 205–213.
27. Rahden-Staroń, I.; Czeczot, H.; Kowalska-Loth, B. The ability of thiram to inhibit eukaryotic topoisomerase

II and to damage DNA. *Acta Biochim. Pol.* 1993, *40*, 51–53.

28. Boros, L.G.; Williams, R.D. Isofenphos induced metabolic changes in K562 myeloid blast cells. *Leuk. Res.* 2001,*25*, 883–890.
29. Williams, R.D.; Boros, L.G.; Kolanko, C.J.; Jackman, S.M.; Eggers, T.R. Chromosomal aberrations in human lymphocytes exposed to the anticholinesterase pesticide isofenphos with mechanisms of leukemogenesis. *Leuk. Res.* 2004, *28*, 947–958.
30. Zhang, X.; Wallace, A.D.; Du, P.; Lin, S.; Baccarelli, A.A.; Jiang, H.; Jafari, N.; Zheng, Y.; Xie, H.; Soares, M.B.; *et al.* Genome-wide study of DNA methylation alterations in response to diazinon exposure *in vitro*. *Environ. Toxicol. Pharmacol.* 2012, *34*, 959–968.
31. Ukpebor, J.; Llabjani, V.; Martin, F.L.; Halsall, C.J. Sublethal genotoxicity and cell alterations by organophosphorus pesticides in MCF-7 cells: Implications for environmentally relevant concentrations. *Environ. Toxicol. Chem.* 2011, *30*, 632–639.
32. Sirma, S.; Agaoglu, L.; Yildiz, I.; Cayli, D.; Horgusluoglu, E.; Anak, S.; Yuksel, L.; Unuvar, A.; Celkan, T.; Apak, H.; *et al.* NAD(P)H:quinine oxidoreductase 1 null genotype is not associated with pediatric *de novo* acute leukemia. *Pediatr. Blood Cancer* 2004, *43*, 568–570.
33. Sanjuan-Pla, A.; Bueno, C.; Prieto, C.; Acha, P.; Stam, R.W.; Marschalek, R.; Menéndez, P. Revisiting the biology of infant t(4;11)/MLL-AF4$^+$ B-cell acute lymphoblastic leukemia. *Blood* 2015, *126*, 2676–2685.
34. Das, P.M.; Singal, R. DNA methylation and cancer. *J. Clin. Oncol.* 2004, *22*, 4632–4642.
35. Kamdar, K.Y.; Krull, K.R.; El-Zein, R.A.; Brouwers, P.; Potter, B.S.; Harris, L.L.; Holm, S.; Dreyer, Z.; Scaglia, F.; Etzel, C.J.; *et al.* Folate pathway polymorphisms predict deficits in attention and processing speed after childhood leukemia therapy. *Pediatr. Blood Cancer* 2011, *57*, 454–460.
36. Sharp, L.; Little, J. Polymorphisms in genes involved in folate metabolism and colorectal neoplasia: A HuGE review. *Am. J. Epidemiol.* 2004, *159*, 423–443.
37. Duncan, T.M.; Reed, M.C.; Nijhout, H.F. The relationship between intracellular and plasma levels of folate and metabolites in the methionine cycle: A model. *Mol. Nutr. Food Res.* 2013, *57*, 628–636.
38. Lightfoot, T.J.; Johnston, W.T.; Painter, D.; Simpson, J.; Roman, E.; Skibola, C.F.; Smith, M.T.; Allan, J.M.; Taylor, G.M.; United Kingdom Childhood Cancer Study. Genetic variation in the folate metabolic pathway and risk of childhood leukemia. *Blood* 2010, *115*, 3923–3929.
39. Franco, R.F.; Simões, B.P.; Tone, L.G.; Gabellini, S.M.; Zago, M.A.; Falcão, R.P. The methylenetetrahydrofolate reductase *C677T* gene polymorphism decreases the risk of childhood acute lymphocytic leukemia. *Br. J. Haematol.* 2001, *115*, 616–618.
40. Garte, S.; Taioli, E.; Crosti, F.; Sainati, L.; Barisone, E.; Luciani, M.; Jankovic, M.; Biondi, A.G. Deletion of parental *GST* genes as a possible susceptibility factor in the etiology of infant leukemia. *Leuk. Res.* 2000, *24*, 971–974.
41. Chokkalingam, A.P.; Metayer, C.; Scelo, G.A.; Chang, J.S.; Urayama, K.Y.; Aldrich, M.C.; Guha, N.; Hansen, H.M.; Dahl, G.V.; Barcellos, L.F.; *et al.* Variation in xenobiotic transport and metabolism genes, household chemical exposures, and risk of childhood acute lymphoblastic leukemia. *Cancer Causes Control.* 2012, *23*, 1367–1375.
42. Buffler, P.A.; Kwan, M.L.; Reynolds, P.; Urayama, K.Y. Environmental and genetic risk factors for childhood leukemia: Appraising the evidence. *Cancer Investig.* 2005, *23*, 60–75.
43. Sherborne, A.L.; Hemminki, K.; Kumar, R.; Bartram, C.R.; Stanulla, M.; Schrappe, M.; Petridou, E.; Semsei, A.F.; Szalai, C.; Sinnett, D.; *et al.* Rationale for an international consortium to study inherited genetic susceptibility to childhood acute lymphoblastic leukemia. *Haematologica* 2011, *96*, 1049–1054.
44. Sedelnikova, O.A.; Redon, C.E.; Dickey, J.S.; Nakamura, A.J.; Georgakilas, A.G.; Bonner, W.M. Role of oxidatively induced DNA lesions in human pathogenesis. *Mutat. Res.* 2010, *704*, 152–159.
45. Esperanza, M.; Cid, Á.; Herrero, C.; Rioboo, C. Acute effects of a prooxidant herbicide on the microalga Chlamydomonas reinhardtii: Screening cytotoxicity and genotoxicity endpoints. *Aquat. Toxicol.* 2015, *165*, 210–221.
46. Guanggang, X.; Diqiu, L.; Jianzhong, Y.; Jingmin, G.; Huifeng, Z.; Mingan, S.; Liming, T. Carbamate insecticide methomyl confers cytotoxicity through DNA damage induction. *Food Chem. Toxicol.* 2013, *53*, 352–358.
47. Muniz, J.F.; McCauley, L.; Scherer, J.; Lasarev, M.; Koshy, M.; Kow, Y.W.; Nazar-Stewart, V.; Kisby, G.E. Biomarkers of oxidative stress and DNA damage in agricultural workers: A pilot study. *Toxicol. Appl. Pharmacol.* 2008, *227*, 97–107.
48. Ojha, A.; Srivastava, N. *In vitro* studies on organophosphate pesticides induced oxidative DNA damage in rat lymphocytes. *Mutat. Res. Genet. Toxicol. Environ. Mutagen.* 2014, *761*, 10–17.
49. Kryston, T.B.; Georgiev, A.B.; Pissis, P.; Georgakilas, A.G. Role of oxidative stress and DNA damage in human carcinogenesis. *Mutat. Res.* 2011, *711*, 193–201.
50. Hernández, A.F.; Lacasaña, M.; Gil, F.; Rodríguez-Barranco, M.; Pla, A.; López-Guarnido, O. Evaluation of pesticide-induced oxidative stress from a gene-environment interaction perspective. *Toxicology* 2013, *307*, 95–102.
51. Mostafalou, S.; Abdollahi, M. Pesticides and human chronic diseases: Evidences, mechanisms, and perspectives. *Toxicol. Appl. Pharmacol.* 2013, *268*, 157–177.
52. Woodbine, L.; Brunton, H.; Goodarzi, A.A.; Shibata, A.; Jeggo, P.A. Endogenously induced DNA double strand breaks arise in heterochromatic DNA regions and require ataxia telangiectasia mutated and Artemis for their repair. *Nucleic Acids Res.* 2011, *39*, 6986–6997.

53. Gupta, S.C.; Mishra, M.; Sharma, A.; Deepak Balaji, T.G.; Kumar, R.; Mishra, R.K.; Chowdhuri, D.K. Chlorpyrifos induces apoptosis and DNA damage in *Drosophila* through generation of reactive oxygen species.*Ecotoxicol. Environ. Saf.* 2010, *73*, 1415–1423.
54. Dillon, L.W. Burrow, A.A.; Wang, Y.H. DNA instability at chromosomal fragile sites in cancer. *Curr. Genom.*2010, *11*, 326–337.
55. Thys, R.G.; Lehman, C.E.; Pierce, L.C.; Wang, Y.H. Environmental and chemotherapeutic agents induce breakage at genes involved in leukemia-causing gene rearrangements in human hematopoietic stem/progenitor cells. *Mutat. Res.* 2015, *779*, 86–95.
56. Dillon, L.W.; Pierce, L.C.; Lehman, C.E.; Nikiforov, Y.E.; Wang, Y.H. DNA topoisomerases participate in fragility of the oncogene RET. *PLoS ONE* 2013, *8*, e75741.
57. Deweese, J.E.; Osheroff, N. The DNA cleavage reaction of topoisomerase II: Wolf in sheep's clothing. *Nucleic Acids Res.* 2009, *37*, 738–748.
58. Nambiar, M.; Raghavan, S.C. How does DNA break during chromosomal translocations? *Nucleic Acids Res.*2011, *39* 5813–5825.
59. Wiemels, J.L.; Greaves, M. Structure and possible mechanisms of *TEL-AML1* gene fusions in childhood acute lymphoblastic leukemia. *Cancer Res.* 1999, *59*, 4075–4082.
60. Greaves, M.F.; Wiemels, J. Origins of chromosome translocations in childhood leukemia. *Nat. Rev. Cancer* 2003,*3*, 639–649.
61. Meissner, B.; Bartram, T.; Eckert, C.; Trka, J.; Panzer-Gruemayer, R.; Hermanova, I.; Ellinghaus, E.; Franke, A.; Moericke, A.; Schrauder, A.; *et al.* Frequent and sex-biased deletion of SLX4IP by illegitimate V(D)J-mediated recombination in childhood acute lymphoblastic leukemia. *Hum. Mol. Genet.* 2014, *23*, 590–601.
62. Lieber, M.R. The mechanism of double-strand DNA break repair by the nonhomologous DNA end-joining pathway. *Annu. Rev. Biochem.* 2010, *79*, 181–211.
63. Murray, J.M.; Messier, T.; Rivers, J.; O'Neill, J.P.; Walker, V.E.; Vacek, P.M.; Finette, B.A. VDJ recombinase-mediated TCR β locus gene usage and coding joint processing in peripheral T cells during perinatal and pediatric development. *J. Immunol.* 2012, *189*, 2356–2364.
64. Pinsonneault, R.L.; Vacek, P.M.; O'Neill, J.P.; Finette, B.A. Induction of V(D)J-mediated recombination of an extrachromosomal substrate following exposure to DNA-damaging agents. *Environ. Mol. Mutagen.* 2007, *48*, 440–450.
65. Ernst, P.; Wang, J.; Korsmeyer, S.J. The role of MLL in hematopoiesis and leukemia. *Curr. Opin. Hematol.* 2002, *9*, 282–287.
66. Marchesi, F.; Girardi, K.; Avvisati, G. Pathogenetic, Clinical, and Prognostic Features of Adult t(4;11)(q21;q23)/MLL-AF4 positive B-cell acute lymphoblastic leukemia. *Adv. Hematol.* 2011, *2011*, 621627.
67. Nanya, M.; Sato, M.; Tanimoto, K.; Tozuka, M.; Mizutani, S.; Takagi, M. Dysregulation of the DNA damage response and KMT2A rearrangement in fetal liver hematopoietic cells. *PLoS ONE* 2015, *10*, e0144540.
68. Strick, R.; Strissel, P.L.; Borgers, S.; Smith, S.L.; Rowley, J.D. Dietary bioflavonoids induce cleavage in the *MLL*gene and may contribute to infant leukemia. *Proc. Natl. Acad. Sci. USA* 2000, *97*, 4790–4795.
69. Sallmyr, A.; Fan, J.; Rassool, F.V. Genomic instability in myeloid malignancies: Increased reactive oxygen species (ROS), DNA double strand breaks (DSBs) and error-prone repair. *Cancer Lett.* 2008, *270*, 1–9.
70. Bueno, C.; Catalina, P.; Melen, G.J.; Montes, R.; Sánchez, L.; Ligero, G.; García-Pérez, J.L.; Menendez, P. Etoposide induces MLL rearrangements and other chromosomal abnormalities in human embryonic stem cells.*Carcinogenesis* 2009, *30*, 1628–1637.
71. Bueno, C.; Montes, R.; Catalina, P.; Rodríguez, R.; Menendez, P. Insights into the cellular origin and etiology of the infant pro-B acute lymphoblastic leukemia with MLL-AF4 rearrangement. *Leukemia* 2011, *25*, 400–410.
72. Eguchi, M.; Eguchi-Ishimae, M.; Knight, D.; Kearney, L.; Slany, R.; Greaves, M. MLL chimeric protein activation renders cells vulnerable to chromosomal damage: An explanation for the very short latency of infant leukemia. *Genes Chromosom. Cancer* 2006, *45*, 754–760.
73. Felix, C.A. Leukemias related to treatment with DNA topoisomerase II inhibitors. *Med. Pediatr. Oncol.* 2001, *36*, 525–535.
74. Menendez, P.; Catalina, P.; Rodríguez, R.; Melen, G.J.; Bueno, C.; Arriero, M.; García-Sánchez, F.; Lassaletta, A.; García-Sanz, R.; García-Castro, J. Bone marrow mesenchymal stem cells from infants with MLL-AF4$^+$ acute leukemia harbor and express the MLL-AF4 fusion gene. *J. Exp. Med.* 2009, *206*, 3131–3141.
75. Spector, L.G.; Xie, Y.; Robison, L.L.; Heerema, N.A.; Hilden, J.M.; Lange, B.; Felix, C.A.; Davies, S.M.; Slavin, J.; Potter, J.D.; *et al.* Maternal diet and infant leukemia: The DNA topoisomerase II inhibitor hypothesis: A report from the children's oncology group. *Cancer Epidemiol. Biomark. Prev.* 2005, *14*, 651–655.
76. Andersson, A.K.; Ma, J.; Wang, J.; Chen, X.; Gedman, A.L.; Dang, J.; Nakitandwe, J.; Holmfeldt, L.; Parker, M.; Easton, J.; *et al.* St. Jude Children's Research Hospital—Washington University Pediatric Cancer Genome Project. The landscape of somatic mutations in infant MLL-rearranged acute lymphoblastic leukemias. *Nat. Genet.* 2015, *47*, 330–337.
77. Driessen, E.M.; van Roon, E.H.; Spijkers-Hagelstein, J.A.; Schneider, P.; de Lorenzo, P.; Valsecchi, M.G.; Pieters, R.; Stam, R.W. Frequencies and prognostic impact of RAS mutations in MLL-rearranged acute lymphoblastic leukemia in infants. *Haematologica* 2013, *98*, 937–944.
78. Dobbins, S.E.; Sherborne, A.L.; Ma, Y.P.; Bardini, M.; Biondi, A.; Cazzaniga, G.; Lloyd, A.; Chubb, D.; Greaves, M.F.; Houlston, R.S. The silent mutational landscape of infant MLL-AF4 pro-B acute lymphoblastic leukemia.*Genes Chromosom.Cancer* 2013, *52*, 954–960.

79. Prelle, C.; Bursen, A.; Dingermann, T.; Marschalek, R. Secondary mutations in t(4;11) leukemia patients. *Leukemia* 2013, *27*, 1425–1427.

80. Prieto, C.; Stam, R.W.; Agraz-Doblas, A.; Ballerini, P.; Camos, M.; Castaño, J.; Marschalek, R.; Bursen, A.; Varela, I.; Bueno, C.; *et al.* Activated KRAS cooperates with MLLAF4 to promote extramedullary engraftment and migration of cord blood CD34+ HSPC but is insufficient to initiate leukemia. *Cancer Res.* 2016. in press.

81. Bardini, M.; Woll, P.S.; Corral, L.; Luc, S.; Wittmann, L.; Ma, Z.; Lo Nigro, L.; Basso, G.; Biondi, A.; Cazzaniga, G.; *et al.* Clonal variegation and dynamic competition of leukemia-initiating cells in infant acute lymphoblastic leukemia with MLL rearrangement. *Leukemia* 2015, *29*, 38–50.

82. Stumpel, D.J.; Schneider, P.; van Roon, E.H.; Pieters, R.; Stam, R.W. Absence of global hypomethylation in promoter hypermethylated *Mixed Lineage Leukemia*-rearranged infant acute lymphoblastic leukemia. *Eur. J. Cancer* 2013, *49*, 175–184.

83. Stam, R.W.; Schneider, P.; Hagelstein, J.A.; van der Linden, M.H.; Stumpel, D.J.; de Menezes, R.X.; de Lorenzo, P.; Valsecchi, M.G.; Pieters, R. Gene expression profiling-based dissection of *MLL* translocated and *MLL*germline acute lymphoblastic leukemia in infants. *Blood* 2010, *115*, 2835–2844.

84. Bhojwani, D.; Yang, J.J.; Pui, C.H. Biology of childhood acute lymphoblastic leukemia. *Pediatr. Clin. N. Am.*2015, *62*, 47–60.

85. Greaves, M. *In utero* origins of childhood leukemia. *Early Hum. Dev.* 2005, *81*, 123–129.

86. Greaves, M. Childhood leukemia. *BMJ* 2002, *324*, 283–287.

87. Papaemmanuil, E.; Rapado, I.; Li, Y.; Potter, N.E.; Wedge, D.C.; Tubio, J.; Alexandrov, L.B.; van Loo, P.; Cooke, S.L.; Marshall, J.; *et al.* RAG-mediated recombination is the predominant driver of oncogenic rearrangement in ETV6-RUNX1 acute lymphoblastic leukemia. *Nat. Genet.* 2014, *46*, 116–125.

88. Teitell, M.A.; Pandolfi, P.P. Molecular genetics of acute lymphoblastic leukemia. *Annu. Rev. Pathol.* 2009, *4*, 175–198.

89. Swaminathan, S.; Klemm, L.; Park, E.; Papaemmanuil, E.; Ford, A.; Kweon, S.M.; Trageser, D.; Hasselfeld, B.; Henke, N.; Mooster, J.; *et al.* Mechanisms of clonal evolution in childhood acute lymphoblastic leukemia. *Nat. Immunol.* 2015, *16*, 766–774.

90. Ma, X.; Does, M.B.; Metayer, C.; Russo, C.; Wong, A.; Buffler, P.A. Vaccination history and risk of childhood leukemia. *Int. J. Epidemiol.* 2005, *34*, 1100–1109.

91. Hosking, F.J.; Leslie, S.; Dilthey, A.; Moutsianas, L.; Wang, Y.; Dobbins, S.E.; Papaemmanuil, E.; Sheridan, E.; Kinsey, S.E.; Lightfoot, T.; *et al.* MHC variation and risk of childhood B-cell precursor acute lymphoblastic leukemia. *Blood* 2011, *117*, 1633–1640.

92. Gilboa-Geffen, A.; Hartmann, G.; Soreq, H. Stressing hematopoiesis and immunity: An acetylcholinesterase window into nervous and immune system interactions. *Front. Mol. Neurosci.* 2012, *5*, 30.

93. Rosas-Ballina, M.; Olofsson, P.S.; Ochani, M.; Valdés-Ferrer, S.I.; Levine, Y.A.; Reardon, C.; Tusche, M.W.; Pavlov, V.A.; Andersson, U.; Chavan, S.; *et al.* Acetylcholine-synthesizing T cells relay neural signals in a vagus nerve circuit. *Science* 2011, *334*, 98–101.

94. Hoogduijn, M.J.; Cheng, A.; Genever, P.G. Functional nicotinic and muscarinic receptors on mesenchymal stem cells. *Stem Cells Dev.* 2009, *18*, 103–112.

95. Stephenson, J.; Czepulkowski, B.; Hirst, W.; Mufti, G.J. Deletion of the acetylcholinesterase locus at 7q22 associated with myelodysplastic syndromes (MDS) and acute myeloid leukemia (AML). *Leuk. Res.* 1996, *20*, 235–241.

96. Grisaru, D.; Pick, M.; Perry, C.; Sklan, E.H.; Almog, R.; Goldberg, I.; Naparstek, E.; Lessing, J.B.; Soreq, H.; Deutsch, V. Hydrolytic and nonenzymatic functions of acetylcholinesterase comodulate hemopoietic stress responses. *J. Immunol.* 2006, *176*, 27–35.

97. Xi, H.J.; Wu, R.P.; Liu, J.J.; Zhang, L.J.; Li, Z.S. Role of acetylcholinesterase in lung cancer. *Thorac. Cancer* 2015, *6*, 390–398.

98. Deutsch, V.R.; Pick, M.; Perry, C.; Grisaru, D.; Hemo, Y.; Golan-Hadari, D.; Grant, A.; Eldor, A.; Soreq, H. The stress-associated acetylcholinesterase variant AChE-R is expressed in human CD34+ hematopoietic progenitors and its C-terminal peptide ARP promotes their proliferation. *Exp. Hematol.* 2002, *30*, 1153–1161.

99. Soreq, H.; Patinkin, D.; Lev-Lehman, E.; Grifman, M.; Ginzberg, D.; Eckstein, F.; Zakut, H. Antisense oligonucleotide inhibition of acetylcholinesterase gene expression induces progenitor cell expansion and suppresses hematopoietic apoptosis *ex vivo*. *Proc. Natl. Acad. Sci. USA* 1994, *91*, 7907–7911.

100. Shapira, M.; Grant, A.; Korner, M.; Soreq, H. Genomic and transcriptional characterization of the human ACHE locus: Complex involvement with acquired and inherited diseases. *Isr. Med. Assoc. J.* 2000, *2*, 470–473.

101. Perry, C.; Sklan, E.H.; Birikh, K.; Shapira, M.; Trejo, L.; Eldor, A.; Soreq, H. Complex regulation of acetylcholinesterase gene expression in human brain tumors. *Oncogene* 2002, *21*, 8428–8441.

102. Johnson, E.; Cotter, F.E. Monosomy 7 and 7q—Associated with myeloid malignancy. *Blood Rev.* 1997, *11*, 46–55.

103. Heerema, N.A.; Nachman, J.B.; Sather, H.N.; La, M.K.; Hutchinson, R.; Lange, B.J.; Bostrom, B.; Steinherz, P.G.; Gaynon, P.S.; Uckun, F.M.; *et al.* Deletion of 7p or monosomy 7 in pediatric acute lymphoblastic leukemia is an adverse prognostic factor: A report from the Children's Cancer Group. *Leukemia* 2004, *18*, 939–947.

104. Xie, J.; Jiang, H.; Wan, Y.H.; Du, A.Y.; Guo, K.J.; Liu, T.; Ye, W.Y.; Niu, X.; Wu, J.; Dong, X.Q.; *et al.* Induction of a 55 kDa acetylcholinesterase protein during apoptosis and its negative regulation by the Akt pathway. *J. Mol. Cell. Biol.* 2011, *3*, 250–259.

105. Zhang, X.J.; Greenberg, D.S. Acetylcholinesterase

involvement in apoptosis. *Front. Mol. Neurosci.* 2012, *5*, 40.

106. Martelli, A.M., Evangelisti, C.; Chiarini, F.; McCubrey, J.A. The phosphatidylinositol 3-kinase/Akt/mTOR signaling network as a therapeutic target in acute myelogenous leukemia patients. *Oncotarget* 2010, *1*, 89–103.

CHAPTER 18

DIG1 PROTECTS AGAINST CELL DEATH PROVOKED BY GLYPHO SATE-BASED HERBICIDES IN HUMAN LIVER CELL LINES

Gasnier C, Benachour N, Clair E, Travert C, Langlois F, Laurant C, Decroix-Laporte C, Séralini GE.

BACKGROUND

Roundup (R) is the most widely used non-selective herbicide worldwide. It is comprised of a mixture of an isopropylamine salt of glyphosate (G) and adjuvants. G is considered as the active ingredient of R, although quantitatively it is a minor constituent, which is not supposed to be toxic alone in mammals [1]. Various adjuvants are present in R as secret of formulations [2], amplifying and thus allowing the G herbicide action, as well as its unintended toxic and endocrine disrupting effects in human placental cells [3]. The adjuvants, which are chosen from a long list that can vary from formulation to formulation [4], stabilize and help G penetration into cells. Among these are benzisothiazolone, isobutene, light aromatic petroleum distillate, methyl pyrrolidinone, polyethoxylated tallowamine or alkylamine (POEA), etc [2]. Some of these compounds may be genotoxic or form adducts with DNA [5]. It is thus important to compare different R formulations when studying this herbicide's toxicity. Moreover R residues are quite stable in rivers and soils [1]. G and its metabolite AMPA (aminomethyl phosphonic acid) are among the primary pollutants of surface waters (IFEN, 2006); they also enter the food chain [6]. These chemicals are found in the urine of agricultural workers [7]. The use of this herbicide is increasing as more than 75% of genetically modified edible plants have been designed to be used in conjunction with R. These plants are engineered to tolerate high intracellular levels of R [8]. We have also shown that the human embryonic kidney 293 cell line was even more sensitive to R, this was dose- and time-dependent [4]; and thus it was hypothesized that this could explain pregnancy outcomes and miscarriages reported for agricultural workers using G-based herbicides [9]. This is consistent with the fact that G-based herbicides have recently been shown to be endocrine disruptors in cell lines [10].

We know that xenobiotics have a main endpoint in the liver, which is the major detoxification organ. Here, we investigated the mechanism of action of R in the human liver cell lines available, HepG2 and Hep3B, which have been used as a model system to study xenobiotic toxicity, most prominently HepG2 [11, 12]. We wanted to compare in the first instance the actions of four R formulations on both cell lines and then to detail the enzymatic pathways activated in HepG2.

Detoxifying mechanisms are frequently enhanced by plant extracts, which can provide additional protection against radicals and electrophilic compounds [13, 14]. We have tested the ability of a new drug described for the first time, Dig1 (D),

Citation: Céline Gasnier, Nora Benachour, Emilie Clair, Carine Travert, Frédéric Langlois, Claire Laurant, Cécile Decroix-Laporte and Gilles-Eric Séralini, Dig1 protects against cell death provoked by glyphosate-based herbicides in human liver cell lines, DOI: 10.1186/1745-6673-5-29

to protect cells from R intoxication. D contains plant extracts from *Taraxacum officinalis*, *Arctium lappa* and *Berberis vulgaris*. These herbal preparations were chosen in particular for their digestive detoxification or hepato-protective effects [15, 16, 17, 18, 19, 20]. It was thus interesting to compare these general findings on plant extracts to some biochemically precise markers that could be modified in human hepatocytes, such as caspases 3/7, cytochromes P450, glutathione S-transferase (GST), and mitochondrial succinate dehydrogenase (SD), in order to detail the pathway(s) of action(s) of these mixtures used as medicinal plants *in vivo*, and thus to explore their cellular protective potential.

METHODS

1. Chemicals

Four main R formulations which have been used in agriculture (Monsanto, Anvers, Belgium) have been chosen in this study: Express® 7.2 g/l of G called glyphosate or N-(phosphonomethyl) glycine, product number 2010321; Bioforce® 360 g/l of G, product number 9800036; GT® 400 g/l of G, product number 8800425; GT+® 450 g/l of G, product number 2020448. The various herbicide formulations were prepared in Eagle›s modified minimum essential medium (EMEM; Abcys, Paris, France), with 10% calf fetal serum from Cambrex (Verviers, Belgium) otherwise specified. G was from Sigma-Aldrich (Saint Quentin Fallavier, France), its called «2% solution» was equivalent in concentration to 2% R Bioforce® and was prepared in serum free-medium, and adjusted to pH 5.8 of 2% R. D is a mixture of diluted plant extracts obtained by Sevene Pharma (Monoblet, France) from original independent macerates corresponding to 1/10 of dried plants in a water-alcohol solution of 45 to 55%. They are afterwards diluted in 70% alcohol with *Taraxacum officinalis* macerate at 10^{-4}, *Arctium lappa* at 10^{-4} and *Berberis vulgaris* at 10^{-5}. D is prepared in the medium at 2% of the mixture in positive controls. The 3-(4,5-Dimethylthiazol-2-yl)-2,5-diphenyl tetrazolium bromide (MTT) and all other compounds, unless otherwise specified, were from Sigma-Aldrich. The MTT stock solution at 5 mg/ml in phosphate-buffered saline was diluted 10-fold in serum-free EMEM and then filtered through a 0.22 μm filter.

2. Cell cultures, Roundup and/or Dig1 exposures

The hepatoma cell lines HepG2 and Hep3B were provided by ECACC, numbers 85011430 and 86062703, respectively. They are from Caucasian and Negroid hepatoma origins (from 15- and 8-year-old children respectively). Cells were grown in flasks of 75 cm² surface from Dutscher (Brumath, France) in phenol red-free EMEM containing 2 mM glutamine, 1% non-essential amino acid, 100 U/ml of antibiotics (mix of penicillin, streptomycin) and 10% fetal calf serum. For treatments, 50,000 cells were plated per well and grown at 37°C (5% CO_2, 95% air) during a period of 48 h to 80% confluence in 48-well plates (except in Figure1, 24-well plates were used). The cells were then exposed (24-72 h) to various concentrations of tested chemicals, which were replaced every 24 h for D studies. D was at 2%. For cytochromes and GST studies, before S9 fractions preparations, cells were treated in 25 ml and in 175 cm² flasks at 80% confluence. In this case after 24 h, another 25 ml was added as the second treatment. In all cases, medium M was used as control and R was present at the LC50, which was 25 ppm for R400 in these conditions, far below doses recommended in agriculture (1-2%, i.e. 10,000-20,000 ppm).

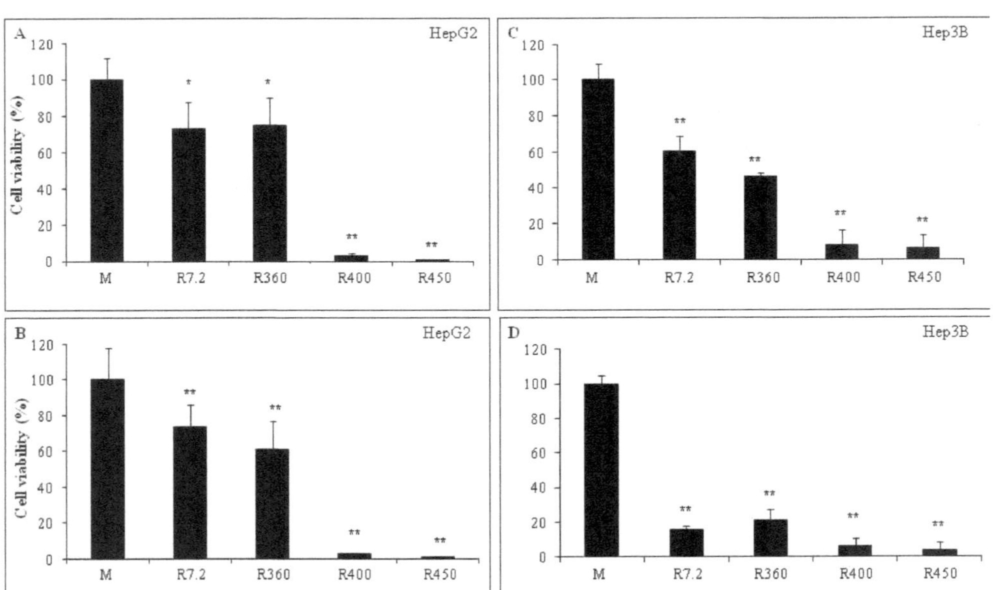

Figure 1: **Time-dependent effects of different Roundup formulations on HepG2 and Hep3B cell viability.** The formulations were applied during 24 h (A and C) or 48 h (B and D). These effects were evaluated by the MTT test (see Methods), measuring mitochondrial succinate dehydrogenase activity. The results are presented in percent compared to non treated cells (M). Cells were grown at 37°C (5% CO_2, 95% air) in medium EMEM with 10% serum during 48 h to 80% confluence in 24-well plates, and then exposed to 4 different Roundup formulations. On x axis, concentrations of G in R in parenthesis: Express® 7.2 g/l of G, Bioforce® 360 g/l of G, GT® 400 g/l of G, GT+® 450 g/l of G, all at 0.5%. All experiments were repeated 3 times in triplicates. Statistically significant differences are calculated in comparison to control by a student *t*-test $p < 0.01$(**) and $p < 0.05$(*).

3. S9 fractions

The medium was removed, and cells dislodged by treatment with 7 ml of trypsin-EDTA (Lonza, France) and washed (PBS, Eurobio, France) twice by centrifugations (70 *g*, 5 min), at room temperature. Cells were then resuspended in 500 µl of 50 mM phosphate buffer pH 7.5 with 0.25 M sucrose, 1 mM DTT, homogenized and centrifuged at 9,000 *g*, 4°C for 30 min. The supernatants corresponding to the S9 fractions (membrane and cytosolic enzymes) were collected and frozen at -80°C until further evaluation for enzyme activities. Protein concentration was determined in each S9 fraction according to the Bicinchoninic Acid Protein Assay (Sigma, France).

4. Cell death measurement

The enzymatic MTT test is based on the cleavage of MTT into blue formazan by the mitochondrial enzyme succinate-dehydrogenase [21, 22], it was used to evaluate human cell viability as described in our group [23]. The optical density was measured using a luminometer (Mithras LB 940, Berthold, France) at 570 nm. The crude protective actions were evaluated at the end of the treatment, by comparing the toxicity of R after treatment by D or not. As R toxicity is induced at the chosen LC50, the relative efficiency of the protective effect (recovering) is the percentage of recovered viability in the presence of D in comparison to the maximal toxic effect at LC50.

5. Caspase 3/7 activity measurement

The Caspase-Glo® 3/7 assay (Promega, Paris, France) in 96-well white plates (Dutscher, France) was a luminescent method designed for automated high-throughput screening of caspases activity, which is a measure of apoptosis. This method can measure caspase-3 and -7 activities in purified enzyme preparations or cultures of adherent or suspended cells [24, 25, 26]. The assay provides a pro-luminescent caspase-3/7 substrate, which contains the tetrapeptide sequence DEVD. This substrate is cleaved to release amino-luciferin, a substrate for luciferase, and the production of light is proportional to the quantity of amino-luciferin released and therefore proportional to caspase. The Caspase-Glo® 3/7 reagent has been optimized for caspase activity, luciferase activity and cell lysis. The addition of the single Caspase-Glo® 3/7 reagent, in an «add-mix-measure» format, results in cell lysis followed by caspase cleavage of the substrate and generation of a «glow-type» luminescent signal. After cell cultures were exposed to 50 µL of various dilutions, an equal volume of Caspase-Glo® 3/7 reagent was added to each well. Plates were then agitated 15 min and incubated 45 min at room temperature in the dark, to stabilize the signal before measuring luminescence. The negative control was the serum-free medium, the positive control was the active Caspase-Glo® 3/7 reagent mixed with cells treated only with serum-free medium to determine the basal activity of the caspases 3/7. Luminescence was measured using the luminometer Mithras LB 940 (Berthold, Thoiry, France) at 565 nm.

6. Cytochrome P450 activity measurement

The cytochrome P450 3A4, 2C9, 1A2 and 1A1 activities were quantified by the P450 Glo™ Assays (Promega, France), as described by Yueh *et al.* [27]. Each Cytochrome P450/1 M KPO_4/Substrate Reaction mixture containing the S9 fractions (duplicate) was pre-incubated at 37°C for 10 min in white 96-well plates (Dutscher, France). The Cytochrome P450 CYP1A1 Reaction mixture contained 135 µg of the human liver S9 fraction as control (Tebu-Bio, France) or cell S9 fraction with 60 µM luciferin-conjugated substrate (luciferin-6›-chloroethyl ether) and 200 mM KPO_4 buffer in a final volume of 25 µl. For CYP1A2 130 µg S9 fractions were used with 200 µM substrate of luciferin-6›-methylether; for CYP2C9 160 µg S9 and 200 µM substrate of 6›-deoxy luciferin but with 50 mM KPO_4 buffer in 25 µl. CYP3A4 was measured with 170 µg S9 with 100 µM substrate of luciferin-6›-benzylether but with 400 mM KPO_4 in 25 µl. The enzymatic reaction was initiated by adding 25 µl of NADPH regenerating system to each well. It contained 2.6 mM $NADP^+$, 6.6 mM glucose-6-phosphate, 0.8 U/ml glucose-6-phosphate dehydrogenase and 6.6 mM $MgCl_2$.

The plate was then incubated at 37°C for 20 min for CYP1A1 and CYP1A2, and, for 30 min for CYP2C9 and CYP3A4. The reconstituted Luciferin Detection reagent (50 µl) was added before mixing for 10 s and incubating at room temperature for 90 min in order to stabilize the luminescent signal. The luminescence was then read with a luminometer (Veritas Turner Biosystems). Three independent experiments were carried out using three independent batches of S9 fractions.

7. GST activity measurement

The protocol was adapted from Habig *et al.* [28]. Briefly, 320 µg (50 µl) of the human liver S9 fraction (positive control) or cell S9 fraction was mixed with 10 µl of 100 mM GSH and 930 µl phosphate buffer in duplicate. Reduced L-glutathione (GSH) was dissolved in deionized water; pH 6.5 buffer was prepared by mixing 0.7 volume of 0.1 M KH_2PO_4 and 0.3 volume of 0.1 M Na_2HPO_4. The reaction was initiated by 10 µl of 100 mM 1-chloro-2,4-dinitrobenzene (CDNB) substrate. The CDNB was dissolved in 95% ethanol at a concentration of 100 mM (20.3 mg/ml). After a 90 s incubation at 37°C, the optical density was measured at 340 nm every 30 s for 90 s with a SmartSpec 3000 Spectrophotometer (Bio-Rad, France). Three independent experiments were carried out using three independent batches of S9 fraction.

8. Statistical analysis

The experiments were repeated 3 times in different weeks in triplicate (n = 9) unless otherwise specified. All data are presented as the mean ± standard error (S.E.M.). Statistical differences were determined by a Student unpaired *t*-test using significant levels of $p < 0.01$ (**) and $p < 0.05$ (*).

RESULTS

Figure 1 presents the different time-dependent effects of various R formulations at 0.5% on viability of liver cell lines HepG2 and Hep3B. The R formulations contained different concentrations of both G and various adjuvants. Both cell lines showed approximately similar growth rates for around 32 h in control medium (M). In both cell lines, growth rate was easily disrupted by any R formulation, but different R formulations had different effects. In the case of R7.2 and R360, Hep3B cells were approximately 3-5 times more sensitive than HepG2 over 48 h. However, in the case of R400 and R450 at 0.5% the two cell lines were roughly equal in sensitivity. These two R formulations were found to be most rapid-acting and toxic. Based on this observation these were chosen for use in subsequent experiments. Cell death was estimated by inhibition of succinate-dehydrogenase and thus of mitochondrial metabolism. In both cell lines, mortality increases with G concentrations and time of exposure to all 4 R formulations, however the increase is not proportional to G concentration (insert Figure 2). The first two formulations demonstrate similar toxicities despite having quite different concentrations of G (7.2 and 360 g/l of G, respectively), along with adjuvants; the two other formulations show higher toxicity as previously explained. This dose-dependent effect is clearly illustrated in Figure 2 with the two groups of decreasing curves with the two families of R (R400 and R450 on one side, first toxic family, and R7.2 and R360 on the other). It also becomes obvious that G has no toxic action alone under the conditions used in this study (empty squares, Figure 2).

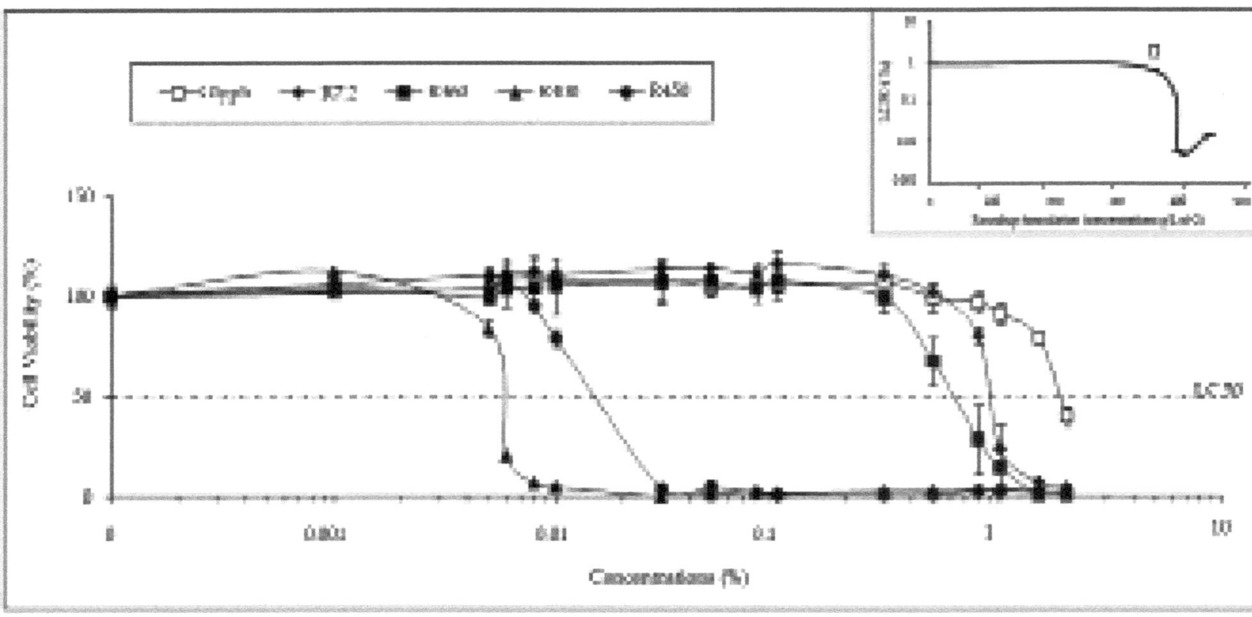

Figure 2: Dose-dependent effects of Glyphosate and different Roundup formulations on HepG2 viability. The formulations were applied during 24 h without serum (even for G) in 48-well plates, after reaching 80% confluence with serum-containing medium. These effects and the formulations with G concentrations (7.2 to 450 g/l) indicated with symbols were evaluated as described in Fig. 1. All experiments were repeated 4 times in triplicates. The curve in frame summarizes the nonlinear dose effects of R formulations on HepG2. The LC50 (%) values are compared for the 4 R and G (in similar conditions) as a function of G concentrations in the formulations. The LC50 for G alone is indicated by the empty square above the curve.

We identified the LC50 of R400 (GT®) in 24 h in 48-well plates as being 40 ppm for Hep3B and 96 ppm for HepG2. No difference was seen between HepG2 and Hep3B cells in their sensitivity to R400 when exposed at relatively high concentrations in Figure 1. Titrations to determine the LC50 of R400 revealed clearly that Hep3B cells were more sensitive to R400 than were HepG2. We then tested the impact of 2% D at these conditions of R intoxication (Figure 3). We confirmed R400 toxicity to hepatocyte-derived cell lines exposed at the LC50 for 24 h, and found that D was able to prevent this toxicity. First, we demonstrated that D alone was not toxic, at 2% for as long as 72 h, nor was it able to inhibit mitochondrial metabolism (data not shown). Then we observed that pre-treatment with D (in comparison to control M) had a time-amplified protective effect from the most toxic R. After 24 h of D exposure and 24 h of R, the efficiency of protective action of D reached 43% for Hep3B, and 55% for HepG2. After 48 h of D and 24 h of R, the efficiency of D reached 62% and 89% respectively. These effects were proportional to time (compare curve DRM to RMM). No curative effect (positive D action after R) was observed under these conditions with these cells since post-treatment with D did not influence R toxicity (curves are superimposed with RMM, see Figure 3, legend).

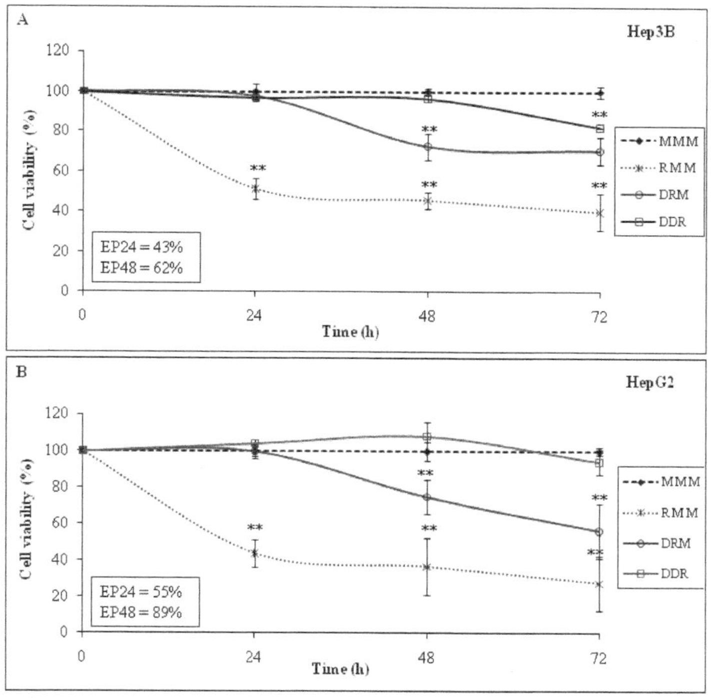

Figure 3: Dig1 general preventive effect of R400 toxicity on Hep3B and HepG2 during 72 h. In frames on the right, each letter (M, R or D) indicates 24 h of successive cell exposures to the corresponding conditions (Medium alone, Roundup, Dig1). The results were evaluated as in Fig. (**1**). To measure preventive effects, D at 2% was applied during 24 or 48 h before R (400 g/l at LC50 in these conditions, 40 ppm for Hep3B and 96 ppm for HepG2): corresponding treatments called DRM or DDR. R was applied alone as negative control during 24 or 72 h (RMM, RRR), or before D to assess curative effects (RDM, RMD or RDD), all these curves are superimposed, and thus only RMM is shown as negative control. No curative effect is evidenced in these conditions. Efficiencies of protection (EP) after 24 or 48 h of treatment by D are indicated in frames.

The mechanism was studied in more detail in HepG2 where the enzymes are better characterized and assessed. First, we evaluated the time-course for onset of the preventive effect of D, by incubating cells with D and removing it before R addition (Figure 4). We show that the efficiency of protection of D is established (53% in this case) at 24 h, but can be observed as early as 6 h after adding D to cells. At this time, protection from the toxicity of R was significant. We then investigated what might be the metabolic target of the protective effect of D. Caspases 3/7 are shown in Figure 5 to be activated up to 156% by 24 h exposure to R and up to 765% by 48 h exposure (comparison was to the control M at 24 h and MM at 48 h). After 24 h of exposure, if R is replaced by M, the caspases recover in 24 h to their initial activity. Figure 5shows that D does not induce caspases itself, but appears to prevent induction of caspases by R (DR). Considering caspases activities as an early sign of apoptosis, these results confirm lack of D toxicity and the ability of D to protect from R toxicity.

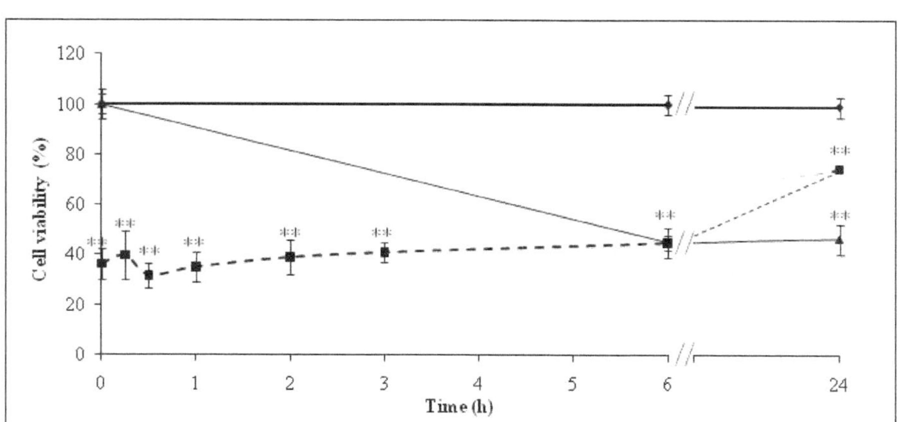

Figure 4: Time necessary for Dig1 pre-incubation to achieve a significant preventive effect of subsequent R intoxication. The study is performed with R400 intoxication on HepG2, cell viability is measured as in Fig. (**1**). First D (2% - dotted line with squares) was applied (time on × axis) 15, 30 min, 1 to 24 h before R400 (96 ppm during 24 h - grey line with triangles), in comparison to M (black line with diamonds). More than 40% viability (R effect in these conditions) is obtained only after at least 6 h of D exposure (increasing dotted line).

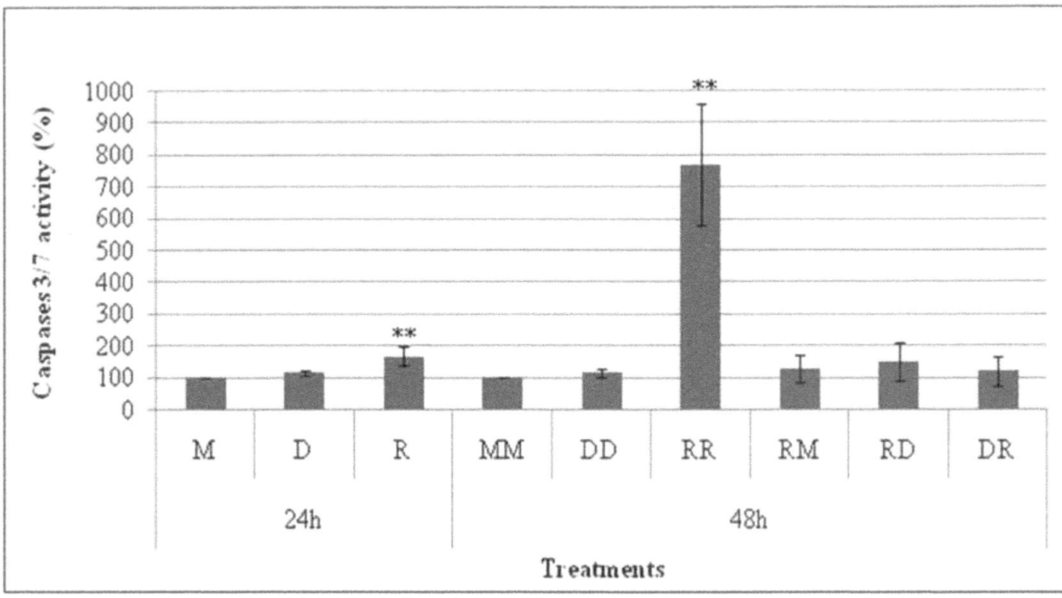

Figure 5: Roundup and Digl on HepG2 caspase 3/7 activity. These effects were evaluated by the caspases Glo® 3/7 assay, the results are presented in percent compared to untreated cells (M). Cells were grown at 37°C (5% $C0_2$, 95% air) in serum containing medium during 48 h to 80% confluence in 96-well plates, and then exposed to different treatments (R450: 60 ppm, D 2%) without serum. The formulation was applied during 24 h (M, D, R) or 48 h (MM to DR).

In addition to caspases, we examined the effects of R on cytochromes, finding that R does not activate all cytochromes but is able to enhance more specifically CYP3A4 (to 240-360%) and to a lesser extent CYP1A2 (to 130-170%, Figure 6). D does not enhance these cytochromes by itself (RD versus RM, Figure 6); but it weakly increases CYP2C9 in combination with R (to 140%), when added after it, even though this is not statistically different from RM treatment (but from control M alone). Once again, based on this additional parameter, D confirmed its ability to block R toxicity: if D is applied before R no cytochrome activity was stimulated, CYP2C9 was even weakly inhibited (40%). By contrast, in Figure 7, it is shown that R inhibits GST almost by half, and D does not modify this effect either before or after R treatment. Figure 8summarizes the results obtained on the different pathways of R and D actions on HepG2.

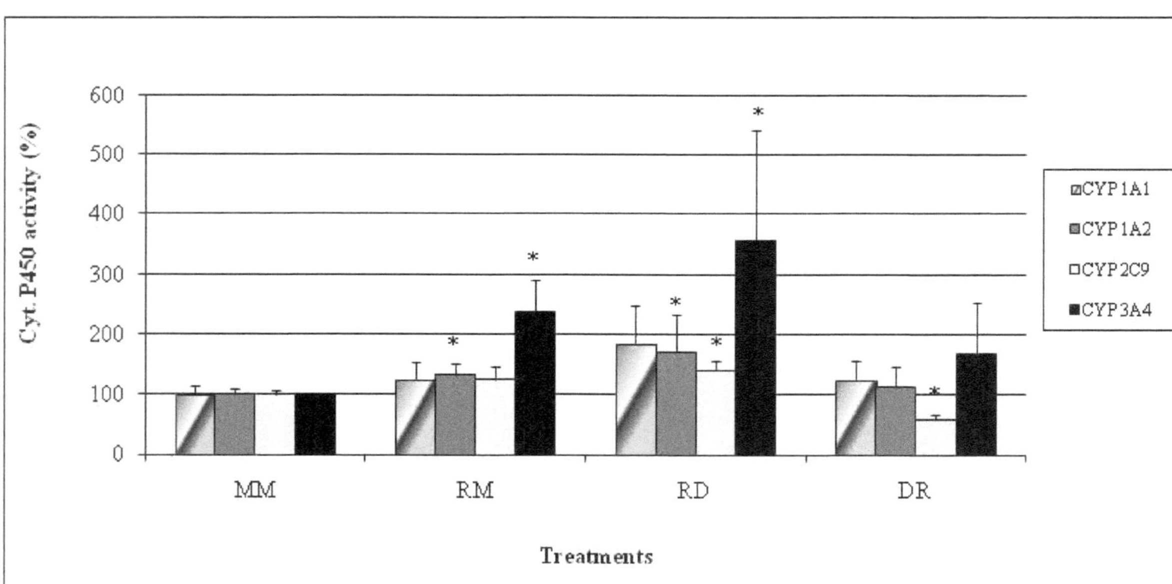

Figure 6: Roundup and Digl on HepG2 Cytochromes P450 activities. These effects were evaluated by the P450 Glo® assay, the results are presented as percent relative to control (MM). Cells were treated before S9 fractions preparations in 25 ml and in 175 cm^2-flasks at 80% confluence. After 24 h of M, R (LC50 of R400, 25 ppm in these conditions) or D (2%), another 25 ml was added as the second treatment.

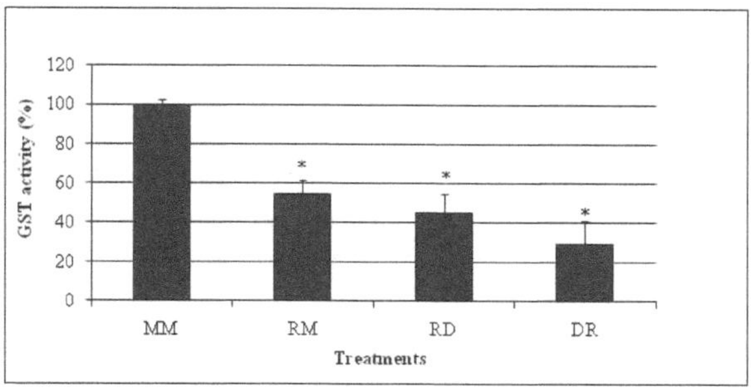

Figure 7: Roundup and Dig1 on HepG2 glutathione-S-transferase activity. The results are presented in percent compared to untreated cells (MM). Cells were treated before S9 fractions preparations in 25 ml and in 175 cm^2-flasks at 80% confluence. After 24 h of M, R (LC50 of R400, 25 ppm in these conditions) or D (2%), another 25 ml was added as the second treatment.

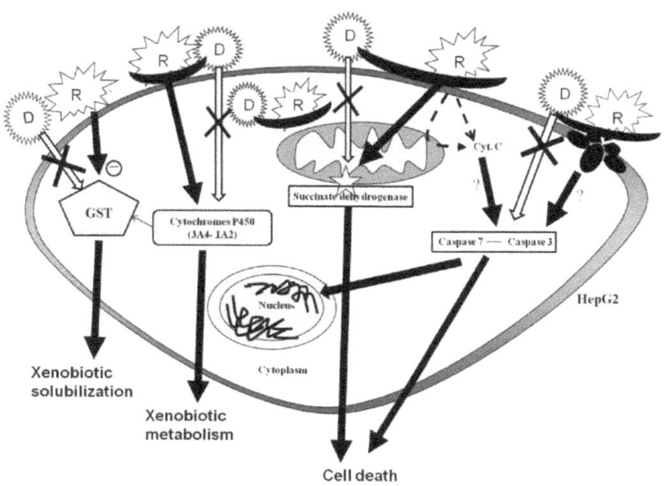

Figure 8: Roundup (R) mechanisms of action and prevention by Dig1 (D) in human hepatocytes HepG2. The different pathways of action identified in this research are summarized with black arrows: action via on mitochondrial succinate dehydrogenase, and action via caspases 3/7 inducing cell death (directly or indirectly through cytochrome C, and possibly via death cell receptors), action via cytochromes CYP3A4 and CYP1A2 stimulating the formation of metabolites, and finally action via the inhibition of Glutathione-S-transferase (GST) blocking metabolites derivatization and excretion. D does not act itself at these levels (crossed empty arrows) but prevents R toxicity (black thick lines).

DISCUSSION

This work evidences for the first time the effects of several formulations of the major herbicide worldwide (R) on human hepatic cell lines available, which are widely recognized as models to study xenobiotic actions. We tested R at sub-agricultural levels; the LC50 measured in this work is 10 times for Hep3B and 4 times for HepG2 below the maximum level of residues authorized in some feed (400 ppm, [29]). We found that the cell sensitivity depended on the nature of the R formulation. Both cell lines have retained the activities of the drug metabolism phase I and phase II enzymes involved in activation and detoxification of genotoxic carcinogens [30, 31]. HepG2 cells are in general considered a better model since they have three-fold higher levels of CYP1A1 and glutathione-S-transferase (GST) than Hep3B [32]. For instance, it was observed that HepG2 are more sensitive than Hep3B to cisplatin [33], to dietary genotoxins [32] and to genotoxicants [12]. In our hands it was the opposite for R, overall in 48 h. In fact, both cell lines are from different genetic origins, from different boys at different ages, and thus have specific enzymatic equipments including cytochromes P450. Greater sensitivity was observed with Hep3B. It was thus important to obtain results in both lines that confirmed R toxicity in all human models tested up to now, including embryonic 293 cells, umbilical cord cells, placental derived JEG3 cells and microsomes from fresh placenta [3, 4, 34]. It was evidenced that cell death increased with time of exposure for all R formulations, this phenomenon shows that the threshold of toxicity depends not only on the dose but also on time, as previously clearly demonstrated on embryonic and placental cells [4]. It was also shown that toxicity was dependent on the nature of the adjuvants present in different R formulations. Moreover, the action of serum only temporarily buffered R toxicity. We found that serum-free culture medium revealed essentially the same xenobiotic impacts that are visible 1-2 days later in serum. Thus, although the timecourse of action is delayed, the pathways of actions appear similar [4].

Indeed, the G cytotoxic effects do not vary linearly with dose; this demonstrates the differential roles of adjuvants in the amplification of toxicity, since G has no toxicity alone at these concentrations. The adjuvants added to G in various R formulations are considered manufacturing secrets, but obviously do not form an inert part of the composition. One mechanism of adjuvant action is most probably to form detergent vesicles that allow cell membrane opening and penetration of G, and that most probably facilitate bioaccumulation of G, metabolites and adjuvants, and gene disruptive effects, which could explain time-amplified effects. A very small quantity of adjuvants combined with G has been already demonstrated to have similar effects to R [3]. It is a recognized fact that mixtures of xenobiotics have synergistic effects [35]. We observed that whatever the nature of the various adjuvants is in the 4 R formulations, the mechanism of toxicity is similar on several crucial endpoints: namely SD, AK, Caspases 3/7 [34]. Only the threshold of toxicity is different.

In this study, we sought to understand the mechanism of toxicity of the two R formulations that have the most rapid toxic effects on hepatic cells. We also evaluated whether it was possible to prevent R toxicity by D. D is a newly described product comprised of a mixture of extracts from *Taraxacum officinalis*, *Arctium lappa* and *Berberis vulgaris*. *Taraxacum* was cited for protective effects in the digestive system [19, 20], also anti-tumoral [36] and anti-oxydant effects [37]. *Arctium lappa* is also found to be hepato-protective [17,18], as well as *Berberis* [16].

First of all, the lack of D impact on cell viability in comparison to controls indicates that it is not cytotoxic at 2%. It was hypothesized first that either D does not penetrate cells without embedding cell-cell interactions, or it is relatively inert on several important markers of cell function at this concentration. Our results are consistent with D penetrating the cells and not just forming a shield that prevents R from penetrating. This is verified since effective protection by D necessitates more than 6 h of contact, and because D modifies enzymatic activities, as detailed below. As a matter of fact, D shows a clear and very strong efficiency of protective action against the toxicity of R in both hepatic cell lines; protection is up to 89% for HepG2 in 48 h. It is not completely excluded that this important action of D can occur by preventing entrance of R into cells, normally helped by adjuvants. However D clearly has intracellular actions, including prevention of caspases 3/7 activation and CYP3A4 enhancement, both provoked by R. CYP 3A4 was induced by Roundup in comparative manner and in similar time than with other xenobiotics Bisphenol A, DDT and phtalates, respectively [38, 39, 40].

Other metabolic/biochemical effects of D components have also been reported, for instance, the protective effects on acute pancreatitis in rats [20] through IL-6 reduction, as well as the suppression of reactive oxygen species, nitric oxide and lipid oxidation [37]. Polyphenolic compounds present in D are considered hepatoprotective [42, 43, 44] but the time-dependent protective effects on the crucial mitochondrial succinate dehydrogenase and caspases 3 and 7 had not been demonstrated before.

Since HepG2 are more resistant and D more preventive on this line, we decided to detail the signalling pathway of R and D actions in these cells. Moreover, the caspases, cytochromes and GST activities are more fully documented in this hepatic cell line [45, 46, 47]. The measurement of caspase 3/7 activity has been recognized as a marker for apoptosis in HepG2 cells [48].

Caspases 3/7 have been rarely measured in HepG2, and found to be induced 200% by 30 μM Tamoxifen in 24 h [48]. Their induction by R in our study (156% in 24 h and 765% in 48 h) confirms the proposed apoptotic mechanism activated by R. Of course, this does not exclude some necrosis as a primary mode of cell death as we previously showed [34]. Our results also show that D alone does not interfere with caspases but may possibly prevent R impact on these enzymes.

At lower levels and even with the buffering effect of serum already documented [4], D also prevents CYP3A4 induction: CYP3A4 is by far the major target of R among the phase I activating enzymes measured. CYP3A4 is the most abundant P450 expressed (60%) in human liver [49]. It is involved in the bioactivation of environmental procarcinogens, such as aflatoxin B1 [50] and benzo[a]pyrene among a number of others [51]. Some organochlorine pesticides can activate the PXR, a nuclear hormone receptor [52] that regulates CYP3A4 gene transcription in particular in liver. R components may also induce this process. The results with CYP1A2 (slight induction by R) show that its action does not depend on a unique pathway, like the results on CYP2C9. Only a few reports are available on CYP2C9, which is inhibited by extracts of other plants such as pineapple [53].

Similarly, only some xenobiotics such as polychlorobyphenyls inhibit GST; this is typical of estrogen-like effects [54] already observed with R on aromatase [3, 4]. The disruption of xenobiotic metabolism by R in our study, which increased some cytochromes P450 and decreased GST, may alter liver detoxification function, leading to the accumulation of toxic reactive oxydated molecules [54] in a manner that could be prevented by D in this study. In fact, GST inhibition, if R intoxication continues, could lead to the accumulation of reactive compounds, due to disruption of xenobiotic excretion.

In conclusion, it is demonstrated and explained that high hepatic cell line mortality is provoked by R, at doses far below those used in agriculture. The mechanism of action on various essential enzymes is detailed in Figure 8. This impact on cell death was observed at doses far smaller than legally allowed residues of G in GM food or feed (400 ppm, [29]), in our study LC50 was in comparison 40 to 96 ppm. Of course G can be metabolized and excreted out of the body but this has to be balanced in regard to its cell penetration and bioaccumulation due to adjuvants. In these conditions, this can be almost totally prevented in HepG2 in 48 h by a specific drug, D, that mostly prevents caspases 3/7 activation and CYP3A4 enhancement, both provoked by R. However it does not prevent GST inhibition by R that could lead to accumulation of toxic reactive compounds. Since the use of cell lines allows longer experiments, and since cell lines may in some instances be less sensitive to xenobiotics than primary cultures [55], this system with R and Dig1 constitutes an interesting tool for studying liver intoxication and detoxification. The activity of Dig1 should be now also tested *in vivo* in animal experiments.

DECLARATIONS

Acknowledgements

This study was supported by Sevene Pharma Company which provided Dig 1. C.G., N.B., E.C. held fellowships from the Conseil Regional de Basse-Normandie and the CRIIGEN (Committee for Independent Research and Information on Genetic Engineering). C.G. fellowship was also supported by the Ethic Committee of Léa Nature Group/Jardin Bio which is gratefully acknowledged here. Part of the work was accomplished in C.RIS Pharma Company (Cytochromes and GST study) and in IMOGERE (University of Caen) for experiments with radioactive compounds. We would like also to thank the Human Earth Foundation and the Denis Guichard Foundation for structural support. We thank John Fagan for the English revision of the manuscript.

Competing Interests

The authors declare that they have no competing interests. The development of Dig1 in Sevene Pharma was performed completely independently of its assessment. The scientists in the University of Caen in charge of the assessment of xenobiotics or plant extracts declare no financial or other interests in the development of these products.

REFERENCES

1. Williams GM, Kroes R, Munro IC: Safety evaluation and risk assessment of the herbicide Roundup and its active ingredient, glyphosate, for human. Regul Toxicol Pharmacol 2000, 31: 117–165. 10.1006/rtph.1999.1371
2. Cox C: Glyphosate. Journal of Pesticide Reform 2004, 24: 10–15.
3. Richard S, Moslemi S, Sipahutar H, Benachour N, Séralini GE: Differential effects of glyphosate and Roundup on human placental cells and aromatase. Environ Health Perspec 2005, 113: 716–720. 10.1289/ehp.7728
4. Benachour N, Sipahutar H, Moslemi S, Gasnier C,

Travert C, Séralini GE: Time- and Dose-dependent effects of Roundup on human embryonic and placental cells. Environ Contam Toxicol 2007, 53: 126–133. 10.1007/s00244-006-0154-8

5. Peluso M, Munnia A, Bolognesi C, Parodi S: 32P-Postlabeling detection of DNA adducts in mice treated with the herbicide Roundup. Environ Mol Muta 1998, 31: 55–59. 10.1002/(SICI)1098-2280(1998)31:1<55::AID-EM8>3.0.CO;2-A
6. Takahashi M, Horie M, Aoba N: Analysis of glyphosate and its metabolite, aminomethylphosphonic acid, in agricultural products by HPLC. Shokuhin Eiseigaku Zasshi 2001, 42: 304–308. 10.3358/shokueishi.42.304
7. Acquavella JF, Bruce H, Alexander BH, Mandel JS, Gustin C, Baker B, Champan P, Bleeke M: Glyphosate biomonitoring for farmers and their families: results from the farm family exposure study. Environ Health Perspec2004, 112: 321–326. 10.1289/ehp.6667
8. James C: Global status of biotech/GM Crops: 2005. ISAAA Brief 2007., 34(1):
9. Savitz D, Arbuckle T, Kaczor DM, Curtis K: Male pesticide exposure and pregnancy outcome. Am J Epidemiol 1997, 146: 1025–1036.
10. Gasnier C, Dumont C, Benachour N, Clair E, Chagnon MC, Séralini GE: Glyphosate-based herbicides are toxic and endocrine disruptors in human cell lines. Toxicology 2009, 262: 184–91. 10.1016/j.tox.2009.06.006
11. Urani C, Doldi M, Crippa S, Camatini M: Human-derived cell lines to study xenobiotic metabolism. Chemosphere1998, 37: 2785–2795. 10.1016/S0045-6535(98)00321-X
12. Knasmüller S, Mersh-Sundermann V, Kevekordes S, Darroudi F, Huber WW, Hoelzl C, Bichler J, Majer BJ: Use of human-derived liver cell lines for the detection of environmental and dietary genotoxicants; current state of knowledge. Toxicology 2004, 198: 315–328. 10.1016/j.tox.2004.02.008
13. Bu-Abas A, Clifford MN, Walker R, Ioannides C: Contribution of caffeine and flavanols in the induction of hepatic phase II activities by green tea. Food Chem Toxicol 1998, 36: 617–621. 10.1016/S0278-6915(98)00019-2
14. Gebhardt R: Antioxydative, antiproliferative and biochemical effects in HepG2 cells of a homeopathic remedy and its constituent plant tinctures tested separately or in combination. Drug Res 2003, 12: 823–830.
15. Fukuda K, Hibiya Y, Mutoh M, Koshiji M, Akao S, Fujiwara H: Inhibition of activator protein 1 activity by berberine in human hepatoma cells. Planta Medica 1999, 65: 381–383. 10.1055/s-2006-960795
16. Janbaz KH, Gilani AH: Studies on preventive and curative effects of berberine on chemical-induced hepatotoxicity in rodents. Fitoterapia 2000, 71: 25–33. 10.1016/S0367-326X(99)00098-2
17. Lin SC, Chung TC, Lin CC, Ueng TH, Lin YH, Lin SY, Wang LY: Hepatoprotective effects of Arctium lappa on carbon tetrachloride- and acetaminophen-induced liver damage. Am J Chi Med 2000, 28: 163–173. 10.1142/S0192415X00000210
18. Lin SC, Lin CH, Lin CC, Lin YH, Chen CF, Chen IC, Wang LY: Hepatoprotective effects of Arctium lappa Linne on liver injuries induced by chronic ethanol consumption and potentiated by carbon tetrachloride. J Biomed Sci 2002, 9: 401–409.
19. TrojanovaI, RadaV, KokoskaL, VlkovaE: Thebifidogenic effect of Taraxacum officinale root. Fitoterapia 2004, 75: 760–763. 10.1016/j.fitote.2004.09.010
20. Seo SW, Koo HN, An HJ, Kwon KB, Lim BC, Seo EA, Ryu DG, Moon G, Kim HY, Kim HM, Hong SH: Taraxacum officinale protects against cholecystokinin-induced acute pancreatitis in rat. World J Gastroenterol 2005, 11: 597–599.
21. Mosmann T: Rapid colorimetric assay for cellular growth and survival: application to proliferation and cytotoxicity assays. J Immunol Meth 1983, 65: 55–63. 10.1016/0022-1759(83)90303-4
22. Denizot F, Lang R: Rapid colorimetric assay for cell growth and survival Modification to the tetrazolium dye procedure giving improved sensitivity and reliability. J Immunol Meth 1986, 89: 271–277. 10.1016/0022-1759(86)90368-6
23. Auvray P, Sourdaine P, Moslemi S, Séralini GE, Sonnet P, Enguehard C, Guillon J, Dallemagne P, Bureau R, Rault S: MR 20492 and MR 20494: two indolizinone derivatives that strongly inhibit human aromatase. J Ster Biochem Mol Bio1999, 70: 59–71. 10.1016/S0960-0760(99)00093-X
24. O'Brien M, Moravec R, Riss T, Promega Corporation: Caspase-Glo(tm) 3/7 Assay: Use Fewer Cells and Spend Less Time with this Homogeneous Assay. Cell Notes 2003, 6: 13–15.
25. Ren YG, Wagner KW, Knee DA, Aza-Blanc P, Nasoff M, Deveraux QL: Differential regulation of the TRAIL death receptors DR4 and DR5 by the signal recognition particle. Mol Bio Cell 2004, 15: 5064–5074. 10.1091/mbc.E04-03-0184
26. Liu JJ, Wang W, Dicker DT, El-Deiry WS: Bioluminescent imaging of TRAIL-induced apoptosis through detection of caspase activation following cleavage of DEVD-aminoluciferin. Cancer Biol Ther 2005, 4(8):885–92. 10.4161/cbt.4.8.2133
27. Yueh MF, Kawahara M, Raucy J: High volume bioassays to assess Cyp3A4-mediated drug interactions: Induction and inhibition in a single cell line. Drug Metab Dispos 2005, 33: 38–48. 10.1124/dmd.104.001594
28. Habig WH, Pabst MJ, Jacoby WB: Glutathione S-transferases. The first enzymatic step in mercapturic acid formation.J Biol Chem 1979, 249: 7130–7139.
29. U.S. EPA. Environmental Protection Agency: Glyphosate; notice of filing a pesticide petition to establish a tolerance for a certain pesticide chemical in or on food. Fedral Register Environment Documents 2006.
30. Wiebel FJ, Lambiotte M, Singh J, Summer KH, Wolff T: Expression of carcinogen-metabolizing enzymes in continuous cultures of mammalian cells. In Biochemicals

Basis of Chemical Carcinogenesis. Raven Press, New York; 1984:77–88.

31. Knasmüller S, Parzefall W, Sanyal R, Ecker S, Schwab C, Uhl M, Mersh-Sundermann V, Williamson G, Hietsch G, Langer T, Darroudi F, Natarajan AT: Use of metabolically competent human hepatoma cells for the detection of mutagens and antimutagens. Mut Res 1998, 402: 185–202.
32. Majer BJ, Mersh-Sundermann V, Darroudi F, Laky B, de Wit K, Knasmüller S: Genotoxic effects of dietary and lifestyle related carcinogens in human derived hepatoma (HepG2 and Hep3B) cells. Mut Res - Fundam Mol Mech Mutagen2004, 551: 153–166. 10.1016/j.mrfmmm.2004.02.022
33. Quin LF: Induction of apoptosis by cisplatin and its effect on cell cycle-related proteins and cell cycle changes in hepatoma cells. Cancer Letters 2002, 175: 27–38. 10.1016/S0304-3835(01)00720-0
34. Benachour N, Séralini GE: Glyphosate formulations induce apoptosis and necrosis in human umbilical, embryonic, and placental cells. Chem Res Toxicol 2009, 22: 97–105. 10.1021/tx800218n
35. Benachour N, Moslemi S, Sipahutar H, Séralini GE: Cytotoxic effects and aromatase inhibition by xenobiotic endocrine disrupters alone and in combination. Toxicol Appl Pharmacol 2007, 222: 129–140. 10.1016/j.taap.2007.03.033
36. Koo HN, Hong SH, Song BK, Kim CH, YOO YH, Kim HM: Taraxacum officinale induces cytotoxicity through TNF-alpha an IL-1alpha secretion in HepG2 cells. Life Sci 2004, 74: 1149–1157. 10.1016/j.lfs.2003.07.030
37. Hu C, Kitts DD: Dandelion (Taraxacum officinale) flower extract suppresses both reactive oxygen species and nitric oxide and prevents lipid oxidation in vitro. Phytomedicine 2005, 12: 588–597. 10.1016/j.phymed.2003.12.012
38. Takeshita A, Koibuchi N, Oka J, Taguchi M, Shishiba Y, Ozawa Y: Bisphenol-A, an environmental estrogen, activates the human orphan nuclear receptor, steroid and xenobiotic receptor-mediated transcription. Europ J Endocrinol2001, 145: 513–517. 10.1530/eje.0.1450513
39. Medina-Diaz IM, Elizondo G: Transcriptional induction of CYP3A4 by o,p'-DDT in HepG2 cells. Toxicol Let 2005, 157: 41–47. 10.1016/j.toxlet.2005.01.003
40. Cooper BW, Cho TM, Thompson PM, Wallace AD: Phtalate induction of CYP3A4 is dependent on glucocorticoid regulation of PXR expression. Toxicol Sci 2008, 103: 268–277. 10.1093/toxsci/kfn047
41. Hu C, Kitts DD: Dandelion (Taraxacum officinale) flower extract suppresses both reactive oxygen species and nitric oxide and prevents lipid oxidation in vitro. Phytomedicine 2005, 12: 588–597. 10.1016/j.phymed.2003.12.012
42. Adzet T, Camarasa J, Laguna JC: Hepatoprotective activity of polyphenolic compounds from Cynara scolymus against CCL4 toxicity in isolated rat hepatocytes. J Nat Prod 1987, 50: 612–617. 10.1021/np50052a004
43. Virtanen P, Lassila V, Njimi T, Mengata DE: Natural protoberine alkaloids from Enantia chlorantha, palmatine, columbamine and jatrorrhizine for thioacetamide-traumatiezd rat liver. Acta Anatomica (Basel) 1988, 131: 166–170. 10.1159/000146507
44. Srinivasan M, Rukkumani R, Ram Sudheer A, Menon VP: Ferulic acid, a natural protector against carbon tetrachloride-induced toxicity. Fundam Clin Pharmacol 2005, 19: 491–496. 10.1111/j.1472-8206.2005.00332.x
45. Aden DP, Vogel A, Plotkin S, Damjanov I, Knowles BB: Controlled synthesis of HBS Ag in a differentiated human liver carcinoma-derived cell line. Nature 1979, 282: 615–616. 10.1038/282615a0
46. Knowles BB, Howe CC, Aden DP: Human hepatocellular carcinoma cell lines secrete the major plasma proteins and hepatitis B surface antigen. Science 1980, 209: 497–499. 10.1126/science.6248960
47. Mersh-Sundermann V, Knasmüller S, Wu XJ, Darroudi F, Kassie F: Use of human-derived liver cell line fort he detection of cytoprotective, antigenotoxic and cogenotoxic agents. Toxicology 2004, 198: 329–340. 10.1016/j.tox.2004.02.009
48. Riss TL, Moravec RA: Use of multiple assay endpoints to investigate the effects of incubation time, dose of toxin, and plating density in cell-based cytotoxicity assays. Assay Drug Dev Technol 2004, 2: 51–62. 10.1089/154065804322966315
49. Shimada T, Yamakasi H, Miruma M, Inui Y, Guengerich F: Interindividual variations in human liver cytochrome P-450 enzymes involved in the oxidation of drugs, carcinogens and toxic chemicals: studies with liver microsomes of 30 Japanese and 30 Caucasians. J Pharmacol Exp Ther 1994, 270: 414–423.
50. Forrester L, Melinkov Z, Nanji A: Evidence for involvement of multiple forms of cytochrome P-450 in aflatoxin B1 metabolism in human liver. Volume 87. Proceedings of the National Academy of Sciences of the United States of America; 1990:8306–8310.
51. Li A, Kaminski D, Rasmussen A: Substrates of human hepatic cytochrome P450 3A4. Toxicology 1995, 104: 1–8. 10.1016/0300-483X(95)03155-9
52. Lehmann J, McKee D, Watson M, Willson T, Moore J, Kliewer S: The human orphan nuclear receptor PXR is activated by compounds that regulate CYP3A4 gene expression and cause drug interactions. J Clin Invest 1998, 102: 1016–1023. 10.1172/JCI3703
53. Hidaka M, Nagata M, Kawano Y, Sekiya H, Kai H, Yamakasi K, Okumura M, Arimori K: Inhibitory effects of fruit juices on Cytochrome P450 2C9 activity in vitro. Biosci Biotech Biochem 2008, 72: 406–411. 10.1271/bbb.70511
54. Mortensen AS, Braathen M, Sandvik M, Arukwe A: Effects of hydroxy-polychlorinated biphenyl (OH-PCB) congeners on the xenobiotic biotransformation gene expression patterns in primary culture of Atlantic salmon (Salmo salar) hepatocytes. Ecotoxicol Environ Saf 2007, 68: 351–360. 10.1016/j.ecoenv.2006.11.019
55. L'Azou B, Fernandez P, Bareille R, Beneteau M, Bourget C, Cambar J, Bordenave L: In vitro endothelial cell

susceptibility to xenobiotics: comparison of three cell types. Cell Biol Toxicol 2005, 21: 127–137. 10.1007/s10565-005-0172-8

56. IFEN: Report on pesticides in waters: Data 2003–2004. In Dossier. Volume 5. Institut Français de l'Environnement, Orléans, France; 2006:15–20.

CHAPTER **19**

CHLORPYRIFOS TOXICITY IN FISH

Nobonita Deb and Suchismita Das

Keywords: CPF, OP, fish, toxic

INTRODUCTION

Chlorpyrifos (O,O-diethyl-O-3,5,6-trichlor-2-pyridyl phosphorothioate; CPF) is a broad spectrum organophosphate insecticide (OP) that is commercially used to control foliar insects that affect agricultural crops[1] and subterranean termites[2] CPF, since it was first introduced into the marketplace in 1965, has been used globally as an insecticide to control pests agriculturally and in the home. It is the second largest selling OP and found to be more toxic to fish than organochlorine compounds[3]. Earlier reports revealed that fish kill incidents in association with chlorpyrifos in water reaching several hundred parts per billion[4]. CPF has an average soil half-life of 30 days and two months in less alkaline soils. It also can persist indoors for weeks to months[5]. CPF passes via air drift or surface runoff into surrounding waters and gets accumulated in different aquatic organisms, particularly fish, adversely affecting them[6]. This OP insecticide is known to inhibit acetylcholinesterase, which plays an important role in neurotransmission at cholinergic synapses by rapid hydrolysis of neurotransmitter acetylcholine to choline and acetate[7]. The inhibitory effects of CPF insecticide is dependent on its binding capacity to the enzyme active site and by its rate of phosphorylation in relation to the behaviour and age[8,9] and is widely used for rapid detection to predict early warning of pesticide toxicity[10]. It is reported to be activated by contact, ingestion and vapour action, causing convulsions and paralysis. CPF can enter the body either by inhalation of air containing CPF, ingestion of contaminated food or by dermal contact with CPF. It can cause acute poisoning and well known symptoms include myosis, increased urination, diarrhoea, diaphoresis, lacrimation and salivation[11]. It is also reported to be involved in multiple mechanisms like causing hepatic dysfunction[12], genotoxicity[13], neurobehavioral and neurochemical changes[14]. CPF intoxication is shown to cause a significant decrease in the reduced glutathione (GSH), catalase (CAT) and glutathione S-transferase (GST) activities[15]. Although the United States Environmental Protection Agency (USEPA) has terminated indoor residential use since 2000, CPF is still one of the most widely used insecticides, and more than 8 million pounds of CPF are used each year for agricultural purposes in the United States[16,17]. CPF is also widely used in agriculture as the substitutes for methamidophos and parathion in China, and has become one of the major pesticides detected in farm products[18,19]. Since agricultural uses on orchards and row crops persist, CPF has been frequently detected in air, food and water. Although various standards exist to minimize its exposure in

Citation: Nobonita Deb and Suchismita Das, Chlorpyrifos toxicity in fish, doi.org/10.12944/CWE.8.1.17.

food and water, CPF is frequently used and bio-accumulates in certain scenarios[6,20].

Fish are probably the most important non-target victims of pesticide over exposure as they have an important role in food chain. The present study thus, aims at reviewing existing literatures on the probable adverse effects of pesticide chlorpyrifos in fish.

Structure of chlorpyrifos

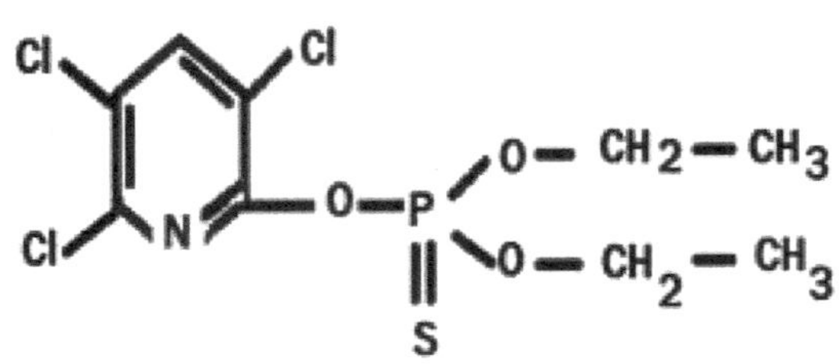

Common name

CPF is also known by its trade names Dursban and Lorsban

Acute toxicity

96 h LC_{50} values for technical grade CPF in Bluegill sun fish, *Lepomis macrochirus,* is 3.3 ppb, in rainbow trout, *Oncorhynchus mykiss* is 3ppb and for channel catfish, *Ictalurus punctatus* is13.4 ppb. 96 h LC_{50} values for 97.0% CPF (active ingredient, a.i.) in lake trout, *Salvelinus namaycush* at pH 6.0 is 140ppb, at pH 7.5 is 98 ppb and at pH 9.0 is 205 ppb while for cutthroat trout, *Salmo clarki,* at pH 7.5 96 h LC_{50} is 18.4 while at pH 9.9 it is 5.4 ppb. 96 h LC_{50} values for 99.9% CPF (a.i.) in fathead minnow,*Pimephales promelas* is 203ppb, while 96 h LC_{50} values for 99.0% CPF (a.i) in golden shiner,*Notemigonus crysoleucas* is 35ppb[21]. The 96 h LC_{50} values of CPF in juvenile and adult of*Oreochromis niloticus* were determined to be 98.67 μgL^{-1} and 154.01 μgL^{-1}, respectively, which reveals that CPF can be rated as highly toxic to fish[22]. The 96 h LC_{50} value of CPF to *Poecila reticulata*was found to be 0.176 ppm/L[23]. LC_{50} for 96 h in mosquito fish, *Gambusia affinis* was found to be 297mg/ L [24] and LC_{50} value of chlorpyrifos in common carp was found to be 580 μg/L[25]. In addition, during toxic stress of CPF, several behavioural anomalies like gulping, increased opercular movement, erractic swimming and subsequent lethargy can be observed[23].

Developmental effects

A variety of studies have shown that exposure to CPF during development can cause persisting neurobehavioural dysfunction, even with low doses that do not elicit acute toxicity. CPF exposure during early development in zebrafish caused long lasting neurobehavioral deficits. Effects of CPF on zebrafish hatchling's swimming behaviour were studied[26]. Results show that a persistent behavioural impairment was caused that lasts into adulthood. This early behavioural effect can be used to help determine which critical molecular mechanisms of CPF underlie the behavioural impairment[26]. Zebrafish, with their clear chorion and extensive developmental information base, provide an excellent model for assessment of molecular processes of toxicant-impacted neurodevelopment[26]. Recently, it was found that embryonic exposure of zebrafish to CPF causes significant impairment in discrimination learning and swimming speed[27] The results of the study indicate that the administration of sub-chronic dose of 1 μM CPF to zebrafish larvae from 0 to 7 day post fertilization significantly impacted body morphology[28]. The results also show that even extremely low sub-chronic doses of CPF administered induced specific behavioural defects or morphological deformities.

Neurotoxic effects

CPF can produce neurotoxic effects. Several studies have assessed the cognitive alterations after acute or chronic exposure to CPF in mammalian models[29,30] but in fish the data available are sparse. CPF causes persistent neurobehavioral impairment in zebrafish, where tests of sensorimotor response (tap startle response and habituation), stress response (novel tank diving test) and learning (3-chamber tank spatial discrimination) were conducted with adult zebra fish after early developmental CPF exposure. The study demonstrated that CPF caused selective long-term neurobehavioral alterations in zebrafish[31]. In another study, a significant decrease in whole brain activity of zebrafish after exposure to CPF has been found[32].

AChE activity

Currently, reports on the toxicity of CPF on AChE activity in aquatic species focused on acute toxicity, but there are few reports on subchronic toxicity of this pesticides on AChE activity in aquatic species. CPF is well known as an AChE inhibitor[33]. Symptoms of high level exposure to OPs include muscle twitching, hyperactivity, paralysis, loss of equilibrium and eventually death[34] whereas low level exposures have been implicated in various behavioural and physiological impairments[34]. Acetylcholinesterase (AChE) and carboxylesterase (CbE) have been used as a specific biomarker for pesticides[24,35]. AChE in fish is mainly cholinergic and its activity is essential for normal behaviour and muscular function[36]. The acute systemic toxicity of CPF is caused by inhibition of cholinesterase through the active metabolite chlorpyrifos oxon, chlorpyrifos is more toxic in immature animals despite their ability to recover rapidly from cholinesterase inhibition. Chlorpyrifos itself, rather than chlorpyrifos oxon is stated, directly targets events that are specific to the developing brain and that are not necessarily related to inhibition of cholinesterase. Acetylcholinesterase is critical to the normal development of the zebrafish nervous system[37], therefore zebrafish studies of the neurobehavioral teratology of acetylcholinesterase inhibitors like CPF are particularly relevant. CPF was a potent inhibitor of AChE activity in fingerling channel catfish[38]. In a study with *Gambusia affinis* exposed to lethal concentration of CPF for 96 h, an inhibition of AChE activity was observed[24]. The inhibition of AChE leading to the accumulation of ACh at synaptic junctions might have been altered the locomotor behaviour of exposed fish. A positive correlation was found between the recovery pattern of AChE activity and locomotor behaviour. The current findings clearly illustrated that the locomotor behaviour of test organism as a promising tool in ecotoxicology, to assess the recovery status of test organism after adverse affects. In a study in *Poecila reticulate*, brain AChE showed dose-dependent inhibition in fish. Exposure to the higher concentrations of CPF showed upto 66% inhibition of AChE[23].

Likewise, CbE is widely distributed in living organisms and its physiological role is still unclear, but it might be related to lipid metabolism and steroidogenesis[39]. Some environmental pollutants found to inhibit AChE activity may also inhibit CbE activity[40-42] demonstrated that muscle ChE of mosquito fish was more sensitive than brain to chlorpyrifos exposure. In a study on carp, CbE activity exhibited a dose–response relationship, with activity decreasing with increasing CPF. Effects of CPF on carp suggest toxic action of low dose CPF on fish recovered after a period of time and toxic action of high dose CPF on fish which was not easily recovered, but the relevant mechanism need further study[43].

Behavioural toxicity

Behaviour is also considered a promising tool in ecotoxicology behaviour[44] is an integrated result of endogenous and exogenous processes and low level of exposures have been implicated in various behavioural and physiological impairments[34]. In a study in zebrafish, persisting behavioral dysfunction after developmental CPF exposure was observed[31,26]. Swimming behaviour of fish is frequently observed as a response in toxicity investigations because altered locomotor activity can indicate effects to the nervous system. In a study, the exposure of *Poecila reticulata* to CPF resulted in the exhibition of aggressive behaviour, rapid gulping of water, increased opercular movement and abnormal and erractic swimming movements. Fish was stressed progressively with time before death. They were lethargic and at the time of death exhibited transient hyperactivity before collapsing[23].

Oxidative stress

For the last decade pesticide induced oxidative stress has also become a very popular of toxicological research as a possible mechanism of toxicity[45,46]. An antioxidant defense system (ADS) is needed to protect biomolecules from the harmful effects of reactive oxygen species (ROS). Fish are endowed with defensive mechanisms to neutralize the impact of reactive oxygen species (ROS) resulting from the metabolism of various chemicals. These include various antioxidant defense enzymes such as superoxide dismutase (SOD), catalase (CAT), glutathione peroxidase (GPOx), glutathione S-transferase (GST), and glutathione reductase (GR). Low molecular weight antioxidants such as glutathione (GSH), ascorbate (vitamin C), and vitamin A are also reported to contribute in the quenching of oxyradicals[47]. ROS which is not neutralized by this antioxidant defense system damages all biomolecules. One of the most important targets of ROS is the membrane lipids which undergo peroxidation (LPO). Thus, LPO estimation has also been successfully employed to signify oxidative stress induced in aquatic animals by such chemicals[48,49]. Pesticides may cause generation of reactive oxygen species (ROS), which may lead to oxidative stress, indicating the role of ROS in pesticide toxicity[50]. Pesticide induced oxidative stress has been also a focus of toxicological research for the last decade as a possible mechanism of toxicity[51,45]. The antioxidants in fish could be used as biomarkers of exposure to aquatic pollutants[52]. Lipid peroxidation (LPO) is one of the molecular mechanisms involved in pesticide toxicity[53]. In *Gambusia affinis* exposed to lethal concentration of CPF for 96 h, an elevated lipid peroxidation level was observed[24]. The same study found decreased levels of antioxidant enzyme (SOD, CAT and GR) activities in the exposed fish can also be effectively used for better assessment of chlorpyrifos toxicity in biomonitoring of aquatic environment. The treatment of *Oreochromis niloticus* with chlorpyrifos results in an increase in GST activity[22]. Inductive effects on GST activity have been observed in studies with *Salmo trutta* after propiconazole exposure [54]. GST-mediated conjugation may be an important mechanism for detoxifying peroxidized lipid breakdown products which have a number of adverse biological effects when it presents in higher amounts[55]. Induced GST activity indicates the role of this enzyme in protection against the toxicity of xenobiotic-induced lipid peroxidation. Elevated GST activity may reflect the possibility of better protection against pesticide toxicity. In guppy, *Poecila reticulate* exposed for 96 h to different sublethal concentrations of CPF,estimated the oxidative stress-induction potential in brain, liver and gill tissues. MDA content is induced in all tissues but maximum rise was observed in gills (153% for CPF). In the same study, with regard to antioxidant defense system (ADS), GSH level showed increase in brain and gills CPF treated (23% and 21% respectively). CAT, GST, GR and SOD levels fluctuated in all treatment groups relative to the control. Collective findings demonstrated that pesticide exposure of fish induced an increase in MDA and fluctuated ADS along with inhibited AChE activity.

Endocrine Function

Chlorpyrifos can interfere with steroid hormone production. CPF is suspected as triggers for harmful effects on the reproductive system in fish. In Tilapia, *Oreochromis niloticus,* CPF exposure decreased serum estrogen and testosterone levels. Estradiol level after 15 days of exposure decreased by 60.45%, 48.65%, 56.93% after 5, 10, 15 ppb chlorpyrifos treatments[22]. Cortisol, a corticosteroid hormone, is considered to be an important physiological effector of homeostasis in all vertebrates, through its effects on metabolism and immune function[56]. Cortisol level in *Oreochromis niloticus*was found to be lower than that of control level after 10 ppb (59.97%) and 15 ppb (39.41) chlorpyrifos treatments[22].

Genotoxicity and Mutagenic Effect

The genotoxic properties of CPF have been studied in a variety of assays in the past, but the results were contradictory[57,58]. Since there is growing a concern over the presence of genotoxins in the aquatic environment, the development of sensitive biomarkers for detection of genotoxic effects in aquatic organisms has gained importance[59]. It has been reported to be genotoxic in *Channa punctatus*[60]. The exposure to 0.08 lg/l of CPF caused reproductive impairment in *Daphnia magna*[61]. In a study on *Channa punctatus*, it was observed that CPF produced a concentration- dependent increase in DNA single-strand breaks in the form of comet induction and a time-dependent decrease in the damage, due to the DNA repair[62]. The decrease in DNA damage has been observed in the tissues of fishes exposed to different concentrations of CPF, although the decrease was non-linear, which may indicate repair of damaged DNA, loss of heavily damaged cells, or both[63]. This inverse relationship between time of exposure and DNA damage may be due to toxicity of contaminants that could disturb the enzymatic processes in the formation of DNA damage[64]. Another possible explanation could be the gene activation of metabolizing enzymes such as cytochrome P450 in various tissues that provides a defensive mechanism against the persistent organic pollutants[65].

Histopathological Changes

Morphological alterations in fish livers and gills are useful biomarkers to indicate prior exposure to environmental stressors or toxicants. Although the liver is the main organ of detoxification, due to their lipophilicity, CPF have a high rate of gill absorption; this could be a contributing factor in the sensitivity of the fish to this pesticide exposure[62]. The aberrant hepatocytes could disturb the normal metabolism of the organisms, thereby inducing diseases or even death. Gills, on the other hand, are extremely important in respiration, osmoregulation, acid–base balance and excretion of nitrogenous wastes in fish, and they are the first area of contact of the animal with the external environment. Therefore, gill morphology is considered a useful indicator in environmental monitoring.

In a study on common carp, CPF altered the structure of the gills and liver. The liver tissue of common carp revealed different degree of hydropic degeneration, vacuolisation, pyknotic nuclei, and fatty infiltration while the gills of common carp displayed varied degrees of epithelial hypertrophy, telangiectasis, oedema with epithelial separation from basement membranes, general necrosis, and epithelial desquamation[66].

CONCLUSION

The present paper reviews the works on effects of CPF in fish. All the workers were of the opinion that widespread use of this pesticide for agricultural as well as domestic purposes can adversely affect the non-target organisms like fish. Investigations on the effects of pesticide on fish have diagnostic significance as the results obtained can be used to predict probable mechanisms of toxicity in human. Besides, fish have proven to be useful experimental models for the evaluation of the health of aquatic ecosystems exposed to environmental pollution and the associated biochemical changes. It was found that the primary toxicity associated with acute exposure to CPF pesticides is acetylcholinesterase inhibition in cholinergic synapses and at neuromuscular junctions. Besides, oxidative stress, disruption of endocrine system, behavioural, neuro and developmental toxicity are some of the probable manifestations of CPF toxicity in fish.

REFERENCES

1. Rusyniak, D.E. and Nanagas, K.A. (2004) Organophosphate poisoning. Semen. Neurol. 24: 197–204, http://dx.doi.org/10.1055/s-2004-830907
2. Venkateswara Rao, J. Parvati, K. Kavitha, P. Jakka, N.M. and Pallela, R. (2005) Effect of chlorpyrifos and monocrotophos on locomotor behaviour and acetylcholinesterase activity of subterranean termites, *Odontotermes obesus*. Pest. Manage. Sci. 61: 417–421,http://dx.doi.org/10.1002/ps.986
3. Tilak, K.S. Veeraiah, K. and Ramanakumari, G.V. (2001) Toxicity and effect of chloropyriphos to the freshwater fish *Labeo rohita* (Hamilton). Neurol Research 20: 438–445.
4. AbdelHalim, K.Y. Salama, A.K. Elkhateeb, E.N. and Barky, N.M. (2006) Organophosphorus pollutants (OPP) in aquatic environment at Damietta Governorate, Egypt: implications for monitoring and biomarker responses. Chemosphere 63: 1491–1498,http://dx.doi.org/10.1016/j.chemosphere.2005.09.019
5. Arcury, T.A. Grzywacz, J.G. Barr, D.B. Tapia, J. Chen, H. and Quandt, S.A. (2007) Pesticide urinary metabolite levels of children in eastern North Carolina farm worker households. Environ Health Perspect.115:1254–60, http://dx.doi.org/10.1289/ehp.9975
6. Varó, I. Serrano, R. Pitarch, E. Amat, F. López, F.J. and Navarro, J.C. (2002) Bioaccumulation of chlorpyrifos through an experimental food chain: study of protein HSP70 as biomarker of sublethal stress in fish. Arch Environ Contam Toxicol. 42:229–235,http://dx.doi.org/10.1007/s00244-001-0013-6
7. Kwong, T.C. (2002) Organophosphate pesticides: biochemistry and clinical toxicology. Ther. Drug. Monit. 24: 144–149, http://dx.doi.org/10.1097/00007691-200202000-00022
8. Richmonds, C.R. and Dutta, H.M. (1992) Effect of malathion on the brain acetylcholinesterase activity of bluegill sunfish *Lepomis macrochirus*. Bull. Environ. Contam. Toxicol. 49: 431- 435,http://dx.doi.org/10.1007/BF01239648
9. Dutta , H.M. Munshi, J.S.D. Dutta, G.R. Singh, N.K. Adhikari, S. and Richmonds, C.R. (1995) Age related differences in the inhibition of brain acetylcholinesterase activity of *Heteropneustes fossillis* (Bloch) by malathion. Comp. Biochem. Physiol. C 111: 331–334,http://dx.doi.org/10.1016/0300-9629(94)00166-Q
10. Dutta, H.M. and Arends, D.A. (2003) Effects of endosulfan on brain acetylcholinesterase activity in juvenile bluegill sunfish. Environ. Res. 91: 157–162, http://dx.doi.org/10.1016/S0013-9351(02)00062-2
11. Samsum, T.E. Hunter, D.L. and Bushnell, P.J. (2005) Effect of chronic dietary and repeated acute exposure to chlorpyrifos on learning and sustained attention in rats, Toxicological Sciences 87: 460–468, http://dx.doi.org/10.1093/toxsci/kfi264
12. Poet, T.S. Wu, H. Kousba, A.A. and Timchalk, C. (2003) In vitro rat hepatic and intestinal metabolism of the organophsophate pesticides chlorpyrifos and diazinon. Toxicological Sciences 72: 193–200, http://dx.doi.org/10.1093/toxsci/kfg035
13. Mehta, A. Verma, R.S. and Srivastava, N. (2008) Oxidative DNA damage induced by chlorpyrifos in rat tissues. Environmental and Molecular Mutagenesis 49: 426–433,http://dx.doi.org/10.1002/em.20397
14. Slotkin, T.A. Olivier, C.A. and Seidler, F.J. (2005) Critical periods for the role of oxidative stress in the developmental neurotoxicity of chlorpyrifos and terbutaline, alone or in combination. Brain Research Development 157: 172–180, http://dx.doi.org/10.1016/j.

devbrainres.2005.04.001

15. Goel, A. Danni, V. and Dhawan, D.K. (2005) Protective effects of zinc on lipid peroxidation Antioxidant enzymes and hepatic histoarchitecture in chlorpyrifos-induced toxicity. Chemico-Biological Interactions 156: 131–140, http://dx.doi.org/10.1016/j.cbi.2005.08.004
16. USEPA (2011a). Chlorpyrifos: Preliminary Human Health Risk Assessment for Registration Review. DP No. D388070.
17. USEPA (2011b). Revised Chlorpyrifos Preliminary Reg Review Drinking Water Assessment. DP No. D368388,389480.
18. Chen, C. Li, Y. Chen, M. Chen, Z. And Qian, Y. (2009) Organophosphorus pesticide residues in milled rice (*Oryza sativa*) on the Chinese market and dietary risk assessment. Food Addit Contam Part A Chem Anal Control Expo Risk Assess. 26:340–7,http://dx.doi.org/10.1080/02652030802524516
19. Sun, F. and Chen, H.S. (2008) Monitoring of pesticide chlorpyrifos residue in farmed !sh: investigation of possible sources. Chemosphere.71:1866–9,http://dx.doi.org/10.1016/j.chemosphere.2008.01.034
20. Jantunen, A.P. Tuikka, A. Akkanen, J. and Kukkonen, J.V. (2008) Bioaccumulation of atrazine and chlorpyrifos to *Lumbriculus variegatus* from lake sediments. Ecotoxicol Environ Saf. 71: 860–8, http://dx.doi.org/10.1016/j.ecoenv.2008.01.025
21. Barron, M.G. and Woodburn, K.B. (1995). Ecotoxicology of chlorpyrifos. Rev. Environ. Contam.Toxicol. 144:1-93, http://dx.doi.org/10.1007/978-1-4612-2550-8_1
22. Oruç, E.O. (2010) Oxidative stress, steroid hormone concentrations and acetylcholinesterase activity in *Oreochromis niloticus* exposed to chlorpyrifos. Pesticide Biochemistry and Physiology 96:160–166, http://dx.doi.org/10.1016/j.pestbp.2009.11.005
23. Sharbidre, A.A. Metkari, V. and Patode, P. (2011) Effect of methyl parathion and chlorpyrifos on certain biomarkers in various tissues of guppy fish, *Poecilia reticulate*. Pesticide Biochemistry and Physiology 10: 132–141, http://dx.doi.org/10.1016/j.pestbp.2011.09.002
24. Kavithaa, P. and Venkateswara Rao, J. (2008). Toxic effects of chlorpyrifos on antioxidant enzymes and target enzyme acetylcholinesterase interaction in mosquito fish, *Gambusia affinis*. Environ. Toxicol. Pharmacol. 26: 192–198, http://dx.doi.org/10.1016/j.etap.2008.03.010
25. Xing, H. Wang, X. Sun, G. Gao, X. Xu, S. and Wang, X. (2011) Effects of atrazine and chlorpyrifos on activity and transcription of glutathione S-transferase in common carp (*Cyprinus carpio* L.). Environ. Toxicol. Pharmacol. 33: 233–244,http://dx.doi.org/10.1016/j.etap.2011.12.014
26. Levin, E.D. Swain, H.A. Donerly, S. and Linney, E. (2004) Developmental chlorpyrifos effects on hatchling zebrafish swimming behaviour. Neurotoxicology and Teratology 26: 719–723,http://dx.doi.org/10.1016/j.ntt.2004.06.013
27. Levin, E. Crysthansis, E. Yacisin, K. and Linney, E. (2003) Chlorpyrifos exposure of developing zebrafish: Effects on survival and long-term effects on response latency and spatial discrimination. Neurotoxicology and Teratology 25: 51– 57, http://dx.doi.org/10.1016/S0892-0362(02)00322-7
28. Richendrfer, H. Pelkowski, S.D. Colwill, R.M. and Créton, R. (2012) Developmental sub-chronic exposure to chlorpyrifos reduces anxiety-related behavior in zebrafish larvae. Neurotoxicology and Teratology 34: 458–465, http://dx.doi.org/10.1016/j.ntt.2012.04.010
29. Braquenier, J.B. Quertemont, E. Tirelli, E. and Plumier, J.C. (2010) Anxiety in adult female mice following perinatal exposure to chlorpyrifos. Neurotoxicol Teratol. 32: 234–9,http://dx.doi.org/10.1016/j.ntt.2009.08.008
30. Middlemore-Risher, M.L. Buccafusco, J.J. Terry, Jr A.V. (2010) Repeated exposures to low-level chlorpyrifos results in impairments in sustained attention and increased impulsivity in rats. Neurotoxicol Teratol 32: 415–24, http://dx.doi.org/10.1016/j.ntt.2010.03.008
31. Sledge, D. Yen, J. Morton, T. Dishaw, L. Petro, A. Donerly, S. Linney, E. and Levin, E.D. (2011) Critical duration of exposure for developmental chlorpyrifos-induced neurobehavioral toxicity. Neurotoxicology and Teratology 33: 742–751, http://dx.doi.org/10.1016/j.ntt.2011.06.005
32. Eddins, D. Cerutti, D. Williams, P. Linney, E. and Levin, E.D. (2010) Developmental chlorpyrifos causes behavioral and neurochemical defects in zebrafish. Neurotoxicol Teratol. 32: 99–108,http://dx.doi.org/10.1016/j.ntt.2009.02.005
33. Taylor, B. and Brown, J.H. (1999). Acetylcholine. In: Siegel, G.J., Agranoff, B.W., Albers, R.W., Fisher, S.K., Uhler, M.D. (Eds.), Basic Neurochemistry: Molecular, Cellular, and Medical Aspects. LippincottRaven, Philadelphia, PA, pp. 213–242.
34. Sandahl, J.F. Baldwin, D.H. Jenkins, J.J. and Scholz, N.L. (2005). Comparative thresholds for acetylcholinesterase inhibition and behavioral impairment in coho salmon exposed to chlorpyrifos. Environ. Toxicol. Chem. 24: 136–145, http://dx.doi.org/10.1897/04-195R.1
35. Leticia, A.G. and Derardo, G.B. (2008). Determination of esterase activity and characterization of cholinesterases in the reef fish *Haemulon plumieri*. Ecotoxicol. Environ. Saf. 71: 787–797, http://dx.doi.org/10.1016/j.ecoenv.2008.01.024
36. Kirby, M.F. Morris, S. Hurst, M. Kirby, S.J. Neall, P. Tylor, T. And Fagg, A. (2000) The use of cholinesterase activity in flounder (*Platichthys flesus*) muscle tissue as a biomarker of neurotoxic contamination in UK estuaries. Mar. Pollut. Bull. 40: 780–791, http://dx.doi.org/10.1016/S0025-326X(00)00069-2
37. Behra, M. Cousin, X. Bertrand, C. Vonesch, J. Biellmann, D. Chatonnet, A. and Strahle, U. (2002) Acetylcholinesterase is required for neuronal and muscular development in the zebrafish embryo, Nature Neuroscience 5: 111– 118, http://dx.doi.org/10.1038/nn788
38. Straus, D.L. and Chambers, J.E. (1995) Inhibition of acetylcholinesterase and aliesterases of fingerling channel catfish by chlorpyrifos, parathion, and S,S,Stributyl

phosphorotrithioate (DEF). Aquat. Toxicol. 33: 311–324, http://dx.doi.org/10.1016/0166-445X(95)00024-X

39. Li, M.H. (2008). Effects of nonylphenol on cholinesterase and carboxylesterase activities in male guppies (*Poecilia reticulata*). Ecotoxicol. Environ. Saf. 71: 781-786,http://dx.doi.org/10.1016/j.ecoenv.2008.02.014

40. Küster, E. (2005) Cholin and carboxylesterase activities in developing zebrafish embryos (*Danio rerio*) and their potential use for insecticide hazard assessment. Aquat. Toxicol. 75: 76–85,http://dx.doi.org/10.1016/j.aquatox.2005.07.005

41. Boone, J.S. and Chambers, J.E. (1997) Biochemical factors contributing to toxicity differences among chlorpyrifos, parathion, and methyl parathion in mosquitofish (*Gambusia affinis*). Aquat. Toxicol. 39: 333, http://dx.doi.org/10.1016/S0166-445X(97)00019-2

42. Carr, R.L. Ho, L.L. and Chambers, J.E. (1997) Selective toxicity of chlorpyrifos to several species of fish during an environmental exposure: biochemical mechanisms. Environ. Toxicol. Chem. 16: 2369, http://dx.doi.org/10.1002/etc.5620161124

43. Xing, H. Wang, J. Li, J. Fan, Z. Wang, M. and Xu, S. (2010) Effects of atrazine and chlorpyrifos on acetylcholinesterase and Carboxylesterasein brain and muscle of common carp. Environmental Toxicology and Pharmacology 30: 26–30,http://dx.doi.org/10.1016/j.etap.2010.03.009

44. Cohn, J. and MacPhail, R.C. (1997) Chlorpyrifos produces selective learning defecits in rats working under a schedule of repeated acquisition and performance. J Pharmacol Exp Ther. 283: 312–20.

45. Abdollahi, M. Ranjbar, A. Shadnia, S. Nikfar, S. and Rezaie, O.E. (2004) Pesticides and oxidative stress: A review. Medical Science Monitoring 10:141– 147.

46. Sharma, Y. Bashir, S. Irshad, M. Gupta, S.D. and Dogra, T.D. (2005) Effects of acute dimethoate administration on antioxidant status of liver and brain of experimental rats, Toxicol. 206: 49–57, http://dx.doi.org/10.1016/j.tox.2004.06.062

47. Orbea, A. Ortiz Zarragoitia, M. Sole, M. Porte, C. and Cajaraville, M.P. (2002) Antioxidant enzymes and peroxisome proliferation in relation to contaminant body burdens of PAHs and PCBs in bivalve molluscs, crabs and fish form the Urdaibai and Plentzia estuaries (Bay of Biscay). Aquat. Toxicol. 58: 75–98, http://dx.doi.org/10.1016/S0166-445X(01)00226-0

48. Favari, L. Lopez, E. Martinez-Tabche, L. and Diaz-Pardo, E. (2002) Effect of insecticides on plankton and fish of Ignacio Ramirez reservoir (Mexico): a biochemical and biomagnification study. Ecotoxicology and Environmental Safety 51:177–186,http://dx.doi.org/10.1006/eesa.2002.2142

49. Monserrat, J.M. Geracitano, L.A. Pinho, G.L.L. Vinagre, T.M. Falerios, M. Alciati, J.C.and Bianchini, A. (2003) Determination of lipid peroxides in invertebrates tissues using the Fe(III) xylenol orange complex formation, Archives of Environmental Contamination and Toxicology 45: 177–183, http://dx.doi.org/10.1007/s00244-003-0073-x

50. Sayeed, I. Parvez, S. Pandey, S. BinHafeez, B. Haque, R. and Raisuddin, S. (2003) Oxidative stress biomarkers of exposure to deltamethrin in freshwater fish *Channa punctatus* Bloch. Ecotoxicol. Environ. Saf. 56: 295–301, http://dx.doi.org/10.1016/S0147-6513(03)00009-5

51. Akhgari, M. Abdollahi, M. Kebryaeezadeh, A. Hosseini, R. and Sabzevari, O. (2003) Biochemical evidence for free radicalinduced lipid peroxidation as a mechanism for subchronic toxicity ofmalathion in blood and liver of rats. Hum. Exp. Toxicol. 22: 205–211,http://dx.doi.org/10.1191/0960327103ht346oa

52. Ahmad, I. Hamid, T. Fatima, M. Chand, H.S. Jain, S.K. Athar, M. and Raisuddin, S. (2000). Induction of hepatic antioxidants in freshwater catfish (*Channa punctatus* Bloch) is a biomarker of paper mill effluent exposure. Biochim. Biophys. Acta 1523: 37–48.

53. Kehrer, J.P. (1993). Free radicals as mediators of tissue injury and disease. Crit. Rev. Toxicol. 23: 21–48, http://dx.doi.org/10.3109/10408449309104073

54. Egaas, E. Sandvik, M. Fleld, E. Kallqvist, T. Goksoyr, A. and Svensen, A. (1999) Some effects of the fungicide propiconazole on cytochrome P450 and glutathione S-transferase in brown trout (*Salmo trutta*). Comp. Biochem. Physiol. 122: 337–344.

55. Leaver, M.J. and George, S.G. (1998) A piscidine glutathione S-transferase which efficiently conjugates the end products of lipid peroxidation, Mar. Environ. Res. 46: 71–74,http://dx.doi.org/10.1016/S0141-1136(97)00071-8

56. Hontela, A. Daniel, C. and Rasmussen, J.B. (1997) Structural and functional impairment of the hypothalomo–pituitary–interrenal axis in fish exposed to bleached kraft mill effluent in the St. Maurice River, Quebec. Ecotoxicology 6: 1–12, http://dx.doi.org/10.1023/A:1018699405158

57. Patnaik, K. and Tripathy, N.K. (1992) Farm grade chloropyrifos (Dermot) is genotoxic in somatic and germ-line cells of Drosophila. Mutat. Res. 279: 15–20,http://dx.doi.org/10.1016/0165-1218(92)90261-W

58. Gollapudi, B.B. Mendrala, A.L. and Linscombe, V.A. (1995) Evaluation of the genetic toxicity of the organophosphate insecticide chloropyrifos. Mutat. Res. 342: 25–36,http://dx.doi.org/10.1016/0165-1218(95)90087-X

59. Hayashi, M. Ueda, T. Uyeno, L. Wada, K. Kinae, N. Saotome, K. Tanaka, N. Takai, A. Sasaki, Y.F. Asano, N. Sifuni, Y. and Ojimma, T. (1998) Development of genotoxicity assay systems that use aquatic organisms. Mutat. Res. 399: 125–133, http://dx.doi.org/10.1016/S0027-5107(97)00251-0

60. Porichha, S.K. Sarangi, P.K. and Prasad, R. (1998) Genotoxic effect of chlorpyrifos in *Channapunctatus*. Pres. Cytol. Genet. 9: 631–638.

61. EPA (1985). Disciplinary review ecological effects profile. Available from US Environ. Protection Agency, Office of Pesticide Programs, 401 M St. S.W., Washington DC 20460, 10p.

62. Ali, D. Nagpure, N.S. Kumar, S. Kumar, R. Kushwaha, B. and Lakra, W.S. (2009) Assessment of genotoxic

and mutagenic effects of chlorpyrifos in freshwater fish *Channa punctatus* (Bloch) using micronucleus assay and alkaline single-cell gel electrophoresis. Food Chem. Toxicol. 47: 650–656, http://dx.doi.org/10.1016/j.fct.2008.12.021

63. Banu, B.S. Danadevi, K. Rahman, M.F. Ahuja, Y.R. and Kaiser, J. (2001) Genotoxic effect of monocrotophos to sentinel species using comet assay. Food Chem. Toxicol. 39: 361–366,http://dx.doi.org/10.1016/S0278-6915(00)00141-1

64. Rank, J. and Jensen, K. (2003) Comet assay on gill and hemocytes from the blue mussel Mytilus edulis. Ecotoxicol. Environ. Saf. 54: 323–329, http://dx.doi.org/10.1016/S0147-6513(02)00006-4

65. Wong, C.K.C. Yeung, H.Y. Woo, P.S. and Wong, M.H. (2001) Specific expression of cytochrome P4501A1 gene in gill, intestine and liver of Tilapia exposed to coastal sediments. Aquatic Toxicol. 54: 69–80, http://dx.doi.org/10.1016/S0166-445X(00)00173-9

66. Xing, H. Li, S. Wang, S. Gao, X. Xu, S. and Wang, X. (2012) Oxidative stress response and histopathological changes due to atrazine and chlorpyrifos exposure in common carp. Pesticide Biochemistry and Physiology 103: 74–80, http://dx.doi.org/10.1016/j.pestbp.2012.03.007

CHAPTER 20

NEUROTOXICITY AND MODE OF ACTION OF N, N-DIETHYL-META-TOLUAMIDE (DEET)

Swale DR, Sun B, tong f and, Bloomquist JR

Keywords: CPF, OP, fish, toxic

INTRODUCTION

The insect repellent *N, N*-diethyl-*meta*-toluamide (DEET) is used more often than any other mosquito repellent, with over 200 million users, worldwide [1]. Because there is deliberate and widespread human exposure to DEET from its use as an insect repellent, questions have arisen regarding its toxicological profile and risk to humans. A recent study [2] suggested the toxic action of DEET may be due to an anticholinesterase effect, with implications for human safety. Large oral doses (blood concentration of 1 mmol/liter) of DEET lead to nausea, vomiting, bradycardia, and seizures [3], [4], as well as cardiotoxicity [5] in exposed humans. Contact exposure to DEET also has the potential for dermal effects, as it can lead to numbness and redness of the affected area [6]. The numbing sensation appears similar to that observed with local anesthetics, such as lidocaine, suggesting DEET might be acting on neuronal ion channels to yield an anesthetic-like effect. DEET has insecticidal properties [7], [8], and was claimed to be synergized in its toxicity to German cockroaches by a compound (eserine) that also synergized the octopaminergic insecticides, chlordimeform (CDM) and amitraz [7]. However, data for DEET synergism by eserine were limited, and based solely upon the observation that 7 of 10 cockroaches were killed in a single combined dose test, making it impossible to assess statistical significance, since 95% confidence limits, slope, and probability values were absent. Moss [7]acknowledged that other mechanisms, such as augmented penetration, might contribute to DEET's synergistic interactions [7], while another study suggested that interaction with mixed function oxidases explained the synergism of DEET and the anticholinesterase insecticide, propoxur [9]. None of these studies [7]–[9] reported any direct mechanistic experiments.

The overall objectives of this study were to determine mechanisms underlying DEET neurotoxicity and compare its effects to known anticholinesterases (propoxur), local anesthetics (lidocaine and toluene), and octopaminergic compounds (octopamine and CDM), having some structural similarity to DEET (Fig. 1). In particular, we investigated the ability of DEET to mimic the neuroexcitatory action of octopamine [10], or the block of sodium or potassium channels by local anesthetics [11] and toluene [12], with the goal of providing insights into the specific targets of DEET underlying its acute toxicity to insects and mammals.

Citation: Swale DR, Sun B, Tong F, Bloomquist JR (2014) Neurotoxicity and Mode of Action of N, N-Diethyl-Meta-Toluamide (DEET). PLoS ONE 9(8): e103713. doi:10.1371/journal.pone.0103713

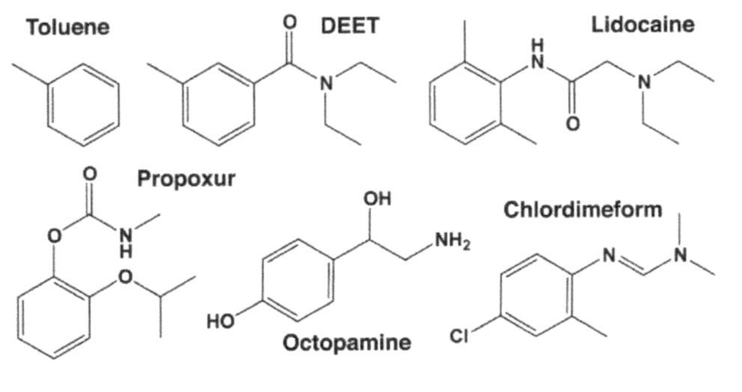

Figure 1: Chemical structures of the pharmacological agents used in this study. http://dx.doi.org/10.1371/journal.pone.0103713.g001

MATERIALS AND METHODS

Compounds, Solvents, and Assay Reagents

DEET, lidocaine, toluene, cesium chloride, 4-aminopyridine (4-AP), and propoxur were all purchased from Sigma-Aldrich (St. Louis, MO, USA) and were ≥98% pure. The solvent dimethyl sulfoxide (DMSO) was used to dissolve agents when needed, and was also purchased from Sigma-Aldrich. Piperonyl butoxide (PBO, 90%) was obtained from Fairfield American Corporation (Frenchtown, NJ, USA) and CDM (97%) was from Nor-Am Chemical Company (Wilmington, DE, USA). Ellman assay [13] reagents are composed of sodium phosphate buffer, the enzyme substrate acetylthiocholine iodide (≥99% purity), and the reactive chromophore 5,5′-dithiobis-(2-nitro) benzoic acid (99% purity), all of which were purchased from Sigma-Aldrich.

Enzymes, Insects, and Neuronal Cells

In vitro biochemical assays utilized five acetylcholinesterase (AChE) enzymes. Recombinant human AChE (*h*AChE) was purchased from a commercial source (lyophilized powder, Sigma C1682, St. Louis, MO, USA). Homogenates to prepare *Anopheles gambiae* AChE (*Ag*AChE) were obtained from the wild type G3 strain and the resistant AKRON strain (BEI Resources;http://www.beiresources.org/). AKRON mosquitoes (from Benin and donated by M. Akogbeto) have both knockdown resistance (*kdr*) to pyrethroids (L1014F sodium channel mutation) and the G119S AChE mutation (*ace*-1R), which confers resistance to carbamates [14], [15]. Both strains were cultured in the Emerging Pathogens Institute, University of Florida, Gainesville, FL, USA from eggs provided by the Center for Disease Control, Atlanta, GA, USA. Homogenates were also used to prepare *Aedes aegypti* AChE (*Ae*AChE) from mosquitoes provided by the CMAVE, USDA-ARS, Gainesville, FL, USA; *Musca domestica* AChE (*Md*AChE) from flies cultured in the Department of Entomology and Nematology, Medical Entomology Laboratory, University of Florida, Gainesville, FL, USA); and *Drosophila melanogaster* AChE (*Dm*AChE) from flies (Oregon-R strain) cultured in the Emerging Pathogens Institute, University of Florida, Gainesville, FL, USA. Homogenate enzymes were prepared from groups of ten non-blood fed adult female mosquitoes, five whole bodied *Drosophila*, or three *Musca* heads homogenized in 1 mL of ice-cold sodium phosphate buffer (0.1 M sodium phosphate, pH 7.8) with an electric motor driven glass tissue homogenizer. The homogenate was centrifuged at 5000×*g* using a Sorvall Fresco refrigerated centrifuge at 4 °C for 5 minutes. The supernatant was used as the enzyme source, and all enzyme preparations contained 0.3% (v/v) triton X-100 and 1 mg/ml BSA. Prior to use, the recombinant human enzyme was diluted 500-fold into sodium phosphate buffer containing triton X-100 and 1 mg/ml BSA.

Insects used for *in vivo* toxicity assays were obtained from the sources listed above. Rat neuronal cortex cells were purchased from Invitrogen (Grand Island, NY, USA), plated on 35 mm glass cover slips, and maintained in primary neuron basal medium without *L*-glutamine at 38 °C until used for patch clamp studies.

Enzyme Inhibition Assays

Inhibition of AChE was determined using the Ellman assay [13] and was based on the method outlined in Carlier et al. [16]. Briefly, enzyme solution (10 µL) was added to each well of a 96-well micro assay plate, along with 20 µL of inhibitor in DMSO/saline suspension, and 150 µL of sodium phosphate buffer. Final concentration of DMSO was 0.1% in all incubations. The plate was incubated at 25 °C for ten minutes. Ellman assay reagents, acetylthiocholine iodide (0.4 mM, final concentration) and 5,5′-dithiobis-(2-nitro)benzoic acid (0.3 mM, final concentration), were prepared fresh and 20 µL was added to the enzyme to initiate the reaction. Changes in absorbance were recorded by a DYNEX Triad spectrophotometer (DYNEX Technologies, Chantilly, VA, USA) at 405 nm. Enzyme concentrations used were within the linear range, therefore eliminating the need for protein quantification. IC_{50} values (inhibitory concentration needed to inhibit 50% of the enzyme activity, negative Hill slope) were calculated using eight inhibitor concentrations by nonlinear regression to a four parameter logistic equation (variable Hill slope) using GraphPad Prism (GraphPad Software, San Diego, CA, USA).

Toxicity Assays

Topical toxicity bioassays on adult female mosquitoes were performed based on the method of Pridgeon et al. [17]. Briefly, insects were chilled on ice for 3 min, during which the appropriate volume (200 nL for mosquitoes, 1 µL for *Musca*) of chemical (dissolved in 95% ethanol) was applied onto the abdomen using a handheld Hamilton microapplicator. For each inhibitor, five doses were applied to groups of ten insects each and repeated three times. An ethanol-only treatment was included in each experiment as a negative control. Insects were transferred into a holding chamber post-treatment and supplied with free access to sugar water for the duration of the experiment. Mortality was recorded at the 24-hour time point, pooled and analyzed by log-probit using Poloplus (LeOra Software Co., Petaluma, CA, USA) to determine 24 hr LD_{50} values (lethal dose needed to kill 50% of treated insects). Three LD_{50} values were obtained and the mean LD_{50} value was calculated and used for statistical analysis.

Diet toxicity assays were performed on mixed sex adult *Drosophila melanogaster* fasted for 8 hours prior to initiating the experiment. Flies were transferred into a container stoppered with a cotton ball infused with 1 ml of a sucrose/

DEET solution containing 20 insects (2–3 day old adults). The assay was run three times on three different days with matched controls. Mortality was recorded at the 24-hour time point.

Contact toxicity bioassays were performed on both strains of *Anopheles gambiae*, G3 (susceptible) and AKRON (pyrethroid and anticholinesterase resistance) according to WHO protocol [18]. Adult female mosquitoes were 2–5 days of age and non-blood fed at the time of experimentation. Five concentrations of inhibitor dissolved in ethanol were prepared and treated by applying 2 mL of each concentration on a 180 cm^2 (12 cm×15 cm) paper. Papers were left to dry for 24 hours prior to use. Mosquitoes were chilled for three minutes on ice, after which 25 females were placed in the WHO kit holding chamber to recover for one hour. Mosquitoes were then moved to the treatment chamber, which contain the treated paper, and exposed for one hour. After the one-hour exposure, the mosquitoes were transferred back to the holding chamber and maintained on 10% sugar solution for 24 hrs. Each concentration was repeated in triplicate. Mortality was recorded 24 hours post treatment and an LC_{50} (lethal concentration needed to kill 50% of exposed insects) was calculated using Poloplus (LeOra Software Company, Petaluma, CA, USA). Three LC_{50} values were obtained and the mean LC_{50} value was used for statistical analysis.

For all toxicity assays, control mortality was corrected for using Abbots formula [19]; where corrected percent mortality = (% alive in control–% alive in treated) /% alive in control.

Electrophysiological Studies in Housefly

Neurophysiological recordings were performed on the central and peripheral nervous systems of larval *Musca domestica*. Glass pipette electrodes were pulled from borosilicate glass capillaries on a P-1000 Flaming/Brown micropipette puller (Sutter Instrument, Novato CA, USA). For CNS recordings [20], it was first excised from the larvae and placed in a separate dish with physiological saline (200 μL) containing: 157 mM NaCl, 3 mM KCl, 2 mM $CaCl_2$, and 4 mM HEPES, pH=7.25. The CNS was manually transected posterior to the cerebral lobes to disrupt the blood-brain barrier and enhance chemical penetration [20]. Any convenient peripheral nerve trunks were pulled into a recording suction electrode. Amplification and digitization of descending electrical activity originating from the CNS were converted on-line into a rate plot, expressed in Hz (MacLab analog to digital converter hardware and LabChart 7 software, ADInstruments, Colorado Springs, CO, USA). Activity was monitored for a ten minute time period to establish a constant baseline firing rate, as the spike frequency typically increased from 0 to 10 minutes before stabilization. After a baseline was established, the CNS preparation was directly exposed to test compound by adding 200 μL of solution to the bath containing 200 μL of saline. The final concentration of solvent in the bath was 0.1% DMSO. Each concentration was recorded for 3–5 min prior to the addition of the next drug concentration. Mean spike frequencies for each concentration were used to construct concentration-response curves to determine EC_{50} values ($EC_{50=}$ concentration of drug to elicit half maximal response, positive Hill slope), and were calculated by nonlinear regression (variable slope) using GraphPad Prism (GraphPad Software, San Diego, CA, USA) in a manner similar to that for AChE inhibition. Each drug concentration was replicated 3-5 times. Neuromuscular recordings of the evoked excitatory postsynaptic potential (EPSP) were performed on third instar housefly larvae, essentially as described previously [21]. In short, the maggot was immobilized with pins, and the nervous and musculature systems were exposed. The preparation was then bathed in saline containing: 140 mM NaCl, 0.75 mM $CaCl_2$, 5 mM KCl, 4 mM $MgCl_2$, 5 mM $NaHCO_3$, and 5 mM HEPES (pH=7.25). The nerves were severed from the base of the CNS, which was removed, and a lateral nerve trunk innervating the longitudinal muscles was drawn into a suction electrode filled with saline. Stimuli were applied at 1 volt and of 0.2 sec duration to elicit a contraction from the longitudinal muscles. The stimulated muscle was then impaled with a recording glass capillary microelectrode filled with 1 M KCl to record effects on the evoked EPSP and membrane potential. Signals from all recordings were amplified and digitized with the use of the MacLab. Chemicals were applied to the preparation directly by hand pipetting 150 μL of solution into the bath volume of 150 μL.

In Vivo Assay for Effects on Firefly Light Organ

Adult firefly beetles (*Photinus sp.*) were collected locally (Nashville, TN) and housed in well-ventilated chambers with tree leaves. The animals had free access to 10% sucrose solution. Chemicals were dissolved in absolute ethanol and 1 μL was topically applied directly to the ventral light organ with the use of a manual pipettor. Prior to DEET application, the beetles were immobilized with molten parafilm and were mounted on corrugated cardboard for the duration of the study. Due to the time required for bioactivation of CDM, insects were treated with 1 μL of CDM and were released back into the holding chamber for three hours. After three hours, they were mounted in the previously described manner and monitored for activation of the lantern. Photographs were captured with a handheld camera (Canon PowerShot SX110 IS). Pictures were captured within five minutes, four hours, and 10 minutes post application for DEET, CDM, and propoxur, respectively. DEET- and propoxur-treated insects were monitored for at least 1 hour post exposure to ensure the response was not slow acting. The original photographs were cropped and background shadows were enhanced to increase detail of the insect using Adobe Photoshop PS5 (Adobe Systems, San Jose, CA, USA). The color or brightness of the light organ was not manipulated in any way during post-processing of the image.

Calcium Fluorescence Assay

The *Sf*21 insect cell line was obtained from a commercial supplier (Invitrogen, Carlsbad, CA, USA) and maintained in log phase culture in *Trichoplusia ni* Medium-Formulation Hink (TNM-FH) from Sigma-Aldrich (St. Louis, MO, USA), supplemented with 10% fetal bovine serum and 100 U/ml penicillin and streptomycin (Sigma-Aldrich). Cells were cultured in a non-humidified environment and maintained at 27°C. *Sf*21 cells were passaged every 3–5 days according to manufacturer's instructions, and maintained for about 30 passes before being replaced by fresh cells.

The FLIPR Calcium 5 Assay Evaluation Kit (Molecular Devices, Sunnyvale, CA, USA) was used to determine calcium fluorescence in *Sf*21 cells, a clonal line of *Sf*9 cells, which are known to possess octopamine receptors [22]. *Sf*21 cells were plated into 96-well black-wall, clear bottom plates 24 h before calcium fluorescence assay. Cell culture medium was carefully removed from each well of the plate, and 100 μL per well of Calcium 5 Assay buffer with 2.5 mM of probenecid and 1.3 mM calcium was then added. After 1 h incubation at room temperature, 100 μM of octopamine, DEET, or propoxur were applied to the assay plate, and fluorescence was measured immediately at 485 and 525 nm wavelengths for excitation and emission, respectively, with slits of 10 nm (excitation) and 20 nm (emission) on a SyntaxMax plate reader (BioTek, Winooski, VT, USA). The octopamine receptor antagonist phentolamine (100 μM) was co-incubated with cells for 1 h before drug challenge. Phentolamine, octopamine, and DEET were dissolved in water, while propoxur was dissolved in 100% DMSO to make a stock solution, and in the assay, DMSO was kept to 0.1%. The experiment was repeated in triplicate with different plates of cells to obtain means and SEMs for each experimental condition.

Patch Clamp Recordings

Rat cortical neurons (purchased from Lonza, Walkersville, MD, USA) were placed on poly-lysine coated glass cover slips in 35 mm dishes, and cultured in primary neuron basal medium with added 2% neural grown factor and 1% glutamine (from Lonza). The medium was half changed every 3 days, and the cells were used at 6–12 days. The neurons had dendrites and axons and the diameters of the somata were about 15–20 μm. Cells were cultured on cover slips and were immersed in 35 mm Petri dishes filled with room temperature extracellular saline. Patch pipettes were pulled from borosilicate glass capillaries with filament (BF150-86-10, Sutter Instrument, Novato CA, USA) on a P-1000 Flaming/Brown micropipette puller (Sutter Instrument). Extracellular solution was the same regardless of the target ion channel and contained: 140 mM NaCl, 5 mM KCl, 2 mM $MgCl_2$, 2 mM $CaCl_2$, 10 mM glucose, and 10 mM HEPES (pH=7.4). Intracellular patch solution for potassium channel recordings consisted of: 140 mM KF, 10 mM NaCl, 2 mM $MgCl_2$, and 10 mM HEPES (pH=7.2). Intracellular patch solution for sodium channel recordings consisted of: 140 mM $CsCH_3SO_3$ 10 mM NaCl, 2 mM $MgCl_2$, 10 mM HEPES (pH=7.2), where $CsCH_3SO_3$ was used to eliminate potassium currents during sodium channel analysis. The patch electrodes had resistances of 5–7 MOhms.

Patch clamp recordings were performed with a 40x/0.80W water immersion objective (working distance 3.5 mm) using a forced-air-cooled Photometrics Evolve 512/CCD97 camera system. Following gigaseal formation, the membrane was ruptured through a brief, manual suction of the electrode, or by a 2 msec long zap pulse. Currents were amplified with the use of a patch-clamp amplifier (Axopatch 200B, Molecular Devices LLC, Sunnyvale, CA, USA) and processed for analysis via A/D-converter (Digidata 1440A, Molecular Devices LLC). Recordings underwent series resistance compensation, low-pass filtering at 1 kHz, and were sampled at 10 kHz or 100 kHz for potassium and sodium currents, respectively. For recording and analyzing data, pClamp 10.0 software (Molecular Devices LLC) was used.

RESULTS

Lethality of DEET

Insect bioassays showed DEET to be moderately toxic via surface contact and topical application (Table 1). No significant differences were observed between mosquito species, but some statistical difference was observed between the G3 and AKRON strains, indicating little species variability and cross-resistance to DEET in the AKRON strain of *An. gambiae* that carries multiple resistance mechanisms [14], [15]. For comparison, the LD_{50} of the carbamate anticholinesterase propoxur to *Aedes aegypti* was 1.4 (95% CI: 0.9–2.1) ng/mg body weight, approximately 1000-fold less than the LD_{50} of DEET. Co-treatment with the cytochrome P450 monooxygenase inhibitor, piperonyl butoxide (PBO, 200 ng) [23] had no statistically significant influence on the topical toxicity of DEET, and synergism ratios were near unity (Table 1). DEET was also toxic to mosquitoes through surface contact (*i.e.*, tarsal) exposure in the WHO paper assay (Table 1). DEET was non-toxic to *Drosophila melanogaster* in a sugar-feeding assay at 1 mg/ml.

Table 1: Toxicity values of DEET to three mosquito strains and the housefly. http://dx.doi.org/10.1371/journal.pone.0103713.t001

Species	[a]LC_{50}, mg/ml (95% CI)	[b]LD_{50}, ng/mg (95% CI)	[c]LD_{50}, ng/ml (+PBO) (95% CI)	[d]SR
A. gambiae. (G3)	1.9 (0.9–2.9)a	1175 (988–1361)a	1021 (829–1231)a	1.2
A. gambiae (AKRON)	2.7 (1.0–4.5)a	1472 (1136–1806)b	1247 (872–1526)a	1.2
Ae. aegypti	2.3 (1.1–3.6)a	1102 (836–1367)a	1082 (841–1310)a	1.0
M. domestica	-	8104 (7026–9000)c	6219 (4405–8563)b	1.3

Letters after 95% confidence intervals (CI) represent statistical significance for LD_{50} or LC_{50} values among species within a given toxicity measurement column. Values not labeled by the same letter represent statistical significance ($P<0.05$) in one-way ANOVA followed by Tukey's multiple comparison test.
[a]LC_{50} in the WHO filter paper assay.
[b]LD_{50} by topical application in ng of compound/mg of mosquito weight.
[c]LD_{50} (same units) by topical application after 4 hr pretreatment with 200 ng PBO.
[d]Synergism ratio = LD_{50} with DEET alone/LD_{50} with DEET + PBO.
doi:10.1371/journal.pone.0103713.t001

Signs of Intoxication

After treatment with lethal doses of DEET, *Aedes aegypti* mosquitoes were found to display both hyperexcitatory and lethargic tendencies. Five minutes after treatment, the mosquitoes were lethargic, with the majority standing with splayed posture or laying ventral side upward. The mosquitoes were unable to rest on the vertical sides of the chamber and collected on the bottom. Agitation induced hyperexcitation, with increased wing beat frequency, spinning on their dorsal side, and erratic movements. Directed flight behavior did not occur. After approximately 10 seconds of hyperexcitation, the mosquitoes resumed lethargic behavior. Control mosquitoes had normal posture (legs not splayed away from the midline), would rest on the sides of the holding chamber versus the bottom, and upon agitation, the mosquitoes would immediately fly from their resting posture to a different location on the container and come to rest.

Mosquitoes intoxicated with propoxur exhibited intense hyperexcitation in the absence of any physical stimulation. Five minutes post-exposure to 1 ng/insect, the mosquitoes were in a supine position and were rapidly beating their wings. This high wing beat frequency caused the mosquitoes to spin on their dorsal side. If the mosquitoes stopped beating their wings, they rapidly twitched and contracted their legs. The mosquitoes continued this behavior until death. Manual agitation caused no change in the behavior of the mosquitoes.

Houseflies presented similar signs of intoxication by DEET, but the flies were mostly lethargic with only occasional bouts of excitation. Unlike *Aedes aegypti*, the flies did not present a change in behavior after agitation, as they remained standing, albeit with splayed posture, and did not begin convulsing. Although the flies presented excitation via twitching and uncoordinated movements, it was not to the same level of intensity as that observed in mosquitoes at toxicologically equivalent doses.

Anticholinesterase Actions of DEET

DEET was found to be a poor inhibitor of *Drosophila melanogaster* AChE (*Dm*AChE), human AChE (*h*AChE), and *Musca domestica* AChE (*Md*AChE) with mean IC_{50} values in the low milliomolar range (Table 2). The mosquito enzymes, wild type *Anopheles gambiae* AChE (*Ag*AChE) and *Aedes aegypti* AChE (*Ae*AChE), were completely insensitive to DEET at concentrations up to 10 mM, but were highly sensitive to propoxur, with IC_{50} values in the 100–500 nanomolar range for all enzymes except AKRON *Ag*AChE (Table 2). The mean $IC_{50}$for propoxur to *Md*AChE was 40,000-fold more potent than the IC_{50} value of DEET to*Md*AChE. Lidocaine was found to have an IC_{50} value for *Md*AChE similar to that of DEET. Toluene was inactive at concentrations up to 10 mM on all enzyme preparations.

Table 2: AChE inhibition data expressed as mean (n=3) IC_{50} values. http://dx.doi.org/10.1371/journal.pone.0103713.t002

	IC_{50}, nM (95% CI)	IC_{50}, mM (95% CI)		
Enzyme	**Propoxur**	**DEET**	**Lidocaine**	**Toluene**
An. gambiae (G3)	447 (420–480)	>10	>10	>10
An. gambiae (AKRON)	>100,000	>10	>10	>10
Aedes aegypti	370 (320–410)	>10	>10	>10
Musca domestica	130 (110–160)	6 (3–8)a	4.9 (3–7)	>10
Drosophila melanogaster	84 (69–110)	10 (6–13)b	9.6 (5–14)	>10
Human	1442 (1255–1629)	12 (7–17)b	–	>10

Inhibition values of *Md*AChE, *Dm*AChE, and hAChE were analyzed by one-way ANOVA followed by Tukey's multiple comparison test. Letters after 95% confidence intervals (CI) represent statistical significance for IC_{50} values among enzymes tested with DEET. IC_{50}s for DEET not labeled by the same letter represent statistical significance ($P<0.05$).
doi:10.1371/journal.pone.0103713.t002

CNS Recordings from Housefly Larvae

House fly larval CNS recordings were performed in an effort to further characterize DEET neurotoxicity (Fig. 2). Figure 2A shows representative plots of neuronal discharge rate over time in response to solvent (0.1% DMSO) and treatments with DEET, toluene, and lidocaine. Concentration-response plots of replicated recordings are shown in Figure 2B. DEET was neuroexcitatory with a threshold concentration of about 50 μM, and had EC_{50} values of 0.12 (0.05–0.29) mM and 0.21 (0.08–0.56) mM on transected and intact CNS, respectively. Despite having documented sodium channel-blocking properties [12], toluene was also found to have excitatory effects on nerve firing, but at concentrations about ten-fold higher than that of DEET (Fig. 2A). The EC_{50} of toluene was 1.0 (0.05–24) mM on the transected CNS (Fig. 2B), where the low potency and efficacy of this compound made quantification difficult. Lidocaine, a prototypical local anesthetic, was found to have an inhibitory effect on the CNS (Fig. 2A) with an EC_{50} of 0.34 (0.22–0.54) mM (Fig. 2B).

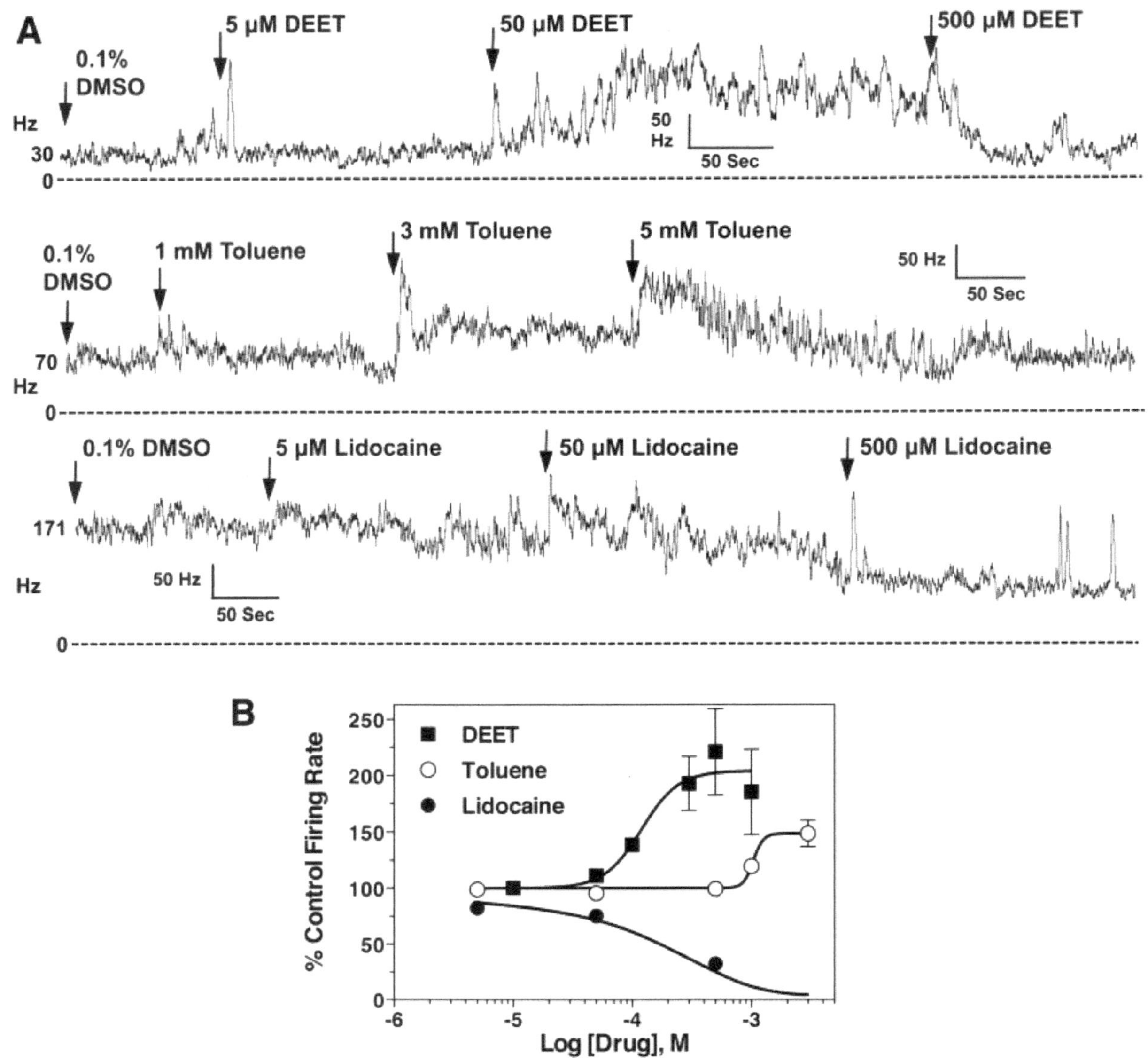

Figure 2: Neurophysiological recordings from the CNS of third instar larvae of *M.*domestica A) Nerve discharges before and after DEET, toluene, and lidocaine treatment across different CNS preparations, as indicated. Initial firing frequencies in spikes/second (Hz) for each experiment are given to the left of each trace. B) Concentration-response curves for DEET, toluene, and lidocaine on CNS nerve discharge of *M. domestica* larvae from replicated recordings (n=4–5 preparations per curve, with each concentration replicated 4 times), as shown in A. Data points represent mean percentage increase of baseline firing rate, and error bars represent SEM of drug concentrations replicated at least 3 times. When error bars are absent, it is because they are smaller than the size of the symbol.http://dx.doi.org/10.1371/journal.pone.0103713.g002

DEET-mediated neuroexcitation and its sensitivity to the octopaminergic antagonist phentolamine was compared to that of octopamine, propoxur, and the potassium channel blocker 4-AP), to assist in the identification of its mode of action. All the compounds increased the maximal firing frequency 2- to 3-fold above control levels (Fig. 3A–C), except for 4-AP, which caused a 6-fold increase (Fig. 3D). Octopamine (Fig. 3B) was found to have an excitatory EC_{50} of 0.11 (0.003–3.8) mM, nearly identical to the EC_{50} found for DEET. Propoxur (Fig. 3C) was used as a positive control for AChE inhibitors, and was found to have an EC_{50} of 344 (251–472) nM for increasing spike frequency in the CNS, 349-fold more potent than that of DEET. The EC_{50} for 4-AP was 13 (0.5–341) μM, and firing declined precipitously at concentrations >1 mM, accounting for the wide confidence limits. Experiments were then performed with phentolamine, an established octopaminergic receptor antagonist [10], to determine its ability to block the neuroexcitation of DEET and test whether neuroexcitation occurred via central octopaminergic pathways. DEET-mediated neuroexcitation (up to 500 μM) was completely blocked by 100 μM phentolamine (Fig. 3A), which also completely blocked octopamine-mediated neuroexcitation at octopamine concentrations up to 3 mM (Fig. 3B). In contrast, 100 μM phentolamine had no effect on the neuroexcitation by propoxur, until the carbamate reached a concentration of 1 μM, where maximal firing declined by 21% compared to propoxur alone (Fig. 3C). This effect was not statistically significant. Similarly, there was no effect of phentolamine on 4-AP mediated neuroexcitation (Fig. 3D).

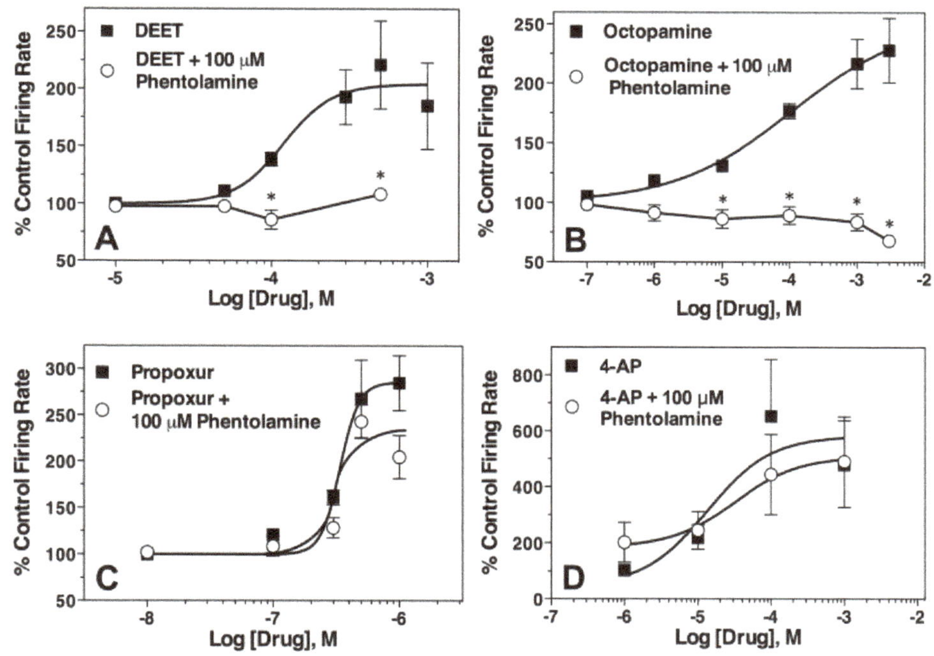

Figure 3: Effect of phentolamine on the activity of DEET (A), octopamine (B), propoxur (C) and 4-AP (D) on discharge rates of housefly larvae CNS preparations (n=3–5 preparations per curve, with each concentration replicated 3–5 times). Data points represent mean percentage increase of baseline firing rate, and error bars represent SEM of drug concentrations replicated at least 3 times. When error bars are absent, it is because they are smaller than the size of the symbol. Data points at each concentration for drug alone were compared to drug + phentolamine, and statistical significance (t-test, P<0.05) is indicated by an asterisk. http://dx.doi.org/10.1371/journal.pone.0103713.g003

Activation of the Firefly Light Organ

An octopaminergic action of DEET was next assessed on the firefly light organ (Fig. 4). Control fireflies (1 µL of absolute ethanol) displayed uniformly dark lanterns with intermittent and brief moments of luminescence. The periods of luminescence of control animals were short in duration (*ca.* one second), involved the whole light organ, and flashed every 45-90 seconds. DEET was found to cause dose-dependent activation of the firefly lantern through increased duration and repeated activation of the lantern every 10–20 seconds. Faint illumination in circumscribed areas of the lantern was observed at 1 and 2.5 µg of DEET (Fig. 4A). Bright and complete illumination of the lantern was observed with DEET concentrations of 5 µg and it typically remained active for periods of 10–60 seconds in the majority of individuals. In two individuals, the lantern stayed illuminated for 5 and 30 min periods. At low doses (1 µg, Fig. 4A), the octopaminergic pesticide CDM showed incomplete activation of the light organ, similar to DEET. At higher doses (5 µg, Fig. 4A), the lanterns of CDM treated insects displayed a bright, constant glow of the entire lantern for approximately four hours, after which it began to fade in brightness. In fireflies treated with 1 µg propoxur, typical anticholinesterase signs of intoxication (e.g., tremors and hyperexcitation) were observed, but there were no changes in lantern illumination and propoxur-treated insects flashed their lanterns the same as controls (Fig. 4A).

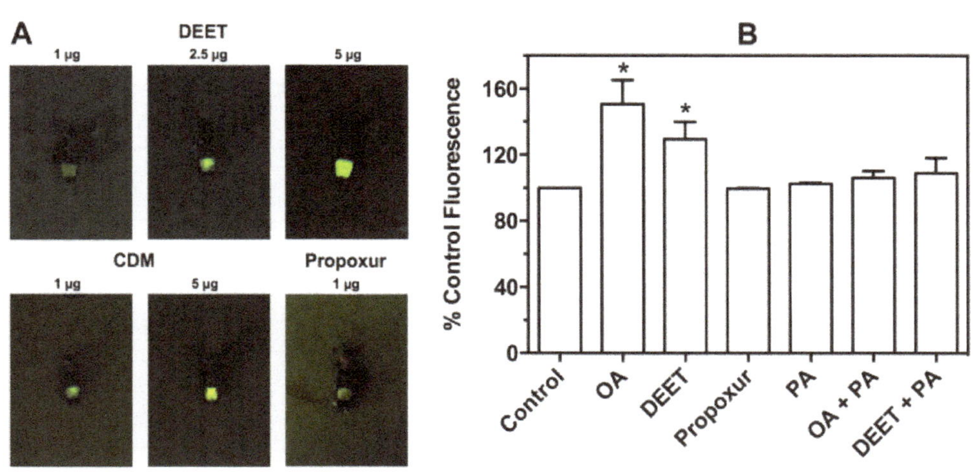

Figure 4: Effects of DEET on octopaminergic systems in firefly and *Sf*21 cells. A) Dose-dependent action of DEET, CDM, and propoxur on the light organ of the firefly,*Photinus pyralis*. See text for explanation. B) Activation of an octopamine receptor in*Sf*21 cells shown by internal calcium fluorescence. Bars represent means of normalized fluorescence with error bars denoting SEM, replicated across individual plates of

cells (n=3). Statistics for each column were determined by a paired t-test against matched control raw fluorescent values, where an asterisk represents statistical significance at P<0.05. For labels, OA= octopamine and PA= phentolamine. All compounds were applied at 100 μM. http://dx.doi.org/10.1371/journal.pone.0103713.g004

Action of DEET at Octopamine Receptor in Sf21 Cells

In order to determine whether DEET had any direct effects on octopamine receptors, it was tested in a cell-based calcium fluorescence assay (Fig. 4B). In these experiments, 100 μM DEET induced a statistically significant (P<0.05) increase of ca. 30% in calcium fluorescence in *Sf*21 cells. Similarly, octopamine caused ca. 50% increase in calcium fluorescence over control cells. For comparison, triton X-100 (0.1%) treatment, expected to flood the cell with calcium via membrane disruption, increased fluorescence 211+12% of control. DEET- and octopamine-mediated activation of calcium fluorescence was abolished by pre-exposure of the cells to phentolamine, yielding fluorescent values not statistically different from controls. These data confirm DEET can activate the octopamine receptor, although it was a weaker agonist than octopamine. As expected, propoxur was shown to have no effect on calcium fluorescence (Fig. 4B).

Neuromuscular Junction Recordings from Housefly

DEET showed a complete and rapid block of the evoked EPSP in the body wall musculature of third instar *Musca domestica* larvae (Fig. 5). The block was found to be an essentially all or none response, with half of the preparations blocked at ca. 7 mM. Complete block was obtained approximately 120 seconds after 10 mM DEET was added to the bath (Fig. 5). Little or no change was observed in the muscle membrane resting potential after the addition of DEET at any concentration. Lidocaine was also an antagonist at the neuromuscular junction and the blocking pattern was an all or none response very similar to DEET (Fig. 5). Toluene was again found to be excitatory at 5 mM (Fig. 5), and the excitatory effects (spontaneous EPSPs and muscle depolarization) were reversed by washing the preparation with drug-free buffer (data not shown). Propoxur behaved as a negative control, and had no effect on the evoked EPSP of *Musca domestica* larvae (Fig. 5).

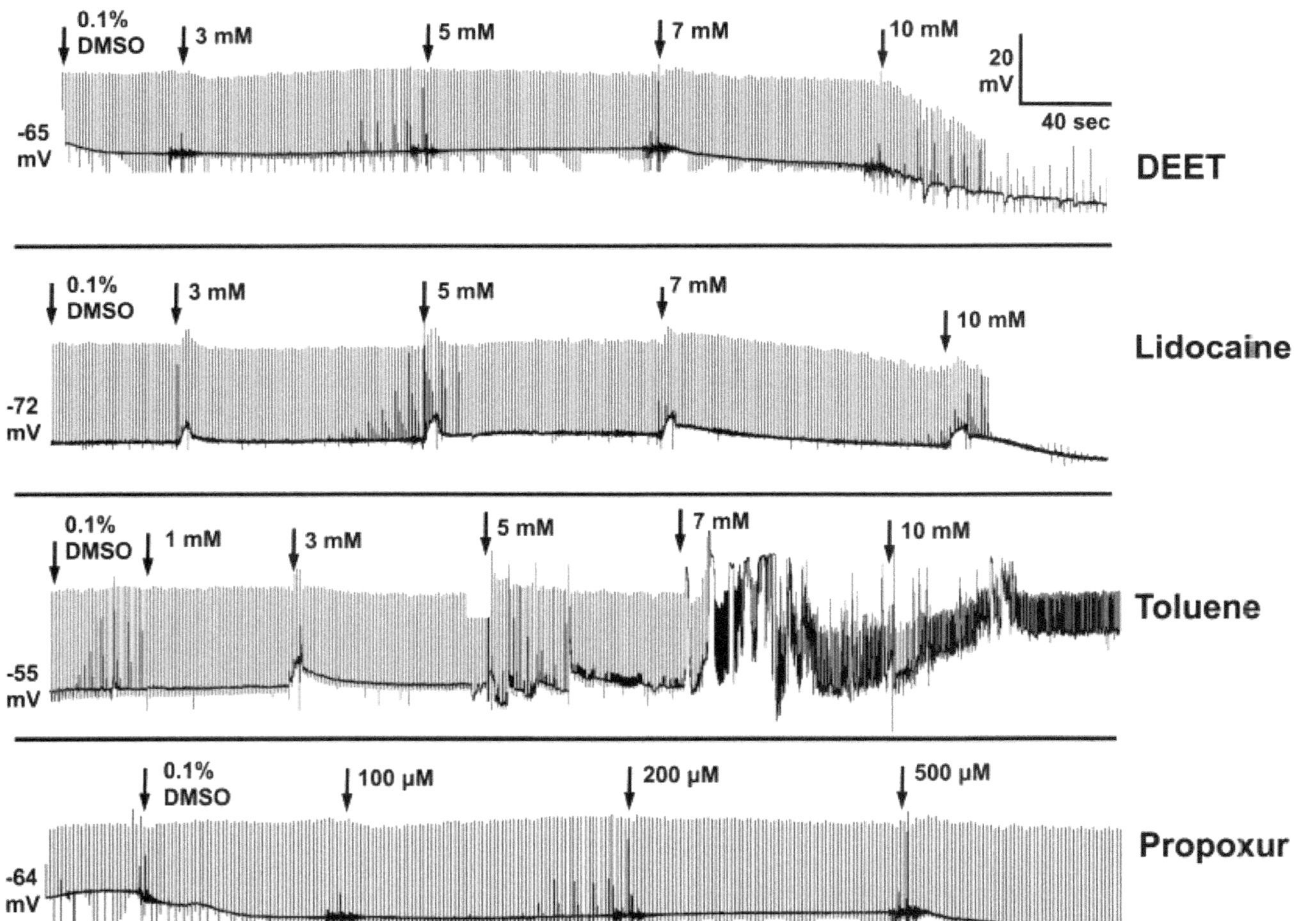

Figure 5: Recordings of the electrically-evoked EPSPs at the neuromuscular junction in *M. domestica* larvae after exposure to DEET (n=11), lidocaine (n=8), toluene (n=8), and propoxur (n=5). In the DEET and lidocaine traces, the remaining transients after block of the EPSP are stimulus artifacts, which are also reflected by any negative excursions from baseline in all traces (artifact amplitudes were truncated from the recordings for clarity of display). http://dx.doi.org/10.1371/journal.pone.0103713.g005

Patch Clamp of Rat Cortical Neurons

Patch clamp recordings of rat cortical neurons found that DEET is a blocker of both sodium and potassium channels in neonatal rat cortical neurons. DEET completely blocked inward sodium currents at 1 mM, and the effect could be washed out to restore approximately 50% of the sodium current amplitude (Fig. 6A). DEET was found to have an IC_{50} against sodium channels of about 0.7 mM. The DEET-mediated inhibition had similar potency as toluene, but was ca. 30-fold less active than lidocaine. Interestingly, lidocaine and toluene had similar Hill slopes values, while the value for DEET was 7- to 10-fold greater (Fig. 6B). DEET-mediated potassium channel block was also concentration-dependent (Fig. 6C). Current-voltage plots consistent with potassium Kv2 delayed rectifier channels were observed, and DEET blockage was capable of being washed out to restore approximately 50% of control current amplitude (Fig. 5D). Potassium channels were more sensitive to DEET compared to sodium channels, as they were blocked with an EC_{50} that was 6-fold lower (Fig. 6E).

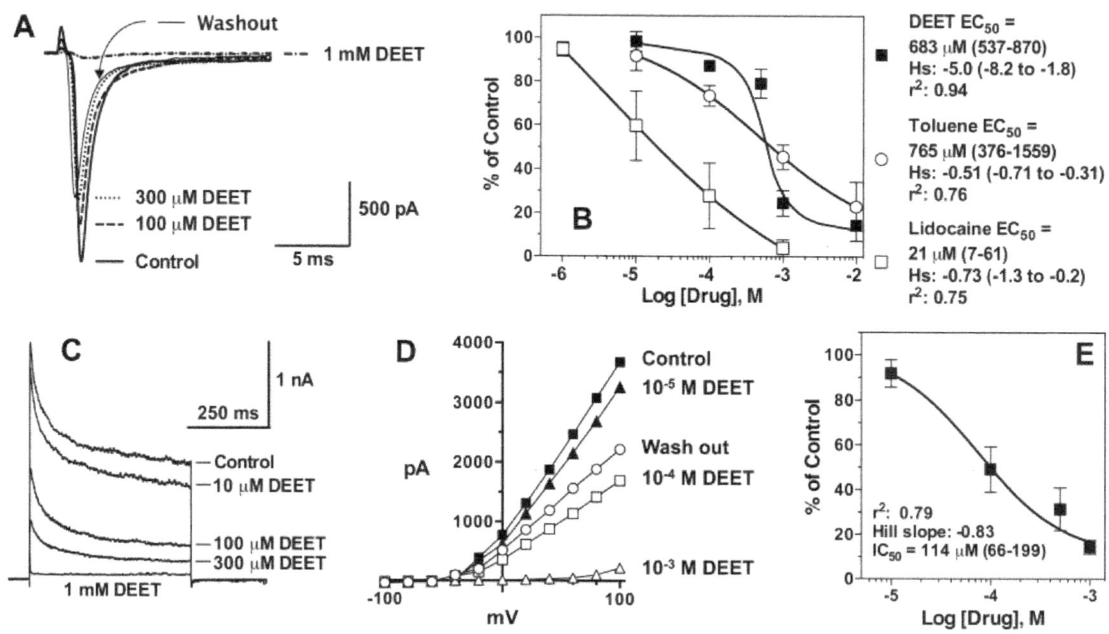

Figure 6: Block of neonatal rat cortical sodium and potassium channels by DEET and related compounds. A) Inward sodium currents activated by a 15 msec pulse to 0 mV from a holding potential of −80 mV. Control is the peak inward sodium current before treatment. Increasing DEET concentrations blocked the current, each trace taken after 1 min incubation in drug, and there was little change thereafter. Each trace is matched in form to treatment: thick line, Control; thin line, Washout; dashed line, 100 μM DEET; dotted line, 300 μM DEET; and dotted/dashed line, 1 mM DEET. B) Concentration-response curves generated from peak sodium currents as shown in A, replicated across different cells treated with DEET (n=3), toluene (n=6), or lidocaine (n=4). Symbols are mean percentage of control current amplitude, with each concentration of blocker replicated 3–6 times. Error bars represent SEM of currents. C) Typical outward currents activated by a 500 msec pulse to +60 mV from a holding potential of −80 mV, and displayed concentration-dependent block by DEET. D) Typical current-voltage relationships and DEET inhibition of potassium currents in rat cortical neurons. Currents were evoked by stepping the membrane voltage between −100 and +100 mV in 20 mV increments from a holding potential of −80 mV. Amplitude of the sustained current was calculated at 200 msec. E) Concentration-response curves for DEET-mediated inhibition of rat neuronal potassium channels from recordings as shown in C, using responses at +60 mV. Symbols are mean percentage of control current amplitude, and error bars represent SEM of currents replicated across different cells (n≥3).
http://dx.doi.org/10.1371/journal.pone.0103713.g006

DISCUSSION

Whole Animal Toxicity

DEET was found to be toxic at low microgram doses to the mosquitoes *Aedes aegypti* and*Anopheles gambiae*, and to the housefly, *Musca domestica*, which is similar to the mosquito toxicity observed by Corbel et al. [2]. Toxicity to the G3 (susceptible) and AKRON (resistant) strains of *Anopheles gambiae* were nearly identical, indicating that the AChE target site mutation does not protect against the toxicity of DEET. Co-administration of PBO also had no significant impact on the toxicity of DEET, demonstrating that DEET toxicity is not sensitive to P450 monooxygenases. Further, there was no inhibition of mosquito AChE and poor inhibition of *Md*AChE, *Dm*AChE, and human AChE by DEET (Table 2), confirming a previous suggestion that DEET is not an anticholinesterase [7]. These data are noteworthy in light of recent literature [2] reporting *in vitro* enzyme kinetic analyses of *Dm*AChE, as well as human AChE and butyrylcholinesterase. In these studies, DEET showed inhibitory effects at 0.1–10 mM concentrations. The fact that DEET is toxic to the mosquito without measurable inhibition of AChE, *in vitro*, suggests that DEET imposes its neurotoxic effect in a manner other than AChE inhibition. The low potency of DEET as an inhibitor of *h*AChE is consistent with the relatively few reports of cholinergic signs of human intoxication following DEET application, and its high LD_{50} value after oral administration to rats (ca. 3000 mg/kg [24]).

Housefly CNS Effects

The excitation of the housefly larval CNS after exposure to DEET was different from the response patterns of toluene and lidocaine (Fig. 2A), and besides propoxur, showed no correlation with inhibition of AChE, *in vitro*. Lidocaine was a blocker in all preparations studied, with EC_{50} values similar to those reported in the literature [25], likely indicating a different action on nerve preparations when compared to DEET, regardless of the similar *Md*AChE inhibition potencies for these two compounds (Table 2). The local anesthetic action of lidocaine on sodium channels apparently negates its anticholinesterase action when measured as descending nerve discharges from the CNS. Toluene was uniformly excitatory in all preparations tested, and had no anesthetic action on the insect nervous system. These findings suggest that the local anesthetic binding site of the insect sodium channel or its interaction with toluene is different from that of the rat Na_v 1.4 channel, as previous studies found toluene blocked these channels at a concentration of 3 mM, *in vitro* [12], well below the concentrations used in our study.

Octopaminergic Pathways and Receptors as Targets for DEET

Because DEET had neuroexcitatory effects on the CNS and a chemical structure somewhat similar to CDM, experiments compared the effects of DEET to compounds acting on octopaminergic systems. CDM and octopamine are neuroexcitatory through activation of octopamine receptors, leading to an increased cyclic AMP concentration that enhances neuronal excitability [10]. Phentolamine, a known octopaminergic antagonist [10], completely blocked the CNS neuroexcitation of DEET and octopamine, but was ineffective against neuroexcitation caused by propoxur or 4-AP. These results provide the first direct evidence that DEET targets octopaminergic nerve pathways as the mechanism of neurotoxicity.

Although there is no documented presence of octopamine receptors in *Sf*21 cells, octopamine receptors coupled to adenylate cyclase are present in *Sf*9 cells and respond positively to the demethylated metabolite of CDM [22]. Our data (Fig. 2B) demonstrate the presence of octopamine receptors on *Sf*21 cells linked to internal calcium fluorescence. Both DEET- and octopamine-mediated fluorescence were antagonized by the receptor antagonist phentolamine, similar to the larval CNS recordings. The action of DEET on calcium fluorescence via an octopamine receptor provides a third piece of evidence suggesting an action on octopaminergic systems. These data, along with the poor anticholinesterase action of DEET, provide strong evidence that DEET is primarily targeting octopamine receptor activation and not acetylcholinesterase to induce insect toxicity.

Activation of the firefly (*Photinus pyralis)* light organ further support that DEET is targeting the octopaminergic system, since it is well documented that octopamine is responsible for induction of luminescence within the light organ [26], [27] via cyclic AMP production [28], [29]. CDM is a potent effector of the firefly light organ [30], but complete activation of the lantern is not observed until four hours post-exposure due to the need for CDM to be demethylated, *in vivo*, to its agonist form [30]. DEET activated the firefly lantern in a dose-dependent manner (Fig. 4A), but its luminescent action was slightly different from that of CDM. DEET-induced illumination was less potent and effective than CDM, perhaps reflecting low receptor affinity, desensitization, or another mechanism(s) of action on the lantern. In contrast, the anticholinesterase propoxur at the intoxicating dose used had no effect on the firefly lantern.

Neuromuscular Actions of DEET

The insect neuromuscular junction was used to assess the action of DEET on the peripheral nervous system and the inactivity of propoxur serves as a negative control for effects of suspected anticholinesterases, as insects lack peripheral cholinergic synapses [31], [32]. DEET blocked the evoked EPSP, an effect consistent with an anesthetic-like action, but was 60–fold less potent than its excitatory action on the CNS. Lidocaine displayed a blocking pattern similar to DEET, indicating a local anesthetic effect and a shared blocking action on the neuromuscular junction. Effects of DEET on the neuromuscular junction were inconsistent with potassium channel block, as there was no evidence of multiple EPSP discharges or any depolarization of the muscle membrane potential, even though four potassium channel subtypes, including calcium-activated, inactivating, and delayed rectifier, are known to exist in these muscles [33]. Perhaps the high concentration of DEET and lidocaine required for block of neurotransmission indicates effects on sodium and potassium channels acting in opposition to each other, or possibly blockage of calcium channels [11], but more experiments would be required to address these possibilities.

Actions of DEET on Mammalian Na^+ and K^+ Channels

Patch clamp studies were performed with rat cortical neurons to determine the mode of action of DEET on mammalian ion channels. DEET was capable of blocking sodium and potassium (Kv2, delayed rectifier type) currents at low- to mid-micromolar concentrations, similar to lidocaine and other local anesthetics. However, for local anesthetics, sodium channel block is more potent than potassium channel block [11], whereas DEET showed the opposite (Fig. 6). In any event, these actions may play a role in the numbing sensation observed when DEET contacts human skin [5]. Local anesthetics have a well characterized numbing effect caused by a blocking action on nerve membrane sodium channels, and this effect is more potent and functionally significant than its ability to block potassium channels, which simply results in a broadening of the action potential [11]. Much further investigation of its ion channel blocking mechanisms is warranted, and should include studies of mammalian sensory nerve conduction in the presence of DEET. DEET blockage of sodium currents had 7- and 10-fold greater Hill slope than lidocaine or toluene, respectively (Fig. 5), but unusually steep Hill slopes were not observed for inhibition of AChE activity or potassium currents. Compounds having steep inhibitory Hill slopes at high concentrations *in vitro*, can occur if there are several inhibitor binding sites on a protein, when [enzyme] >> than inhibitor K_d, or phase transitions/precipitation/colloid formation occurs for some compounds in high throughput screening situations [34]. Additional research is required to address these different possible mechanisms.

With regard to insect toxicity, it is unlikely that sodium or potassium channel blockage is the primary mechanism of DEET toxicity, since excitatory effects on the CNS are much more potent, and the effects of 4-AP, a classical potassium channel blocker, are not inhibited by phentolamine. This line of reasoning supports the idea that splayed posture and hyperexcitation after toxic doses of DEET arise because of a combination of central octopaminergic hyperexcitation complexed with incomplete suppression of peripheral neurotransmission.

CONCLUSIONS

DEET is of relatively low acute toxicity to insects and mammals. It is unlikely that DEET exerts its toxicity through anticholinesterase action because of its low potency for enzyme inhibition and the complete block of its neuroexcitation in housefly CNS by phentolamine, which does not occur with propoxur or 4-AP. DEET toxicity to houseflies, and likely mosquitoes, is mediated by central octopaminergic pathways via activation of octopamine receptors. The poisoning signs caused by DEET reflect an excitatory octopaminergic effect in combination with peripheral neurosuppressive actions. The low potency of DEET for inhibiting human acetylcholinesterase makes it unlikely to cause toxicity by this mechanism. Numbness of mammalian mucous membranes is explained through anesthetic-like effects of DEET on nerve conduction.

ACKNOWLEDGMENTS

We thank Dr. Phil Kaufman (University of Florida, Department of Entomology and Nematology) for providing *Musca domestica* larvae, and Dr. Dan Kline (USDA-ARS) and Mr. Paul Howell (CDC) for providing *Aedes aegypti* and *Anopheles gambiae* mosquitoes, respectively.

REFERENCES

1. Moore S, Debboun M (2007) History of insect repellents. In: Debboun M, Frances S, Strickman D, editors.Insect repellents: Principles, methods, and uses.Boca Raton: CRC Press. pp. 3–30.
2. Corbel V, Stankiewicz M, Pennetier C, Fournier D, Stojan J, et al. (2009) Evidence for inhibition of cholinesterases in insect and mammalian nervous systems by the insect repellent deet. BMC Biol 7: 47 Available: http://www.biomedcentral.com/1741-7007/7/47 Accessed 16 July 2014.
3. Ellenhorn M (1997) Ellenhorn's medical toxicology: Diagnosis and treatment of human poisoning, 2nd edition. Baltimore:: William and Wilkins. 2300 pp. doi: 10.1001/jama.1997.03550140095052
4. Lipscomb J, Kramer J, Leikin J (1992) Seizure following brief exposure to the insect repellent N,N Diethyl-m-toluamide. Ann Emerg Med 21: 315–317. doi: 10.1016/s0196-0644(05)80896-0
5. Clem J, Havemann D, Raebel M (1993) Insect repellent (N,N-Diethyl-m-toluamide) cardiovascular toxicity in an adult. Ann Pharacother 27: 289–293.
6. Reuveni H, Yagupsky P (1982) Diethyltoluamide-containing insect repellent: Adverse effects in worldwide use. Arch Dermatol 18: 582–583. doi: 10.1001/archderm.1982.01650200050015
7. Moss J (1996) Synergism of toxicity of N,N Diethyl-m-toluamide to German cockroaches (Orthoptera: Blattellidae) by hydrolytic enzyme inhibitors. J Econ Entomol 89: 1151–1155.
8. Licciardi S, Herve J, Darriet F, Hougard J, Corbel V (2006) Lethal and behavioral effects of three synthetic repellents (DEET, IR3535, and KBR 3023) on *Aedes aegypti*mosquitoes in laboratory assays. J Med Vet Entomol 20: 288–293. doi: 10.1111/j.1365-2915.2006.00630.x
9. Bonnet J, Pennetier C, Duchon S, Lapied B, Corbel V (2009) Multi-function oxidases are responsible for the synergistic interactions occurring between repellents and insecticides in mosquitoes. Parasites & Vectors 2: 17 doi:10.1186/1756-3305-2-17.
10. Hollingsworth R, Lund A (1982) Biological and neurotoxic effects of amidine pesticides. In: Coats J editor.Insecticide Mode of Action. Academic Press, New York. Chap. 7, pp. 189–227.
11. Scholz A (2002) Mechanisms of (local) anaesthetics on voltage-gated sodium and other ion channels. Br J Anaesthesia 89: 52–61. doi: 10.1093/bja/aef163
12. Scior T, Martinez-Morales E, Cruz S, Salinas-Stefanon E (2009) In silico modeling of toluene binding site in the pore of voltage-gate sodium channel. J Receptor Ligand Channel Res 2: 1–9.
13. Ellman G, Courtney K, Andres V, Featherstone R (1961) A new and rapid colorimetric determination of acetylcholinesterase activity. Biochem Pharmaco 7: 88–95. doi: 10.1016/0006-2952(61)90145-9
14. Djogbenou L, Weill M, Hougard J, Raymond M, Akogbeto M, et al. (2007) Characterization of insensitive acetylcholinesterase (ace-1R) in *Anopheles gambiae*(Diptera: Culicidae): Resistance levels and dominance. J Med Entomol 44: 805–810. doi: 10.1603/0022-2585(2007)44[805:coiaai]2.0.co;2
15. Yadouleton A, Asidi A, Djouaka R, Braima J, Agossou C, et al. (2009) Development of vegetable farming: a cause of the emergence of insecticide resistance in populations of Anopheles gambiae in urban areas of Benin. Malar J 8, 103 Available:http://www.malariajournal.com/content/8/1/103. Accessed 16 July 2014.
16. Carlier P, Anderson T, Wong D, Hsu D, Hartsel J, et al. (2008) Towards a species-selective acetylcholinesterase inhibitor to control the mosquito vector of malaria,*Anopheles gambiae*.. Chem Biol Interact 175: 368–75. doi: 10.1016/j.cbi.2008.04.037
17. Pridgeon J, Pereira R, Becnel J, Allan S, Clark G, et al. (2008) Susceptibility of *Aedes aegypti, Culex quinquefasciatus Say*, and *Anopheles quadrimaculatus* to 19pesticideswithdifferentmodesofaction.JMedEntomol 45: 82–87. doi: 10.1603/0022-2585(2008)45[82:soaacq]2.0.co;2
18. World Health Organization (1981) Instructions for determining the susceptibility or resistance of adult mosquitoes to organochlorine, organophosphorus and

carbamate insecticides. World Health Organization, WHO/VBC 81.805 and WHO/VBC 81.806

19. Abbot W (1925) A method of computing the effectiveness of an insecticide. J Econ Entomol 18: 265–267.

20. Bloomquist J, ffrench-Constant R, Roush R (1991) Excitation of central neurons by dieldrin and picrotoxinin in susceptible and resistant Drosophila melanogaster (Meigen). Pestic Sci 32: 463–469. doi: 10.1002/ps.2780320408

21. Bloomquist J, Kinne L, Deutsch V, Simpson S (1996) Mode of action of an insecticidal peptide toxin from the venom of a weaving spider (*Diguetia canities*). Toxicon 34: 1072–1075. doi: 10.1016/0041-0101(96)00028-1

22. Orr N, Orr G, Hollngworth R (1992) The Sf9 cell line as a model for studying insect octopamine-receptors. Insect Biochem Molec Biol 22: 591–597. doi: 10.1016/0965-1748(92)90036-e

23. Casida J (1970) Mixed-function oxidase involvement in the biochemistry of insecticide synergists. J Agric Food Chem 18: 753–772. doi: 10.1021/jf60171a013

24. Macko J, Weeks M (1980) Phase 6: Acute toxicity evaluation of N,N-diethyl-meta-toluamide (M-Det.). U.S. Army Environmental Hygiene Agency Study No.71-51-0034-81.

25. Jaffe R, Rowe M (1996) Differential nerve block. Direct measurements on individual myelinated and unmyelinated dorsal root axons. Anesthesiology 84: 1455–1464. doi: 10.1097/00000542-199606000-00022

26. Robertson H, Carlson A (1976) Octopamine: presence in firefly lantern suggests a transmitter role. J Exp Zoo 195: 159–164. doi: 10.1002/jez.1401950116

27. Copeland J, Robertson H (1982) Octopamine as the transmitter at the firefly lantern: presence of an octopamine-sensitive and a dopamine-sensitive adenylate cyclase. Comp Biochem Physiol 72: 125–127. doi: 10.1016/0306-4492(82)90217-9

28. Nathanson J (1979) Octopamine receptors, adenosine 3', 5'-monophosphate, and neural control of firefly flashing. Science 203: 65–68. doi: 10.1126/science.214856

29. Nathanson J, Hunnicutt E (1979) Neural control of light emission in *Photuris* larvae: identification of octopamine-sensitive adenylate cyclase. J. Exp. Zool 208: 255–262. doi: 10.1002/jez.1402080213

30. Hollingworth R, Murdock L (1980) Formamidine Pesticides: octopamine-like actions in a firefly. Science 208: 74–76. doi: 10.1126/science.208.4439.74

31. Calhoun E (1963) The physiological significance of acetylcholine in insects and observations upon other pharmacologically active substances. In: Beament J, Treherne J, Wigglesworth V, editors.Advances in insect physiology.London: Academic Press, Vol. 1 , pp. 1–45.

32. Booth G, Lee A (1971) Distribution of cholinesterase in insects. WHO Bull 44: 91–98.

33. Salgado VL (1992) Block of voltage-dependent K^+ channels in insect muscle by the diacylhydrazine insecticide RH-5849, 4-aminopyridine, and quinidine. Arch Insect Biochem Physiol 21: 239–252. doi: 10.1002/arch.940210307

34. .Shoichet B (2006) Interpreting steep dose-response curves in early inhibitor discovery. J Med Chem 49: 7274–7277. doi: 10.1021/jm061103g

CHAPTER 21 CANTHARIDIN IMPEDES ACTIVITY OF GLUTATHIONE S-TRANSFERASE IN THE MIDGUT OFHELICOVERPA ARMIGERA HÜBNER

Rashid Ahmed Khan, Ji Yuan Liu , Maryam Rashid, Dun Wang, and Ya Lin Zhang

Keywords: glutathione S-transferases; Helicoverpa armigera; cantharidin; mRNA; molecular docking simulations

INTRODUCTION

Glutathione *S*-transferase (GST EC 2.5.1.18) is an important family of multifunctional isozymes found in all eukaryotes. One of the main metabolic functions of GST is to catalyse xenobiotics, including pesticides in the mercapturic acid pathway leading to the elimination of toxic compounds [1]. GSTs also convert a reactive lipophilic molecule into a water-soluble, non-reactive conjugate which may easily be excreted [2]. This family of enzymes has been implicated as one of the major mechanisms for neutralizing the toxic effects of insecticides in insects [3,4].

In recent years, the management of *Helicoverpa armigera*, the American bollworm, has become increasingly difficult due to the development of resistance to various groups of insecticides, particularly pyrethroids and cyclodyienes [5].*H. armigera* is an important polyphagous pest of cotton and many other crops of agricultural importance all over the world. In insects, GSTs provide an important defense mechanism against plant allelochemicals [6] as well as insecticides [7]. An increased level of GSTs has been regarded as causing organochlorine and organophosphorus insecticide resistance [8–14].

The active constituent of mylabris, cantharidin is produced by as many as 1500 different species of blister beetles, with the Spanish fly *Cantharis vesicatoria* probably being the best known source [15,16]. Cantharidin was first isolated by Robiquet, a French chemist in 1810. It has an important role in the ecology of different kinds of insects that use or produce it as a defense to preserve their eggs from predators [17].

Recently this defensive tool has been developed into a bio-pesticide and one of the formulations as an emulsifiable concentrate (EC) has been registered for the control of lepidopteran pests while other formulations of cantharidin and its analogues are under field trial for registration. Cantharidin as 1.0% EC has been tested for its environmental safety and toxicity was found to be within safe limits for ladybugs, quail and soil microorganisms [18]. The antifeedant activity of cantharidin and its toxicity was earlier established against armyworm, *Mythimna separata*[19]. Furthermore, inhibitory effect of cantharidin on GSTs was reported in *M. separata*[20]. However, its toxicity and inhibitory effect on GSTs in *H. armigera* have not yet been investigated in detail.

At present there is very little information about the toxicity mechanism of cantharidin to insects and its interaction with metabolizing enzymes, especially GSTs. In the present study,

Citation: Rashid Ahmed Khan, Ji Yuan Liu, Maryam Rashid , Dun Wang and Ya Lin Zhang, Cantharidin Impedes Activity of Glutathione S-Transferase in the Midgut of Helicoverpa armigera Hübner, doi:10.3390/ijms14035482

our aim was to investigate the effect of cantharidin on mRNA transcript of HaGST (GenBank accession no EF033109) and also its putative role in the inhibition of GSTs in *H. armigera* both *in vivo* and *in vitro*. For this purpose, we cloned a model *H. armigera* GST gene (HaGST) which was previously reported for its role in insect defense mechanism [21] and prokaryotically expressed it to get soluble recombinant protein, rHaGST. Homology modeling and molecular docking simulation techniques were employed to rationalize our experimental results.

RESULTS AND DISCUSSION

Bioassay

Bioassay results showed an increase in levels of *H. armigera* mortality with time after feeding on cantharidin-treated artificial diet. The artificial diet incorporated cantharidin of 250 μg g^{-1} at 12, 24, 48, 72 h after treatment caused significant larval mortality of 23%, 41% and 69% and 98%, respectively (Figure 1).

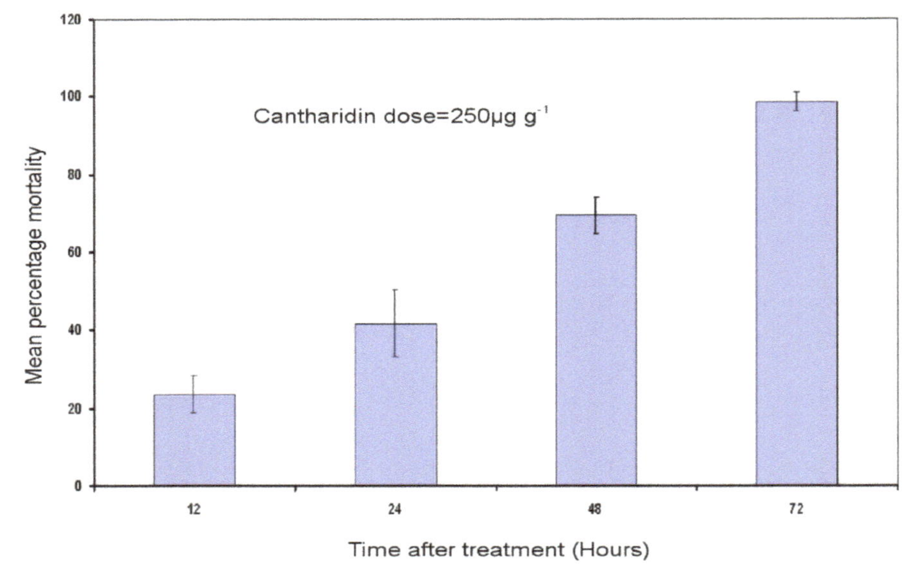

Figure 1. Mean percentage mortalities of *H. armigera*. Third-instar larvae were subjected to bioassay. Error bars show ± SD among three replications. Number of third-instar larvae tested per treatment (n = 72).

SDS-PAGE Analysis

The positive clones were transformed in BL-21 (DE-3) and protein expression induced by the addition of IPTG was detected initially by SDS-PAGE using standard protein molecular weight marker. The expected band was detected at 27 kDa as the MW of the HaGST is about 24 kDa and the pET-28a tag is about 3 kDa (Figure 2). The expression of recombinant protein was detected by 6× His mouse monoclonal primary antibody on a PVDF membrane.

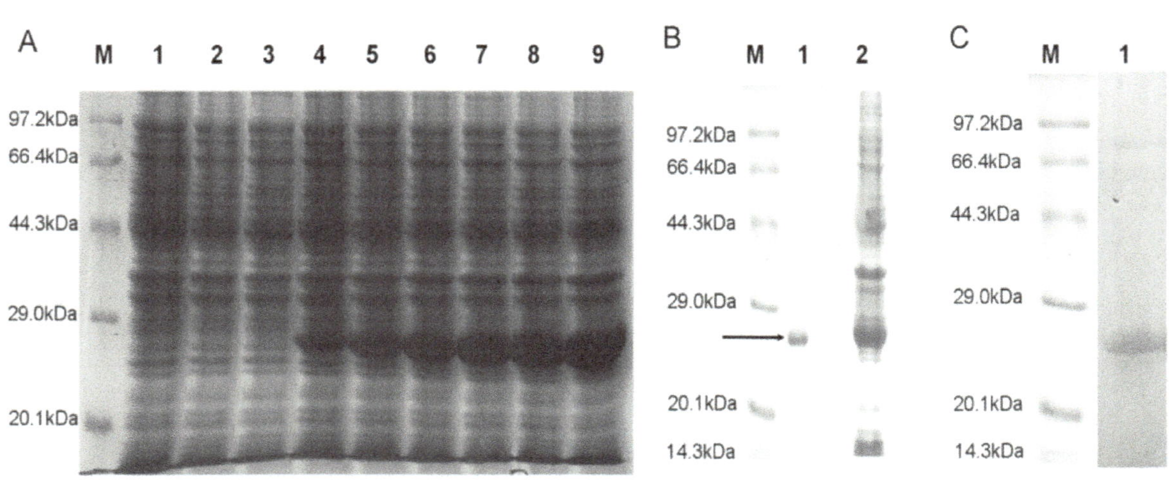

Figure 2. SDS-PAGE analysis of fusion protein. (A) Lane M, Protein weight marker; Lane1, DE-3; Lane 2, DE-3 + pET28a; Lane 3, DE-3 + pET28a-HaGST (without IPTG); Lane 4–6, expression level of the soluble fusion protein at 1–6 h; (B) Purified soluble rHaGST. Lane M, Protein weight marker; Lane 1, Purified rHaGST by Ni^{2+}-nitrilotriacetate (NTA) column; Lane 2, non purified protein; (C) Immunoblotting of rHaGST with 6× His mouse monoclonal primary antibody. Lane M, Molecular weight marker; Lane 1, rHaGST detected by peroxidase conjugated goat anti-mouse IgG secondary antibody.

Specific Activity of HaGST

The inhibitory effects of cantharidin *in vivo* on GSTs enzyme within midguts dissected from larvae treated with sub-lethal dose of cantharidin is shown in Figure 3. A sub-lethal dose of 25 μg g^{-1} exerted inhibitory effects on the GSTs in midgut as compared to the untreated control. Data showed that the specific activity of the GSTs tended to decrease in treatment from 24 to 96 h, whereas specific activity tended to increase in untreated controls. The inhibitory effect on the activity at 96 h after treatment was 22.8 compared to 48.32 μM min^{-1} mg^{-1} of control.

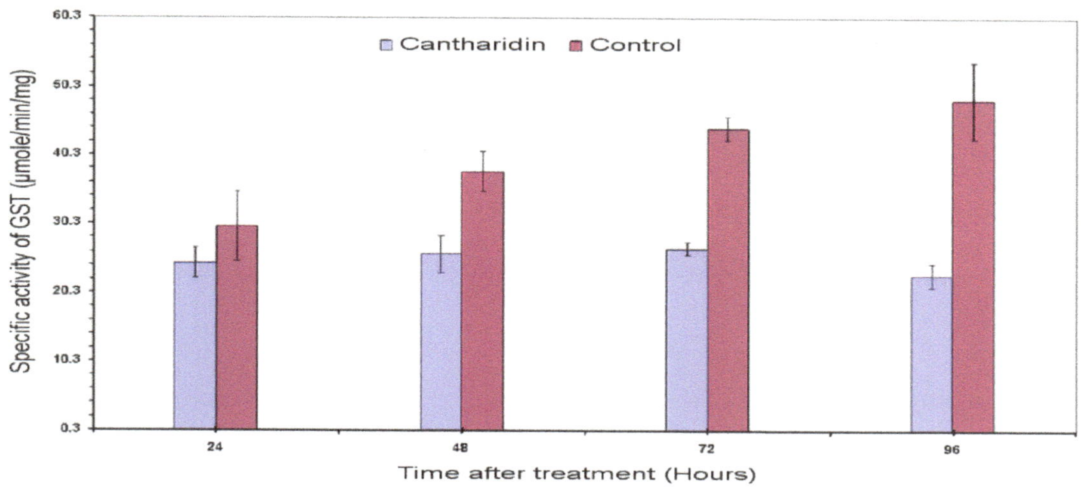

Figure 3: Specific activity of the GSTs in larval midgut of *H. armigera* subjected to sub-lethal dose of cantharidin using glutathione (GSH) and 1-chloro-2,4-dinitrobenzene (CDNB) secondary substrate. The activity of the GSTs was measured at 340 nm both in treated and control samples.

Kinetic Properties of GSTs

The inhibitory effects of cantharidin on the GSTs enzyme extract activity using GSH as substrate is shown in Figure 4. To find out the kind of cantharidin inhibition of the GSTs enzyme extract by cantharidin, the GSTs activity was calculated with variable concentrations of GSH. A Lineweaver-Burk plot with GSH as the variable substrate and for the type of inhibition by cantharidin is shown in Figure 4A. The Lineweaver-Burk plot revealed that cantharidin inhibited GSTs non-competitively as V_{max} lowered down, whereas Km remained unchanged with respect to GSH.

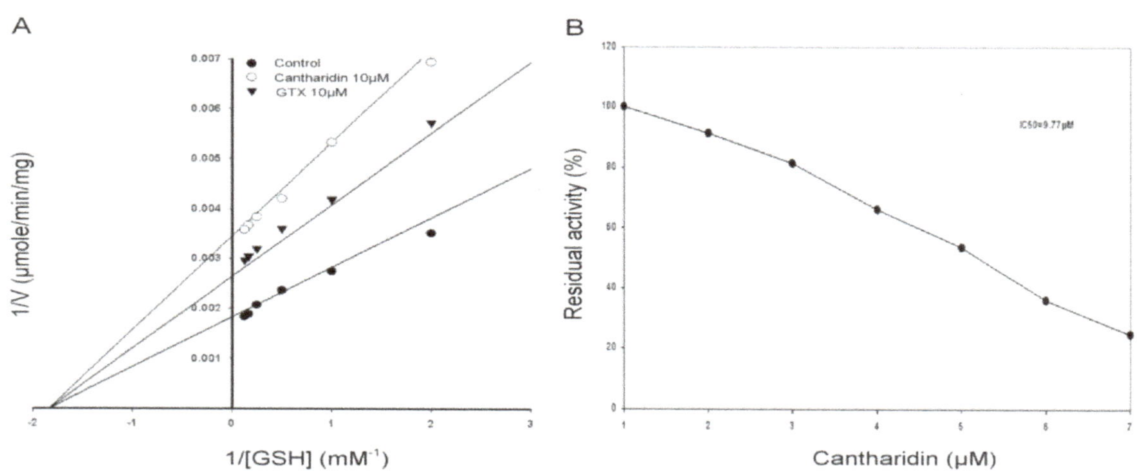

Figure 4: Lineweaver-Burk plot of the GSTs activity in crude enzyme extract. (A) Specific activity of GSTs with and without cantharidin. IC50 value of cantharidin for the GSTs using glutathione (GSH) and 1-chloro-2,4-dinitrobenzene (CDNB) secondary substrate; (B) IC50 value was obtained using a plot of percent activities *vs.* varying concentrations of cantharidin. *S*-Hexylglutathione (GTX) was used as positive control.

Kinetic Properties of Purified rHaGST

The inhibitory effects of the cantharidin on the affinity of the column purified soluble rHaGST activity using GSH as substrate is shown in Figure 5. To determine the type of inhibition of the rHaGST by cantharidin, the rHaGST activity was calculated under different concentrations of GSH. The Lineweaver-Burk plot for GSH as the variable substrate and type of inhibition is shown in Figure 5A. The Lineweaver-Burk plot revealed that cantharidin inhibited rHaGST non-competitively as V_{max} lowered, whereas Km remained unchanged with respect to GSH.

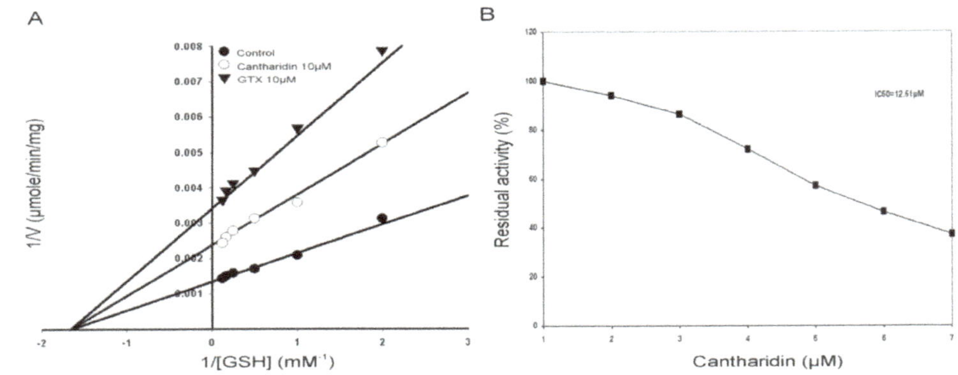

Figure 5: Lineweaver-Burk plot of the purified soluble rHaGST. (A) Specific activity of GSTs with and without cantharidin. IC50 value of cantharidin for GSTs using glutathione (GSH) and 1-chloro-2,4-dinitrobenzene (CDNB) secondary substrate; (B) IC50 value was obtained using a plot of percent activities *vs.* varying concentrations of cantharidin. *S*-Hexylglutathione (GTX) was used as positive control.

IC50 of Cantharidin

To calculate IC50 of cantharidin for the GSTs and the soluble purified rHaGST, variable concentrations of cantharidin were used using GSH as substrate. Results showed that cantharidin inhibited activity of the GSTs and the purified rHaGST in a dose-dependent manner with 50% inhibitory concentration at 9.77 μM (Figure 4B) and 12.5 μM (Figure 5B), respectively.

Time Course Expression Profile of the HaGST Gene by Real-Time qPCR

Real-time qPCR was carried out to investigate the effect of cantharidin on the mRNA transcript of the HaGST based on time after treatment. Results showed that the HaGST was down-regulated at 24, 48, 72 and 96 h after treatment. Normalized expression results revealed that the HaGST was down regulated by 2.5, 8.3, 9.09 and 12.5 folds after 24, 48, 72 and 96 h, respectively (Figure 6).

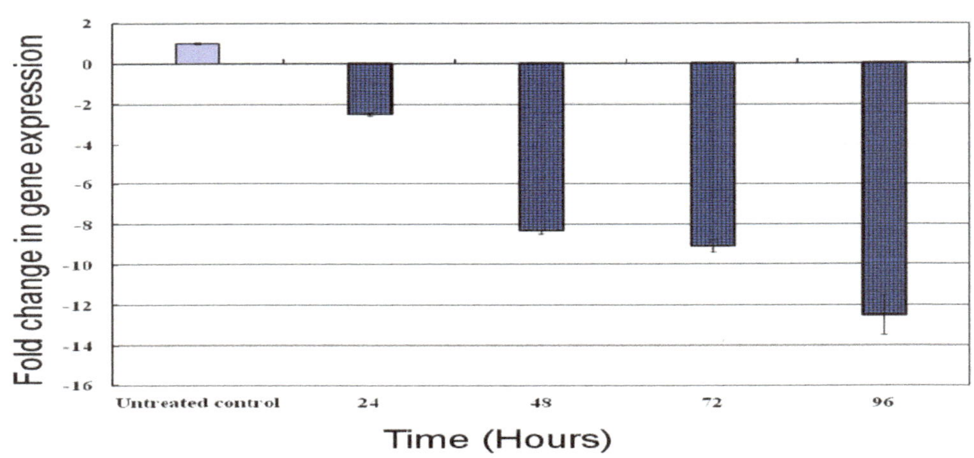

Figure 6. The real-time q-PCR analysis of the HaGST mRNA transcript at different time intervals from 24 to 96 h. Target gene expression was normalized by comparing ΔΔCT to an untreated control. Error bars show standard deviation using three replications.

Homology Modeling of HaGST

In order to study the binding of cantharidin with HaGST, a better crystallographic *R*-factor (20.9%) and higher overall sequence identity (57%) was considered (Figure 7). We finally selected the complete crystal structure of an insect delta-class glutathione *S*-transferase from a DDT-resistant strain of the malaria vector *Anopheles gambiae* in complex with its inhibitor named *S*-hexylglutathione (GTX) as the template (PDB:1PN9) [22] at a resolution of 2.0 Å. The best model was selected with the lowest value of DOPE assessment score (−27,127.846). The analysis of the Ramachandran plot showed that 97.2% (212/218) of all residues were in favored (98%) regions, and 99.1% (216/218) of all residues were in allowed (>99.8%) regions. Only two amino acids GLU66 and ALA212 were found in the disallowed region of the Ramachandran plot. The resultant 3D structure of the HaGST is shown in Figure 8. The active site is located in a deep cleft formed at the interface of the two domains.

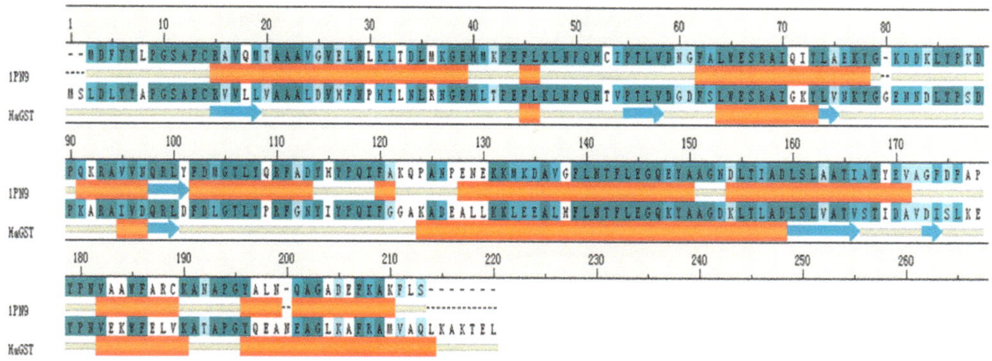

Figure 7: Sequence alignment results. The target protein HaGST and template protein, IPN9. Deep green color indicates conserved residues in both the sequences. Red bands show α helices while blue arrows show β sheets.

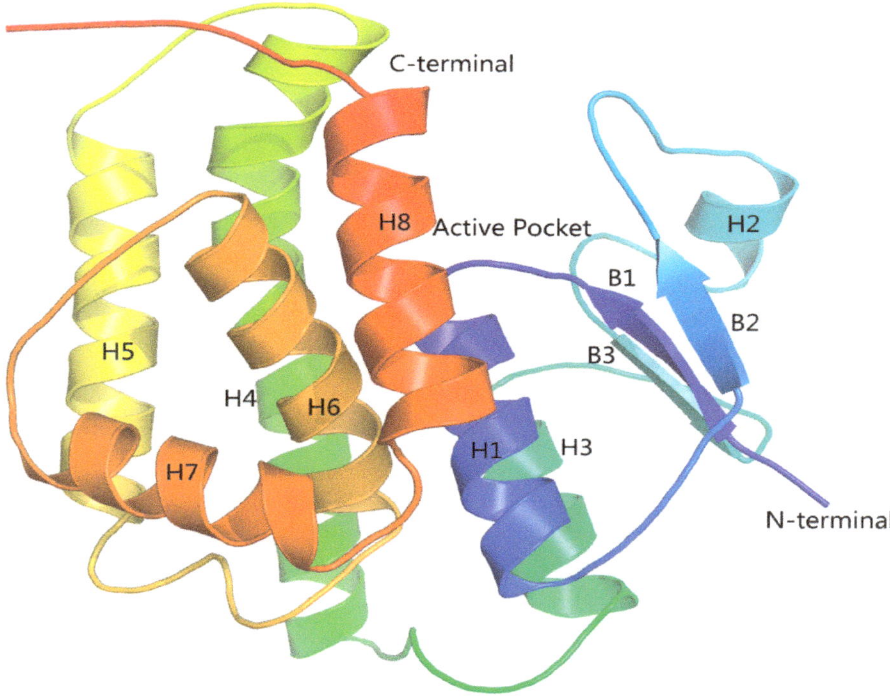

Figure 8: The ribbon representation of the 3-D model of the HaGST. Blue and red colors represent a chain trace from the *N*-terminus to *C*-terminus, respectively. α helices and β sheets are represented by H and B, respectively. The active site is located in the cleft formed at the interface of H8, H3 and between loops of H2, B3.

Molecular Docking Simulations

As shown in Figure 9 the final binding mode of the GTX-HaGST was obtained by molecular docking and superimposition (RMSD of only 0.210Å) of the conformations of the GTX in the 1PN9 and HaGST. The O26 atom in the GTX and the NH atom of the HIS52 side chain formed hydrogen bonds having a distance of 2.2 Å between atoms. The NH and the O atoms, which are derived from the VAL54 backbone, interact with the O13 atom and the H8 atom in the GTX by hydrogen bonds respectively, having distances of 1.8 Å and 2.0 Å between them. The NH atom of SER67 backbone also interacts with the O5 atom of GTX with a hydrogen bond distance of 1.9 Å between atoms. The hydrogen bonds are formed between the H2 atom of the GTX and the O atom from GLU66 side chain whose distance is 2.4 Å (Figure 10). While comparing the schematic representation of residual-ligand hydrogen bond interactions, only one interaction site in insect delta class GST, ILE52 in *Anopheles gambiae* may have mutated to VAL54 in *Helicoverpa armigera*. Although the VAL54 and the ILE52 are non-polar hydrophobic amino acids, the NH atom derived from the backbone of ILE52 only interacts with the O13 atom of the GTX. Based on our findings, it could be assumed that the hydrogen bond network is more stable in the GTX-HaGST 3D model complex than those in the crystal structure named 1PN9. Based on the docking work mentioned above, the accurate binding mode of the HaGST 3D model with the cantharidin was obtained as shown in Figure 11.

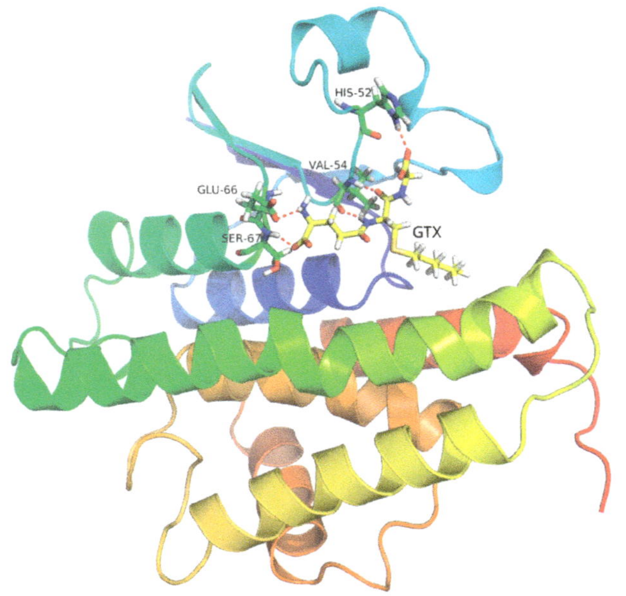

Figure 9: The binding model of GTX with the HaGST. Red dotted lines show hydrogen bonding among the corresponding atoms of amino acid residues of the active site and GTX.

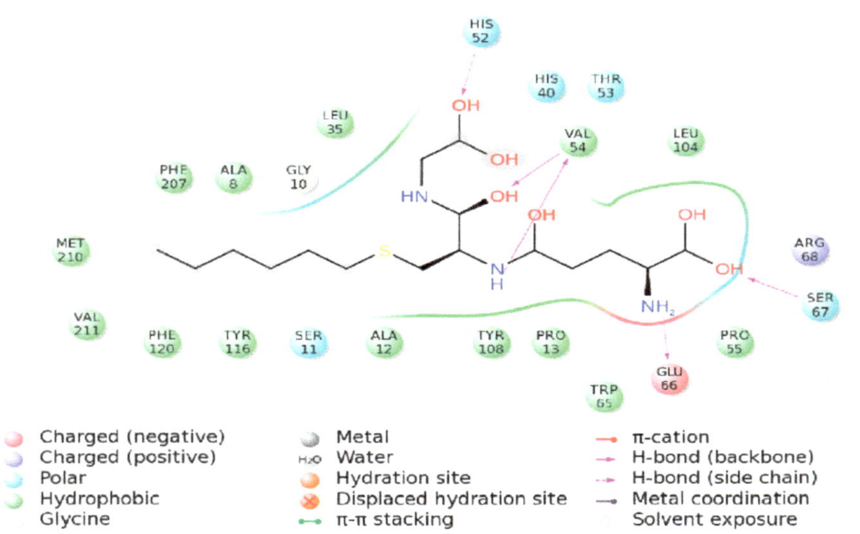

Figure 10: The interaction diagram of the insect delta-class HaGST from *Helicoverpa armigera* with its inhibitor, GTX.

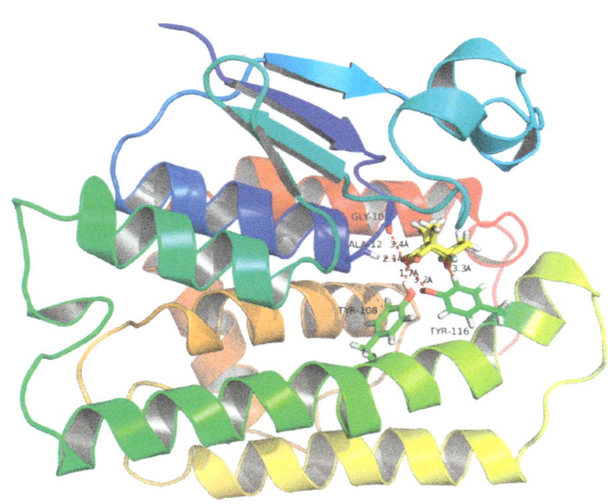

Figure 11: Binding mode of the cantharidin-HaGST complex. Red dotted lines show hydrogen bonding between the amino acid residues of the active site and atoms of cantharidin. The O atom of GLY10 and NH atom of ALA12 interact with the cantharidin O3 atom, simultaneously by hydrogen bonding. The OH atom of TRY116 also interacts with the O3 atom of cantharidin. A OH atom of TRY108 forming a hydrogen bond with O1 of cantharidin plays an important role in binding affinity based on its lowest inter-atomic distance.

The schematic representation of residue-ligand interactions for cantharidin is shown in Figure 12. The cantharidin docks inside the active site formed by amino acid residues TYR116, PHE120, SER11, ALA8, GLY10, ALA12, ARG15, PRO13, TYR108, LEU35, VAL54. The O atom of GLY10 and the NH atom of ALA12 which are both derived from the backbone of the HaGST 3D model simultaneously interact with the O3 atom of the cantharidin by hydrogen bonds, whose distances are 3.4 Å and 2.1 Å, respectively. The OH atom from the side chain of TYR116 also interacts with the O3 atom of the cantharidin by hydrogen bonds. The hydrogen bonds are formed between the OH atom of TYR108 and the O1 atom of the cantharidin which are only1.7 Å apart. The smaller distance of 1.7 Å between the OH atom of TYR108 and the O1 atom of the cantharidin may have a profound impact on their binding affinity. The hydrogen bond network occupying the active site of HaGST allows the formation of the stable complex with cantharidin.

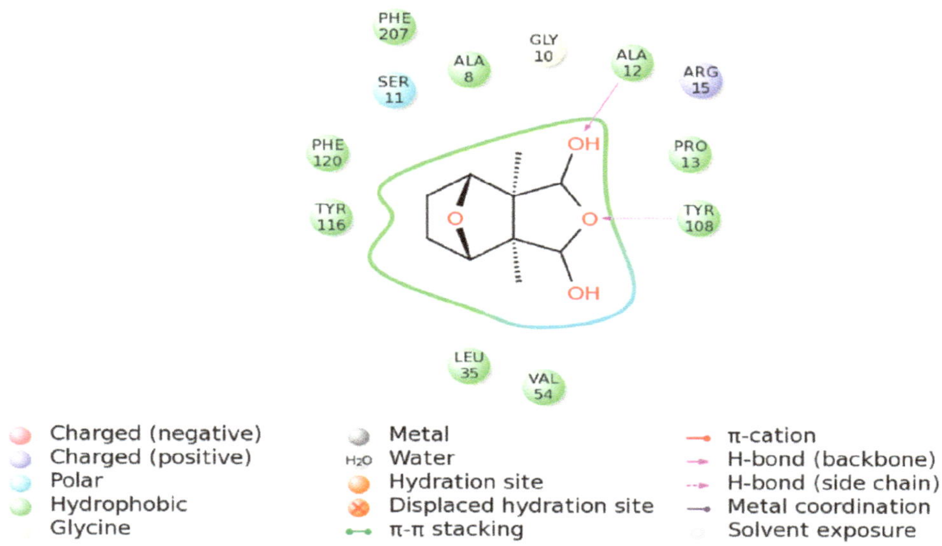

Figure 12: The Interaction diagram of the delta class HaGST with cantharidin. ALA12 and TRY108 are mainly responsible for making hydrogen bonds with the O atoms of cantharidin.

Binding Energy Calculations

As shown in Table 1, the calculated binding energy delta G (DG) indicates that cantharidin has a higher binding affinity than the GTX.

Table 1: Delta G values of compounds, GTX and cantharidin against the HaGST 3D model. A ChemScore function was applied to measure affinity data by ranking according to ChemScore delta value.

Molecule	Score	DG	S (hbond)	S (lipo)	H (rot)	DE (clash)	DE (int)
GTX	16.76	−19.65	3.87	142.65	6.04	0.10	2.79
Cantharidin	21.58	−21.86	1.80	88.77	0.00	0.28	0.00

In our current research we have used GST as a molecular target of cantharidin since GSTs plays an important role in defense against plant allelochemicals [6] as well as insecticides [7].

Earlier studies have suggested the increased level of GSTs as one of the major reasons for the development of resistance using metabolic detoxification of insecticides. Many researchers have documented the development of insecticide resistance caused by increased levels of GSTs especially in diamondback moth (DBM) and *H. armigera*which are phylogenetically related. In one report, indiscriminate use of insecticides, multiple generation of DBM per annum and year round availability of host crops have been mentioned as reasons for development of resistance in this pest to all kinds of insecticides [23,24]. There is a clear correlation between resistance and level of GSTs in insects. Likewise, there is higher activity of GST in the DBM-R population by a 3 to 4 fold increase in enzyme activity over susceptible strains of *Plutella xylostella* [25]. Similarly, a 1.5 to 2 fold increase in parathione selected DBM was observed [26]. Higher activity of GSTs in pyrethroid resistant strain has established that GST plays an important role as a detoxifying mechanism in DBM [27]. There are earlier reports of resistance in *H. armigera* to synthetic and nonsynthetic pyrethroid insecticides in China, with resistance to deltamethrin, cyhalothrin, fenpropathrin, esfenvalerate, cyfluthrin and methomyl ranging between 10 and 50-fold [28]. GST could provide passive protection by binding pyrethroid molecules in a sequestration mechanism in resistant field strains of *H. armigera*[29]. Detoxifying GSTs are a family of enzymes that catalyze the conjugation of glutathione with electrophilic substrates including insecticides

[30]. The GSTs are involved in *O*-dealkylation or dearylation of OPs [31]. High frequencies of profenofos resistance were moderately correlated with GST activity toward 1-chloro-2,4-dinitrobenzene in larvae of *H. virescens* that were collected in Louisiana cotton fields during the 1995 cotton growing season [32]. A recent study suggests that GSTs act as an antioxidant-defense agent and confer pyrethroid resistance in *Nilaparvata lugens* and possibly in other insects [33]. Enhanced activities of GSTs that confer insecticide resistance result from both quantitative and qualitative alterations in gene expression. First, there is evidence for over-expression of one or more GST isoforms in resistant insects. For example, the highest activity found in an insecticide-resistant strain of *M. domestica* is correlated with a high level of GST1 transcript [12].

Our investigations revealed that cantharidin is an effective inhibitor of the GSTs and the HaGST in the midgut of *H. armigera* with IC50 of 9.77 and 12.5 μM, respectively. The low value of IC50 *in vivo* suggests that it may be a general inhibitor of GSTs. Enzyme kinetics studies were carried out to detect the inhibitory mechanism of GSTs in enzyme extract and soluble purified rHaGST by cantharidin with respect to GSH. Results revealed that cantharidin was non-competitive inhibitor of the GSTs and the HaGST with respect to GSH, suggesting that cantharidin binding to GSTs may have caused conformational changes consequently leading to the enzyme inactivation. Furthermore, cantharidin has the potential to bind to GSTs through hydrogen a bond causing steric obstruction leading to inactivation of catalytic activity.

Homology modeling and molecular docking simulations were employed to rationalize our results more precisely. Our docking results confirmed putative binding of cantharidin to the catalytic active site residues, ALA12 and TRY108, resultantly causing conformational changes that lead to the inactivation of enzyme catalytic activity.

EXPERIMENTAL SECTION

Insects

Helicoverpa armigera larvae were procured from Henan Jiyuan Baiyun Industry Co., Ltd. China and reared on artificial diet [34] until F1 were available for use in the experiments. Groups of 24 larvae were placed into 24 chamber plastic boxes obtained from the company. The boxes were placed in an incubator at 27 + 1 °C and 40% to 50% RH with a 12 h photoperiod.

Bioassay

Diet incorporation bioassay was used to determine the toxicity of cantharidin. Batches of healthy homogeneous third-instar larvae were selected for bioassay. A homogeneous group comprising 24 larvae per replication was subjected to bioassay. The bioassay experiment was replicated thrice. Cantharidin dissolved in acetone was added to the semisolid artificial diet at the rate of 250 μg $g^{-1}$and mixed well. Acetone was allowed to evaporate for 1 h before allowing insects to feed. The larvae were starved for 8 h before their introduction to treated diet. One larva of third-instar was introduced to each cell of the 24-cell plastic bioassay tray. The mortality data were recorded at 12, 24, 48 and 72 h.

Larval Treatment

Cantharidin used in the experiment was extracted in the laboratory. The third-instar larvae were selected for this study. The insects were starved for 8 h before their introduction to the cantharidin-treated artificial diet containing 25 μg g^{-1} cantharidin. Afterward, larvae were collected at an interval of 24, 48, 72 and 96 h. The collected larvae were flash frozen in liquid nitrogen for storage at −80 °C and subsequently used for extraction of enzyme extract and total RNA for synthesis of cDNAs.

Total RNA Preparation and Synthesis of cDNAs Template for Real-Time qPCR

A total of 10 × 3 larvae per time interval (10 larvae per replication), treated as mentioned above were used for extraction of total RNA. At first midguts were dissected from the larvae stored at −80 °C and homogenized using liquid nitrogen before addition of RNAiso Plus (TaKaRa, Dalian, China). RNA was extracted under the guidelines of the manufacturer's instructions. The quality of the RNA samples was examined by running on 1% (*w*/*v*) agarose gel. DNA contamination was removed by DNaseI (Fermentas, Beijing, China). The cDNAs were synthesized by reverse transcription using RevertAid™ Reverse Transcriptase (Fermentas, Beijing, China) in a 20 μL reaction containing 5 μL total RNA having 1 μg RNA, oligo $(dT)_{18}$ primer 1 μL, 5× Reaction Buffer 4 μL, 10 mM dNTP Mix 2 μL and RevertAid™ M-MuLV Reverse Transcriptase (200 U μL^{-1}) 1 μL. The reaction mixture was incubated for 60 min at 42 °C. The reaction was terminated by heating at 70 °C for 10 min. The product of the reverse transcription reaction was stored at −80 °C.

Cloning of Glutathione S-Transferase Gene from H. armigera

Glutathione *S*-transferase (GenBank accession no. EF033109) was amplified from cDNA by polymerase chain reaction (PCR) using a pair of sense and antisense primers, respectively (Table 2). The *Bam*HI restriction site was incorporated to sense primer, whereas *Hind*III restriction site was incorporated to antisense primer for double restriction digestion reaction. The amplification reaction was performed by the PCR program: first step denaturation for 3 min at 95 °C followed by 34 cycles of 95 °C for 30 s, 55 °C 30 s, 72 °C for 1 min and final extension of 5 min at 72 °C. The PCR product was run on 1% (*w*/*v*) agarose gel and visualized by ethidium bromide using the BioRad imaging system. Target gene amplified product was gel purified by a gel extraction kit (Biomiga, San Diego, CA, USA). Gel purified PCR product was then ligated to pMD-19T vector (TaKaRa, Dalian, China) and transformed into *Escherichia coli* DH5α. The transformants were selected on LB agar plates containing 50 μg mL^{-1} kanamycin after overnight incubation at 37 °C. The resultant PCR clones were sequenced by Shanghai Sunny Biotech, Shanghai, China.

Table 2: Oligonucleotide primer sequences for the reverse transcription and the real-time qPCR used in this study.

Name (bp)	Sequence (5-3)	Usage	T_m a	Corresponding cDNA region
HaGST-F (29)	CGGATCCATGTCCTTAGACTTGTATTACG	RT	59.2	43–705
HaGST-R (30)	CGAAGCTTTTACAATTCAGTTTTAGCTTTT	RT	56.6	
HaGST-Fq (19)	ACGCTTTACCCAAGATTTG	Real-time qPCR	60	316–430
HaGST-Rq (19)	GGAATGTGTTGAGGAAGTG	Real-time qPCR	60	
HaBA-Fq (18)	GTATTGCTGACCGTATGC	Real-time qPCR	59.7	11–s152
HaBA-Rq (18)	ATCTGTTGGAAGGTGGAG	Real-time qPCR	60	

[a]Melting temperature (T_m) of the primers was calculated by Beacon Designer 7 software.

Construction of Recombinant Expression Plasmid

The pMD19T-HaGST was subjected to double restriction digestion by *Bam*HI and *Hind*III. The digested fragments were gel purified and ligated into the prokaryotic expression vector, pET-28a (Novagen, Darmstadt, Germany) using TaKaRa quick ligation kit to secure the recombinant plasmid, rHaGST. The ligation reaction was transformed into BL-21 (DE-3) competent cells. The transformed Bl-21 cells were cultured in LB media containing kanamycin (50 μg mL^{-1}) at 37 °C with 220 rpm shaking until the absorbance at OD_{600} reached 0.5 nm, then isopropyl-β-D-thiogalactopyranoside (IPTG) was added to the culture in final concentration of 1 mM at 30 °C for expression of recombinant protein.

SDS-PAGE Analysis of Recombinant Protein and Immunoblotting

The expressed recombinant protein of 29.81 kDa was confirmed and visualized by 12% SDS-PAGE using a standard protein marker (TaKaRa, Dalian, China). After running the recombinant protein on 12% SDS-PAGE, the gel was subjected to Coomassie brilliant blue R250 staining and proteins were transferred to a polyvinylidene fluoride membrane (PVDF). Immunoblotting was done [35] with 6-His monoclonal primary antibody and peroxidase-conjugated goat anti-mouse IgG secondary antibody.

Prokaryotic Expression and Purification of the Soluble Recombinant Protein, rHaGST

The *E. coli* strain Bl-21 (DE-3) cells with the rHaGST were grown at 37 °C in 50 mL LB media containing 50 μg mL^{-1}kanamycin until the OD_{600} reached 1. The media was then added 0.5 mM IPTG and cells were grown at 28 °C for 6 h with shaking at 200 rpm. The cells were harvested at 10,000 rpm for one min. The resultant pellet was washed with sterile water three times and finally mixed with the binding buffer containing 20 mM imidazol in equilibration buffer. Lysozyme was added to the mixture at the rate of 1 mg mL^{-1}. After incubation for 30 min on ice, cells were lysed by gentle vortexing. The lysate was subjected to centrifugation at 12,000 rpm for 10 min to remove the cellular debris. The supernatant was passed through a 0.45 nM syringe filter for removal of any remaining debris. The protein extract obtained was passed through a Ni^{2+}-nitrilotriacetate (NTA) chromatographic column. The column was washed with equilibration buffer containing, 300 mM NaCl, 50 mM sodium phosphate buffer, 10 mM imidazol and 0.01 M Tris-Cl (pH 8.0). Protein was eluted with a linear imidazole gradient of 50, 100, 150 and 200 mM. The eluted protein was desalted using a dialysis membrane against 50 mM sodium phosphate buffer, pH 7.2 for 24 h at 4 °C.

Enzyme Extract Preparation

A total of 10 × 3 larvae per time interval (10 larvae per replication), treated as mentioned above were used for enzyme extraction. The midguts dissected from the larvae were washed with 1× phosphate buffer and homogenized in 0.1 M potassium phosphate buffer, pH 6.5 on ice using a glass homogenizer. The homogenates were centrifuged at 10,000*g* for 15 min at 4 °C. The supernatants were used as an enzyme extract solution.

GST Activity Determination Assay

Glutathion *S*-transferase activity was determined by an earlier method with little modifications [36]. Ten microliters of ten-times diluted enzyme extract solution was added to a total volume of 200 μL in microplate wells. The reaction mixture was incubated with 10 mM glutathione at 25 °C for 10 min and added 10 μL 10 mM 1-chloro-2,4-dinitrobenzene (CDNB). Enzyme activity was measured spectrophotometrically at 340 nm using a TECAN™ Infinite® 200 PRO multimode micro-plate reader. The enzyme activity was determined using the extinction coefficient of 9.6 mM^{-1} cm^{-1} for CDNB.

Kinetic Properties of GST

The enzyme extract solution was prepared as mentioned above. Ten microliters of 10 μM cantharidin dissolved in acetone was added to the reaction mixture as an inhibitor. *S*-Hexylglutathione (GTX) in a concentration of 10 μM was used as a positive control. The reaction was started by the addition of 10 mM glutathione and the reaction mixture was incubated at 25 °C for 10 min and finally added 10 μL of 10 mM CDNB. The enzyme activity was measured spectrophotometrically at 340 nm using a TECAN™ Infinite® 200 PRO multimode micro-plate reader. The enzyme activity was determined using the extinction coefficient of 9.6 mM^{-1} cm^{-1} for CDNB.

Kinetic Properties of Purified Soluble rHaGST

In this assay the purified rHaGST as mentioned above was used as the enzyme source. Ten microliters of 10× diluted purified GST enzyme solution was added to the reaction mixture. Ten microliters of 10 μM cantharidin dissolved in acetone was added to the reaction mixture as an inhibitor. *S*-Hexylglutathione (GTX) in a concentration of 10 μM was used as a positive control. The reaction was started by the addition of 10 mM glutathione and the reaction mixture was incubated at 25 °C for 10 min and added 10 μL 10 mM CDNB. Enzyme activity was measured spectrophotometrically at 340 nm using the TECAN™ Infinite® 200 PRO multimode micro-plate reader. The enzyme activity was determined using the extinction coefficient of 9.6 mM^{-1} cm^{-1} for CDNB. The enzyme kinetics module of the SigmaPlot computer package was used to analyze enzyme kinetics data (SigmaPlot, Systat Software, San Jose, CA. USA).

Determination of IC50

To calculate the concentration of inhibitor that inhibits 50% activity of enzyme (IC50), variable concentration of cantharidin dissolved in acetone were added to the mixture containing 170 μL GST buffer, 10 μL enzyme extract and 10 μL of 10 mM GSH solution at 25 °C. No inhibitor was added to the control. The inhibition reaction was carried out at 25 °C. The value of IC50 was calculated by percent inhibitory activity *vs.* concentration of inhibitor using Microsoft Excel 2003.

Real-Time qPCR Analysis of Gene Expression

The real-time qPCR was performed by a BioRad iQ™ 5 cycler. The real-time qPCR reaction was carried out in PCR strips. SYBR Green was used to detect an amplification signal. The reaction mixture consisted of 1 μL 10× diluted cDNA templates, 0.5 μL of 10 μM forward/reverse primers and Maxima™ SYBR Green/ROX qPCR Master Mix (Fermentas, Beijing, China) in a final volume of 25 μL. Forward and reverse primers were used as mentioned above. The real time PCR condition used: initial denaturing at 95 °C for 30 s., forty cycles of 95 °C for 10 s, 60 °C for 30 s and 72 °C for 30 s. The real time data were acquired at 72 °C. Three replicate for each sample were used for real time PCR analysis. The quantification of the relative transcript levels was performed using the comparative CT method. The expression ratio (*R*) was calculated as recommended by the manufacturer and corresponds to $2^{-\Delta\Delta CT}$, where:

$$\text{Ratio} = \frac{(E_{\text{target}})^{\Delta C_T \text{ target (calibrator} - \text{test)}}}{(E_{\text{reference}})^{\Delta C_T \text{ target (calibrator} - \text{test)}}} \quad (1)$$

Relative quantification relies on the comparison between expression of a target gene *versus* a reference gene (*Helicoverpa armigera* β-actin) and the expression of the same gene in the target sample *versus* the reference sample [37].

Homology Modeling of HaGST

In this study, we used glutathione *S*-transferase of *Helicoverpa armigera* (HaGST) (ABK40535) obtained from the GenBank database [21] having 220 amino acid residues as a model sequence. All Homology Modeling computations were performed using the Modeller 9.10 [38] on a Linux High performance workstation based on 2 Intel Xeon 5680 processors (Super Micro Computer Inc., San Jose, CA, USA).

Using our model HaGST sequence as a probe, the PDB95 database was searched for non-redundant PDB sequences to select the most appropriate template for our query sequence. In order to visualize differences among 12 similar structures selected at 95% sequence identity as the candidate template, we compared all of the structures in the dendrogram, which can generate the weighted pair-group average clustering based on a distance matrix. The best template was picked according to the crystallographic *R*-factor and overall sequence identity. The sequence alignment between the HaGST sequence and the best template was generated by Align2D and also identified by ClustalX with the Blosum scoring function [39]. The best alignment was selected according to both the alignment score and the reciprocal positions of the conserved residues, especially those in or close to the GTX-binding sites of the template.

Once the target template alignment was constructed, it calculated 100 3D models of the target automatically by the automodel of Modeller using the optimization and refinement protocol. Each model was first optimized with the variable target function method (VTFM) with conjugate gradients (CG), and was then refined using molecular dynamics (MD) with simulated annealing (SA). We also used the loop model class in Modeller to refine the conformation of the loop between residues. To measure the relative stability of the protein conformation, GA341 and Discrete Optimized Protein Energy (DOPE) scores were employed and credible structure of HaGST was selected based on the lowest DOPE energy. MolProbity was used to generate the Protein Main-Chain dihedral Ramachandran map to identify the rationality of the stereo chemical for the structure [40].

Molecular Docking Simulations

All the simulations and docking work was performed using the software, GOLD 5.1 [41]. GTX is bound tightly inside the active-site pocket formed by residues Leu6, Ser9, Ala10, Pro11, Leu33, Met34, His38, His50, Ile52, Glu64, Ser65, Arg66, Tyr105, Phe108, Tyr113, Ile116, Phe117, Phe203 and Phe207 as observed from the crystal structure. This pocket was selected as a binding site for cantharidin, so we aligned the 3D model of HaGST to the crystal structure by the superimposition in pymol 1.3r1 edu [42], saved the coordinates of the 3D model of HaGST, then used the coordinates of the CA2 atom in GTX to define a centroid close to the center of the active site with the radius of 10 Å. In order to adopt the best sets of docking parameters and obtain the reliability of the docking results, the GTX was first docked into the binding pocket. The chemical structure of the cantharidin was derived from PubChem [43] and directly used the structure of GTX from 1PN9. Mercury 3.0 software [44] was used to add hydrogen atoms and the coordinates were saved as MOL2 files. Hydrogen atoms were added to the 3D model structure of HaGST and correct ionization and tautomeric states of residues such as Asp, Glu and His were defined, allowing serine, threonine and tyrosine hydroxyl groups, as well as lysine NH^{3+} groups to rotate during docking. All torsion angles in each ligand were allowed to rotate freely. An accurate GTX-GST complex possessing the smallest root-mean-square deviation of the docked conformation of GTX from its conformation in the crystal structure named 1PN9 was obtained first by docking using Goldscore and then by Chemscore after tuning parameters of Gold software several times. Similar docking parameters were adopted for cantharidin and GTX.

Binding Energy Calculations

In order to compare the binding affinity between the cantharidin and GTX with the HaGST model, a ChemScore function was applied to measure the affinity data by a ranking made according to delta value. ChemScore estimates of the total free energy change that occurs on ligand binding were estimated:

$$\Delta G_{binding} = \Delta G_O + \Delta G_{hbond} + \Delta G_{metal} + \Delta G_{lipo} + \Delta G_{rot} \quad (2)$$

CONCLUSIONS

In brief, the results from our investigations revealed that the cantharidin is a potent inhibitor of the GSTs *in vivo*and the HaGST *in vitro*. We therefore suggest the use of cantharidin based bio-insecticides directly or as a synergist where insecticide resistance is related to the over expression of GSTs.

ACKNOWLEDGMENTS

We sincerely appreciate Schrock, J.R. (Emporia State University, USA) for revising the manuscript. This study was supported by the Special Fund for the Public Interest (Agriculture) (200903052) by The Ministry of Science and Technology, The Ministry of Agriculture, China. The NSFC grants (31270691, 31170609) and the "13115" Sci-Tech Innovation Project of Shaanxi Province (2007ZDKG-14).

CONFLICT OF INTEREST

The authors declare no conflict of interest.

REFERENCES

1. Hayes, J.D.; Pulford, D.J. The glutathione *S*-transferase supergene family-regulation of GST and the contribution of isozymes to cancer chemoprotection and drug resistance. *Crit. Rev. Biochem. Mol. Biol* 1995, *30*, 445–600.
2. Habig, W.H.; Pabst, M.J.; Jakoby, W.B. Glutathione *S*-transferases. *J. Biol. Chem* 1974, *249*, 7130–7141.
3. Grant, D.F.; Dietze, E.C.; Hammock, B.D. Glutathione *S*-transferase isozymes in *Aedes aegypti*: Purification, characterization and isozyme specific regulation. *Insect Biochem* 1991, *21*, 421–433.
4. Huang, H.S.; Hu, N.T.; Yao, Y.E.; Wu, C.Y.; Chiang, S.W.; Sun, C.N. Molecular cloning and heterologous expression of glutathione *S*-transferase involved in insecticide resistance from the diamondback moth, *Plutella xylostella*. *Insect Biochem. Mol. Biol* 1998, *28*, 651–658.
5. Armes, N.J.; Jadhav, D.R.; Bond, G.S.; King, A.B.S. Insecticide resistance in *Helicoverpa armigera* in South India.*Pestic. Sci* 1992, *34*, 355–364.
6. Yu, S.J. *Molecular Aspects of Insect—Plant Association*; Brattsten, L.B., Ahmad, S., Eds.; Plenum: New York, NY, USA, 1986; p. 153.
7. Motoyama, N.; Dauterman, W.C. Glutathione *S*-transferases: Their role in the metabolism of organophosphorus insecticides. *Rev. Biochem. Toxicol* 1980, *20*, 49–70.
8. Motoyama, N.; Dauterman, W.C. Inter-strain comparison of glutathione dependent reactions in susceptible and resistant houseflies. *Pestic. Biochem. Physiol* 1975, *5*, 489–493.
9. Clark, A.G.; Shamaan, N.A.; Dauterman, W.C.; Hayaoka, T. Characterization of multiple glutathione transferases from the housefly, *Musca domestica*. *Pestic. Biochem. Physiol* 1984, *22*, 51–59.
10. Hemingway, J.; Malcolm, C.A.; Kissoon, K.E.; Boddington, R.G.; Curtis, C.F.; Hill, N. The biochemistry of insecticide resistance in *Anopheles sacharovi*: Comparative studies with a range of insecticide susceptible and resistance *Anopheles* and *Culex* species. *Pestic. Biochem. Physiol* 1985, *24*, 68–71.
11. Grant, D.F.; Matsumura, F. Glutathione *S*-transferase 1 and 2 in susceptible and insecticide resistant *Aedes aegypti*. *Pestic. Biochem. Physiol* 1989, *33*, 132–140.
12. Fournier, D.; Bride, J.M.; Poire, M.; Berge, J.B.; Plapp, F.W. Insect glutathione *S*-transferases: Biochemical characteristics of the major forms from houseflies susceptible and resistant to insecticides. *J. Biol. Chem* 1992,*267*, 1840–1845.
13. Legadic, L.; Cuany, A.; Berge, J.B.; Echaubard, M. Purification and partial characterization of glutathione *S*-transferases from insecticide resistant and lindane-induced susceptible *Spodoptera littoralis* (Boisd.) larvae. *Insect Biochem. Mol. Biol* 1993, *23*, 467–474.
14. Zibaee, A.; Jalali, S.J.; Alinia, F.; Ghadamyari, M. Diazinon resistance in different selected strains of *Chilo suppressalis* Walker (Lepidoptera: Pyralidae), rice striped stem borer, in the north of Iran. *J. Econ. Entomol* 2008,*102*, 1189–1196.
15. Wang, G.S. Medical uses of *Mylabris* in ancient China and recent studies. *J. Ethnoparmacol* 1989, *26*, 147–162.
16. Oaks, W.W.; diTunno, J.F.; Magnam, T.; Levy, H.A.; Mills, L.C. Cantharidin Poisoning. *Arch. Intern. Med* 1960,*105*, 574–582.
17. Robiquet, P.J. Expériences sur les cantharides. *Ann. Chim* 1810, *76*, 302–322.
18. Cui, F.L.; Li, X.; Ma, Z.Q.; Zhang, Y.L. Safety evaluation of animal-origin pesticide cantharidin against some non-target organisms. *J. Environ. Entomol* 2009, *31*, 143–149.
19. Zhang, Y.L.; Zhou, Y.; Zhang, Z.Y. Effect of cantharidin on the midgut of oriental armyworm (*Methimna. seperata*) and diamond moth *Plutella xylostella*. *Acta Entomol. Sin* 2003, *46*, 272–276.
20. Ma, Y.; Liu, R.R.; Ma, Z.Q.; Zhang, Y.L. Effects of cantharidin on four metabolizing enzymes and PPO in*Mythimna separata* (Walker) (Lepidoptera Noctuidae). *Acta Entomol. Sin* 2010, *53*, 870–875.
21. Mao, YB.; Cai, W.J.; Wang, J.W.; Hong, G.J.; Tao, X.Y.; Wang, L.J.; Huang, Y.P.; Chen, X.Y. Silencing a cotton bollworm P450 monooxygenase gene by plant mediated RNAi impairs larval tolerance to gossypol. *Nat. Biotechnol.* 2007, *25*, 1307–1313.
22. Chen, L.; Hall, P.R.; Zhou, X.E.; Ranson, H.; Hemingway, J.; Meehan, E.J. Structure of an insect delta-class

glutathione *S*-transferase from a DDT-resistant strain of the malaria vector *Anopheles gambiae*. *Acta Crystallogr. D* 2003, *D59*, 2211–2217.

23. Furlong, M.J.; Wright, D.J. Examination of stability of resistance and cross resistance patterns to acylurea insect growth regulators in field populations of diamond back moth, *Plutella xylostella* from Malaysia. *J. Pestic. Sci* 1994, *42*, 315–326.
24. Mohan, M.; Gujar, G.T. Local variation in susceptibility of diamondback moth, *Plutella xylostella* (L.) to insecticides and role of detoxifying enzymes. *Crop Prot* 2003, *2*, 495–504.
25. Balabaskaran, S.; Chuen, S.S.; Muniandy, S. Glutathione *S*-transferase from the diamondback moth. *Insect Biochem* 1989, *19*, 435–443.
26. Kao, C.H.; Hung, C.F.; Sun, C.N. Parathion and methyl parathion resistance in diamond back moth (Lepidoptera: Plutellidae) larvae. *J. Econ. Entomol* 1989, *82*, 1299–1300.
27. Yu, S.J.; Nguyen, S.N. Detection and biochemical characterization of insecticide resistance in the diamond back moth. *Pestic. Biochem. Physiol* 1992, *44*, 74–81.
28. Wu, Y.; Shen, D.J. Character of Fenvalerate resistance in *Helicoverpa arraigera* (Hubner) from China. *Resistant Pest Manag. Newsl* 1996, *8*, 25–27.
29. Kostaropoulos, I.; Papadopoulos, A.I.; Metaxakis, A.; Boukouvala, E.; Papadopoulou-Maurkidou, E. Glutathione *S*-transferase in the defense against pyrethroids in insects. *Insect Biochem. Mol. Biol* 2001, *31*, 313–319.
30. Soderlund, D.M.; Hessney, C.W.; Helmuth, D.W. Pharmacokinetics of *cis*- and *trans*-substituted pyrethroids in the American cockroach. *Pestic. Biochem. Physiol* 1983, *20*, 161–168.
31. Hayes, J.D.; Wolf, C.R. Role of Glutathione Transferases in Drug Resistance. In *Glutathione Conjugation: Mechanisms and Biological Significance*; Sites, H., Ketter, B., Eds.; Academic Press: London, UK, 1988; pp. 3150–355.
32. Harold, J.A.; Ottea, J.A. Toxicological significance of enzyme activities in profenofos-resistant tobacco budworms, *Heliothis virescens* (F.). *Pestic. Biochem. Physiol* 1997, *58*, 23–33.
33. Vontas, J.G.; Small, G.J.; Hemingway, J. Glutathione *S*-transferases as antioxidant defense agents confer pyrethroid resistance in *Nilaparvata lugens*. *Biochem. J* 2001, *357*, 65–72.
34. Ahmed, M.; McCaffery, A.R. Elucidation of detoxification mechanisms involved in resistance to insecticides against third instar larvae of a field selected strain of *Helicoverpa armigera* with the use of synergists. *Pestic. Biochem. Physiol* 1991, *41*, 41–52.
35. Sambrook, J.; Russel, D.W. *Molecular Cloning: A Laboratory Manual*; Cold Spring Harbor Laboratory Press: New York, NY, USA, 1989; pp. 18:1–18:85.
36. Booth, G.M.; Connor, J.; Metcalf, R.A.; Larsen, J.R. A comparative study of the effects of selective inhibitors on esterase isozymes from the mosquito *Anopheles punctipennis*. *Comp. Biochem. Physiol. B* 1973, *44*, 1185–1195.
37. Pfaffl, M.W. A new mathematical model for relative quantification in real-time RT-PCR. *Nucleic Acids Res* 2001,*29*, 2002–2007.
38. Sali, A.; Blundell, T.L. Comparative protein modelling by satisfaction of spatial restraints. *J. Mol. Biol* 1993, *234*, 779–815.
39. Thompson, J.D.; Gibson, T.J.; Plewniak, F.; Jeanmougin, F.; Higgins, D.G. The ClustalX windows interface: Flexible strategies for multiple sequence alignment aided by quality analysis tools. *Nucleic Acids Res* 1997, *24*, 4876–4882.
40. Chen, V.B.; Arendall, W.B., 3rd; Headd, J.J.; Keedy, D.A.; Immormino, R.M.; Kapral, G.J.; Murray, L.W.; Richardson, J.S.; Richardson, D.C. MolProbity: All-atom structure validation for macromolecular crystallography. *Acta Crystallogr. D* 2010, *D66*, 12–21.
41. GOLD*, version 5.1*; The Cambridge Crystallographic Data Centre (CCDC): Cambridge, UK, 2012.
42. DeLano, W.L. *The PyMol Molecular Graphics System*; DeLano Scientific: Palo Alto, CA, USA, 2010.
43. Ivetic, T.V.; Hrvacic, B.; Bosnar, M.; Cuzic, S.; Bosnjak, B.; Erakovic, H.V.; Glojnaric, I. Cantharidin-induced inflammation in mouse rar model for translational research of novel anti-inflammatories. *Tranl. Res* 2012, *160*, 137–145.
44. Macrae, C.F.; Bruno, I.J.; Chisholm, J.A.; Edgington, P.R.; McCabe, P.; Pidcock, E.; Rodriguez-Monge, L.; Taylor, R.; Van de streek, J.; Wood, P.A. Mercury CSD 2.0—New features for the visualization and investigation of crystal structures. *J. Appl. Cryst* 2008, *41*, 466–470

CHAPTER 22 DICHLOROVOS TOXICITY IN FISH

Suchismita Das

Keywords: dichlorvos, toxic, acute, chronic, fish

INTRODUCTION

Use of pesticide has become a necessary evil for developing countries like India where it is estimated that approximately 30% of its crop yield valued at Rs.60,000 crores are lost due to pest attack each year[1]. Amongst others, organophosphorus pesticides (OPs) are the most commonly used pesticides in the world due to their quick degradation[2]. Unfortunately, OPs lack target specificity and can cause severe, long lasting population effects on terrestrial and aquatic non-target species, particularly vertebrates[3]. Quick degradation is probably the reason why, irrespective of reports of health hazardous, developing countries especially, in the Asia-Pacific region, use these chemicals for agricultural and public health purposes [4,5].

Dichlorvos (2, 2-dichlorovinyl dimethyl phosphate) was first introduced in 1961[6]. It has a molecular formula $C_4H_7Cl_2O_4P$ and molecular weight to be 220.98 (Fig 1). It is also known by its trade name DDVP, Dedevap, Nogos,Nuvan, phosvit or Vapona[7]. It is one of the most commonly used organophosphate pesticides in developing countries[8]. It is classified by the WHO as a Class IB, 'highly hazardous'chemical[9]. Dichlorvos is usually used as an agricultural insecticide on crops and stored products but is also used as an anti-helminthic (worming agent) for dogs, swine, and horses, as a botacide; agent that kills fly larvae[10]. It is poisonous if swallowed, inhaled, or absorbed through the skin[11]. It is extremely toxic pesticides to aquatic organisms and hampers fish health through impairment of metabolism sometimes leading to death. As one of the few organophosphates still registered for use, dichlorvos has elicited worldwide concern for many reasons. Although dichlorvos serves as a contact and stomach insecticide for food and non-food crop pests, it is also toxic to fish and other aquatic organisms[12-14]. Dichlorvos is also commonly used in fish farming to eradicate crustacean ectoparasites. It is specially used in the treatment of sea lice (*Lepophtheirus salmonis* and*Caligus elogatus*) on commercial salmon farms. But this pesticide often ends up producing both lethal and sub-lethal effects on the fish[15] and even zooplanktons[16]. At only 1 ppm, dichlorvos, showed both acute and chronic toxicity in fish[17]. Some other workers have also noted adverse effects of dichlorvos in fish[18-20]. The present study is an attempt to review the potential adverse effects of dichlorvos in fish.

Citation: Das S. Dichlorvos toxicity in fish. Curr World Environ 2013;8(1). doi : http://dx.doi.org/10.12944/CWE.8.1.08.

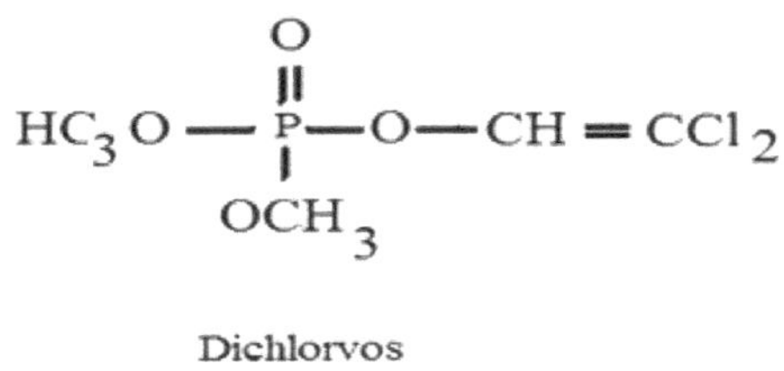

Fig. 1 Dichlorvos (2, 2-dichlorovinyl dimethyl phosphate)

ACUTE TOXICITY OF DICHLORVOS ON FISH

The acute toxicity of dichlorvos to fish has been previously determined by a number of researchers. Its toxicity for freshwater and estuarine fish is moderate to high, and it does not bioaccumulate in fish[21]. For freshwater and estuarine fish, 96h-LC_{50} values range from 0.2 to 12 mg/L[22]. For marine fish, the toxicity was estimated to be more than 4 mg/L for adults and pre-adults of Atlantic salmon (*Salmo salar*)[23]. The 96h-LC_{50} value of dichlorvos obtained for fingerlings of European sea bass (*Dicentrarchus labrax*) was 3.5 mg/L[15]. A comparison of the 96h-LC_{50} values published for several teleost fish species[22] indicates that fingerlings of the European sea bass are more resistant to dichlorvos exposure than the most part of the other species of estuarine and freshwater fish studied. However, the comparison with fathead minnow (*Pimephales promelas*) or with mosquito fish (*Gambusia affinis*) of similar size indicates that sea bass fingerlings are more sensitive to dichlorvos, since 96h-LC_{50}-values of 12 and 5.3 mg/L have been reported[22] for both species, respectively. In a study, it was found that 100% of 100 g salmon (*Salmon salar*) survived after 24 h of exposure to 1, 3, and 5 mg/L of dichlorvos[24]. The 96h-LC_{50} value of dichlorvos obtained for *Labeo rohita* was 16.71ppm. The fish in the same study exhibited erratic swimming, copious mucus secretion, loss of equilibrium and hitting to the walls of test tank prior to mortality in acute toxicity tests[25]. The 96-h LC_{50}values of Dichlorvos has been reported in *Cirrhinus mrigala* to be 9.1ppm[26], in Zebra fish, the 24-hpost fertilization LC_{50} value of dichlorvos in the semi static test was 39.75 mg/L[27] and48-h LC_{50}values to be 0.5-10mg/L of dichlorvos formulations in carp[28]. A study report indicated that 96-h LC_{50}value in rainbow trout was 0.93 mg/L[29] and on golden orfe was 0.45mg/L[30]. In another study, 100% lethality at 10 mg/L in fry of rainbow trout was found[31]. In *Tilapia mossambica* with three size groups, 96-h LC_{50} values were found to be 1.4-1.9mg/L, the smaller sizes being more sensitive[32]. 24, 48 and 96-h LC_{50} values of dichlorvos in common carp to be 3.8, 2.7, 2.3mg/L respectively and 4.1, 4.0 and 3.7 mg/L in Java carp respectively.[33] In harlequin fish found 24-h LC_{50} value to be 12mg/L and 48-h LC_{50} value to be 7.8mg/L[34] while 24 and 48-h LC_{50} in bluegill sunfish to be 1 and 0.7mg/L respectively[35]. Again, 96-h LC_{50} in bluegill and spots were reported to be 0.48 and 0.55mg/L respectively[36].

CHRONIC TOXICITY OF DICHLORVOS ON FISH

Effects on Choline esterase activity:

Dichlorvos is an organophosphorus insecticide reported to be neurotoxic due to its irreversible inhibitory effect on AChE[37]. The enzyme AChE degrades the neurotransmitter acetylcholine in cholinergic synapses. The inhibition provokes an accumulation of acetylcholine in synapses with disruption of the nerve function that can end in the death of the organism. Several authors have been reporting significant inhibition of ChE activity in fish at sub-lethal concentrations of dichlorvos[38-41]. In sea bass, dichlorvos significantly inhibited the activity of ChE in the selected tissues, both in vitro and in vivo conditions. Differences in ChE sensitivity were found in relation to the age of the fish and the tissue analysed. Sea bass fingerlings are able to tolerate high levels of head and muscle ChE inhibition before death[15]. Similar results were obtained for pinfish (*Lagodon rhomboides*)[42] and European eel (*Anguilla anguilla*)[43]. Brain tissue showed higher ChE activity than muscle, whole blood or plasma tissues. On the contrary, in fingerlings, the highest ChE activity was obtained in muscle. This is in agreement with the results obtained by other researchers[44-46]. Skeletal muscle presented higher ChE activity than brain tissue in juveniles of goldfish (*Carassius auratus*) of size ~5 g exposed to three different pesticides[47]. Chronic dichlorvos exposure impaired mitochondrial energy metabolism and neuronal apoptotic cell death in brain[48]. AChE activity of *Tilapia mossambica* in relation to the interacting effects of aging and sub-lethal concentrations of dichlorvos was studied[49]. The enzyme activity of brain and liver decreased with increasing size (and age) and dichlorvos exposed fish showed considerable inhibition of brain and liver AChE. There was a positive correlation between dichlorvos concentration and the time of exposure when the degree of enzyme inhibition was considered. Brain exhibited a higher degree of enzyme inhibition in all age groups of fish as compared to liver. Small fish were more susceptible to the insecticide with respect to AChE activity. When transferred to clean water, most of the exposed fishes recovered their AChE activity and the recovery was greater in liver than in brain[49].

Effects on Antioxidants:

It has now been established that OP pesticides induced oxidative stress[50]. An antioxidant defence system (ADS) is needed to protect biomolecules from the harmful effects of ROS. Fish are endowed with defensive mechanisms to neutralize the impact of reactive oxygen species (ROS) resulting from the metabolism of various chemicals. These include various antioxidant defence enzymes such as superoxide dismutase (SOD), catalase (CAT), glutathione peroxidase (GPOx), glutathione S-transferase (GST), and glutathione reductase (GR). Low molecular weight antioxidants such as glutathione (GSH), ascorbate (vitamin C), vitamin A and E are also reported to contribute in the quenching of oxy radicals[51]. ROS which is not neutralized by this antioxidant defense system damages all biomolecules. One of the most important targets of ROS is the membrane lipids which undergo peroxidation (LPO). Thus, LPO estimation has also been successfully employed to signify oxidative stress induced in aquatic animals by such chemicals[52]. Decreased GSH levels and also decreased MnSOD activity were observed, in the brain mitochondria isolated from low-level chronic dichlorvos treated rat[43]. Also, in fish exposed to dichlorvos for 24 h, at concentrations of 1 or 5 mg/L, a dose-dependent increase was noted in the activities of SOD and CAT in the liver and brain. A rise was also observed in the level of

GSH and changes were noted in MDA level in these organs. The increase in GSH was noted mainly in the brain and was accompanied by a decrease in MDA level. The decrease was greater at the exposure to the higher dose of the compound[53].

Chromosomal aberrations and carcinogenic effects:

Dichlorvos concentration of 0.01 ppm caused chromosomal aberrations in the form of centromeric gaps, chromatid gaps, chromatid breaks, sub-chromatid breaks, attenuation, extra fragments, pycnosis, stubbed arms etc in kidney cells of *Channa punctatus* after exposure periods of 24, 48, 72 and 96 h[54]. Interestingly, there was an inverse relationship between duration of exposure and aberration frequency. Longer exposures to dichlorvos were associated with lower frequencies of aberrations. The toxicity of dichlorvos has also been related to alterations in DNA replication, which causes mutations[55] and cellular hyperproliferation as a result of local irritation[56-58].

Dichlorvos has carcinogenic potential, which has been reviewed on several earlier occasions by several workers[59-62].

Immune response:

Dichlorvos has the potential to induced altered immune response in fish and it was reviewd by Dunier *et al.* 1991[63].

Developmental effects:

Dichlorvos exposure during early development in Zebra fish caused clear behavioural impairments detectable during the post hatching period. It also showed mortality and developmental abnormalities[27].

Histopathology

Histopathology is an important tool in assessing pesticide toxicity[64]. The histopathological effects of liver tissues in *Cirrhinus mrigala* chronically exposed to dichlorvos showed hepatic lesions in the liver tissues were observed which were characterized by cloudy swelling of hepatocytes, congestion, vacuolar degeneration, karyolysis, karyohexis, dilation of sinusoids and nuclear hypertrophy. In the same study, changes in gills such as hyperplasia, desquamation, and necrosis of epithelial, epithelial lifting, oedema, lamellar fusion, collapsed secondary lamellae, curling of secondary lamellae and aneurism in the secondary lamellae were observed after exposure to dichlorvos[26]. The effects of sub-lethal doses of dichlorvos on lipid composition and metabolism of rainbow trout skin cells in primary culture were investigated and it was suggested that dichlorvos may have direct effects on fish skin that could have important consequences for fish health in general[65]. In another study in air-breathing catfish *Clarias batrachus* exposed to lethal and sublethal concentrations of the dichlorvos, significant cytoarchitectural changes in the oocytes, including pronounced vacuolation, degeneration and deformation were observed[66]. Clumping of the cytoplasm and karyohypertrophy were also evident and rupture of the cell wall, with extrusion of the cytoplasm and the nuclei, was observed in the same study[66]. Pesticides are also reported to cause changes in structure and functions of fish gonads[67]. Although the studies with dichlorvos are scarce, the effects of sublethal concentrations of dichlorvos (0.65 mg/l, 0.90 mg/l and 1.17 mg/l) on the gonadosomatic index of the fish, *Cyprinus carpio communis* was studied[68]. The Ganadosomatic index decreased with the increase in concentration, whereas it increased with increase in exposure at all concentrations[68].

CONCLUSION

Dichlorvos toxicity in fish has been studied by several workers who have shown that at chronic level, it causes diverse effects including oxidative damage, inhibition of AchE activity, histopathological changes as well as developmental changes, mutagenesis and carcinogecity. With reports of dichlorvos usage and its adverse effects on non-target organisms like fish, it has become essential to formulate stringent rules against indiscriminate use of this pesticide. Since dichlorvos is present in the environment with other similar organophosphate compounds, additive responses to organophosphate compounds may induce lethal or sublethal effects in fish. It is, therefore, a matter of great public health significance to regularly monitor the pesticide residues in foods and humans in order to assess the population exposure to this pesticide. Besides, for a safe use of this insecticide more experimental work should be performed to determine the concentration and time of exposure that do not induce significant sub-lethal effects on fish.

REFERENCES

1. http://www.nabard.org/modelbankprojects/land_development.asp retrieved on 11 January, 2013.
2. Eto, M. (1974) Organophosphorus Pesticides: Organic and Biological Chemistry, CRC Press.
3. Rahimi, R. Nikfar, S. and Abdollahi, M. (2006) Increased morbidity and mortality in acute human organophosphate-poisoned patients treated by oximes: a metaanalysis of clinical trials. Hum. Exp. Toxicol. 25: 157–162, http://dx.doi.org/10.1191/0960327106ht602oa
4. Dave, P.P. (1996) India: A generic giant. Farm Chem Int., 10, 36–37.
5. Li, Y. Mcmillan, A. and Scholtz, M.T. (1996) Global HCH usage with 1° _1° longitude/latitude resolution. Environ. Sci. Technol., 30: 3525–3533, http://dx.doi.org/10.1021/es960312v
6. Mennear, J.H. (1998) Dichlorvos: A Regulatory Conundrum. Regulatory Toxicology and Pathology 27: 265–272, http://dx.doi.org/10.1006/rtph.1998.1217
7. http://en.wikipedia.org/wiki/Dichlorvos retrieved on 11 January, 2013.
8. Binukumar, B.K. and Gill, K.D. (2010) Cellular and Molecular mechanisms of dichlorvos neurotoxicity: Cholinergic, noncholinergic, cell signaling, gene expression and therapeutic aspects. Indian journal of experimental biology. 48: 697-709.
9. World Health Organisation (WHO) (1992) International Programme on Chemical Safety, WHO Recommended Classification of Pesticide by Hazard and Guidelines to Classification 1994-1995, UNEP/ILO/WHO.
10. USEPA: United States Environmental Protection Agency (1994) Integrated Risk Information System (IRIS) on Dichlorvos. Environmental Criteria and Assessment

Office, Office of Health and Environmental Assessment, Office of Research and Development, Cincinnati, OH.

11. Musa, U. Hati, S.S. Mustapha, A. and Magaji, G. (2010). Dichlorvos oncentrations in locally formulated pesticide (*Ota-piapia*) utilized in northeastern Nigeria. Scientific Research and Essay. 5: 49-54.
12. Suntio, L.R. Shiu, W.Y. Glotfelty, D. MacKay, D. and Seiber, J.N. (1988) Critical review of Henry's Law constants for pesticides. Rev. Environ. Contam. Toxicol. 103: 1–59,http://dx.doi.org/10.1007/978-1-4612-3850-8_1
13. Naqvi, S.M. and Vaishnavi, C. (1993) Mini review. Bioaccumulative potential and toxicity of dichlorvos insecticide to non-target animals. Comp. Biochem. Physiol. C 105: 347–361,http://dx.doi.org/10.1016/0742-8413(93)90071-R
14. Toledo, M.C.F. and Jonsson, C.M. (1992) Bioaccumulation and elimination of endosulfan in zebra fish (*Brachydanio rerio*). Pesticide Sci. 36: 207–211,http://dx.doi.org/10.1002/ps.2780360306
15. Varo, I. Navarro, J.C. Amat, F. and Guilhermino, L. (2003) Effect of dichlorvos on cholinesterase activity of the European sea bass (*Dicentrarchus labrax*). Pesticide Biochemistry and Physiology 75: 61–72, http://dx.doi.org/10.1016/S0048-3575(03)00019-1
16. Gupta, A. K.. Verma, G.P. and Jain, K.L. (2008) Acute toxicity of organophosphate insecticide, dichlorvos in relation to selected water hardness for the freshwater zooplankters. J Env Biol. 29: 837-839.
17. Roberts, R.J. and Sheperd, C.J. (1986) Handbook of trout and salmon diseases. FishingNew Book, 2nd edition.
18. Horsberg, T.E. Hoey, T. and Nafstad, I. (1989) Organophosphate poisoning of Atlantic salmon in connection with treatment against salmon lice. Acta Vet. Scand. 30: 385-390.
19. Rajeswari, K. Reddy, S.J. Reddy, D.C. and Ramamurthi, R. (1989) Effect of dichlorvos on certain blood parameters of the fish *Clarias batrachus*. Environ. Ecol. 7: 933-934.
20. Demael, A. Dunier, M. and Siwicki, A.R. (1990) Some effects of dichlorvos on carp metabolism. Comp. Biochem. Physiol. 95C: 237-240.
21. Howard, P.H. (1991) Pesticides, Lewis Publisher, Chelsea, MI.
22. World Health Organisation (WHO) (1989) Environmental health criteria for dichlorvos. Series, No. 79. Geneva, Italy.
23. Roth, M. (2000) The availability and use of chemotherapeutic sea lice control products, Contribut. Zool. 69:109-118.
24. Sievers, G. Palacios, P. Inostroza, R.and D'olz, H. (1995) Evaluation of the toxicity of 8 insecticides in *Salmo salar* and the in vitro effects againts the isopode parasite, *Ceratothoa gaudichaudii.* Aquaculture 134: 9-16, http://dx.doi.org/10.1016/0044-8486(95)00026-X
25. Bhat, B.A. Bhat, I.A. Vishwakarma, S. Verma, A. and Saxena, G. (2012) A Comparative Study on the Toxicity of a Synthetic Pesticide, Dichlorvos and a Neem based Pesticide, Neem-On to *Labeo rohita* (Hamilton). Current World Environment. 7: 157-161.
26. Velmurugan, B. Selvanayagam, M. Cengiz, E.I. and Unlu, E. (2009) Histopathological changes in the gill and liver tissues of freshwater fish, *Cirrhinus mrigala* exposed to dichlorvos. Brazilian Archives of Biology and Technology 52: 1291-1296, http://dx.doi.org/10.1590/S1516-89132009000500029
27. Sisman, T. (2010) Dichlorvos-induced developmental toxicity in Zebrafish. Toxicol Ind Health. 26: 567-573, http://dx.doi.org/10.1177/0748233710373089
28. Nishiuchi, Y. (1981) Toxicity of pesticides to some aquatic organisms – I Toxicity of pesticides to some aquatic insects. English translation from Seitai Kagaku 4: 31-46.
29. Bayer (1980). Toxicity to fish. Report No. FF-110. Crop Protection Application Technology, Chemical Product Development and Ecobiology, Bayer AG, Leverkusen, Germany. Bayer Australia Ltd Agricultural Division, Dichlorvos TGAC Submission to the Technical Committee on Agricultural Chemicals. Book X, Part 7: Environmental toxicology, pp 7:058-060. Unpublished Report.
30. Bayer (1981). Toxicity to fish. Report No. FO-373. Crop Protection Application Technology, Chemical Product Development and Ecobiology, Bayer AG, Leverkusen, Germany. Bayer Australia Ltd Agricultural Division, 60 Dichlorvos TGAC Submission to the Technical Committee on Agricultural Chemicals. Book X, Part 7: Environmental toxicology, pp 7:065-068. Unpublished Report.
31. Lewallen, L.L. and Wilder, W.H. (1962) Toxicity of certain organophosphorus and carbamate insecticides to rainbow trout. Mosquito News 22: 369-372.
32. Rath, S. and Misra, B.N. (1981) Toxicological effects of dichlorvos (DDVP) on brain and liver acetylcholinesterase (AChE) activity of *Tilapia mossambica,* Peters. Toxicology. 19: 239-45,http://dx.doi.org/10.1016/0300-483X(81)90133-5
33. Koesoemadinata, S. (1983) Lethal toxicity of 24 insecticide formulations commonly used for rice pest control in irrigated rice field to two Indonesian freshwater fish species, *Cyprinus carpio*and *Puntius gonionotus*. Badan Pelelitian dan Pengembangan Pertanian, Balai Penelitian Perikanan Darat (Research Institute for Inland Fisheries, Bogor, Indonesia).
34. Alabaster, J.S. (1969) Survival of fish in 164 herbicides, insecticides, fungicides, wetting agents and miscellaneous substances. Intern. Pest Control 11: 25-35.
35. Pimentel, D. (1971). Ecological effects of pesticides on non-target species. Executive Office of the President, Office of Science and Technology. US Government Printing Office, Washington DC, USA, Stock No. 4106-0029 (excerpt only).
36. Kenaga, E.E. (1979) Acute and chronic toxicity of 75 pesticides to various animal species. Down to Earth 35: 25-31.
37. Wang, H.H. Chou, Y.C. Liao, J.F. and Chen, C.F. (2004)

The effect of insecticide dichlorvos on esterase activity extracted from the Psocids *Liposceids bostrychophila* and *L. entomophilila*. J. Insect Sci. 4: 1–5.

38. Galgani, F. and Bocquene, G. (1990) In vitro inhibition of acetylcholinesterase from four marine species by organophosphates and carbamates. Bull. Environ. Contam. Toxicol. 45: 243-249, http://dx.doi.org/10.1007/BF01700191

39. Bocquene, G. Bellanger, C. Cadiou, Y. and Galgani, F. (1995) Join action of combinations of pollutants on the acetylcholinesterase activity of several marine species. Ecotoxicology 4: 266-279, http://dx.doi.org/10.1007/BF00116345

40. Sturm, A. Wogram, J. Hansen, P.D. and Liess, M. (1999) Potential use of cholinesterase in monitoring low levels of organophosphates in small streams: natural variability in three-spined stickleback (*Gasterosteus aculeatus*) and relation to pollution. Environ. Toxicol. Chem. 18: 194-200.

41. Sturm, A. Wogram, J. Segner, H. and Liess, M. (2000) Different sensitivity to organophosphates of acetylcholinesterase and butyrylcholinesterase from threespined stickleback (*Gasterosteus aculeatus*): application in biomonitoring, Environ. Toxicol. Chem. 19: 1607-1615.

42. Coppage, D.L. and Matthews, E. (1975) Head acetylcholinesterase inhibition in a marine teleost during lethal and sublethal exposures to 1-dichloroethyl dimethyl phosphate (Naled) in seawater. Toxicol. Appl. Pharmacol. 31: 128-133, http://dx.doi.org/10.1016/0041-008X(75)90060-5

43. Sancho, E. Ferrando, M.D. and Andreu-Moliner, E. (1997). Response and recovery of head acetylcholinesterase activity in the European eel, *Anguilla Anguilla*. Ecotoxicol. Environ. Safe. 38: 205-209, http://dx.doi.org/10.1006/eesa.1997.1579

44. Ceron, J.J. Ferrando, M.D. Sancho, E. Gutierrez- Panizo, C. and Andreu-Moliner, E. (1996) Effects of diazinon exposure on cholinesterase activity in different tissues of european eel (*Anguilla anguilla*). Ecotoxicol. Environ. Safe. 35: 222-.225.

45. Straus, D.L. and Chambers, J.E. (1995) Inhibition of acetylcholinesterase and aliesterases of fingerling channel catfish by chlorpyrifos, parathion, and s,s,s-tributyl phosphorotrithioate (DEF). Aquat. Toxicol. 33: 311-324, http://dx.doi.org/10.1016/0166-445X(95)00024-X

46. Sancho, E. Ceron, J.J. and Ferrando, M.D. (2000). Cholinesterase activity and hematological parameters as biomarkers of sublethal molinate exposure in *Anguilla anguilla*, Ecotoxicol. Environ. Safe. 46: 81-86, http://dx.doi.org/10.1006/eesa.1999.1888

47. Bretaud, S. Toutant, J.P. and Saglio, P. (2000) Effects of carbofuran, diuron, and nicosulfuron on acetylcholinesterase activity in goldfish (*Carassius auratus*). Ecotoxicol. Environ. Safe. 47, 117-124, http://dx.doi.org/10.1006/eesa.2000.1954

48. Kaur, P. Radotra, B. Minz, R.W. and Gill, K.D. (2007) Impaired mitochondrial energy metabolism and neuronal apoptotic cell death after chronic dichlorvos (OP) exposure in rat brain. Neurotoxicology 28, 1208–1219, http://dx.doi.org/10.1016/j.neuro.2007.08.001

49. Rath, S. and Misra, B.N. (1979). Relative toxicity of dichlorvos (DDVP) to *Tilapia mossambica*Peters of 3 different age groups. Exp. Gerontol. 14: 307-309, http://dx.doi.org/10.1016/0531-5565(79)90042-1

50. Lukaszewicz-Hussain, A. (2010) Role of oxidative stress in organophosphate insecticide toxicity – Short review. Pesticide Biochemistry and Physiology 98: 145–150,http://dx.doi.org/10.1016/j.pestbp.2010.07.006

51. Kalender, S. Ogutcu, A. Uzunhisarcikli, M. Acikgoz, F. Durak, D. Ulusoy, Y. and Kalender, Y. (2005) Diazinon-induced hepatotoxicity and protective effect of vitamin E on some biochemical indices and ultrastructural changes. Toxicology 211, 197–206,http://dx.doi.org/10.1016/j.tox.2005.03.007

52. Lukaszewicz-Hussain, A. and Moniuszko-Jakoniuk, J. (2004) Chlorfenvinphos, an organophosphate insecticide, affects liver mitochondria antioxidative enzymes, glutathione and hydrogen peroxide concentration. Pol. J. Environ. Stud. 13: 397–401.

53. Hai, D.Q. Varga, S. I. and Matkovics, B. (1997) Organophosphate effects on antioxidant system of Carp (*Cyprinus carpio*) and Catfish (*Ictalurus nebulosus*). Comp. Biochem. Pharmacol. 117C, 83–88.

54. Rishi, K.K. and Grewal, S. (1995) Chromosomal aberration test for the insecticide, dichlorvos, on fish chromosomes. Mutation research, 344: 1-4, http://dx.doi.org/10.1016/0165-1218(95)90032-2

55. Gilot-Delhalle, J. Colizzi, A. Moutshen, J. and Moutshen-Dahmen, M. (1983) Mutagenicity of some organophosphorus compounds at the ade6 locus of *Schizosaccharomyces pombe*. Mutat. Res. 117: 139-148, http://dx.doi.org/10.1016/0165-1218(83)90161-1

56. Mirsalis, J.C. Tyson, C.K.. Steinmetz, K.L. Loh, E.K.. Hamilton, C.M. Bakke, J.P. and Spalding, J.W. (1989) Measurement of unscheduled DNA synthesis and S phase synthesis in rodent hepatocytes following in vivo treatment: testing of 24 compounds. Environ. Mol. Mutagen. 14: 155-164,http://dx.doi.org/10.1002/em.2850140305

57. Oshiro, Y. Piper, C.E. Balwierz, P.S. and Soelter, S.G. (1991) Chinese hamster ovary cell assays for mutation and chromosome damage: data from non-carcinogens. J. Appl. Toxicol. 11: 167-177,http://dx.doi.org/10.1002/jat.2550110304

58. Benford, D.J. Price, S.C. Lawrence, J.N. Grasso, P. and Bremmer J.N. (1994). Investigations of the genotoxicity and cell proliferative activity of dichlorvos in mouse forestomach. Toxicology 92: 203-215, http://dx.doi.org/10.1016/0300-483X(94)90178-3

59. Bremmer, J.N. Walker, A.I.T. and Grasso, P. (1988) Is dichlorvos a carcinogenic risk for human? Mutation research 209, 39-44, http://dx.doi.org/10.1016/0165-7992(88)90108-X

60. Mennear, J. H. (1994) Dichlorvos carcinogenicity: An assessment of the weight of experimental evidence. Regul. Toxicol. Pharmacol. 20: 354–361,http://dx.doi.org/10.1006/rtph.1994.1080

61. International Agency for Research on Cancer (IARC) (1987). Overall Evaluations of Carcinogenicity: An Updating of IARC Monographs, Volumes 1 to 42. IARC Monographs on the Evaluation of Carcinogenic Risks to Humans, Supplement 7.

62. National Toxicology Program (NTP) (1989). Toxicology and carcinogenesis studies of dichlorvos in F344/N rats and B6C3F1 mice. U.S. Dept. of HHS, PHS, NIH, NTP Technical Report No. 334.

63. Dunier, M. Siwicki, A.K. and Demael, A. (1991) Effects of organophosphorus insecticides: effects of trichlorfon and dichlorvos on the immune response of carp (*Cyprinus carpio*).III. In vitro effects on lymphocyte proliferation and phagocytosis and in vivo effects on humoral response. Ecotoxicol. Environ. Safety 22: 79-87, http://dx.doi.org/10.1016/0147-6513(91)90049-U

64. Das, S. and Gupta, A. (2012) Effect of Malathion (EC_{50}) on Gill Morphology of Indian Flying Barb, *Esomus danricus* (Hamilton-Buchanan). World Journal of Fish and Marine Sciences 4: 626-628.

65. Ghioni, C. Tocher, D. R. and Sargent, J. R. (1998) Effects of dichlorvos and formalin on fatty acid metabolism of rainbow trout (Oncorhynchus mykiss) skin cells in primary culture. Fish Physiol biochem, 18: 241-252, http://dx.doi.org/10.1023/A:1007730730655

66. Benarji, G., and Rajebdranath, T. (1991) Dichlorvos-induced histoarchitectural changes in the oocytes of a freshwater fish. Funct Dev. Morphol. 1: 9-12.

67. Singh, H. and T.P. Singh, 1982. Effect of pesticides on fish reproduction. Ichthyologia, 15: 71-81.

68. Mir, F.A. Shah, G.M. Jan, U. and Mir, J.I. (2012) Studies on Influences of Sublethal Concentrations of Organophosphate Pesticide; Dichlorvos (DDVP) on Gonadosomatic Index (GSI) of Female Common Carp, *Cyprinus carpio communis.* American-Eurasian Journal of Toxicological Sciences 4: 67-71.

CHAPTER 23

ORGANOCHLORINATED PESTICIDE MIXTURE

Brandon D. Gaytán, Alex V. Loguinov, Xenia Peñate, Jan-Michael Lerot, Sebastián Chávez, Nancy D. Denslow, Chris D. Vulpe

Keywords: dichlorvos, toxic, acute, chronic, fish

INTRODUCTION

Toxaphene is a complex mixture of polychlorinated camphenes and bornanes primarily used to control insects on cotton during the 1960-80s (Figure 1A) [1]. After the ban of DDT in 1972, toxaphene became the most heavily applied pesticide in the United States, but all registered uses were cancelled by the U.S. Environmental Protection Agency (EPA) in 1989 over concerns related to its toxicity and persistence [2]. Today, toxaphene remains a problematic environmental contaminant, ranking 32nd on the Agency for Toxic Substances and Disease Registry (ATSDR) Priority List of Hazardous Substances, a list of compounds that possibly threaten human health via their toxicity and possibility for exposure at EPA National Priorities List hazardous waste sites. Toxaphene's most persistent congeners and degradation products have been detected in water, air, and sediment, and are known to bioaccumulate in wildlife and humans [1]. Animal studies have deemed toxaphene a neuro-, nephro-, immuno-, and hepatotoxicant, an endocrine disruptor, and a carcinogen, with the International Agency for Research on Cancer (IARC) classifying toxaphene as Group 2B (possibly carcinogenic to humans) [1,3]. Epidemiological analyses have linked toxaphene to leukemia [4], non-Hodgkin's lymphoma [5], melanoma [6], and more recently, amyotrophic lateral sclerosis [7]. However, the cellular and molecular processes that toxaphene perturbs to result in these toxicities and disease states remain unclear.

The eukaryotic yeast Saccharomyces cerevisiae is a valuable model in which to conduct toxicological studies. First, basic cellular processes, along with metabolic and signaling pathways, are conserved to higher organisms. Second, a close human homolog has been identified for a significant portion of yeast genes, with several hundred of the conserved genes linked to disease in humans [8]. Finally, the availability of deletion mutant collections, overexpression libraries, and genetic and physical interaction data provide unmatched resources for inquiries into potential cellular and molecular mechanisms of toxicity. With the deletion mutant collection [9], functional toxicogenomic analyses (also known as functional profiling) can be conducted by examining, in parallel, the sensitivity or resistance of each mutant strain to a compound of interest. Such investigations, through the identification of yeast genes required for chemical tolerance, have discovered molecular mechanisms for numerous drugs and toxicants [10,11], with several studies confirming results in human cells [12-14].

Citation: Gaytán BD, Loguinov AV, Peñate X, Lerot J-M, Chávez S, Denslow ND, et al. (2013) Organochlorinated Pesticide Mixture. PLoS ONE 8(11): e81253. doi:10.1371/journal.pone.0081253.

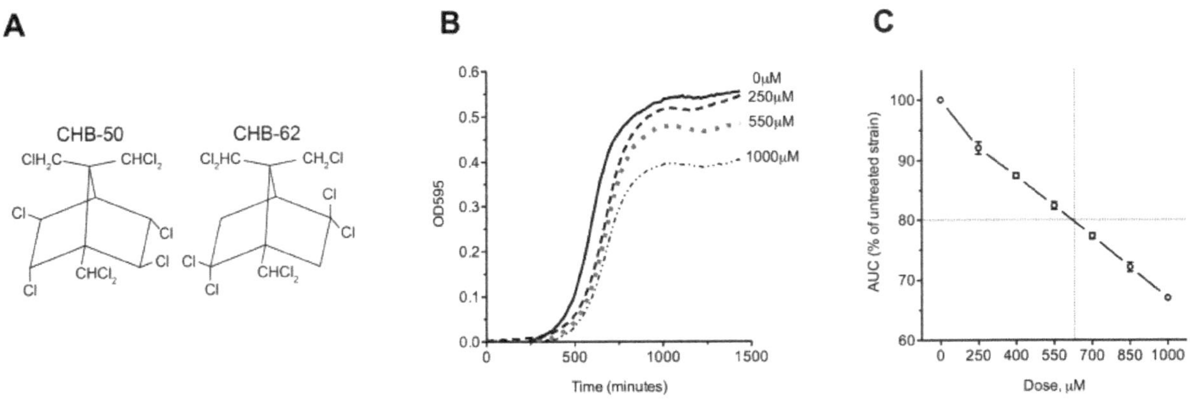

Figure 1: Determining the toxaphene IC20 for functional profiling. (A) The structure of two chlorinated congeners present in the toxaphene technical mixture. (**B**) Representative growth curves in YPD media for the BY4743 wild-type strain treated with toxaphene. For clarity, only the 250, 550, and 1000µM toxaphene doses are shown, although additional curves were performed at 400, 700, and 850µM. (**C**) The area under the curve (AUC) was calculated at each dose for three independent experiments, expressed as the mean and SE, and plotted as a percentage of the untreated control. The toxaphene IC20 was determined to be 640µM, as indicated by the dashed lines. http://dx.doi.org/10.1371/journal.pone.0081253.g001

Here we present the results of a functional screen devised to identify yeast genes necessary for growth in the presence of toxaphene. It is the first known genome-wide study in any organism to examine the genetic requirements for toxaphene tolerance. Our results demonstrate that similar to the known transcription elongation inhibitors mycophenolic acid (MPA) and 6-azauracil (6-AU), mutants defective in processes linked to transcription elongation are sensitive to toxaphene. While toxaphene does display synergism with MPA, it apparently exhibits a mechanism of action distinct from that of MPA/6-AU and additionally does not appear to directly affect transcription elongation. Many yeast genes required for toxaphene resistance have human homologs that may play a role in human toxicity.

MATERIALS AND METHODS

Yeast strains and culture

The diploid non-essential yeast deletion strains used for functional profiling and confirmation analyses were of the BY4743 background (MATa/MATα his3Δ1/his3Δ1 leu2Δ0/leu2Δ0 lys2Δ0/LYS2 MET15/met15Δ0 ura3Δ0/ura3Δ0, Life Technologies). Yeast growth was performed in liquid rich media (1% yeast extract, 2% peptone, 2% dextrose, YPD) at 30°C with shaking at 200 revolutions per minute (rpm). For the elongation assays, the GAL1-YLR454strain [15] was grown in rich media containing galactose (1% yeast extract, 2% peptone, 2% galactose, YPGal).

Dose-finding and growth curve assays

Dose-finding and growth curves were performed as in [16]. Toxaphene and MPA (Sigma Aldrich) solutions were prepared in dimethylsulfoxide (DMSO) and added to the desired final concentrations (1% or less by volume) with at least three technical replicates per dose. The area means and standard error (SE) for the growth of each strain (as measured by the area under the curve) was derived from three independent cultures.

Functional profiling of the yeast genome

The functional screen and differential strain sensitivity analysis (DSSA) were performed as previously described [17]. Briefly, pools of deletion mutants (n = 4607) were cultured for 15 generations in YPD at various toxaphene concentrations. Following extraction of genomic DNA with the YDER kit (Pierce Biotechnology), DNA sequences unique to each strain were amplified by PCR and subsequently hybridized to TAG4 arrays (Affymetrix). Arrays were incubated overnight, stained, and scanned at 560 nm with a GeneChip Scanner (Affymetrix). Data files are available at the Gene Expression Omnibus database (http://www.ncbi.nlm.nih.gov/geo/).

Over-enrichment and network mapping analyses

The Functional Specification (FunSpec) resource [18] identified significantly overrepresented Gene Ontology (GO) and MIPS (Munich Information Center for Protein Sequences) categories within the DSSA data using a p value cutoff of 0.002 and Bonferroni correction. Gene interaction networks were generated in Cytoscape [19] by mapping fitness scores for toxaphene-sensitive strains onto the BioGrid Saccharomyces cerevisiae functional interaction network. The jActiveModules Cytoscape plugin identified sub-networks enriched with fitness data, within which the BiNGO plugin discovered overrepresented GO categories.

Analysis of relative strain growth by flow cytometry

Analyses of relative strain growth were performed as described [16]. Briefly, green fluorescent protein (GFP)-tagged wild-type and untagged deletion strains were mixed in approximately equal numbers and cultured for 24 hours at 30°C in the presence of toxaphene. At least 20,000 cells were analyzed at T=0 and T=24 hours using a FACSCalibur flow cytometer. A ratio of growth was calculated for untagged cells in treated versus untreated samples using the percentages of wild-type

GFP and untagged mutant cells present. Statistically significant differences between the means of three independent DMSO-treated and toxaphene-treated cultures were determined with Student's t-test.

Analyses of transcription elongation

Gene Length Accumulation of mRNA (GLAM) assays were performed as described [20]. Chromatin immunoprecipitation experiments were performed as described [21], except mouse monoclonal anti-Rpb3 (1Y26, Abcam) antibody was used. Immunoprecipitated DNA was measured by quantitative PCR in a LightCycler (Roche), using the primers listed. Normalizations required for RNA polymerase II processivity comparisons were applied as described [15].

RESULTS

Functional profiling in yeast identifies genes required for toxaphene tolerance

The IC20, the concentration at which growth is inhibited by 20%, is a dose frequently utilized in functional screens, as it elicits a response without being overly toxic [17]. After performing growth curve analyses for wild-type yeast treated with increasing concentrations of toxaphene (Figure 1B), the toxaphene IC20 was calculated as 640μM (Figure 1C). Pools of yeast homozygous diploid deletion mutants (n = 4607) were grown for 15 generations at the toxaphene IC20 (640μM), 50% IC20 (320μM), and 25% IC20 (160μM) to identify genes important for growth in toxaphene. DSSA deemed 130 strains sensitive and 542 strains resistant to at least one dose of toxaphene. Sensitive strains were the focus of this study, with the top 30 displaying growth defects shown in Table 1.

Table 1: Fitness scores for the top 30 deletion strains identified as significantly sensitive to toxaphene after 15 generations of growth.

	Log_2 values				
Deleted Gene	**25% IC20 160μM**	**50% IC20 320μM**	**100%IC20 640μM**	**Function of deleted gene**	**Confirmed**
PDR5	-6.30	-5.80	-6.05	Plasma membrane multidrug transporter	S
RPN4	-3.15	-3.05	-2.55	Transcription factor; stimulates expression of proteasome genes	S
DAL81	-3.10	-3.50	-3.00	Positive regulator of genes in nitrogen degradation pathways	S
TRP4	-2.90	-4.50	-4.70	Anthranilate phosphoribosyl transferase for tryptophan biosynthesis	S
SWF1	-2.90	-3.20	-3.00	Palmitoyltransferase; acts on various SNAREs	NS
URE2	-2.75	-2.45	-2.95	Nitrogen catabolite repression transcriptional regulator	S
STP1	-2.50	-3.10	-3.00	Transcription factor for amino acid permease genes	S
YGR153W	-2.50	-2.60	-2.60	Putative protein of unknown function	
YDR008C	-2.30	-2.80	-3.10	Dubious ORF; partially overlapsTRP1 tryptophan biosynthetic enzyme	
SEC 66	-2.30	-2.60	-2.40	Subunit of Sec63 complex; involved in ER protein translocation	
YEL045C	-2.20	-2.60	-2.40	Dubious ORF	
PDR1	-2.15	-2.25	-2.70	Transcriptional regulator of multidrug resistance genes	S
SPT4	-2.00	-1.85	-1.95	Regulates Pol I and Pol II transcription	S
IRS4	-1.75	-2.50	-2.00	Regulates phosphatidylinositol 4,5-bisphosphate levels and autophagy	S
YKL077W	-1.75	-1.45	-1.20	Putative protein of unknown function	

THP2	-1.65	-2.00	-2.50	Subunit of the THO complex; involved in transcription elongation	S
YDR203W	-1.60	-1.90	-2.20	Dubious ORF; partially over-lapsRAV2	
ICE2	-1.50	-1.50	-2.20	Integral ER membrane protein	
TKL1	-1.50	-1.40	-1.70	Transketolase in the pentose phosphate pathway	S
COG7	-1.50	-1.40	-1.40	Component of the COG golgi transport complex	
COX20	-1.45	-1.85	-2.05	Mitochondrial inner mem-brane protein	
IMG2	-1.40	-1.70	-2.60	Mitochondrial ribosomal pro-tein of the large subunit	
YDR455C	-1.40	-1.50	-1.30	Dubious ORF; partially over-lapsNHX1	
URA2	-1.30	-1.40	-1.55	Involved in de novobiosynthe-sis of pyrimidines	NS
SIW14	-1.30	-1.30	-1.30	Tyrosine phosphatase	
GYP1	-1.25	-1.55	-1.50	cis-golgi GTPase-activating protein (GAP) for the Rab family	NS
YSP1	-1.25	-1.50	-1.75	Mitochondrial protein; poten-tial role in programmed cell death	S
YJL120W	-1.25	-1.30	-1.35	Dubious ORF; partially over-laps RPE1	
CUE1	-1.20	-1.00	-1.15	ER membrane protein; regu-lates ubiquitination	
PBP1	-1.20	-0.90	-1.10	Component of glucose depri-vation induced stress granules	

Fitness scores, defined as the normalized $\log_2$ ratio of strain growth in the presence versus absence of toxaphene, quantify the requirement of a gene for growth. The confirmed column indicates whether the strain was confirmed as sensitive (S) or not sensitive (NS- a false positive) by growth curve assays. The DSSA used to identify altered strain growth is semi-quantitative, as variations in individual strain growth along with initial deletion pool strain counts can impact relative $\log_2$ ratios. Contains a list of all mutants displaying altered growth in the functional screen.

Overrepresentation analyses identify biological attributes needed for toxaphene resistance

All toxaphene-sensitive strains identified by DSSA (n = 122;) were analyzed with FunSpec for significantly overrepresented biological attributes at a corrected p value of 0.002 (Table 2). Transcription elongation and aerobic respiration were enriched in both GO and MIPS categories, indicating that mutants lacking genes associated with these processes are sensitive to toxaphene. Other overrepresented GO classifications included mitochondrial respiratory chain complex IV biogenesis and aromatic amino acid biosynthesis. To supplement the FunSpec evaluation, network mapping was performed with Cytoscape to identify additional attributes required for toxaphene tolerance. The BiNGO plugin revealed that transcription elongation, aerobic respiration, and aromatic amino acid biosynthesis were overrepresented within the network data (Figure 2). Other categories uncovered were cell death and metabolic salvage.

Table 2: Genes required for toxaphene tolerance and their associated GO or MIPS categories.

GO Biological Process	*p*value	Genes identified	k[a]	f[b]
mitochondrial respiratory chain complex IV biogenesis (GO:0097034)	3.14E-004	PET122, PET54, PET494	3	8
regulation of ER to Golgi vesicle-mediated transport (GO:0060628)	3.33E-004	UBP3, BRE5	2	2
transcription elongation from RNA polymerase II promoter (GO:0006368)	4.21E-004	DST1, SPT4, THP2, ELF1, CDC73, MFT1	6	54

Group I intron splicing (GO:0000372)	6.56E-004	PET54, CBP2, MRS1	3	10
aerobic respiration (GO:0009060)	8.16E-004	COX20, QCR9, QCR8, COQ9, COX11, MRPL51	6	61
response to arsenic-containing substance (GO:0046685)	8.90E-004	RPN4, GET3, TIM18	3	11
heme a biosynthetic process (GO:0006784)	9.87E-004	COX15, COX10	2	3
ribophagy (GO:0034517)	9.87E-004	UBP3, BRE5	2	3
aromatic amino acid family biosynthetic process (GO:0009073)	1.17E-003	ARO3, TRP4, ARO2	3	12
MIPS Functional Classification	***p* value**	***Genes identified***	**k[a]**	**f[b]**
transcription elongation (11.02.03.01.04)	1.69E-005	DST1, SPT4, THP2, ELF1, CDC73, MFT1	6	31
aerobic respiration [02.13.03)	4.85E-004	COX20, QCR9, COX23, QCR8, COQ9, COX11, MRPL51	7	77

Strains exhibiting sensitivity to three doses of toxaphene in the functional screen were entered into FunSpec and analyzed for overrepresented biological attributes (see Materials and Methods section). [a] Number of genes in category identified as sensitive to toxaphene. [b] Number of genes in GO or MIPS category.

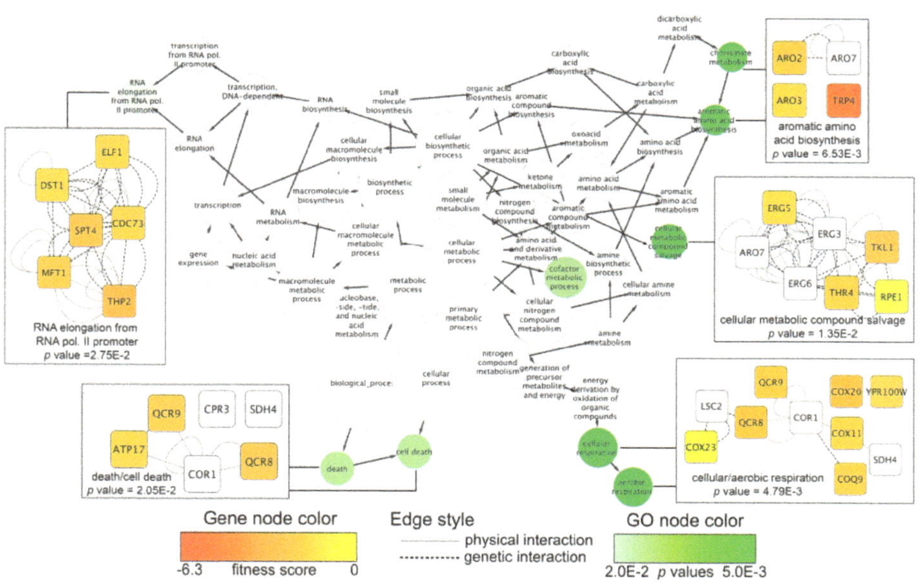

Figure 2: Biological attributes required for toxaphene tolerance are identified by network mapping. Cytoscape was used to map fitness scores (the ratio of the $\log_2$ hybridization signals between DMSO and toxaphene exposures) for toxaphene-sensitive strains onto theSaccharomyces cerevisiae BioGRID interaction dataset. A subnetwork (n = 104) containing genetic and physical interactions between the sensitive, non-sensitive, and essential genes was created and significantly overrepresented (p value cutoff of 0.03) GO categories were identified. The green node color corresponds to the GO p-value while the node size correlates to the number of genes in the category. Edge arrows indicate hierarchy of GO terms. Networks for various GO categories are shown, where node color corresponds to deletion strain fitness score and edge defines the type of interaction between the genes. http://dx.doi.org/10.1371/journal.pone.0081253.g002

Mutants defective in transcription elongation associated processes are sensitive to toxaphene

FunSpec and Cytoscape analyses indicated enrichment of transcription elongation mutants within the functional profiling data. Accordingly, growth curves were obtained for the transcription elongation mutants identified in the screen and compared to the BY4743 wild-type strain, with five out of the six (cdc73Δ, dst1Δ , mft1Δ, thp2Δ, and spt4Δ, but not elf1Δ) confirmed as sensitive to toxaphene (Figure 3). Considering two of these mutants (mft1Δ andthp2Δ) lacked components of THO, a complex required for efficient transcription elongation [22] and mRNA export [23], we tested strains harboring deletions of the two additional THO subunits (hpr1Δ and tho2Δ), finding growth defects (Figure 3). Many of these confirmed strains are also sensitive to the transcription elongation inhibitors MPA and 6-AU [24], therefore, we examined whether toxaphene affected a set of MPA- or 6-AU-sensitive mutants known to exhibit transcription elongation defects. Indeed, strains lacking subunits of the SAGA histone acetyltransferase (spt20Δ), the Paf1p complex (rtf1Δ), and the TREX-2 transcriptional export machinery (sac3Δ and thp1Δ) were sensitive to toxaphene (Figure 3). Additionally, a gene encoding an RNA polymerase II subunit (RPB9), along with genes implicated in RNA polymerase II activation (CTK3, RAD6, and SNF6) or reactivation through deubiquitylation (BRE5 and UBP3) were required for toxaphene tolerance (Figure 3).

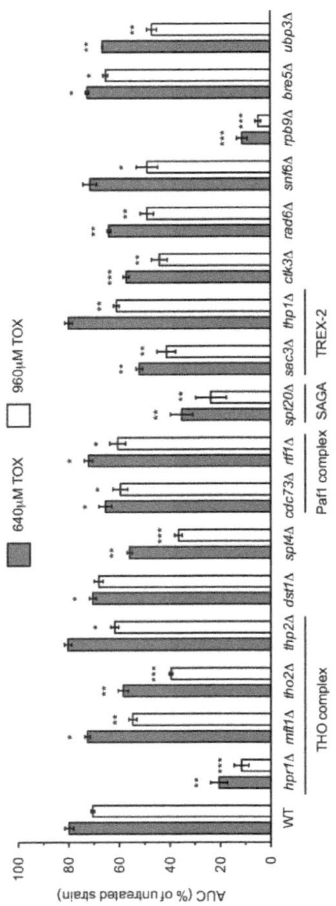

Figure 3: Transcription elongation mutants are sensitive to toxaphene. Growth curves for three independent cultures were obtained for the indicated strains and toxaphene concentrations. Mutants with known defects in transcription elongation are sensitive to toxaphene, including members of the THO, Paf1p, SAGA, and TREX-2 complexes. Additional mutants lacking genes implicated in transcription elongation exhibit sensitivity as well. The AUC was calculated for each curve and is shown as a percentage of the untreated strain. Statistical significance between the wild-type and mutant strains was calculated with Student's t-test, where ***p<0.001, **p<0.01, and *p<0.05. http://dx.doi.org/10.1371/journal.pone.0081253.g003

Nitrogen utilization and aromatic amino acid biosynthesis mutants are sensitive to toxaphene

The dal81Δ, stp1Δ, and ure2Δ nitrogen utilization mutants identified in the functional screen (Table 1) were confirmed by growth curve analyses to exhibit severe growth defects in presence of toxaphene (Figure 4). For unknown reasons, the growth of these mutants is also hindered by the transcription elongation inhibitors MPA and 6-AU [24,25]. Additionally, in agreement with enrichment analyses (Figure 2 and Table 2), mutants deficient in aromatic amino acid biosynthesis were toxaphene-sensitive, with the TRP4 tryptophan biosynthesis gene implicated as the pathway component furthest downstream (Figure 4). However, neither tryptophan supplementation of YPD media nor titration into defined media altered growth of the BY4743 wild-type strain in toxaphene (data not shown).

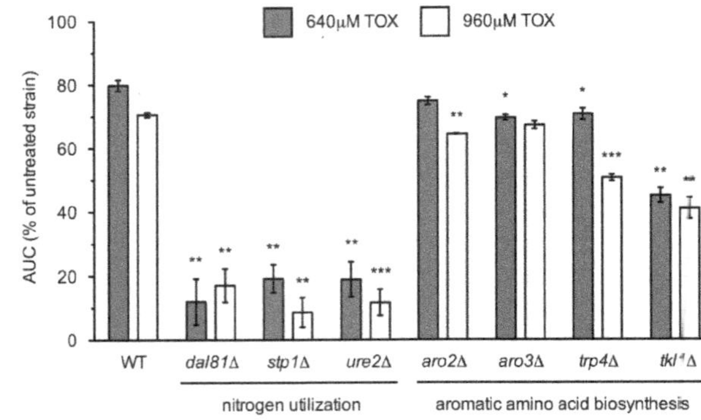

Figure 4: Nitrogen utilization and aromatic amino acid synthesis genes are required for toxaphene tolerance. The AUC was calculated for strains treated with 640μM or 960μM toxaphene and expressed as a percentage of the AUC for the untreated strain. Bars signify the mean and SE for three independent cultures. http://dx.doi.org/10.1371/journal.pone.0081253.g004

Toxaphene exhibits synergy with MPA, but its mechanism of action is not similar

Similarities between the mutant sensitivity profiles for toxaphene and the transcription elongation inhibitors MPA and 6-AU prompted us to examine whether the compounds shared a mechanism of action. Both MPA and 6-AU inhibit the guanosine monophosphate (GMP) synthesis enzyme inosine monophosphate dehydrogenase (IMPDH), which reduces ribonucleotide levels and increases dependence on transcription elongation factors for transcriptional efficiency [26,27]. As a first step, we assessed synergy between toxaphene and MPA by obtaining growth curves for each condition as well as the mixture. We also considered 4-nitroquinoline-N-oxide (4-NQO), a model carcinogen whose DNA adducts may be repaired by transcription-coupled nucleotide excision repair [25], and tunicamycin, an endoplasmic reticulum stressor [28]. Both MPA and 4-NQO displayed additive inhibitory growth effects with toxaphene, while the general stressor tunicamycin did not (Figure 5). Second, we examined whether guanine or uracil supplementation could reverse toxaphene sensitivity, as both can rescue the growth of transcription elongation mutants in the presence of either MPA or 6-AU [24,26]. A flow cytometry assay, in which relative growth of a mutant strain to a wild-type GFP-expressing strain was compared under the indicated conditions, confirmed that neither guanine nor uracil reversed toxaphene sensitivity of transcription elongation mutants (Figures 6A and B). Third, we tested a strain deleted for IMD2, the only yeast IMPDHhomologue that provides resistance to MPA [29], for toxaphene sensitivity. Although hypersensitive to MPA, the imd2Δ strain did not display altered growth in toxaphene (data not shown). Finally, we found toxaphene did not affect strains deleted for URA2 or URA4, enzymes involved in the de novo biosynthesis of pyrimidine ribonucleotides [30] (data not shown). Collectively, these data suggest that toxaphene's mechanism is not analogous to MPA/6-AU, i.e., it does not alter nucleotide pools or target the IMPDH family of enzymes.

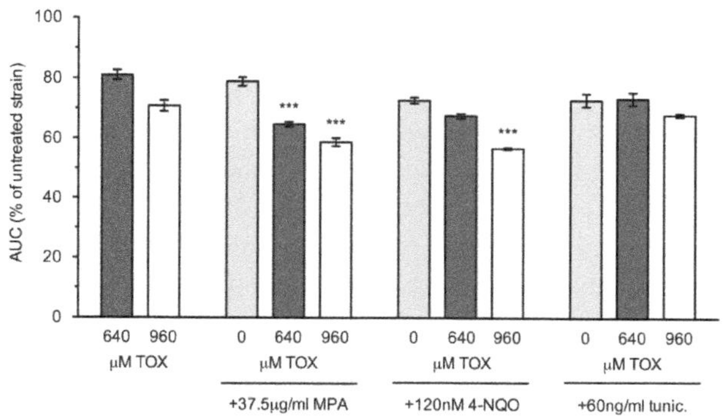

Figure 5: Toxaphene exhibits synergy with MPA and 4-NQO.

Growth curve assays were performed for three independent cultures of the BY4743 wild-type strain with the indicated compounds. Both MPA (a transcription elongation inhibitor) and 4-NQO (a genotoxicant) displayed synergy with toxaphene, while tunicamycin (an endoplasmic reticulum stressor) did not. Statistical significance was determined with one-way ANOVA with a Tukey post-test. *** represents significance observed at p<0.001 between both toxaphene/toxaphene+synergist and synergist/toxaphene+synergist comparisons.

http://dx.doi.org/10.1371/journal.pone.0081253.g005

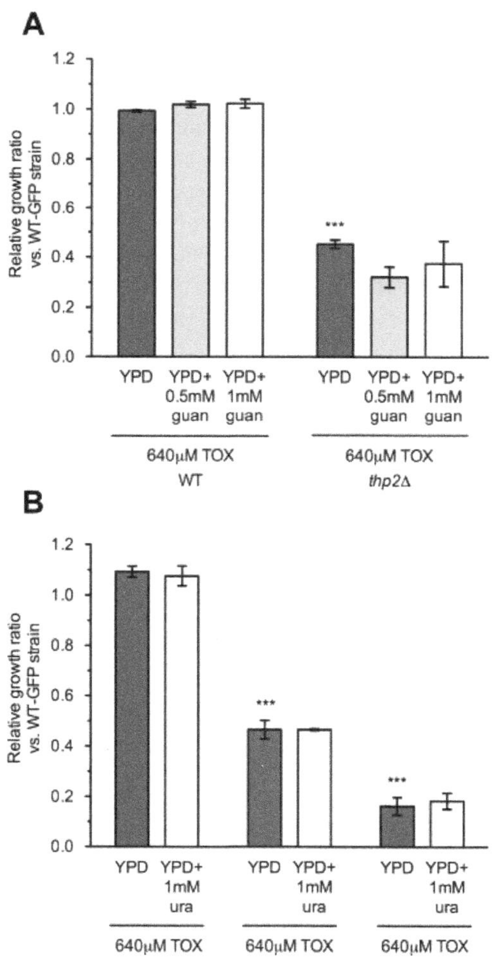

Figure 6: Neither guanine nor uracil rescues toxaphene sensitivity of transcription elongation mutants. Relative growth ratios (treatment vs. control) to a GFP-expressing wild-type strain were obtained for three independent cultures and the means and SEs are shown. One-way ANOVA followed by a Bonferroni post-test determined statistical significance. ***p<0.001 for wild-type/mutant comparisons. (**A**) The toxaphene sensitivity of thethp2Δ strain cannot be rescued by guanine. YPD media was supplemented with the indicated concentrations of guanine and toxaphene. (**B**) Uracil cannot reverse the toxaphene sensitivity of the mft1Δ or thp2Δ strains. Uracil and toxaphene were added to YPD media at the indicated concentrations. The impact of toxaphene on mft1Δ andthp2Δ was stronger in these relative growth experiments versus growth curve assays (see Figure 3). Most likely, this is due to the competitive nature of the relative growth assays, where even in control experiments, deletions with intrinsic growth defects are outcompeted by wild-type. Exposure to toxaphene likely magnified the relative growth defects between mft1Δ or thp2Δ and the wild-type strain in this assay. http://dx.doi.org/10.1371/journal.pone.0081253.g006

Toxaphene does not affect transcription elongation

We next examined toxaphene's potential to obstruct transcription elongation, reasoning that inhibition of this process could still occur via a mechanism distinct from that of MPA/6-AU. The GLAM assay has been developed to indirectly examine defects in transcription elongation [20], using the premise that mutants impaired in elongation are less able to transcribe long versus short transcription units. The toxaphene-sensitive transcription elongation mutants identified in this study have previously exhibited low scores when assayed for GLAM [20,25]. We measured the GLAM-ratios of acid phosphatase activity for a long (PHO5-lacZ or PHO5-LAC4) versus short transcription unit (PHO5) for BY4743 wild-type cells in the presence or absence of toxaphene, but did not find altered ratios upon toxaphene exposure (Figure 7A).

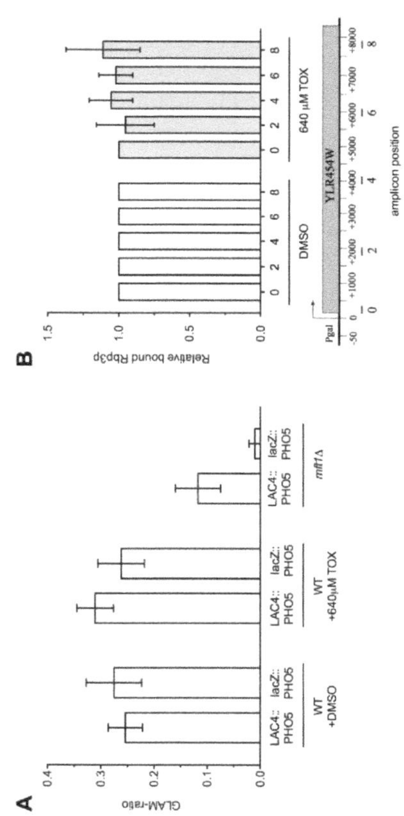

Figure 7: Toxaphene does not inhibit transcription elongation. (**A**) GLAM-ratios are not altered upon toxaphene treatment. The acid phosphatase activity of long (PHO5-lacZ or PHO5-LAC4) versus short (PHO5) transcriptional units was

measured and the means and SE are shown for three independent experiments. The mft1Δ strain was used as a positive control. (**B**) Toxaphene does not affect RNA processivity. Levels of RNA polymerase II bound to different regions of a long gene were measured by chromatin immunoprecipitation. http://dx.doi.org/10.1371/journal.pone.0081253.g007

Since GLAM is an indirect measurement of transcription elongation that may not recognize all transcription elongation defects, we directly assessed RNA polymerase II elongation by performing an RNA polymerase II processivity assay [15], where levels of RNA polymerase II bound to different regions of a long gene are measured. If transcription elongation were compromised under toxaphene treatment, the profile of RNA polymerase II would change in comparison to a non-treated sample, as seen in the case of 6AU and most transcription elongation mutants detected in this study [15]. However, the patterns of the toxaphene-treated and DMSO-treated samples were very similar, indicating that toxaphene does not affect RNA polymerase II processivity during transcription elongation (Figure 7B).

DISCUSSION

While the complex mixture of chlorinated terpenes known as toxaphene was once the most widely applied pesticide in the United States, its congeners are now considered persistent, bioaccumulative, and toxic. In 2004, these unfavorable characteristics resulted in toxaphene's addition to the Stockholm Convention on Persistent Organic Pollutants treaty as a member of the original "dirty dozen" compounds designated for international elimination or restriction. Those most at risk for exposure include Arctic populations who eat aquatic mammals and people consuming sport-caught fish from the Great Lakes [2]. Although toxaphene has been linked to diseases such as cancer and amyotrophic lateral sclerosis [4-7], cellular and molecular toxicity data associated with exposure are severely lacking.

To discover potential mechanisms of toxicity, we screened the S. cerevisiae homozygous diploid non-essential deletion mutant collection to identify strains with altered growth in the presence of toxaphene. The majority of yeast genes confirmed as required for toxaphene tolerance are implicated in transcription elongation and associated processes (Figure 3), with additional resistance genes involved in nutrient utilization, drug transport, and various other cellular functions (Figures 4). Our results regarding nutrient utilization mutants are congruous with a report in which the toxicity of toxaphene was approximately 3-fold greater in rats fed a protein deficient diet [34]. Both results point to a need of a fully functional catabolic environment to resist toxaphene. Enrichment analyses indicated aerobic respiration mutants were sensitive to toxaphene (Table 2), which is consistent with toxaphene's ability to inhibit ATPases [31-33]. However, this group of strains was not studied to a large extent herein, as (1) the qcr8Δ strain (which has an electron transport chain defect) was a false positive (data not shown) and (2) most are petite and/or slow growing, which causes inherent competitive fitness defects during pool screens and may thus misinform further analyses. Future studies may elucidate the effects, if any, of toxaphene on aerobic respiration in yeast. The most sensitive strain identified by DSSA (and confirmed by growth curve assays) was pdr5Δ, which, not unexpectedly, lacks a drug resistance transporter involved in detoxification. Many yeast genes described in this study are conserved (Table 3) and may thus play a role in human toxicity. As the technical toxaphene mixture utilized in this investigation is comprised of hundreds of related chlorinated compounds, the congener(s) responsible for the observed toxic effects in yeast remain unknown. Moreover, both human metabolism and environmental weathering of toxaphene [3] may produce derivatives of differing toxicological relevance than those present in the technical mixture.

Table 3: Human orthologs of yeast genes required for toxaphene tolerance.

Yeast gene	Human ortholog(s)	Human protein description
CDC73	CDC73	Tumor suppressor; involved in transcriptional/post-transcriptional pathways
DST1	TCEA1	Transcription elongation factor A (SII)
HXK2	HK2	Hexokinase 2
IRA2	NF1	Neurofibromin 1, tumor suppressor
PDR5	ABCG2	ATP-binding cassette protein
RAD6	UBE2A/UBE2B	Ubiquitin-conjugating enzyme E2A
RPB9	POLR2I	DNA-directed RNA pol. II subunit RPB9
RTF1	RTF1	Role in transcription-coupled histone modification
SAC3	GANP	Synonym MCM3AP, minichromosome maintenance protein 3
SPT4	SUPT4H1	Regulates mRNA processing and transcription elongation by RNA pol. II
STP1	ZNFN1A4	Zinc finger protein, subfamily 1A, 4 (Eos)
THO2	THOC2	Component of the THO subcomplex of the TREX complex
THP1	PCID2	PCI domain containing 2
TKL1	TKTL1/2, TKT	Transketolase
UBP3	USP10	Ubiquitin specific peptidase 10

Deletion of any of these yeast genes caused sensitivity to toxaphene (listed in alphabetical order).

Although various -omics approaches have been utilized to examine the molecular effects of toxaphene, its mechanism(s) of toxicity remain ambiguous and findings directly related to transcription elongation have not been reported. Perhaps most relevant to this study is a report indicating that toxaphene altered expression of transcription termination genes in largemouth bass (Mehinto et al., in preparation). Woo and Yum [35] performed gene expression analyses in marine medaka, showing that toxaphene affected regulation of cytoskeletal, developmental, metabolic, nucleic acid/protein binding, and signal transduction genes. Increased expression of homocysteine methyltransferase, a zinc metalloenzyme involved in the metabolism of various amino acids [35], may indicate a link to the nutrient utilization genes described in this study (Figure 4). Toxaphene perturbed hepatic expression of one carbon metabolism and ribosomal biogenesis genes in adult male largemouth bass [36], while another study in the same organism could not establish changes in neuroendocrine signaling or neurotransmitter synthesis transcripts [37]. Proteomic analyses in the livers of largemouth bass identified differentially expressed proteins following toxaphene exposure, including an ion channel, a component of the pentose phosphate pathway, and a glutathione S-transferase [38]. Functional profiling in yeast has been performed with the related organochlorine pesticide dieldrin, but its toxic mechanism (altered leucine availability) is different from that of toxaphene [16].

Toxaphene-sensitive mutants also experience growth defects in MPA and 6-AU two compounds that diminish transcription elongation by inhibiting GMP synthesis [26,27]. By decreasing nucleotide availability, MPA and 6-AU reduce RNA polymerase II elongation rate and processivity [15], with transcription elongation mutant sensitivity ascribed to the deleterious combination of transcriptional defects [39]. Although toxaphene and MPA synergistically inhibit yeast growth (Figure 5), two different elongation assays did not detect any effect of toxaphene on transcription elongation (Figure 7), unlike results seen with MPA and 6-AU [15]. Intriguingly, several toxaphene tolerance genes, such asSAC3, SPT4, THP1, and those encoding components of the THO complex, are associated with other processes tightly coupled to transcription elongation, such as mRNA processing, mRNA nuclear export, or transcription-coupled nucleotide excision repair [23,40-44]. The possibility that one of these cellular operations is required for toxaphene resistance led us to examine mRNA export in presence of toxaphene using in situ hybridization, however, our findings were inconclusive (data not shown). Alternatively, toxaphene sensitivity of transcription elongation mutants may be attributed to defective expression of yet to be defined toxaphene tolerance protein(s). This type of indirect effect occurs in elongation mutants exhibiting sensitivity to the nucleotide depleting compound 6-AU; these deletions cannot sufficiently induce Imd2p, the protein that combats 6-AU toxicity by restoring nucleotide levels [45].

By identifying mutants with altered growth in toxaphene, our study advances understanding of the genetic requirements for the toxaphene response in yeast. Despite evidence indicating transcription elongation mutants exhibit sensitivity to toxaphene, our data suggest toxaphene does not affect transcription elongation itself. Instead, we propose toxaphene tolerance requires a yet to be identified cellular process closely associated with transcription elongation, as toxaphene synergism with MPA indicates a likely effect along this pathway. Using data provided in this study, further pathway-specific investigations in yeast or humans may elucidate the distinct mechanism of toxaphene toxicity.

ACKNOWLEDGMENTS

We thank Vanessa De La Rosa and Mani Tagmount of the Vulpe laboratory (University of California, Berkeley) for helpful discussions and Daniel Reines (Emory University) for the imd2Δ strain. BDG is a trainee in the Superfund Research Program at the University of California, Berkeley.

REFERENCES

1. Agency for Toxic Substances and Disease Registry (ATSDR) (2010) Toxicological profile for toxaphene. Atlanta, GA, USA: US Dept of Health and Human Services, ATSDR.
2. National Toxicology Program (NTP) (2011) Report on carcinogens, twelfth edition. Research Triangle Park, NC, USA: US Dept of Health and Human Services, NTP.
3. De Geus HJ, Besselink H, Brouwer A, Klungsøyr J, McHugh B et al. (1999) Environmental occurrence, analysis, and toxicology of toxaphene compounds. Environ Health Perspect 107: 115–144. doi:10.2307/3434478. PubMed: 10229713.
4. MillsPK,YangR,RiordanD(2005)Lymphohematopoietic cancers in the United Farm Workers of America (UFW), 1988-2001. Cancer Causes Control 16: 823–830. doi:10.1007/s10552-005-2703-2. PubMed: 16132792.
5. Schroeder JC, Olshan AF, Baric R, Dent GA, Weinberg CR et al. (2001) Agricultural risk factors for t(14;18) subtypes of non-Hodgkin's lymphoma. Epidemiology 12: 701–709. doi:10.1097/00001648-200111000-00020. PubMed: 11679800.
6. Purdue MP, Hoppin JA, Blair A, Dosemeci M, Alavanja MCR (2007) Occupational exposure to organochlorine insecticides and cancer incidence in the Agricultural Health Study. Int J Cancer 120: 642–649. doi:10.1002/ijc.22258. PubMed: 17096337.
7. Kamel F, Umbach DM, Bedlack RS, Richards M, Watson M et al. (2012) Pesticide exposure and amyotrophic lateral sclerosis. Neurotoxicology 33: 457–462. doi:10.1016/j.neuro.2012.04.001. PubMed: 22521219.
8. Steinmetz LM, Scharfe C, Deutschbauer AM, Mokranjac D, Herman ZS et al. (2002) Systematic screen for human disease genes in yeast. Nat Genet 31: 400–404. PubMed: 12134146.
9. Giaever G, Chu AM, Ni L, Connelly C, Riles L et al. (2002) Functional profiling of theSaccharomyces cerevisiae genome. Nature 418: 387–391. doi:10.1038/nature00935. PubMed: 12140549.
10. dos Santos SC, Teixeira MC, Cabrito TR, Sá-Correia I (2012) Yeast toxicogenomics: genome-wide responses to chemical stresses with impact in environmental health, pharmacology, and biotechnology. Front Genet. p. 3. Available: .http://www.ncbi.nlm.nih.gov/pmc/articles/PMC3329712/ . Accessed 16 July 2013.

11. North M, Vulpe CD (2010) Functional toxicogenomics: mechanism-centered toxicology. Int J Mol Sci 11: 4796–4813. doi:10.3390/ijms11124796. PubMed: 21614174.

12. Blackman RK, Cheung-Ong K, Gebbia M, Proia DA, He S et al. (2012) Mitochondrial electron transport is the cellular target of the oncology drug elesclomol. PLOS ONE 7: e29798. Available:http://www.plosone.org/article/info%3Adoi%2F10.1371%2Fjournal.pone.0029798/. Accessed 16 July 2013 doi:10.1371/journal.pone.0029798. PubMed: 22253786.

13. Jo WJ, Ren X, Chu F, Aleshin M, Wintz H et al. (2009) Acetylated H4K16 by MYST1 protects UROtsa cells from arsenic toxicity and is decreased following chronic arsenic exposure. Toxicol Appl Pharmacol 241: 294–302. doi:10.1016/j.taap.2009.08.027. PubMed: 19732783.

14. Skrtić M, Sriskanthadevan S, Jhas B, Gebbia M, Wang X et al. (2011) Inhibition of mitochondrial translation as a therapeutic strategy for human acute myeloid leukemia. Cancer Cell 20: 674–688. doi:10.1016/j.ccr.2011.10.015. PubMed: 22094260.

15. Mason PB, Struhl K (2005) Distinction and relationship between elongation rate and processivity of RNA polymerase II in vivo. Mol Cell 17: 831–840. doi:10.1016/j.molcel.2005.02.017. PubMed: 15780939.

16. Gaytán BD, Loguinov AV, Lantz SR, Lerot J-M, Denslow ND et al. (2013) Functional profiling discovers the dieldrin organochlorinated pesticide affects leucine availability in yeast. Toxicol Sci 132: 347–358. doi:10.1093/toxsci/kft018. PubMed: 23358190.

17. Jo WJ, Loguinov A, Wintz H, Chang M, Smith AH et al. (2009) Comparative functional genomic analysis identifies distinct and overlapping sets of genes required for resistance to monomethylarsonous acid (MMAIII) and arsenite (AsIII) in yeast. Toxicol Sci 111: 424–436. doi:10.1093/toxsci/kfp162. PubMed: 19635755.

18. Robinson MD, Grigull J, Mohammad N, Hughes TR (2002) FunSpec: a web-based cluster interpreter for yeast. BMC Bioinformatics 3: 35. doi:10.1186/1471-2105-3-35. PubMed: 12431279.

19. Shannon P, Markiel A, Ozier O, Baliga NS, Wang JT et al. (2003) Cytoscape: a software environment for integrated models of biomolecular interaction networks. Genome Res 13: 2498–2504. doi:10.1101/gr.1239303. PubMed: 14597658.

20. Morillo-Huesca M, Vanti M, Chávez S (2006) A simple in vivo assay for measuring the efficiency of gene length-dependent processes in yeast mRNA biogenesis. FEBS J 273: 756–769. doi:10.1111/j.1742-4658.2005.05108.x. PubMed: 16441662.

21. Rodríguez-Gil A, García-Martínez J, Pelechano V, Muñoz-Centeno MdeL, de la C, Geli V et al. (2010) The distribution of active RNA polymerase II along the transcribed region is gene-specific and controlled by elongation factors. Nucleic Acids Res 38: 4651–4664. doi:10.1093/nar/gkq215. PubMed: 20385590.

22. Chávez S, Beilharz T, Rondón AG, Erdjument-Bromage H, Tempst P et al. (2000) A protein complex containing Tho2, Hpr1, Mft1 and a novel protein, Thp2, connects transcription elongation with mitotic recombination in Saccharomyces cerevisiae. EMBO J 19: 5824–5834. doi:10.1093/emboj/19.21.5824. PubMed: 11060033.

23. Strässer K, Masuda S, Mason P, Pfannstiel J, Oppizzi M et al. (2002) TREX is a conserved complex coupling transcription with messenger RNA export. Nature 417: 304–308. doi:10.1038/nature746. PubMed: 11979277.

24. Desmoucelles C, Pinson B, Saint-Marc C, Daignan-Fornier B (2002) Screening the yeast "disruptome" for mutants affecting resistance to the immunosuppressive drug, mycophenolic acid. J Biol Chem 277: 27036–27044. doi:10.1074/jbc.M111433200. PubMed: 12016207.

25. Gaillard H, Tous C, Botet J, González-Aguilera C, Quintero MJ et al. (2009) Genome-wide analysis of factors affecting transcription elongation and DNA repair: a new role for PAF and Ccr4-not in transcription-coupled repair. PLOS Genet 5: e1000364. Available:http://www.plosgenetics.org/article/info%3Adoi%2F10.1371%2Fjournal.pgen.1000364. Accessed 16 July 2013 PubMed: 19197357.

26. Exinger F, Lacroute F (1992) 6-Azauracil inhibition of GTP biosynthesis inSaccharomyces cerevisiae. Curr Genet 22: 9–11. doi:10.1007/BF00351735. PubMed:1611672.

27. Hedstrom L (2009) IMP dehydrogenase: structure, mechanism and inhibition. Chem Rev 109: 2903–2928. doi:10.1021/cr900021w. PubMed: 19480389.

28. Elbein AD (1981) The tunicamycins – useful tools for studies on glycoproteins. Trends Biochem Sci 6: 219–221. doi:10.1016/0968-0004(81)90080-3.

29. Hyle JW, Shaw RJ, Reines D (2003) Functional distinctions between IMP dehydrogenase genes in providing mycophenolate resistance and guanine prototrophy to yeast. J Biol Chem 278: 28470–28478. doi:10.1074/jbc.M303736200. PubMed:12746440.

30. Denis-Duphil M (1989) Pyrimidine biosynthesis in Saccharomyces cerevisiae: the ura2 cluster gene, its multifunctional enzyme product, and other structural or regulatory genes involved in de novo UMP synthesis. Biochem Cell Biol 67: 612–631. doi:10.1139/o89-094. PubMed: 2679804.

31. Mourelle M, Garcia M, Aguilar C (1985) Adenosine triphosphatase activities in plasma liver membranes of rats treated with DDT and toxaphene. J Appl Toxicol 5: 39–41. doi:10.1002/jat.2550050108. PubMed: 2985682.

32. Trottman CH, Desaiah D (1979) Adenosine triphosphatase activities in brain, kidney and liver of mice treated with toxaphene. J Environ Sci Health B 14: 393–404. doi:10.1080/03601237909372137. PubMed: 224087.

33. Trottman CH, Prasada Rao KS, Morrow W, Uzodinma JE, Desaiah D (1985) In vitro effects of toxaphene on mitochondrial calcium ATPase and calcium uptake in selected rat tissues. Life Sci 36: 427–433. doi:10.1016/0024-3205(85)90254-1. PubMed:3155819.

34. Boyd EM, Taylor FI (1971) Toxaphene toxicity in protein-deficient rats. Toxicol Appl Pharmacol 18: 158–167. doi:10.1016/0041-008X(71)90325-5. PubMed: 5100790.

35. Woo S, Yum S (2011) Transcriptional response of marine medaka (Oryzias javanicus) on exposure to toxaphene. Comp Biochem Physiol C 153: 355–361. PubMed:21220043.

36. Sanchez BC, Carter B, Hammers HR, Sepúlveda MS (2011) Transcriptional response of hepatic largemouth bass (Micropterus salmoides) mRNA upon exposure to environmental contaminants. J Appl Toxicol 31: 108–116. PubMed: 20589742.

37. 37.Martyniuk CJ, Sanchez BC, Szabo NJ, Denslow ND, Sepúlveda MS (2009) Aquatic contaminants alter genes involved in neurotransmitter synthesis and gonadotropin release in largemouth bass. Aquat Toxicol 95: 1–9. doi:10.1016/j.aquatox.2009.06.009. PubMed: 19781795.

38. Sanchez BC, Ralston-Hooper KJ, Kowalski KA, Dorota Inerowicz H, Adamec J et al. (2009) Liver proteome response of largemouth bass (Micropterus salmoides) exposed to several environmental contaminants: potential insights into biomarker development. Aquat Toxicol 95: 52–59. doi:10.1016/j.aquatox.2009.08.002. PubMed: 19717195.

39. Kaplan CD (2013) Basic mechanisms of RNA polymerase II activity and alteration of gene expression in Saccharomyces cerevisiae. BBA-Gene Regul Mech 1829: 39–54.

40. Ding B, LeJeune D, Li S (2010) The C-terminal repeat domain of Spt5 plays an important role in suppression of Rad26-independent transcription coupled repair. J Biol Chem 285: 5317–5326. doi:10.1074/jbc.M109.082818. PubMed: 20042611.

41. Fischer T, Strässer K, Rácz A, Rodriguez-Navarro S, Oppizzi M et al. (2002) The mRNA export machinery requires the novel Sac3p-Thp1p complex to dock at the nucleoplasmic entrance of the nuclear pores. EMBO J 21: 5843–5852. doi:10.1093/emboj/cdf590. PubMed: 12411502.

42. Gaillard H, Wellinger RE, Aguilera A (2007) A new connection of mRNP biogenesis and export with transcription-coupled repair. Nucleic Acids Res 35: 3893–3906. doi:10.1093/nar/gkm373. PubMed: 17537816.

43. Lei EP, Stern CA, Fahrenkrog B, Krebber H, Moy TI et al. (2003) Sac3 is an mRNA export factor that localizes to cytoplasmic fibrils of nuclear pore complex. Mol Cell Biol 14: 836–847. doi:10.1091/mbc.E02-08-0520. PubMed: 12631707.

44. Saguez C, Schmid M, Olesen JR, Ghazy MAE-H, Qu X et al. (2008) Nuclear mRNA surveillance in THO/sub2 mutants is triggered by inefficient polyadenylation. Mol Cell 31: 91–103. doi:10.1016/j.molcel.2008.04.030. PubMed: 18614048.

45. Shaw RJ, Reines D (2000) Saccharomyces cerevisiae transcription elongation mutants are defective in PUR5 induction in response to nucleotide depletion. Mol Cell Biol 20: 7427–7437. doi:10.1128/MCB.20.20.7427-7437.2000. PubMed: 11003640.

CHAPTER 24

EFFECTS OF SPINOSAD ON HONEY BEES

Mark J. Miles, Anne Alix, Chloe Bourgouin, Stephan Schmitzer

Keywords: honey bee, pesticide, risk assessment, risk management, spinosad

INTRODUCTION

Spinosad is an insect control agent derived by fermentation of the Actinomycete bacterium, Saccharopolyspora spinosa. The active ingredient is composed of two metabolites, spinosyn A and spinosyn D. Spinosyns (such as spinosad and spinetoram) have a novel mechanism of activity on nicotinic acetylcholine receptors which is identified as the primary cause of death.1 The action of spinosyns on nicotinic receptors is unique in comparison with other insecticides and is at a different site from that of nicotine and imidacloprid.

In common with other insecticides spinosad is intrinsically toxic to honey bees. In laboratory tests worker honey bees were exposed orally (in sugar water diet) or to doses topically applied. LD_{50} values for technical material of 0.057 and 0.0036 µg a.s. bee^{-1} for oral and contact routes of administration respectively were recorded. Similar levels of toxicity were exhibited for a 480 g a.s. L-1 SC formulation containing spinosad with LD50 values of 0.049 and 0.050 µg a.s. bee-1 for oral and contact routes of administration respectively.[2]

Citation: Mark J. Miles, Anne Alix , Chloe Bourgouin , Stephan Schmitzer, Effects of spinosad on honey bees, doi: 10.5073/jka.2012.437.032.

Spinosad achieved its first registration 1998 in the US for control of bollworms in cotton. Since then it has been registered globally on over 150 crops in North America, Latin America, Asia, Europe and Australasia under a variety of trademarks (such as Tracer, SpinTor, Entrust, and Success; registered trademarks of Dow Agro Sciences LLC.). Spinosad is used in vegetables, fruit trees, turf, viticulture and ornamental cultivation to control lepidopteron larvae, thysanopteran some dipteran, coleopteran and hymenoptera pest species.

It is important that plant protection products (PPPs) are authorised for use only in ways that do not pose an unacceptable risk of harm to honeybees. Data should be obtained to enable the safety to be evaluated. An evaluation of the risks to honey bees has thus been undertaken in every country where the product is authorized based on the data available at this time.[3,4] Rules for risk evaluation have been updated since, in Europe as well as in the United States, which require that potential effects on the development of larvae and the behaviour of adults are considered at earlier steps of the risk assessment process.[5,6,7] Beside the regulatory risk assessment, it is useful to look at the feedback from public research and from field surveys of apiaries in the countries where the product is used.8,9

This paper summarises the effects of spinosad to the honeybee (Apis mellifera) and updates the current knowledge on this substance. Data come from a range of Dow AgroSciences reports conducted to meet regulatory requirements. This dataset has been complemented with a survey of literature data and feedback from surveys on incidents, if any, involving honey bees in the countries where the product is authorized from the past 10 years of use.

EXPERIMENTAL METHODS

Semi-field studies were re-analyzed with regard to mortality data with the aim to characterize and address uncertainties on this parameter as a function of the application rate. Ten trials performed in France, UK and Germany were used. These studies (tunnel + cages) were conducted according to CEB method n°129 and EPPO guideline 170.[10,11] Application rates were ranging from 10 to 540 g a.s./ha, depending on the pest, sprayed onto flowering crops. The crops (Phacelia, oilseed rape, wheat with sugar solution) were selected to maximize foraging and exposure. These ten trials were analyzed for mortality rates at the key use rate of 96 g a.s./ha. These studies are summarized in table 1.

Table: 1 Description of the semi-field trials used for the analysis of mortality rates at 96 g a.s./ha.

Year	Site type	Country	Crop	Application type	Rate (g a.s./ha)	Number bees/hive	Replicates
2004	Tunnel	France	*Phacelia*	During bee activity	144 96	10,000	1 2
2002	Tunnel	France	Winter wheat with sugar	During bee activity	96 144	10,000	2 1
2003	Tunnel	France	*Phacelia*	During bee activity	144	10,000	1
				Evening	144		
2006	Tunnel	France	Rape seed	During bee activity	96	10,000-15,000	1
				During bee activity	50		
				During bee activity	10		
				During bee activity	20		
				Evening	96		
2006	Tunnel	France	Rape seed	Evening	96	10,000-15,000	1
2010	Tunnel	Germany	*Phacelia*	Evening	96 76	3,500-4,000	3
2010	Tunnel	Germany	*Phacelia*	During bee activity	76	3,500-4,000	3
				Evening	96		
				During bee activity	76	3,500-4,000	3
				Evening	96		
2010	Tunnel	Germany	*Phacelia*	Evening	76 96	3,500-4,000	3
2002	Tunnel	France	*Phacelia*	During bee activity	96 144	10,000	2 1
2000	Tunnel	United Kingdom	*Phacelia*	Morning	144 540	3,500-4,000	1 1

To allow for a comparison across the studies a mortality index was calculated according to the CEB method: tox = Ma/Mb x Cb/Ca.

With Ma: mortality in test substance after treatment, Mb: mortality in test substance before treatment, Ca: mortality in control after treatment, Cb: mortality in control before treatment. The Itox index was analyzed over time, per day and up to one week after treatment as well as the influence of the time of application i.e. when bees are present and when bees are not present (early in the morning or late in the evening). A toxic reference treatment (dimethoate) and a water treated control were included.

New tunnel tests were analyzed as well, with the aim to further describe effects of spinosad applied at 76 and 96 g a.s./ha. These studies were conducted according to EPPO guideline 170 and OECD.10,12 Parameters relating to these studies are summarized in table 2.

Table 2: Description of the semi-field trials used for the analysis of effects on bees at 96 g and 76 g a.s./ha.

Test description		Test 1	Test 2	Test 3
Application rate		**76 and 96 g a.s./ha**	**76 and 96 g a.s./ha**	**76 and 96 g a.s./ha**
Application time	During bee activity	✓		
	Out of bee activity	✓	✓	✓
Assessment	Mortality	✓	✓	✓
	Foraging	✓	✓	✓
	Brood development	✓	✓	✓
	Behavior	✓	✓	✓
	Colony strength at 28 days		✓	✓
	Colony strength at 60 days	✓		

RESULTS

Results of the semi-field studies are presented in figures 1 to 5. Mortality records expressed as Itox index 1 day after treatment (1DAT) as a function of the application rate and the activity of honey bees at the time of treatment were calculated. Itox index values were comparable (mean ranging from 1.10 to 2.41) in honey bees for treatments performed out of foraging activity, for all application rates i.e. from 76 g a.s./ha to 540 a.s./ha. For sprays during foraging activity, Itox index ranged from 1.25 to 3.12 (mean values) for application rates ranging from 10.08 g a.s./ha to 76 g a.s./ha. Spray at 96 g a.s./ha lead to a higher mean Itox index value (4.01) but the median of 11 values was slightly below 2. Both the mean (6.26) and median Itox value for honey bees exposed to a spray with 144 g a.s./ha were ca 6. When applied out of bee activity at 96 g a.s./ha Itox values less than 2.0 were observed daily from one to seven days after exposure. In contrast, dimethoate (400 – 600 g a.s./ha) applied during bee flight resulting in an Itox value of 20, by one day after application (figure 1).

Mortality in honey bees exposed to a spray application spinosad performed out of bee flight are reproduced in figure 2, and expressed as the mean number of dead bees after a spray of 76 or 96 g a.s./ha. Mortality records were comparable to the water treatment control before and after treatment for both application rates. Peaks of mortality were recorded in bees exposed to the acute toxic standard (Perfekthion: dimethoate) on the day of 1 day after treatment, and mean mortality was significantly higher than in the control up to 3 days after treatment.

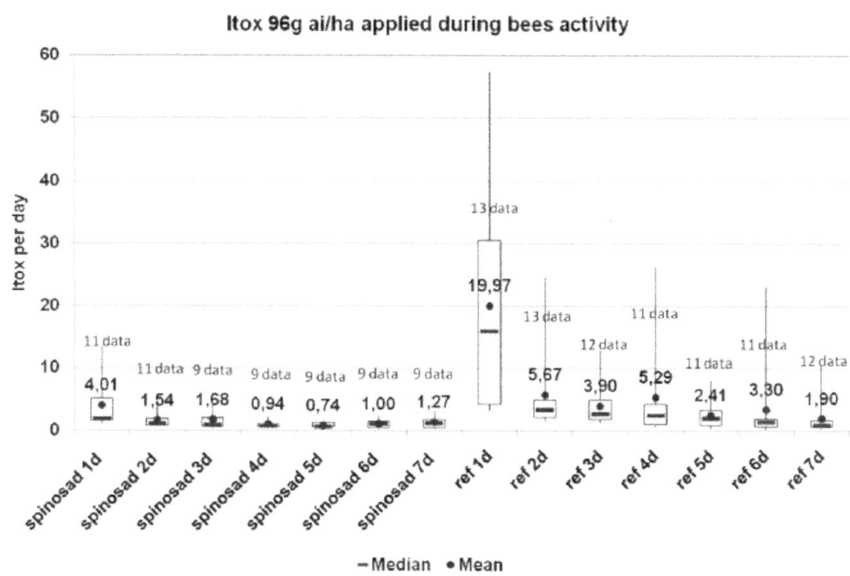

Figure 1: Effects of spinosad on honey bees in tunnel tests when applied out of bee flight. Daily mortality expressed as a toxicity index (Itox). The ref(erence) is dimethoate. See text for explanation and calculation.

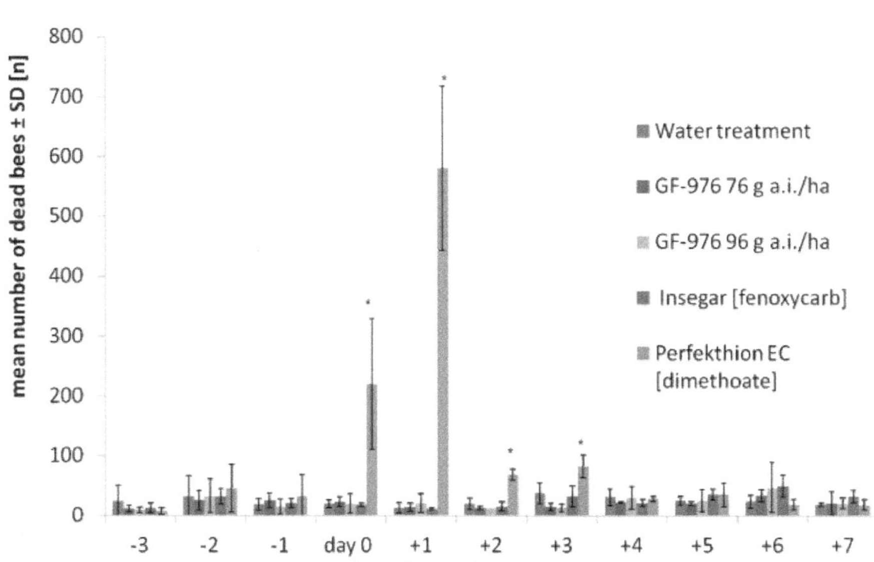

Figure 2: Mortality to honey bees after exposure to applications of spinosad (GF-976) at 76 and 96 g a.s./ha applied out of bee flight under tunnel test conditions.

Foraging activity in honey bees exposed in the trials described in table 2 are reproduced in figure 3, and expressed as the mean number of bees /m2 flowers. All records followed a similar trend with an increase in bee presence on flowers from day 3 pre-treatment to day 3 after treatment.

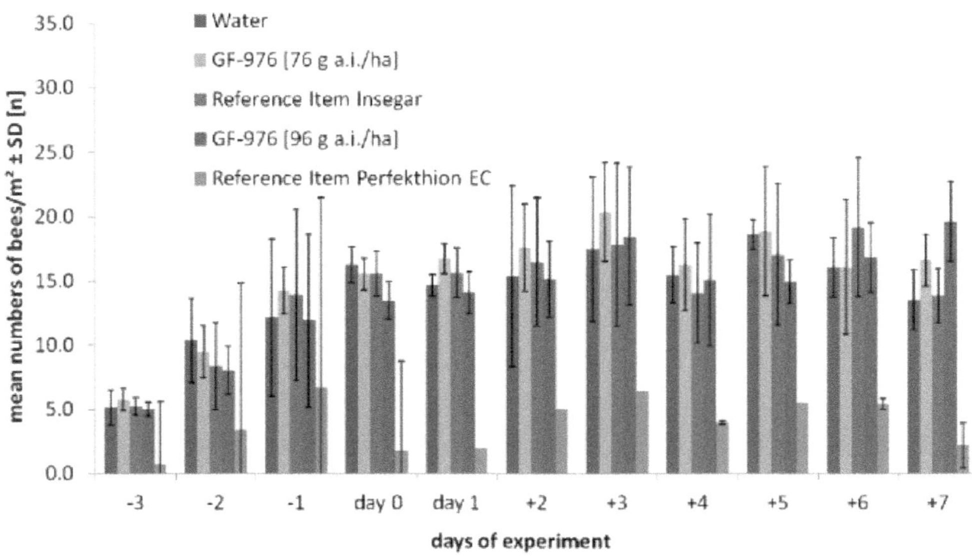

Figure 3: Foraging activity of honey bees after exposure to applications of spinosad (GF-976) at 76 and 96 g a.s./ha applied out of bee flight under tunnel test conditions.

Effects on brood were expressed as brood compensation index from day 6 to day 21 post brood fixing date. Results are reproduced on figure 4. The brood compensation index in honey bees exposed to a spray of spinosad at 76 or 96 g a.s./ha was comparable to the brood compensation index in honey bees of the water control, and as for the control it slightly increased within time. Both reference items Insegar and Perfekthion lead to a reduced brood compensation index at all assessment dates.

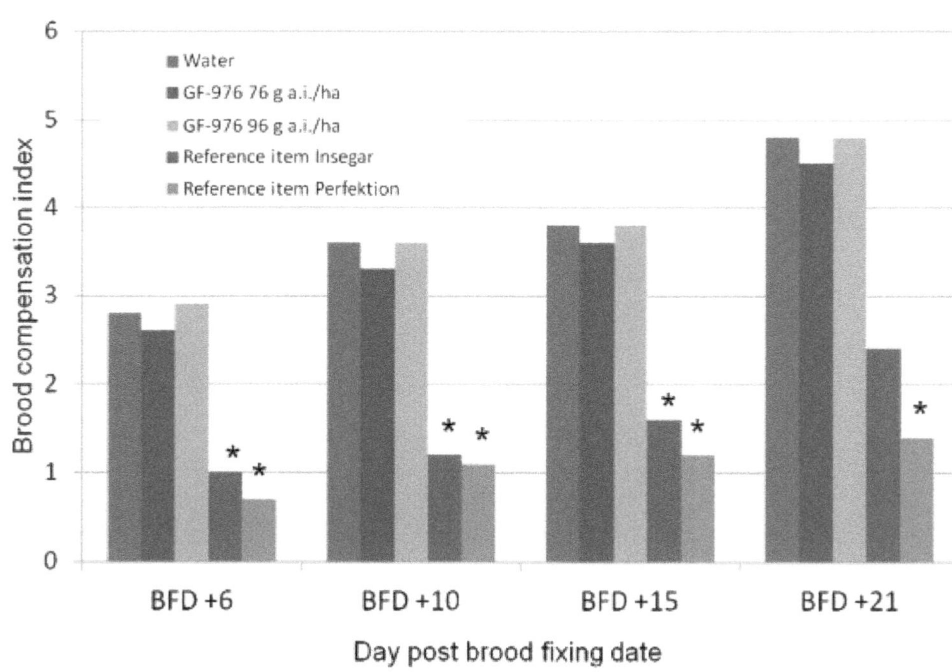

Figure 4: Impact on brood of honey bees after exposure to applications of spinosad (GF-976) at 76 and 96 g a.s./ha applied out of bee flight under tunnel test conditions.

Finally, honey bee colony strength was measured as the mean number of bees/colony throughout the study, i.e. from day 6 before treatment to day 60 post treatment. Results are represented in figure 5. Colony strength was comparable in all treatments, with ca 3,000 bees/colony.

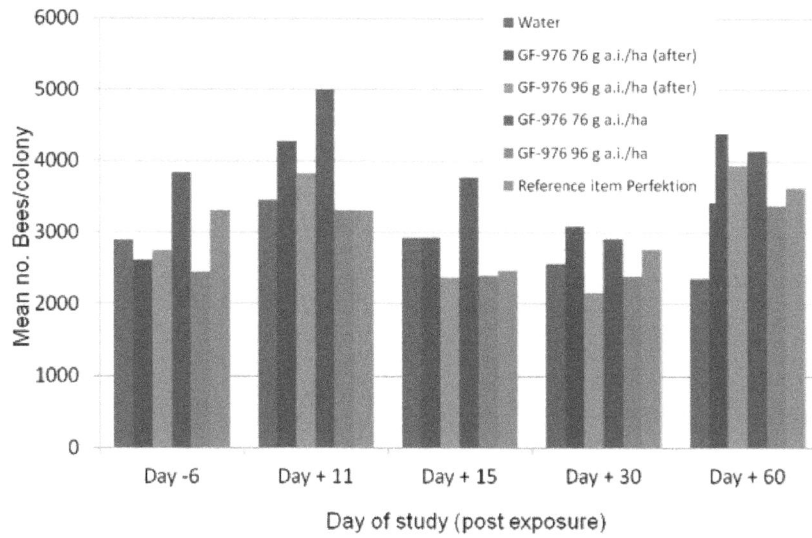

Figure5: Colony development and strength of honey bees after exposure to applications of spinosad (GF- 976) at 76 and 96 g a.s./ha applied out of bee flight under tunnel test conditions.

DISCUSSION

As previously stated, spinosad is intrinsically toxic to honey bees when tested in standard laboratory studies where worker honey bees are exposed orally (in sugar water diet) or topically to the test material. These laboratory tests are used in the screening step which is performed as an entry point in most risk assessment processes, as for example in the U.S or in Europe.[5,6] In the European risk assessment process, the screening step necessitates the calculation of Hazard Quotients (HQ), that compare toxicity to the application rate (HQ = application rate / LD_{50}). HQ values above the trigger value of 50 indicate a need for a refined risk assessment, which could involve higher tier testing (e.g. semi-field or field tests). In the case of spinosad, an application rate of 96 g a.s./ha results in HQ values ranging from 1,920 (oral HQ) to 1,950 (contact HQ) and thus indicate, in accordance with European regulation, a potential risk to honey bees "unless it is clearly established through an appropriate risk assessment that under field conditions there are no unacceptable effects on honeybee larvae, honeybee behaviour, or colony survival and development after use of the plant protection product according to the proposed conditions of use".[13]

The studies undertaken in tunnels on various crops, application periods and application rates aim at investigating the level of effects that are expected on honey bees under field conditions, as recommended by the European regulation. Accordingly, effects on honeybee survival, honeybee larvae, honeybee behaviour, and colony survival and development are monitored. The protocols used in the tunnel studies with spinosad allow for a more realistic appreciation of the level of acute effects that can be expected. The selection of cropped plants being attractive to honey bees and sprayed at flowering maximizes interactions of bees with the treated plants and any avoidance behavior can be observed and recorded. The inclusion of a water control and reference items allow to check that bees behaved as expected during the course of the experiment, and that effects of the product of well-known toxicity are appropriately displayed during the course of the study. These tests may or may not reproduce a direct contact of bees with spray droplets, depending on whether the spray is performed during or out of bee activity. However in any case, they reproduce the conditions of exposure of bee colonies that could be placed close to crops treated during flowering and can be considered as worse case with bees being forced to collect their food from the treated flowers. With regards to the acute effects of fresh and dried residues of spinosad products on honeybees, Itox values indicated a dose – effect relationship when direct contact to spray droplets was allowed. In this analysis a threshold application rate for lethal effects of around 96 g a.s./ha was observed. When allowed to dry, residues of spinosad on flowers do not induce significant levels of honey bee mortality up to and including the highest application rate of 540 g a.s./ha. Assessments performed up to 7 days after treatment made during bee activity confirm the absence of mortality to foragers visiting treated flowers at 96 g a.s./ha. Therefore, this exposure rate can be considered as a threshold for immediate acute toxicity, but at which no long lasting acute toxicity is expected at this application rate or higher. Such differences of honeybee responses in acute laboratory tests compared to tunnel test can be common and can be explained by the reduced availability of product residues on natural surfaces compared to direct contact in laboratory tests and due to the highly conservative nature of the tier I risk assessment. This phenomenon is well addressed for other non target arthropods and has lead to the development of laboratory tests exposing insects through natural substrates such as leaf discs, seedlings or soil samples as an intermediate experimental step between laboratory tests and semifield/field tests.[14] For the two standard species used in the risk assessment procedure for non target arthropods, the parasitic wasp Aphidius rhopalosiphi and the predatory mite Typhlodromus pyri, moving from an inert surface to a natural surface reduces the residual toxicity by a factor of 9.8. Similarly, moving from inert surface exposure conditions to semi-field testing results in 45.1-fold lower residual toxicity (both factors assessed as the geometrical mean ratio of LR_{50} measured in laboratory testing on either inert or natural support and semi-field tests).[15] Spinosad is not systemic and its rapid dissipation from plant surfaces and exposure on natural surfaces (leaves and flowers) may explain the reduced residual toxicity observed.

Effects of a spinosad spray on the parameters representing sublethal effects on honey bees i.e. foraging behavior, brood and colony strength were also very limited in tunnel studies at the two application rates tested in detail (76 and 96 g a.s./ha). These observations are consistent with the mode of action of the substance. Spinosad acts by causing excitation of the insect nervous system, leading to involuntary muscle contractions, prostration with tremors, and finally paralysis. In addition, dissipation data indicate no persistence in environmental media and thus limited exposure duration. This is confirmed through the limited duration of residual toxicity in honey bees and other non target arthropods. Finally, the dissipation of spinosad does not lead to the formation of any active degradation products, which also limits the residual toxicity potency of the product.

The conclusions of the risk assessment appear to be confirmed by the very limited number of published data describing the potential effects of spinosad in pollinating species exposed in field conditions. With only three articles recorded in the last ten years. This could reflect the limited level of concern raised by the frequency of incidents and by the profile of the substance itself, for which the likeliness of long term or delayed effects that could have been missed in the studies having been performed in the context of the regulatory assessments is very limited.

CONCLUSIONS

The data presented address the potential effects of spinosad, applied as a spray to control various pests, on pollinators and more particularly to the honey bee. The analysis of higher tier studies on attractive crops having been performed for regulatory risk assessment purposes confirm the absence of significant impacts on honey bees even for treatments during flowering, provided that a delay allowing for droplets to dry is respected. Spinosad has been used all over the world for more than ten years in a wide range of crops without a recorded incident to pollinators. The feedback from field surveys is of particular importance as it reflects the potential impact of products on pollinators in realistic exposure conditions, which include interactions with other factors. Therefore the confirmation of risk assessment outcome through survey data appears as a strong evidence of the actual limited impact of the product and its suitability for sustainable crop protection.

REFERENCES

1. Salgado V. L., 1997.- The modes of action of spinosad and other insect control products.- Down to Earth, Dow AgroSciences, 52 (1): 35-43.
2. SANCO/1428/2001 –rev. final 14 July 2006.
3. Mayes MA, Thompson GD, Husband B and Miles MM. Spinosad toxicity to pollinators and associated risk. Rev Environ Contam Toxicol. 179:37-71 (2003).
4. COMMISSION DIRECTIVE 2007/6/EC of 14 February 2007 amending Council Directive 91/414/EEC to include metrafenone, Bacillus subtilis, spinosad and thiamethoxam as active substances. Official Journal L43/13 of 15.02.2007 (2007).
5. EPPO, 2010. Environmental risk assessment scheme for plant protection products, Chapter 10. Risk assessment to honey bees, PP 3/10 (3), OEPP/EPPO, Bulletin OEPP/EPPO Bulletin 40, 1–9.
6. USEPA. Interim guidance on honey bee data requirements. Draft USEPA OPP guidance (www.epa.gov oppefed1 ecorisk_ders honeybee_data_interim_guidance.htm) (2011).
7. Fischer D and Moriarty T. Pesticide Risk Assessment for Pollinators: Summary of a SETAC Pellston Workshop. Summary of the SETAC Pellston Workshop on Pesticide Risk Assessment for Pollinators 15–21 January 2011, Pensacola, Florida, USA, (http://www.setac.org/node/265).(2011).
8. Thompson H, Thorbahn D. Review of honeybee pesticide poisoning incidents in Europe – evaluation of the hazard quotient approach for risk assessment. Hazards of pesticides to bees – 10th International Symposium of the ICP-Bee Protection Group. Julius-Kühn-Archiv 423 (2009).
9. Mineau P, Harding, KM, Whiteside, M, Fletcher, MR, Garthwaite, D, Knopper, LD Using reports of honeybee mortality in the field to calibrate laboratory derived pesticide risk indices. Environ Entomol 37(2): 546-554 (2008).
10. EPPO Guideline on test methods for evaluating the side-effects of plant protection products on honeybees.- EPPO Bulletin No. 170: 22 (1992).
11. CEB, Commission des Essais Biologiques - Méthode d'évaluation des effets de toxicité aiguë et a court terme des préparations phytopharmaceutiques sur l'abeille domestique (Apis mellifera L.). ANPP, méthode no. 230: 8 – 21 (2003).
12. OECD. Guidance document on the honey bee (Apis mellifera L.) brood test under semi-field conditions. Series on Testing and Assessment No. 75. ENV/JM/MONO(2007)22 (2007).
13. Council Directive of 15 July 1991 concerning the placing of plant protection products on the market (91/414/EEC). Official Journal L 230, 19.8.1991 (1991).
14. Candolfi MP, Barrett KL, Campbell PJ, Forster R, Grandy N, Huet MC, Lewis G, Oomen PA, Schmuck R, and Vogt H. Guidance document on regulatory testing and risk assessment procedures for plant protection products with non-target arthropods, in ESCORT 2 workshop (European Standard Characteristics of non-target arthropod Regulatory Testing), Wageningen, The Netherlands. SETAC Publication, ISBN 1-880611-52-x, 46 pp. (2001).
15. Grimm C., Schmidli H., Bakker F., Brown K., Campbell P., Candolfi M.P., Chapman P., Harrison E.G., Mead-Briggs M., Schmuck R. and Ufer A: Use of standard toxicity tests with Typhlodromus pyri and Aphidius rhopalosiphi to establish a dose-response relationship. J. Pest Science, 74 (3), 72-84, (2001).

CHAPTER 25

A PRELIMINARY INVESTIGATION INTO THE IMPACT OF A PESTICIDE COMBINATION ON HUMAN NEURONAL AND GLIAL CELL LINES IN VITRO

Michael D. Coleman, John D. O'Neil, Elizabeth K. Woehrling, Oscar Bate Akide Ndunge, Eric J. Hill, Andre Menache, and Claude J. Reiss

INTRODUCTION

Pesticide use is integral in world agriculture. In the Californian wine industry, over twenty thousand tonnes of pesticide are used per annum, including more than 150 different agents [1]. Although pesticides can improve yields and restrict dietary threats to human health such as mycotoxins [2], there remains a long-standing concern over the impact of the sheer quantity of pesticide usage on the environment [3], [4]. There also appears to be some association between human toxicity and the weight of pesticide application, as commercially farmed areas in the wine industry increase in size [1].

Amongst the various pesticides deployed, fungicides are particularly important in the wine grape industry and their usage in various guises has been documented since Roman times [5], [6]. The application of combinations of different pesticides and especially those with novel modes of action has been largely driven by widespread fungal resistance; this has resulted from the pressure of historical biocidal usage, as well as increased efficacy against pests and the promotion of better yields [7], [8]. In the wine industry, the persistence of biocides, leading to detectable contamination of the finished product, is highly variable and depends on many factors [9]–[11]. The process of wine production generally reduces pesticide contamination in comparison with that of grapes, although this depends on the physiochemical properties of the agents used [9] and it is now apparent that wines sourced from Europe contain multiple residues of many different pesticide agents in measurable quantities [12], [13]. Indeed, some combinations of agents such as fludioxonil and cyprodinil can be resistant to destruction during wine processing [14]. There are concerns that these levels of contamination might exceed published European Union maximum residue levels (MRL; [9], [15]), although these limits are not strictly enforced [16].

Considerable research has been carried out on the impact of pesticides on various non-target flora and fauna [17], [18] and there is evidence that many biocidal agents lack specificity. Indeed, they can exert significant mammalian toxicity that may be synergistic where combinations of different agents are deployed [19]–[21]. There is also evidence that pesticide exposure can increase the risk of genotoxicity and this may result in specific malignancies [22], [23]. In addition, pesticide exposure can be neurotoxic [24] and is even considered a risk factor in the development of neurodegenerative conditions such as Parkinsonism [25], [26]. However, in view of the use of many combinations of biocides, their known persistence through foodstuff processing and their potential neurological

Citation: Coleman MD, O'Neil JD, Woehrling EK, Ndunge OBA, Hill EJ, Menache A, et al. (2012) A Preliminary Investigation into the Impact of a Pesticide Combination on Human Neuronal and Glial Cell Lines In Vitro. PLoS ONE 7(8): e42768. doi:10.1371/journal.pone.0042768

human impact, there has been little investigation into the possible synergistic biological effects on human neuronal and glial cellular systems. In the present study, we have utilized two cell lines, gliomal U251 and neuroblastomal SH-SY5Y cells, which model the basic cell types of the human central nervous system, the astrocytes and neurones. In this preliminary study, we have explored the effects of a combination of three commonly used biocides (pyrimethanil, ciprodinil and fludioxonil) on cell viability, mitochondrial health and generation of oxidative stress, alone and in combination.

METHODS

Materials and Reagents

Tissue culture flasks, pipettes and 96-well microtitre plates were obtained from Corning Costar (Lowell, MA, USA). All types of cell culture media, as well as foetal bovine serum (FBS) and L-glutamine were purchased from Invitrogen (Paisley, UK). Penicillin and streptomycin, as well as the biocidal agents cyprodinil, fludioxonil and pyrimethanil were supplied by Sigma-Aldrich (Poole, Dorset, UK). The CellTiter Blue™ viability assay was purchased from Promega (Southampton, UK).

Cell Culture

SH-SY5Y (human neuroblastoma) cells (ECACC no. 94030304; [27] were maintained in Roswell Park Memorial Institute 1640 containing Glutamax I® (Invitrogen), supplemented with 10% (v/v) FBS, 1% non-essential amino acids (NEAA) and 1% (v/v) penicillin/streptomycin (100 units penicillin- G/ml and 10 mg/ml streptomycin). U251-MG cells [28] were maintained in and Hams F10 medium with 25 mM HEPES, supplemented with 10% heat-inactivated FBS, 2 mM l-glutamine and 1% (v/v) PenStrep solution. The cells were passaged using 0.25% Trypsin, 0.1 mM EDTA when they had reached approximately 80–90% of confluency.

Study Design

The pesticides were dissolved completely in stock DMSO solutions and serially diluted in media prior to addition to the cells. The agents were studied singly in the various assays and in combination across a concentration range of 0–1 mM. in 100 µl phenol red free DMEM (containing 2 mM L-Glutamine, 10% v/v FBS, 1% (v/v) PenStrep solution, in triplicate wells, for 48 hours at 37°C, 5% CO_2. Cells were incubated with increasingly cytotoxic concentrations of pesticides with the aim of the calculation of IC_{50} values for the various assays. In the combination studies, all three agents were added so that the same net weight of pesticide was present in the incubations as those containing single agents. The vehicle controls contained DMSO alone.

Cell Viability Assay in the presence of Pesticides

Pyrimethanil, ciprodinil and fludioxonil effects on cell general viability were evaluated initially through the CellTiter Blue™ (resazurin assay; Promega) viability assay singly and in combinations. Prior to toxin treatment, SHSY5Y and U251 cells were plated in 96-well microtitre plates at concentrations of 4 or 5×10^5cells/ml respectively, in a 100 µl volume. After incubation overnight, the medium was removed and the cells were maintained in the presence of 100 µl medium supplemented with increasing concentrations of pesticides. After a 48-hour incubation period, the cell culture medium was completely replaced with phenol red free DMEM to which 1% v/v CellTiter-Blue™ (Promega) solution was added. Cultures were incubated for 4 hours at 37°C/5% CO_2 and then read at 620 nm. Untreated negative controls were run together with the treated cells. Plates with reagent only served as background controls. Reciprocal absorbance values were calculated and the percent viability was expressed as the value in the presence of toxicant as a percentage of that in the medium only control (which was set as 100%).

JC-1 Mitochondrial Membrane Potential Assay

The mitochondrial membrane potential (MMP) decrease may be determined using JC-1 dye which only enters cells possessing healthy mitochondria with polarised membranes, where it forms aggregates which exhibit a fluorescent shift from green to red. The JC-1 assay was performed according to Gartlon *et al.*[29]. Briefly, following a 48 hour exposure to the test chemicals, the cell culture medium in each well was completely replaced with 100 µl phenol red free DMEM containing 5 µM JC-1 (Sigma, UK), prepared from a 1 mM JC-1 stock in DMSO. Following incubation of the plates for 30 min at 37°C, 5% CO_2, the medium was removed, the cells washed three times with PBS and 100 µl PBS was added to each well. The red substrate fluorescence intensity was then read at 544 nm/590 nm (excitation/emission). The results were expressed as a percentage of the fluorescence value from the medium only control well (which was set as 100%).

Total Glutathione Assay

The total glutathione assay was performed according to as described by Schuglia *et al.*, [30]. Briefly, following a 48 hour exposure to increasingly cytotoxic concentrations of test chemical, the cell culture medium in each well was completely replaced with 25 µl/well of a 5% (w/v) sulfosalicylic acid (SSA) solution and the plates subjected to three freeze-thawing steps. A working solution of 0.2 mM NADPH and 0.52 mM DTNB was prepared in sodium dihydrogen phosphate assay buffer (0.1 M sodium dihydrogen phosphate, pH 7.5 with 0.15 mM EDTA) and a 5 U/ml GSR enzyme solution was prepared by dilution of glutathione reductase from baker›s yeast (500 U in 3.6 M ammonium sulphate; Sigma, UK) with assay buffer. Aliquots of 10 µl from each SSA treated well were removed in triplicate to a new 96-well plate and 165 µl of NADPH/ DTNB working solution was added to each well, followed by incubation at 37°C for 15 min. GSR enzyme solution at 40 µl was added, the plate incubated at room temperature for 5 min whilst protected from light and the A_{405} was then measured. The total glutathione content of samples was determined from standard curves generated with known amounts of GSH using the same procedure and expressed as a percentage of the medium only control well (which was set as 100%).

ATP Assay

ATP levels were determined using the ATP luminescence assay kit from Invitrogen (Paisley, UK), as per the manufacturer's protocol. Briefly, following a 48 hour exposure increasingly cytotoxic concentrations of test chemical, a 10 µl aliquot from each well was transferred to a black 96-well plate and 90 µl of an ATP standard solution (containing 1 mM dithiothreitol, 0.5 mM D-luciferin, and 2.5 µl of 5 mg/ml firefly luciferase stock solution per 10 ml of the 1X reaction buffer provided) added. The plate was then incubated for 15 min at 37°C, 5% CO_2 and then the luminescence was measured. The ATP content of samples was determined from standard curves generated with known amounts of ATP using the same procedure and expressed as a percentage of the medium only control well (which was set as 100%).

Data Analysis

If applicable, GraphPad Prism was used to define the concentration that gave a 50% reduction in assay response (IC_{50} value) and standard error of the mean (SEM) for each pesticide and the combination. All experiments were conducted on three separate occasions in quadruplicate and one-way ANOVA followed by the relevant post-hoc test was used to assess for differences between IC_{50} values, with significance accepted at the 5% level ($p<0.05$). All figures and tables are presented as mean ± SEM.

Real-Time PCR

Total RNA was extracted using Tri® Reagent, quantified by spectrophotometry and treated with DNase and an RNase inhibitor (Promega, Southampton, UK). 1 µg of total RNA was reverse transcribed using AMV reverse transcriptase (Promega, Southampton UK) and oligo dT_{15} primers (Promega, Southampton, UK). Real-Time PCR: cDNAs were amplified in a standard 40-cycle SYBR® green real-time PCR reaction using optimised sequence specific primers for caspase-3, superoxide dismutase (SOD) and glutathione peroxidase (GSHPx) supplied by PrimerDesign Ltd (Southampton UK), according to the manufacturer's instructions.

GAPDH was selected as a stably expressed gene for normalisation of test gene expression after GeNorm analysis (PrimerDesign Ltd, Southampton UK). The comparative CT method was used to calculate the relative quantification of gene expression. The following formula was used to calculate the relative amount of the transcripts in the chemical treated samples (treat) and the vehicle-treated samples (control), both of which were normalized to the endogenous controls. ΔΔCT=ΔCT (treat) – ΔCT (control) for biological RNA samples or ΔΔCT=ΔCT (HBRR) – ΔCT (UHRR) for reference RNA samples. ΔCT is the difference in CT between the target gene and endogenous controls by subtracting the average CT of controls from each replicate. The fold change for each treated sample (relative to the control sample (or UHRR)=$2^{-\Delta\Delta CT}$. Fold changes in gene expression using the comparative CT method and statistical analysis were determined using the freely available Relative Expression Software Tool (REST 2009, www.qiagen.com).

RESULTS AND DISCUSSION

Impact of the agents alone and in combination on cell viability

These studies are summarized on Table 1. In terms of the CellTiter Blue™ results, both cell lines exhibited similar levels of sensitivity with regard to the combination of pesticides, as well as to fludioxonil and cyprodinil alone, although pyrimethanil was significantly more toxic in the U-251 line compared with the SH-SY5Y cells ($P<0.001$). For both cell lines, the combination was the most toxic, followed by cyprodinil and either fludioxonil (SH-SY5Y) or pyrimethanil (U-251; $P<0.001$). There was a marked significant difference between the CellTiter Blue™ assay IC_{50}'s and those of the JC-1 assay in the SH-SY5Y cells ($P<0.001$), but not in the U251 cells with the exception of the cyprodinil measurements. With the JC-1 assay, in both cell lines, cyprodinil and the combination were the most toxic ($P<0.001$). In order of descending toxicity, fludioxonil in the SH-SY5Y cells and pyrimethanil on the U251 cells were the next most potent, followed by pyrimethanil in the neuronal and fludioxonil in the glial line were the least toxic ($P<0.001$). All the pesticides showed an extremely potent reduction in ATP levels, which was approximately ten-fold greater than their effects in the CellTiter Blue™ viability assay ($P<0.001$). However, ATP reductions were not significantly different with regard to cell line or individual agent, with the minor exception of cyprodinil values, which were significantly lower ($P<0.05$) than those of pyrimethanil in the SH-SY5Y cells.

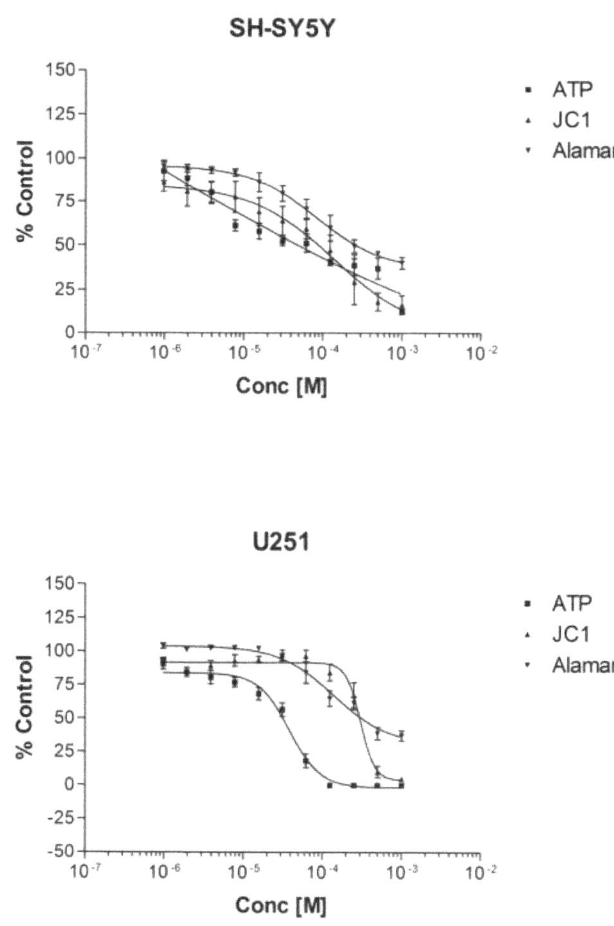

Figure 1: CellTiter Blue™ viability, ATP and JC-1 determinations expressed as a percentage of control values after the incubation of SH-SY5Y and U251 cells with a mixture of pyrimethanil, cyprodinil and fludioxonil over 1–1000 **µM** over 48 ...

From Figure 1, it is apparent that the pattern of toxicity of the pesticide combination, with respect to the mitochondrial effects (JC-1 and ATP assays) differed markedly between the neuronal and glial cell lines. Whilst the viability, ATP and JC-1 data assumed an approximately linear increase in toxicity (Figure 1), the U251 cells appeared to demonstrate a more sigmoidal appearance in terms of the ATP and JC-1 data, with the glial lines exhibiting apparently greater resistance to mitochondrial membrane attrition compared with the SH-SY5Y cells ($P<0.001$).

Table 1: Respective IC_{50} values (μM) after exposure of U251 and SH-SY5Y cell lines to pyrimethanil, cyprodinil and fludioxonil singly and in combination using three viability assays (CellTiter Blue™, JC-1 and ATP).

Assay	Pesticide	U251 (μM IC_{50})	±SEM	SH-SY5Y (μM IC_{50})	±SEM
CellTiter Blue	Pyrimethanil	$598.1^{a***, c*** \&}$	22.5	$822.3^{a***, b***, c*** \&}$	14.2
	Cyprodinil	$332.3^{b**, c***}$	28.8	$304.4^{b***, c***}$	28.2
	Fluodioxonil	$801.5^{a***, c***}$	46.7	$708.1^{a***, b***, c***}$	42.6
	Combination	**257.2**	26.8	**269.9**^{b***}	26.2
JC-1	Pyrimethanil	526.3^{a***}	47.6	144.3^{a***}	9.6
	Cyprodinil	203.7	18.5	40.5	1.7
	Fluodioxonil	877.2^{a***}	13.5	100.6^{a***}	23.6
	Combination	**273.6**	20.3	**63.9**	13.9
ATP	Pyrimethanil	31.8	2.2	44.5@	6.3
	Cyprodinil	28	3.4	33@	2.2
	Fluodioxonil	32.7	1.3	34.2	6.1
	Combination	**30.9**	2.8	**39.3**	2.7

* $P<0.05$,
** $P<0.001$,
*** $P<0.001$.
[a)] denotes significant difference between single pesticide and combination IC50 values for each of the 3 assays.
[b)] denotes significant difference between respective CellTiter Blue™ and JC-1 IC50 values.
[c)] denotes significant difference between respective CellTiter Blue™ and ATP IC50 values.
[@] denotes $P<0.05$.
[&] denotes $P<0.001$.
doi:10.1371/journal.pone.0042768.t001

Studies on GSH cellular content (Figure 2) indicated that the presence of the individual pesticides caused significant reductions in both cell lines at low agent concentrations; (cyprodinil and pyrimethanil in the SH-SY5Y cells and cyprodinil and fludioxonil in the U251 cells; $P<0.05$; 0.01). However, the pesticide combination showed significant reductions in GSH at low and high agent concentrations in both cell lines ($P<0.001$). Interestingly, cyprodinil at 62.5 μM appeared to show a net increase in GSH levels with respect to control ($P<0.01$). Overall, with the U251 cells even at the highest concentrations tested, GSH levels did not actually fall to 50% so an IC_{50} could not be calculated. With these cells, IC_{50} values for individual determinations for pyrimethanil, cyprodinil and fludioxonil ranged from 63.7–59.1%, although for the combination, an IC_{50} was determined to be 653+/−57.3 μM. In contrast, in terms of thiol depletion, the SH-SY5Y cells were more vulnerable than the glial cell line. IC_{50}'s for thiol depletion for pyrimethanil and fludioxonil were not significantly different (770.1+/−66.5; and 849.9+/−49.9 μM), however, the values for combination (476.7+/−34.6 μM) as well as cyprodinil alone (535.8+/−54.8 μM) were not significantly different from each other, but they were significantly lower than the values for pyrimethanil and fludioxonil ($P<0.001$).

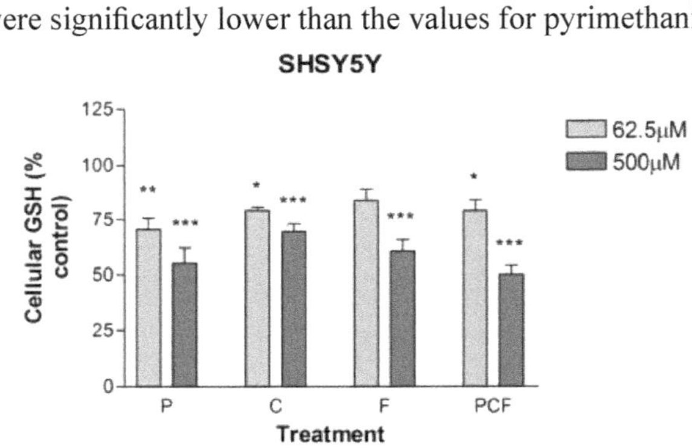

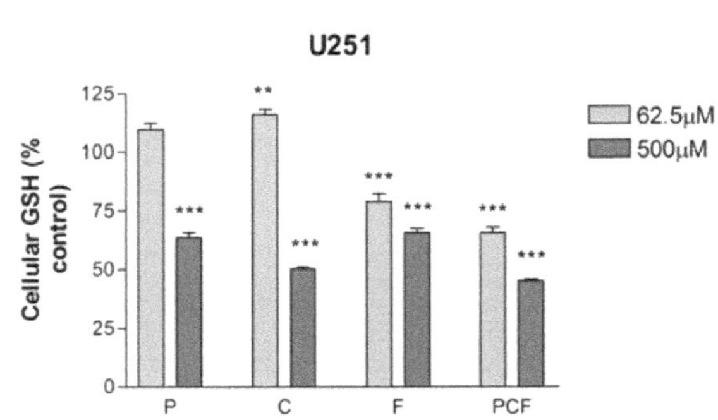

Figure 2: GSH determinations expressed as a percentage of control values after the incubation of SH-SY5Y and U251 cells with pyrimethanil, cyprodinil and fludioxonil used singly and in combination, over 1–1000 **μM** over 48 h (n=3 ...

qPCR gene changes

Three enzymes that are strongly associated with oxidative stress, namely caspase-3, superoxide dismutase (SOD) and glutathione peroxidase (GSHPx), were studied using qRT-PCR. From Figure 3 it is clear that there was a marked difference between the two cell lines investigated, with the U251 cells demonstrating the most significant responses to the toxicants. With the U251 cells, cyprodinil and pyrimethanil treatment at both concentrations resulted in a marked decrease in the expression of GSHPx (P<0.05), whilst treatment with both concentrations of fludioxonil resulted in enhanced gene expression (P<0.05). In contrast, SOD expression was elevated to varying degrees by both concentrations of the individual compounds, with the most marked increase being 19.93-fold with the higher concentration of cyprodinil (P<0.05). Caspase-3 expression was enhanced by 11.53-fold and 4.1-fold in the presence of 500 µm cyprodinil and 62.5 µm fludioxonil, respectively (P<0.05). Whereas, treatment with the higher dose of pyrimethanil resulted in a marked decrease in expression (0.62 relative to control). In contrast to the varying increases and decrease in gene expression found with the compounds tested individually, the high dose of the compounds in combination resulted in a robust increase in the expression of GSHPx, SOD and caspase-3 by 28.54, 18.46 and 13.21-fold, respectively.

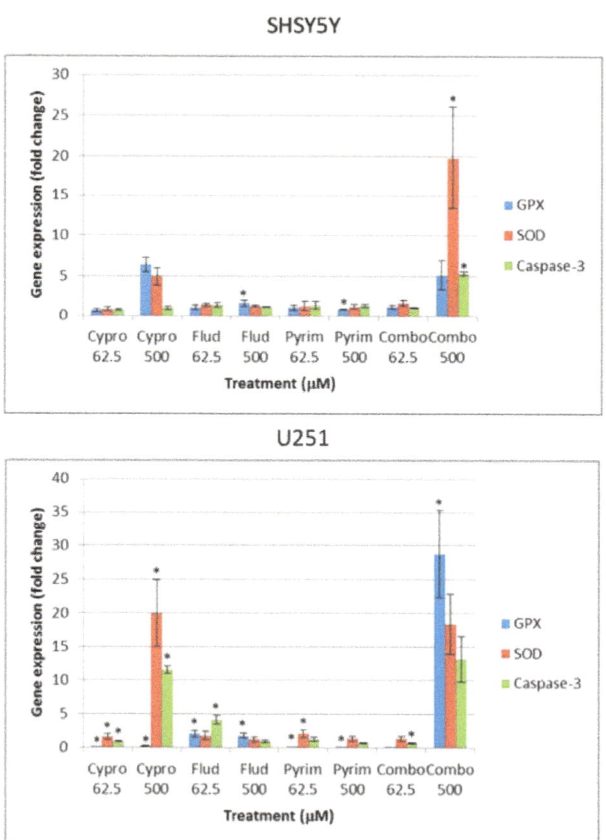

Figure 3: Fold changes in the expression of GSH peroxidase, superoxide dismutase and caspase-3 after the incubation of SH-SY5Y and U251 cells with pyrimethanil, cyprodinil and fludioxonil singly and in a mixture at a low (62.5 **µM**) and high (500 **µM**) ...

With the SH-SY5Y cells, fludioxonil and pyrimethanil showed only modest significant increases in expression at the higher concentration studied (P<0.05), although a 19.79 fold increase was recorded in SOD expression in the neuronal line in the presence of the combination (P<0.05). In the neuronal cells, a significant 5.3-fold increase in caspase-3 expression was also recorded (P<0.05). GSHPx expression was also found to be elevated in the presence of the higher concentration of the combination (5.12-fold), although this increase in gene expression was not found to be statistically significant.

Pesticide Effects on Energy Metabolism

The most striking aspect of the effects of cyprodinil, pyrimethanil and fludioxonil in this study, was that their toxicity towards the cell lines appeared to be directly linked with their potent impact on ATP production; this was in turn connected with their detrimental effects on the mitochondrial membrane potential, as indicated by the JC-1 assay. ATP production has a critical effect on cell viability and whether cell death is either necrotic or apoptotic and it is strongly dependent on the level of cellular ATP depletion [31]. In the human CNS, ATP depletion is a known route of neurotoxicity linked with several agents [32], [33]. In addition, all three pesticides are sufficiently lipophilic (log P's range from 2.8–4) to penetrate the human blood brain barrier and reach the CNS.

Negative effects on energy metabolism may also damage cell defence against reactive species. In this regard, the pesticides impacted cellular reducing power capability, but significantly, they also influenced the expression of several key protective enzymes. Such effects may be either direct, in terms of suppression or induction of a specific gene's expression, or they may be a cellular response to a secondary effect on cellular metabolism or health, such as oxidative stress and/or reduction in ATP levels. Although it is not always possible to distinguish between the two possible effects, in this report with the U251 cell line, cyprodinil and pyrimethanil directly impaired the expression of a major antioxidant defence enzyme (GSHPx) at low and high concentrations, whilst negatively affecting mitochondrial performance, an effect that should in itself lead to an increase in GSHPx expression. This impact on GSHPx occurred at pesticide concentrations that did not significantly impact thiol levels, or in the case of cyprodinil, when they were actually increased. It is conceivable that such an increase may have been linked with the absence of thiol demand that resulted from the fall in GSHPx expression. Although the pesticides caused some cellular response to increases in reactive species to occur, such as the increase in SOD expression, in both cell lines, the suppression of GSHPx expression in this report suggests that in the U251 line, cell defence could potentially be partially undermined by the pesticides. This effect was not apparent in the neuronal cells, where fludioxonil and pyrimethanil alone were associated with increases in GSHPx expression.

Pesticide effects on Caspase-3 and detoxification response

Regarding caspase-3 activation, which is essential for the execution of apoptosis [34], cyprodinil and fludioxonil alone caused this effect, although the combination of pesticides with the U251 line showed very significant increases in the three key protective enzyme systems, GSHPx, SOD and caspase-3. Whilst this suggests that the combination of these agents was responsible for sufficient oxidative stress generation to elicit appropriate cellular defence gene responses in the U-251 cells, such a response to the combination was not evident in the SH-SY5Y line. At higher pesticide concentrations, it was apparent that thiol levels were also eroded in both cell lines and it is likely that this was a consequence of the combination of oxidative stress, attenuation of the ATP supply and mitochondrial toxicity. Although high consumption of thiols usually triggers a 'thermostatic' increase in thiol synthesis [35], this requires both reducing power and ATP to recycle GSH through GSSG reductase and *de novo* synthesis [36]. The impact of the pesticides on energy metabolism and antioxidant protection may have amplified the toxic effects of the pesticides alone and in combination.

Context of findings in terms of modes of action and application

The effects of the pesticides seen in this report do not immediately appear to be linked with their mode of action in fungal control. The anilinopyrimidine pyrimethanil is a dual action fungicide, as it inhibits methionine synthesis and also perturbs cell wall degradation enzymes, thus retarding fungal invasion [37], [38]. Interestingly, although significantly more toxic than pyrimethanil in our hands, cyprodinil is actually a closely related structural anilinopyrimidine analogue. Indeed, cyprodinil is often mixed with fludioxonil, in such products as 'Switch®' which are used extensively in the wine industry [39]. Fludioxonil is a phenylpyrrole derivative of the antibiotic pyrrolnitrin [6] and is a potent phenylpyrrole protein kinase inhibitor; it can also interfere with signal transmission of osmoregulatory control in fungi [40]. Interestingly, the three antifungals are not perceived as especially toxic to mammals; oral LD_{50}'s for these agents in rodents exceed 2–5 g/kg [41], [42] and their toxicity when used individually towards many benign species is often relatively low [43]. Overall, the toxicity of the agents singly and in combination seen in this report may be linked with commonality in basic cellular function between mammalian and other target species and this may have significantly eroded these agents' fungal specificity. Indeed, it is known that concerning mitochondrial structure and function, there are many similarities between mammalian and fungal systems [44]. In addition, a recent report has shown both cyprodinil and fludioxonil to inhibit human erythrocytic SOD, an effect that may also promote oxidative stress and cellular attrition [45].

Pesticide cell-specific effects

The responses of the two cell lines explored in this study to the toxic impact of the pesticides differed markedly. The U251 line possesses considerable biotransformational activity [46] and is widely used as a cytotoxic model for a range of disparate agents such as ethanol and trimethyl tin chloride at concentrations which were within the range shown in human and other mammalian cellular systems [47]–[50]. The U251 line is also a relevant model of human astrocytes, demonstrating comparable susceptibility to glial toxins such as 6-hydroxydopamine in other models [47], [51]. The antioxidant responses in terms of protective enzyme expression and relatively higher resistance to thiol depletion compared with the SH-SY5Y cells, to some extent reflects the role of the astrocyte *in vivo*. Neurones are acutely vulnerable to damage caused by reactive oxygen and nitrogen-derived species and astrocytes play a key role in the oxidative defence of neurones and the preservation of their functionality [52].

The SH-SY5Y neuroblastoma line is used to model dopaminergic human neurones in several disease contexts [53], [54], as well as in the exploration of toxic cellular mechanisms and neurotoxin screening [55], [56]. The SH-SY5Y line has been reported as more sensitive to neurotoxins in comparison with hepatic and breast cancer lines [57]. However, these neurone-like cells are less robust than other transformed lines [57] and this was to some extent reflected in their greater degree of susceptibility to the pesticides in this report compared with the glioma cells.

Findings in context of pesticide usage

The persistence of some of these agents is highly variable and is related to their immediate environment. With cyprodinil, this can range for a few days in vegetable crops [58], to several weeks along with fludioxinil in grape juice stored at 4°C [39]. Refrigeration of produce significantly extends their half-lives and can lead to breach of EU maximum residue limits [59]. Cyprodinil is also resistant to destruction in the vinification process [14] and only charcoal treatment will eliminate these agents from wine [60]. This leads to significant concentrations of these agents in wines and foodstuffs. In a study in Italian 'ready meals', there was an average of 2.4, but up to ten pesticides in every meal. Whilst this contamination, which included pyrimethanil and cyprodinil, did not exceed acceptable daily intakes (ADI) in adults, evidence was found that contamination was higher in children and teenagers and in some cases in these latter groups, the ADI's were actually exceeded [61].

Although pyrimethanil concentrations in some wines can range from about 0.6 to just over one micromolar [15], [62], this is well short of the levels required in the present study to cause mitochondrial toxicity in the two human cell lines. However, pyrimethanil and other related pesticides are found in some water supplies [63] as well as in many other foodstuffs. Therefore, in view of this report, further studies are necessary to determine the impact of individual pesticides and combinations of these agents on human cellular energy metabolism and oxidative stress production, particularly with regard to their potential ability to reach the human CNS.

ACKNOWLEDGMENTS

Dedicated to the memory of Mark J. Winn, Ph.D.

FUNDING STATEMENT

This study received financial support from The Marchig Animal Welfare Trust Edinburgh, United Kingdom (www.marchigtrust.org), as well as the Union Belge pour l'Abolition de l'Expérimentation sur Animaux Vivants (UBAEAV, Rue H. van Zuylen 21, 1180 Bruxelles Tél: 02/376 82 83 Bruxelles, Belgium. In addition, Generations Futures, Paris, France (http://www.mdrgf.org)also contributed to the funding of the work. The funders had no role in study design, data collection and analysis, decision to publish, or preparation of the manuscript.

REFERENCES

1. Li W, Qin ZH, Zhang MH, Browde J (2011) An index method to evaluate growers' pesticide use for identifying on-farm innovations and effective alternative pest management strategies: a case study of winegrape in Madera County, California. J Zhejiang Uni-SCIENCE B (Biomedicine & Biotechnology) 12: 226–246
2. LoCurto R, Pellicano T, Vilasi F, Munafo P, Dugo G (2004) Ochratoxin A occurrence in experimental wines in relationship with different pesticide treatments on grapes. Food Chem 84: 71–75
3. Thrupp LA (1990) Entrapment and escape from fruitless insecticide use: lessons from the banana sector of Costa Rica. Int J Environ Stud 36: 173–189
4. Reus J, Leendertse P, Bockstaller C, Fomsgaard I, Gutsche V, et al. (2002) Comparison and evaluation of eight pesticide environmental risk indicators developed in Europe and recommendations for future use. Agric Ecosyst Environ 90: 177–187
5. González-Rodríguez RM, Cancho-Grande B, Gándara JS (2009) Multiresidue determination of 11 new fungicides in grapes and wines by liquid–liquid extraction/clean-up and programmable temperature vaporization injection with analyte protectants/gas chromatography/iontrap mass spectrometry. J Chromatogr A 1216: 6033–6042
6. Rosslenbroich HJ, Stuebler D (2008) *Botrytis cinerea* history of chemical control and novel fungicides for its management. J Plant Dis & Prot 115: 208–213
7. Engelmeier D, Hadacek F (2006) Antifungal natural products: assays and applications. Rai and Carpinella (eds.) in Naturally Occurring Bioactive Compounds. Elsevier B.V.
8. Wing KD, Sacher M, Kagaya Y, Tsurubuchi Y, Mulderig L, et al. (2000) Bioactivation and mode of action of the oxadiazine indoxacarb in insects. Crop Protect 19: 537–545
9. Likas DT, Tsiropoulos NG (2011) Fate of three insect growth regulators (IGR) insecticides (flufenoxuron, lufenuron and tebufenozide) in grapes following field application and through the wine-making process. Food Add Contam 28: 189–197
10. Anli E, Vural N, Vural H, Gucer Y (2007) Application of solid-phase micro-extraction (SPME) for determining residues of chlorpyrifos and chlorpyrifos-methyl in wine with gas chromatography (GC). J Inst Brew 113: 213–218
11. Tsiropoulos NG, Miliadis GE, Likas DT, Liapis K (2005) Residues of spiroxamine in grapes following field application and their fate from vine to wine. J Ag Food Chem 53: 10091–10096
12. Oliva J, Payá P, Cámara MA, Barba AJ (2007) Removal of famoxadone, fluquinconazole and trifloxystrobin residues in red wines: Effects of clarification and filtration processes. Environ Sci Health Part B-Pesticides Food Contaminants & Agricultural Wastes 42: 775–781
13. Jiménez JJ, Bernal JL, de Nozal MJ, Bernal J, Toribio L (2007) Persistance and degradation of metalaxyl, lindane fenvalarate and deltamethrin during the wine making process. Food Chem 104: 216–223
14. Cuš F, Cesnik HB, Bolta SV, Gergorcic A (2010) Pesticide residues in grapes and during vinification process. Food Control 21: 1512–1518
15. Anonymous, Pesticide Action Network Website, Available: http://pan-europe.info/Resources/Briefings/Message_in_a_Bottle.pdf Accessed 2012 July 13.
16. European Food Safety Authority (2009) Reasoned Opinion of EFSA prepared by the Pesticides Unit on MRLs of concern for the active substance procymidone (revised risk assessment). EFSA Scientific Report 227: 1–26 Available: http://www.efsa.europa.eu/en/scdocs/doc/227r.pdf Accessed 2012 July 13.
17. Ensminger M, Bergin R, Spurlock F, Goh KS (2008) Pesticide concentrations in water and sediment and associated invertebrate toxicity in Del Puerto and Orestimba Creeks, California, 2007–2008. Env Mon Assess 4: 573–587
18. Caceres TP, Megharaj M, Naidu R (2011) Toxicity and transformation of insecticide fenamiphos to the earthworm, *Eisenia fetida*. Ecotoxicology 20: 20–28
19. Sidiropoulou E, Sachana M, Flaskos J, Harris W, Hargreaves AJ, et al. (2011) Fipronil interferes with the differentiation of mouse N2a neuroblastoma cells. Toxicol Lett 201: 86–91
20. Zhao Q, Ren QA, Chen JA, Qiu ZQ, Cao J (2011) Reproductive Toxicity in Male Mice Caused by Organic Extracts in Tap Water from the Jialing River in Ciongqing. China Birth Def. Res. Part B; Dev. Reproduct. Toxicol 92: 1–9
21. Tuzmen MN, Candan N, Kaya E (2007) The evaluation of altered antioxidative defense mechanism and acetylcholinesterase activity in rat brain exposed to chlorpyrifos, deltamethrin, and their combination. Toxicol Mech Methods 17: 535–40
22. Alavanja MCR, Samanic C, Dosemeci M, Lubin J, Tarone R, et al. (2003) Use of agricultural pesticides and prostate cancer risk in the Agricultural Health Study Cohort. Am J Epidemiol 157: 800–814
23. Band PR Abanto Z, Bert J, Lang B, Fang R (2011) Prostate Cancer Risk and Exposure to Pesticides in British Columbia Farmers. The Prostate 71: 168–183
24. Kimura H, Tsukagoshi NA, Yamaguchi T, Iijima A, Aoyama Y (2010) Relationships between cellular events and signaling pathways in various pesticide-affected neural cells. Toxin Rev 29: 43–50
25. Franco R, Li S, Rodriguez-Rocha R, Burn M, Panayiotidis MI (2010) Molecular mechanisms of pesticide-induced neurotoxicity: Relevance to Parkinson's disease. Chemico-Biological Interactions 188: 289–300
26. Tanner CM, Kamel F, Ross GW, Hoppin JA, Goldman SM (2011) Rotenone, Paraquat and Parkinson's Disease. Environ Health Perspect 119: 866–872
27. Ross RA, Spengler BA, Biedler JL (1983) Coordinate morphological and biochemical interconversion of human neuroblastoma cells. J Natl Cancer Inst 71: 741–747
28. Wikstrand CJ, Bigner DD (1981) Hyperimmunization of

non-human primates with bcg-cw and cultured human glioma-derived cells - production of reactive antisera and absence of induction. J Neuroimmunol 1: 249–260

29. Gartlon J, Kinsner A, Bal-Price A, Coecke S, Clothier RH (2006) Evaluation of a proposed *in vitro* test strategy using neuronal and non-neuronal cell systems for detecting neurotoxicity. Toxicol In Vitro 20: 1569–1581
30. Schuliga M, Chouchane S, Snow ET (2002) Upregulation of glutathione-related genes and enzyme activities in cultured human cells by sublethal concentrations of inorganic arsenic. Toxicol Sci 70: 183–192
31. McConkey DJ (1998) Biochemical determinants of apoptosis and necrosis. Toxicol Lett 99: 157–168
32. Marini AM, Nowak TS (2000) Metabolic effects of 1-methyl-4-phenylpyridinium (MPP+) in primary neuron cultures. Journal of Neuroscience Research 62: 814–820
33. Gabryel B, Adamek M, Pudelko A, Malecki A, Trzeciak HI (2002) Piracetam and vinpocetine exert cytoprotective activity and prevent apoptosis of astrocytes *in vitro* in hypoxia and reoxygenation. Neurotoxicol 23: 19–31
34. Brecht S, Gelderblom M, Srinivasan A, Mielke K, Dityateva G (2001) Caspase-3 activation and DNA fragmentation in primary hippocampal neurons following glutamate excitotoxicity. Molecular Brain Research 94: 25–34
35. Anderson ME (1985) Determination of glutathione and glutathione disulphide in biological samples. Methods in Enzymol 113: 548–555
36. Coleman MD (2000) Use of *in vitro* methaemoglobin generation to study antioxidant status in the diabetic erythrocyte. Biochem Pharmac 60: 1409–1416
37. Fritz R, Lanen C, Colas V, Leroux P (1997) Inhibition of methionine biosynthesis in *Botrytis cinerea*by the anilinopyrimidine fungicide pyrimethanil. Pest Sci 49: 40–46
38. Daniels A, Lucas JA (1995) Mode of action of the anilinopyrimidine fungicide pyrimethanil. 1. In-vivo activity against *Botrytis fabae* on broad bean (*Vicia faba*) leaves. Pest Sci 45, 33–41
39. Pose-Juan AE, Rial-Oteroa R, Paradelob M, López-Periagob JE (2011) Influence of the adjuvants in a commercial formulation of the fungicide "Switch" on the adsorption of their active ingredients: Cyprodinil and fludioxonil, on soils devoted to vineyard. J Hazard Mat 193: 288–295.
40. Pillonel CH, Meyer T (1997) Effect of phenylpyrroles on glycerol accumulation and protein kinase activity of *Neurospora crassa*. Pest Sci 49: 229–236
41. FAO/WHO (2005) Report of the joint meeting of the FAO panel of experts on pesticide residues in food and the environment and the WHO core assessment group on pesticide residues. Switzerland: Geneva. Available: http://whqlibdoc.who.int/publications/2006/9241665211_eng.pdf Accessed 2012 July 13.
42. United States Environmental Protection Agency: Pesticide Fact Sheet Cyprodinil: July 1998.
43. Gradish AE, Scott-Dupree CD, Shipp L, Harris CR, Ferguson G (2010) Effect of reduced risk pesticides for use in greenhouse vegetable production on *Bombus impatiens* (Hymenoptera: Apidae). Pest Manag Sci 66: 142–146
44. Ragan CI (1987) Structure of NAH-Ubiquinone reductase (complex-1). Curr Top Bioenerget 15: 1–161
45. Karadag H, Bilgin R (2010) Effect of Cyprodinil and Fludioxonil Pesticides on Human Superoxide Dismutase. Asian J Chem 22: 8147–8154
46. Wang W, Ghandi A, Liebes L, Louie SG, Hofman FM (2011) Effective conversion of irinotecan to SN-38 after intratumoral drug delivery to an intracranial murine glioma model *in vivo* Laboratory investigation. J Neurosurg 114: 689–694
47. Holden LJ, Coleman MD (2007) Assessment of the astrogliotic responses of three human astrocytoma cell lines to ethanol, trimethyltin chloride, and acrylamide. Toxicology 241: 75–83
48. Holden LJ, Coleman MD (2008) Further preliminary assessment of three human glioma cell lines as models of human astrocytic toxicity *in vitro*. Env Toxicol Pharmacol 26: 290–296
49. Reali C, Scintu F, Pillai R, Donato R, Michetti F (2005) S100B counteracts effects of the neurotoxicant trimethyltin on astrocytes and microglia. J Neurosci Res 81: 677–686
50. Figiel I, Fiedorowicz A (2002) Trimethyltin-evoked neuronal apoptosis and glia response in mixed cultures of rat hippocampal dentate gyrus: a new model for the study of the cell type-specific influence of neurotoxins. Neurotoxicology 23: 77–86
51. Raicevica N, Mladenovica A, Perovica M, Harhajia L, Miljkovica D (2005) Iron protects astrocytes from 6-hydroxydopamine toxicity. Neuropharmacol 48: 720–731
52. Fernandez-Fernandez S, Almeida A, Bolanos JP (2012) Antioxidant and bioenergetic coupling between neurons and astrocytes. Biochem J 443: 3–11
53. Koprivica V, Regardie K, Wolff C, Fernall DR, Murphy JJ (2011) Aripiprazole protects cortical neurons from glutamate toxicity. Eur J Pharmacol 651: 73–76
54. Zou DJ, Wang G, Liu JC, Dong MX, Li XM (2011) Beta-asarone attenuates beta-amyloid-induced apoptosis through the inhibition of the activation of apoptosis signal-regulating kinase 1 in SH-SY5Y cells. Pharmazie 66: 44–51
55. Jaworska-Feil L, Jantas D, Leskiewicz M, Budziszewska B, Kubera M (2010) Protective effects of TRH and its analogues against various cytotoxic agents in retinoic acid (RA)-differentiated human neuroblastoma SH-SY5Y cells. Neuropeptides 44: 495–508
56. Yang W, Tiffany-Castiglione E, Lee MY, Son IH (2010) Paraquat induces cyclooxygenase-2 (COX-2) implicated toxicity in human neuroblastoma SH-SY5Y cells. Toxicol Lett 199: 239–246
57. Coleman MD, Zilz TR, Griffiths HR, Woehrling EK (2008) A Comparison of the Apoptotic and Cytotoxic Effects of Hexanedione Derivatives on Human Non-

Neuronal Lines and the Neuroblastoma Line SH-SY5Y. Basic & Clin Pharmacol Toxicol 102: 25–31

58. Liu C, Wang S, Li L, Zhao H, Jiang S (2011) Analysis of cyprodinil in leek and pepper and its decline under field conditions. Environ Monit Assess 179: 209–215
59. Marian A, Oliva J, Garcia C, Navarro SN, Barba A (2003) Dissipation Rates of Cyprodinil and Fludioxonil in Lettuce and Table Grape in the Field and under Cold Storage Conditions. J. Agric. Food Chem. 51: 4708–4711
60. Cabras P, Angioni A, Garau VL, Melis M, Pirisi FM (1997) Fate of Some New Fungicides (Cyprodinil, Fludioxonil, Pyrimethanil, and Tebuconazole) from Vine to Wine. J Agric Food Chem 45: 2708–2710
61. Lorenzin M (2007) Pesticide residues in Italian Ready-Meals and dietary intake estimation. J Environ Sci Health Part B 42: 823–833.
62. Ravelo-Pérez LM, Hernández-Borges J, Cifuentes A. Rodríguez-Delgado MA (2007) Multiple pesticide analysis in wine by MEKC combined with solid-phase microextraction and sample. Electrophoresis 28: 4072–4081.
63. Ravelo-Pérez LM, Hernández-Borges J, Cifuentes A (2007) Rodríguez-Delgado MA. MEKC combined with SPE and sample stacking for multiple analysis of pesticides in water samples at the ng/L level. Electrophoresis 28: 1805–1814.

CHAPTER 26

ACUTE HUMAN LETHAL TOXICITY OF AGRICULTURAL PESTICIDES

Andrew H. Dawson, Michael Eddleston, Lalith Senarathna, Fahim Mohamed, Indika Gawarammana, Steven J. Bowe
Gamini Manuweera, Nicholas A. Buckley

EDITORS' SUMMARY

Background

Suicide is a preventable global public health problem. About 1 million people die each year from suicide and many more harm themselves but survive. Although many people who commit suicide have a mental illness, stressful events (economic hardship or relationship difficulties, for example) can sometimes make life seem too painful to bear. Suicide attempts are frequently impulsive and use methods that are conveniently accessible. Strategies to reduce suicide rates include better treatment of mental illness and programs that help people at high risk of suicide deal with stress. Suicide rates can also be reduced by limiting access to common suicide methods. The single most important means of suicide worldwide is agricultural pesticide poisoning. Every year, between 250,000 and 370,000 people die from deliberate ingestion of pesticides (chemicals that kill animal pests or unwanted plants). Most of these suicides occur in rural areas of the developing world where high levels of pesticide use in agriculture combined with pesticide storage at home facilitate this particular method of suicide.

Why Was This Study Done?

To help reduce suicides through the ingestion of agricultural pesticides, the Food and Agriculture Organization of the United Nations recommends the withdrawal of the most toxic pesticides—World Health Organization (WHO) class I pesticides—from agricultural use. This strategy has proven successful in Sri Lanka where a ban on class I pesticides in 1995 and on the class II pesticide endosulfan in 1998 has reduced pesticide deaths by 50% over the past 20 years without decreasing agricultural output. Further reductions in suicides from pesticide ingestion could be achieved if regulatory restrictions on the sale and distribution of the most toxic class II pesticides were imposed. But such restrictions must balance agricultural needs against the impact of pesticides on public health. Unfortunately, the current WHO pesticide classification is based on toxicity in rats. Because rats handle pesticides differently from people, there is no guarantee that a pesticide with low toxicity in rodents is safe in people. Here, the researchers try to determine the relative human toxicity of agricultural pesticides in a prospective cohort study (a study in which people who share a characteristic—in this case,

Citation: Dawson AH, Eddleston M, Senarathna L, Mohamed F, Gawarammana I, Bowe SJ, et al. (2010) Acute Human Lethal Toxicity of Agricultural Pesticides. PLoS Med 7(10): e1000357. doi:10.1371/journal.pmed.1000357

deliberate pesticide ingestion—are enrolled and followed to see how they fare).

What Did the Researchers Do and Find?

The researchers examined the case fatality (the proportion of patients dying after hospital admission) of different agricultural pesticides among patients who presented with pesticide self-poisoning at two Sri Lankan referral hospitals. Between April 2002 and November 2008, 9,302 people were admitted to the hospitals after swallowing a single pesticide. The researchers identified the pesticide ingested in 7,461 cases by asking the patient what he/she had taken or by identifying the container brought in by the patient or relatives. 10% of the patients died but there was a large variation in case fatality between pesticides. The herbicide paraquat was the most lethal pesticide, killing 42% of patients; several other pesticides killed no one. Compounds in the same chemical class and/or the same WHO toxicity class sometimes had very different toxicities. For example, dimethoate and malathione, both class II organophosphate insecticides, had case fatalities of 20.6% and 1.9%, respectively. Similarly, pesticides used for similar agricultural purposes sometimes had very different case fatalities.

What Do These Findings Mean?

These findings provide a toxicity ranking for pesticides that deviates markedly from the WHO toxicity classification based on rat toxicity. Although the findings are based on a study undertaken at just two Sri Lankan hospitals, they are likely to be generalizable to other hospitals and to other parts of rural Asia. However, because the study only included patients who were admitted to hospital after ingesting pesticides, the actual case fatalities for some pesticides may be somewhat different. Nevertheless, these findings have several important public health implications. For example, they suggest that the decision taken in January 2008 to withdraw paraquat, dimethoate, and fenthion from the Sri Lankan market should reduce deaths from pesticide poisoning in Sri Lanka by a further 33%–65% (equivalent to about 1,000 fewer suicides per year). More generally, they suggest that basing the regulation of pesticides on human toxicity has the potential to prevent hundreds and thousands of intentional and accidental deaths globally without compromising agricultural needs.

Additional Information

- Please access these Web sites via the online version of this summary at http://dx.doi.org/10.1371/journal.pmed.1000357.
- This study is further discussed in a *PLoS Medicine* Perspective by Matt Miller and Kavi Bhalla
- The World Health Organization provides information on the global burden of suicide and on suicide prevention (in several languages) and on its classification of pesticides
- The US Environmental Protection Agency provides information about all aspects of pesticides (in English and Spanish)
- Toxtown, an interactive site from the US National Library of Science, provides information on environmental health concerns including exposure to pesticides (in English and Spanish)
- The nonprofit organization Pesticide Action Network UK provides information about all aspects of pesticides
- The US National Pesticide Information Center provides objective, science-based information about pesticides (in several languages)
- The Food and Agriculture Organization of the United Nations leads international efforts to reduce hunger; as part of this effort, it has introduced pesticide policy reforms (in several languages)
- MedlinePlus provides links to further resources about suicide and about pesticides (in English and Spanish)

INTRODUCTION

Suicide and deliberate self-harm using pesticides is a major but under-recognised public health problem in the developing world. Each year 250,000–370,000 thousand people die from deliberate ingestion of pesticides [1],[2]. These deaths are responsible for about a third of suicides globally [1]; the World Health Organization (WHO) now recognizes pesticide poisoning to be the single most important means of suicide worldwide [3].

Within the rural developing world, high levels of pesticide use with storage at home increases the risk of acute poisoning [4]. One strategy to reduce mortality is to restrict access to more toxic pesticides [5]. As a first line, countries should follow Food and Agriculture Organization (FAO) advice [6] and withdraw the most toxic WHO/US Environmental Protection Agency (EPA) class I pesticides (see Table 1 for description of toxicity classifications) from agricultural practice. Further efforts can range from educating farmers in the use of safer pesticides to imposing regulatory restrictions on the sale and distribution of the most toxic class II pesticides [7],[8]. These strategies would be aided if countries developed pesticide policies that balanced agricultural and economic needs against the public health impact of acute and chronic human toxicity [9]. The development of such a policy should be iterative and based on evidence about which pesticides are major public health concerns [1].

Table 1: WHO classification of toxicity [18]. http://dx.doi.org/10.1371/journal.pmed.1000357.t001

Class	Description	LD_{50} for the Rat (mg/kg Body Weight)			
		Oral		Dermal	
		Solids	Liquids	Solids	Liquids
Ia	Extremely hazardous	≤5	≤20	≤10	≤40
Ib	Highly hazardous	5–50	20–200	10–100	40–400
II	Moderately hazardous	50–500	200–2,000	100–1,000	400–4,000
III	Slightly hazardous	>500	>2,000	>1,000	>4,000

doi:10.1371/journal.pmed.1000357.t001

Unfortunately, at present, regulatory decisions are based on a classification of pesticide toxicity that is largely based upon rat oral LD50s. The scientific basis for extrapolating this classification to human poisoning with class II pesticides is weak. Rodents handle xenobiotics differently to humans [10]; as an example, they have greater capacity for metabolic detoxification of organophosphates [11]. And unlike human patients receiving intensive care, they do not receive any treatment in the toxicity studies. It is therefore not clear that a pesticide with low toxicity in rodents should be safe in humans and vice versa.

Information on the acute human toxicity of a wide range of pesticides is needed to complement the animal toxicity data. We therefore set up a prospective cohort of intentional pesticide-poisoned patients admitted to two Sri Lankan hospitals to study the relative toxicity of formulated pesticides in humans. Sri Lanka is an ideal location for this research. Ahead of the FAO recommendations, it has banned all WHO/EPA class I pesticides leaving just class II and III pesticides in agricultural use. Other Asian countries are slowly following suit—within a few years class I pesticides will no longer be used. Therefore, the current situation in Sri Lanka represents the future situation in other Asia countries. Furthermore, because only class II and III pesticides are used in Sri Lanka, the great majority of deaths from pesticide poisoning occur in the secondary referral study hospitals [12],[13]. Bias from prehospital deaths is minimized.

METHODS

Ethics Statement

Ethics approval for this data collection has been obtained from Oxfordshire Clinical Research Ethics Committee, Oxford Tropical Medicine Ethics Committee, Colombo University Faculty of Medicine Ethics Committee, Sri Lankan Medical Association, University of Peradeniya, and the Australian National University.

Patients

This was a prospective observational cohort study of patients aged greater than 12 y with deliberate ingestion of a single pesticide who presented to two Sri Lankan rural referral hospitals for an agricultural provincial district of 1.1 million people. The poison ingested was determined from the history given by the patient or relatives, the hospital transfer letter, or from the pesticide bottle if it accompanied the patient. Patients who deliberately ingested more than one substance (except for alcohol) were excluded from this study. Patients were either direct admissions to the study hospital or transfers from smaller primary hospitals. Patient recruitment commenced on 31 March 2002 in Anuradhapura Hospital and 4 June 2002 in Polonnaruwa Hospital. Details of the referring hospital name were documented from 1 June 2006. Data analysis was performed on all patients who had been enrolled up until 17 November 2008.

All patients were enrolled into the cohort at admission by full-time study doctors employed as clinical research assistants. Clinical care followed a standard protocol that emphasized identifying patients poisoned by pesticides that would likely respond to antidotes, in particular organophosphorus (OP) and carbamate insecticides [14]. All patients were seen regularly at least every 4 h. Significant events (intubation, seizures, death) were recorded prospectively. Patients were also seen on a study ward round twice each day and their condition over the previous 12 h recorded. Patients remained under the care of the hospital consultant physicians. Decisions about medical treatment, intubation, and transfer of patients to intensive care were made solely by the hospital staff on the basis of the patient's clinical condition, and independently of the research team.

Statistics

Case fatality was defined as the proportion of deaths over admissions for any given pesticide. Odds ratios (ORs) and the 95% confidence intervals (CIs) of the proportions were calculated using the binomial exact method [15]. The binomial exact method will generate a one-sided CI (97.5% CI) when the proportion of deaths over admissions for a given pesticide is zero.

Logistic regression was used to calculate unadjusted and adjusted (for age and gender) ORs for death relative to the pesticide most commonly ingested (chlorpyrifos).

The potential effect of recently implemented pesticide bans was examined assuming proportional redistribution based upon existing distribution of poisoning across the class after excluding patients who had taken unidentified pesticides. Sensitivity analyses were undertaken by assuming complete redistribution to the next most toxic substitute and to the least toxic substitute.

RESULTS

During the study period, 9,302 patients were admitted following deliberate ingestion of a single pesticide. The pesticide ingested could be identified by history in 7,461 patients; a further 1,841 had ingested an unknown pesticide. Within the unknown group, 497 were considered to have taken a cholinesterase inhibitor (either an OP or carbamate insecticide) on the basis of a typical anticholinesterase clinical syndrome, significant atropine requirement, and/or measured cholinesterase inhibition. A total of 808 patients, whose ingested pesticide was identified by history, had admission samples assayed for other nested studies; history correctly identified the ingested poison in 94.7% of these patients, the other 5.3% were not necessarily misclassifications (more likely to be simply below the level of assay detection). In a subset of the cohort we have also previously shown that analytical assay confirmed history in 92% of symptomatic patients with organophosphate poisoning [16].

The patients were predominately male (67%) and young; the median age was 28 y (interquartile range [IQR] 21–40). The median time to admission to the study hospitals following ingestion was 4 h (IQR 3–7).

The case fatality for the most commonly ingested pesticides is presented in Table 2. The overall mortality for pesticide self-poisoning (including patients who had ingested an unidentified pesticide) was 10.1% (CI 9.5–10.8). From 1 June 2006, 2,608 patients were admitted with a single pesticide ingestion; mortality was 8.9% (61/678) for direct study hospital admissions compared with 7.8% in patients transferred from primary rural hospitals. As 12% of all primary hospital deaths occur in the primary hospitals, there was no clear difference in overall mortality for patients who first presented to a primary rural hospital compared with those presenting to a referral study hospital. Anticholinesterase insecticides and the herbicides paraquat, MCPA, propanil, and glyphosate accounted for 94% of admissions and 98% of deaths. For those ingesting an identified pesticide, just three compounds with relatively high case fatality (paraquat, dimethoate, fenthion) were responsible for 17.6% of total admissions but 47% of the total deaths.

Table 2: Case fatality of any pesticide with more than ten admissions or any death. http://dx.doi.org/10.1371/journal.pmed.1000357.t002

Pesticide	Deaths	*n* Patients	Percent Case Fatality	95% CI Binomial Exact	Rat Oral LD50 (mg/kg)	WHO Tox Class
OPs						
Chlorpyrifos	104	1,376	7.6	6.2–9.1	135	II
Diazinon	4	84	4.8	1.3–11.7	1,000	II
Dimethoate	172	833	20.6	17.9–23.6	c.150	II
Fenthion	35	237	14.8	10.5–19.9	215	II
Malathion	4	209	1.9	0.5–4.8	2,100	III
Methamidophos	1	8	12.5	0.3–52.7	30	Ib
Oxydemeton-methyl	1	8	12.5	0.3–52.7	65	Ib
Phenthoate	11	168	6.5	3.3–11.4	c.400	II
Pirimiphos-methyl	0	12	0.0	0.0–26.5[a]	2,018	III
Profenofos	16	146	11.0	6.4–17.2	358	II
Prothiofos	1	13	7.7	0.2–36.0	925	II
Quinalphos	15	124	12.1	6.9–19.2	62	II
Other OPs[b]	0	38	0.0	0.0–9.3[a]	—	—
Summary	**364**	**3,256**	**11.2**	**10.1–12.3**	—	—
Carbamates						
Carbaryl	1	18	5.6	0.1–27.3	c.300	II
Carbofuran	5	479	1.0	0.3–2.4	8	Ib
Carbosulfan	37	345	10.7	7.7–14.5	250	II
Fenobucarb	6	104	5.8	2.1–12.1	620	II
Methomyl	1	7	14.3	0.4–57.9	17	Ib
Propoxur	0	16	0.0	0.0–20.6[a]	95	II
Other carbamates[c]	0	7	0.0	0.0–41.0[a]	—	—
Summary	**50**	**976**	**5.1**	**3.8–6.7**	—	—
Pyrethroids						
Deltamethrin	0	11	0.0	0.0–28.5[a]	c.135	II
Esfenvalerate	1	12	8.3	0.2–38.5	87	II
Etofenprox	1	121	0.8	0.0–4.5	>10,000	IV
Permethrin	0	13	0.0	0.0–24.7[a]	c.500	II
Other pyrethroids[d]	0	46	0.0	0.0–7.7[a]	—	—
Summary	**2**	**203**	**1.0**	**0.1–3.5**	—	—
Organochlorines						
Endosulfan	2	9	22.2	2.8–60.0	80	II
Lindane	0	3	0.0	0.0–70.8[a]	88	II
Summary	**2**	**12**	**16.7**	**2.1–48.4**	—	—
Other noncholinesterase						
Abamectin	2	18	11.1	1.4–34.7	650	IV
Acetamiprid	0	11	0.0	0.0–28.5[a]	146	NC
Chlorfluazuron	1	45	2.2	0.1–11.8	8,500	IV
Fipronil	0	26	0.0	0.0–13.2[a]	92	II
Imidacloprid	0	70	0.0	0.0–5.1[a]	450	II
Other insecticides[e]	0	12	0.0	0.0–26.5[a]	—	—
Summary	**3**	**182**	**1.6**	**0.3–4.7**	—	—
Herbicides						
Alachlor	1	9	11.1	0.3–48.2	930	III
Bispyribac-sodium	3	103	2.9	0.6–8.3	2,635	IV
Fenoxaprop-p-ethyl	0	74	0.0	0.0–4.9[a]	2,357	U
Glyphosate	21	887	2.4	1.5–3.6	4,230	IV
MCPA	33	681	4.8	3.4–6.7	700	III

Pesticide	Deaths	*n* Patients	Percent Case Fatality	95% CI Binomial Exact	Rat Oral LD50 (mg/kg)	WHO Tox Class
Oxyfluorfen	0	15	0.0	0.0–21.8[a]	>5,000	II
Paraquat	243	569	42.7	38.6–46.9	150	II
Pretilachlor	0	11	0.0	0.0–28.5[a]	6,100	U
Propanil	45	412	10.9	8.1–14.3	c.1,400	III
Other herbicides[f]	0	22	0.0	0.0– 15.4[a]	—	—
Summary	**346**	**2,783**	**12.4**	**11.2–13.7**	—	—
Fungicides						
Edifenphos	2	17	11.8	1.5–36.4	150	Ib
Propamocarb	1	1	100	2.5–100	2,000–2,900	IV
Other fungicides[g]	0	31	0.0	0.0–11.2	—	—
Summary	**3**	**49**	**6.1**	**1.3–16.9**	—	—
Unknown pesticides	173	1,841	9.4	8.1–10.8	—	—

Detail of pesticides included in "Other" groupings, the number of cases in parenthesis following each pesticide.
[a]Denotes one sided 97.5% CI.
[b]Acephate (10), coumaphos (4), fenitrothion (2), formothion (1), monochrotophos (10), phoxim (10), terbufos (1).
[c]Thiodicarb (6), methylcarb (1).
[d]Cyfluthrin (5), cypermethrin (7), d-trans allethrin (4), fenvalerate (4), flumethrin (6), unspecified pyrethroid (20).
[e]Azadirachtin (5), chromafenozide (1), flufenoxuron (1), tebufenozide (3), thiacloprid (1), novaluron (1).
[f]Dinitroaniline (1), ethoxysulfuran (1), methyl 3,4-dichlorocarbanilate (1), dinitroaniline (1), oxadiazon (1), pendimethalin (9), propachlor (1), quinclorac (7).
[g]Binapacryl (1), carbendazim (2), chlorothalonil (4), dithiocarbamate (7), ethoxysulfan (1), hexaconazole (4), isoprothioline (1), mancozeb (5), propiconazole (1), propineb (1), tebuconazole (2), thiophanate (1), triazole (1).
c., cutaneous; NC Not classified.
doi:10.1371/journal.pmed.1000357.t002

There was a very wide range of lethal toxicity for compounds within the same pesticide classes (e.g., OP insecticides) or with the same agricultural indication (e.g., nonselective herbicides). For example the risk ratio for death after ingestion of the OP insecticides dimethoate versus chlorpyrifos was 2.7 (CI 2.2–3.4) and for the herbicides paraquat versus glyphosate was 18.1 (CI 11.7–27.6). These risk ratios confirm significant differences in pesticides that are in the same WHO class for risk (Figure 1; Table 2) and have comparable agricultural efficacy. There was marked variation in case fatality for OPs with similar LD_{50}s, emphasizing the limited usefulness of animal toxicity data to drive human regulatory decisions (Table 2).

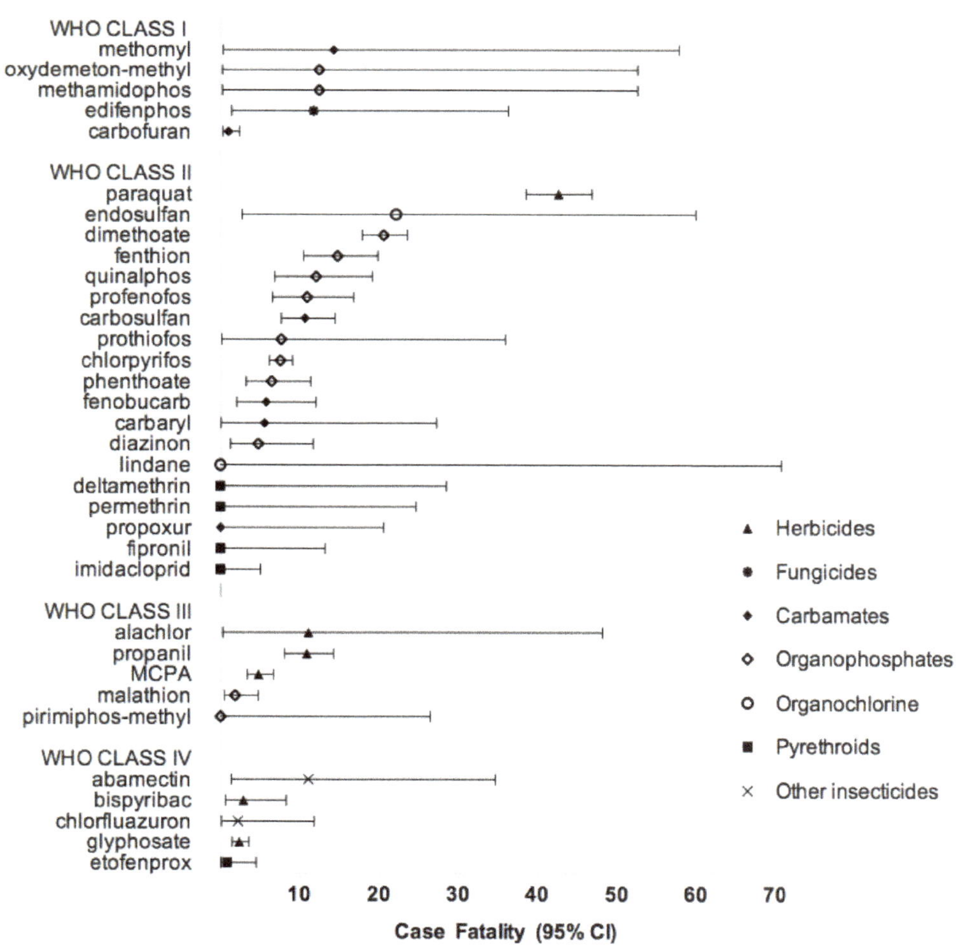

Figure 1: Plot of case fatality for different pesticides grouped by WHO class. http://dx.doi.org/10.1371/journal.pmed.1000357.g001

Increasing age and male sex was significantly associated with a fatal outcome. However, adjustment for these factors did not result in any major changes in the relative toxicity assessment. For example, the odds of dying from paraquat ingestion was 9.1 (95% CI 7.0–11.8) times that of chlorpyrifos (reference group). When adjusted for age and gender the relative risk of dying from paraquat was moderately greater (OR 15.4; 95% CI 11.6–20.4). Similar moderate increases in ORs were seen for dimethoate and fenthion after adjustment (Table 3).

Table 3: Logistic regression of odds of a fatal outcome for each pesticide before and after adjustment for gender and age. http://dx.doi.org/10.1371/journal.pmed.1000357.t003

Factor	Unadjusted $n=8{,}883$[a]		Adjusted $n=8{,}883$	
	Odd Ratio	95% CI	Odd Ratio	95% CI
Females	—	—	1.00	—
Males	—	—	1.49	1.24–1.80
<25 y	—	—	1.00	—
25–34 y	—	—	1.48	1.18–1.85
35–44 y	—	—	2.39	1.90–3.02
45–64 y	—	—	5.86	4.69–7.33
>64 y	—	—	19.10	13.45–27.12
Chlorpyrifos	1.00	—	1.00	—
Abamectin	1.53	0.35–6.74	1.74	0.38–7.99
Alachlor	1.53	0.19–12.34	3.00	0.34–26.85
Bispyribac-sodium	0.37	0.11–1.18	0.41	0.12–1.35
Carbaryl	0.72	0.09–5.46	0.78	0.09–6.64
Carbofuran	0.13	0.05–0.32	0.14	0.05–0.34
Carbosulfan	1.47	0.99–2.18	1.93	1.28–2.92
Chlorfluazuron	0.28	0.04–2.04	0.23	0.03–1.74
Diazinon	0.61	0.22–1.70	0.58	0.20–1.69
Dimethoate	3.18	2.45–4.13	3.97	3.01–5.23
Edifenphos	1.63	0.37–7.23	1.62	0.32–8.24
Endosulfan	3.49	0.72–17.04	2.39	0.43–13.25
Esfenvalerate	1.11	0.14–8.70	1.65	0.20–13.48
Fenobucarb	0.75	0.32–1.75	1.20	0.50–2.84
Fenthion	2.12	1.41–3.20	2.91	1.89–4.49
Glyphosate	0.30	0.18–0.48	0.42	0.26–0.69
Malathion	0.24	0.09–0.65	0.32	0.11–0.89
MCPA	0.62	0.42–0.93	0.75	0.49–1.13
Methamidophos	1.75	0.21–14.34	1.23	0.14–10.46
Methomyl	2.04	0.24–17.09	2.71	0.32–23.15
Paraquat	9.12	7.03–11.82	15.42	11.63–20.44
Phenthoate	0.86	0.45–1.63	0.92	0.47–1.79
Profenofos	1.51	0.86–2.63	1.37	0.76–2.46
Propanil	1.50	1.04–2.17	2.06	1.40–3.04
Prothiofos	1.02	0.13–7.92	0.88	0.11–7.06
Quinalphos	1.68	0.95–2.99	2.18	1.19–3.99
Unknown pesticides	1.27	0.98–1.64	1.40	1.08–1.83
Oxydemeton methyl	1.75	0.21–14.34	2.42	0.28–21.20
Etofenprox	0.10	0.01–0.74	0.08	0.01–0.58

Note of caution: Large OR and wide 95% CI due to small number of deaths in subgroup.
[a] $n=419$ omitted from model since no deaths occurred for some categories of pesticide.
doi:10.1371/journal.pmed.1000357.t003

The potential effect on mortality of banning the three most lethal pesticides and assuming best and worst case substitutions suggests a reduction in overall pesticide case fatality of between 33% and 65%. The actual fall in case fatality seen after withdrawal of these pesticides will therefore depend substantially on which pesticides replace them in the market (Table 4).

Table 4: Modeling the potential effect of dimethoate, fenthion, and paraquat bans in an equal size cohort (7,461 patients with known pesticide[a] ingestion). http://dx.doi.org/10.1371/journal.pmed.1000357.t004

Type of Model	Deaths	Case Fatality	95% CI
No bans (history repeats)	769	10.3%	9.6–11.0%
Proportionate redistribution to other OPs or herbicides[a]	423	5.7%	5.2–6.2%
Least toxic class substitute[b]	351	4.7%	4.2–5.2%
Most toxic class substitute[c]	516	6.9%	6.4–7.5%

[a] Excludes unknown pesticides.
[b] Substitution of glyphosate for paraquat as it is the only nonspecific herbicide. Substitution of dimethoate and fenthion with the "Other pesticides" group (using the pooled case fatality).
[c] Substitution of propanil for paraquat and oxydemeton-methyl for dimethoate and fenthion. Propanil would be an unlikely substitute as it is a selective herbicide.
doi:10.1371/journal.pmed.1000357.t004

DISCUSSION

This study demonstrates major differences in human case fatality between pesticides that are used for similar agricultural indications. These are the first systematically collected prospective human data, to our knowledge, that allow estimates of relative toxicity for pesticides. The data are much more directly relevant to human risk assessment than the existing animal data from which the WHO/EPA classifications of toxicity used in regulation are derived. Moreover, it provides evidence of very large differences in acute human toxicity within these widely used classifications. These data provide a basis for refining further public health, regulatory, and clinical responses to the problem of acute pesticide poisoning.

Public Health Implications

In regions where pesticide poisoning is a public health problem, pesticide use must be considered in the context of a societal need that balances agricultural benefits with the costs related to human toxicity. Ideally, this requires human toxicity data to be incorporated into regulatory decision making.

This study supports previous observations of the mismatch of human toxicity with animal LD_{50}s for OP insecticides [16],[17]. The current WHO/EPA classification is linked to a number of regulatory mechanisms designed to minimize human risk from pesticides on the basis of occupational or unintentional exposure to pesticides [18]. However, the most important current public health problem of pesticides is deliberate rather than unintentional exposure [19]. There is also an overlap between the two in terms of plausible exposure, and therefore acute self-poisoning data also provide substantial information for risk assessment in unintentional exposure.

The criteria for the classifications have provision for the inclusion of other data to supplement the existing standard means of determining classification based on animal data: "Provision is made for the classification of a particular compound to be adjusted if, for any reason, the acute hazard to man differs from that indicated by LD_{50} assessments alone" [18]. The data reported here provide a strong argument for utilizing acute human toxicity data in the existing classification scheme that would be a better guide for national regulatory and promotional policy.

The societal and policy question is what threshold should be adopted to move compounds from a class II (moderately hazardous) status to class 1a (extremely hazardous) or class 1b (highly hazardous) status at which point these compounds would fall under the scrutiny of international regulatory guides and agreements. We have previously suggested that a human case fatality of less than 10% using treatments that are widely available and inexpensive could be the threshold for classification of a pesticide formulation into class II [8].

Alternatively, rather than arbitrarily setting a threshold, benchmarking could utilize data on a range of class I agents. In a retrospective Indian study, class I pesticides had case fatality ranging from 17% to 60%, and no class II pesticides were in this range [17]. Thus one might set the threshold at a human case fatality of less than 15% to remain in class II. From a public health perspective it seems irrational for pesticide formulations with estimated case fatalities of 21% (dimethoate EC40), 22% (endosulfan EC35), and 47% (paraquat 20%) to be in the same (moderately hazardous) WHO class as many pesticides with a 20-fold lower human case fatality (see Table 2, case fatality for other class II pesticides cluster in the range 0% to 12.5%).

The public health impact of such a change in classification is supported by past experience of pesticide restriction. In Sri Lanka, the withdrawal of all class I pesticides in the years leading up to 1995 and withdrawal of endosulfan in 1998 coincided with a halving of the number of suicides and even greater reduction in fatal poisonings [7],[20]. These pesticide restrictions were introduced without any adverse effects on agricultural costs or output [21]. In January 2008, the data presented within this paper combined with other studies [22] underpinned a Sri Lankan government policy decision to withdraw paraquat, dimethoate, and fenthion from the Sri Lankan market. Our analysis (Table 3) suggests the decision to withdraw these three pesticides is likely to lead to a further 33% to 65% reduction in deaths from acute poisoning. On the basis of Sri Lankan 2005 figures for deaths from poisoning, this action should translate to a reduction in suicide deaths by about 1,000 lives per year [7]. Similar regulatory activities across Asia would likely reduce the suicide rate in the region by more than 30% contributing to a substantial fall in the global number of suicides.

Clinical Implications

The large variation in mortality within OP and carbamate pesticides suggests variation in toxicokinetics and/or dynamics for compounds that are often regarded as requiring the same medical management [16]. Clinical implications of significant variability within a toxicological class include the need for a more complex risk assessment for individual patients and perhaps specific treatment protocols for individual agents [16]. Previous analysis of the relative toxicity of just three OP insecticides (chlorpyrifos, dimethoate, and fenthion) demonstrated large difference in the time course of toxicity, kinetics and dynamics of the pesticide, and mode of death [16]. Better understanding of factors that are associated with higher mortality will allow clinicians to triage and manage patients more effectively. While this analysis has focused simply upon differences in case fatality, further studies are required to provide more detail on the clinical course of high risk poisonings.

Effects of Resource Limitations in Rural Asian Hospitals

The limited treatment resources in Sri Lankan primary referral hospitals might have increased case fatality [23]. However, such limitations are the norm throughout the developing world. For example, propanil's case fatality of 11% is unexpectedly high for an agent whose toxicity is largely due to methaemoglobinaemia and haemolysis, complications that should be relatively easily treated [24]. However, the difficulty in monitoring treatment response without cooximeters and problems with access to and dose adjustment of the antidote have all been suggested as major contributory causes to the high case fatality [24]. Previous studies have also documented high complication rates from gastrointestinal decontamination in rural hospitals that may increase mortality [25]. Other issues identified in primary hospitals that could impact on care include lack of medication, equipment, and staffing [23]. Resource restrictions are less likely to have an effect on case-fatality estimates for highly toxic pesticides such as paraquat that have no proven effective treatment [22],[26].

These two study hospitals received additional resources in the form of medically qualified research assistants and additional monitoring equipment. These and standardized treatment protocols would be expected to have contributed to a generally lower case fatality than other rural hospitals [27],[28], and thus we believe the estimates of actual lethality and the potential impact of further regulation are both conservative. In addition, for 3 y of this study, dimethoate and fenthion were banned in approximately 25% of the province, contributing to an underestimate of the effects of more widespread pesticide restriction.

Effect of Pesticide Formulation

For some pesticides in particular, mortality may not be just related to the intrinsic toxicity and whether effective antidotes have been developed. Formulation differences can be important. The acute toxicity of the class I agent carbofuran is far higher (rat oral LD_{50}, 8 mg/kg) than the related carbosulfan (250 mg/kg). However, carbofuran has remained on the market as it is sold as 3% granules and therefore has significantly lower case fatality than carbosulfan that is formulated as a 25% emulsifiable concentrate liquid. The benefits of this formulation change have been attenuated by farmers using the granules "off label" to produce a solution. The OP quinalphos has the highest acute rat toxicity of any OP sold in Sri Lanka; as a result, it is formulated at a lower concentration (25%) than most other OPs (40%–50%) to bring its predicted toxicity down. Unfortunately, changes in formulation for paraquat have not led to clinically significant reductions in case fatality [22]. Formulation changes have not yet been attempted for other pesticides.

Comparison with Other Research Studies

There are no other comparable prospective studies of pesticide mortality but previous retrospective studies support our key conclusion that pesticides used for the same agricultural need have very important differences in acute human toxicity.

A retrospective study in South India of 8,040 pesticide ingestion showed an overall mortality from OP insecticides of 22% [17] compared to 11.1% in this study (Table 2). The majority of deaths were due to the class I OP monocrotophos, which had a case fatality of 35%. Similar data have been reported from a retrospective poison center study in Taiwan [29]. Class I OPs in these studies showed higher mortality than all of the class II or III OPs in our study with the exception of dimethoate. While the overall mortality in our cohort was much lower, the results for the few pesticides that were common to these studies were similar despite the different setting; the case fatality in the Indian study was chlorpyrifos (6%), quinalphos (12%), and endosulfan (28%), and in the Taiwan study was chlorpyrifos (4.4%), dimethoate (16.6%), and fenthion (15.3%).

These studies provide strong support for our contention that these results are representative of typical poisonings in the region. However, since relatively few pesticides overlapped, there is a clear need for more large, prospective cohort studies in the region to inform pesticide regulation across the full range of pesticides in agricultural use.

Limitations

The most important limitation of our data is that they were collected from just two rural referral hospitals in one country. However, these hospitals are likely to be representative for many rural hospitals in the developing world where resources may be restricted. Although data were collected from within one country, the pattern of agriculture and related pesticide requirements within the study area are similar to much of rural Asia [30].

Since Sri Lanka has already banned some pesticides (notably all WHO class I pesticides [31]), these data do not include some WHO class I pesticides (such as parathion and monocrotophos) that are still manufactured and available in other countries of the region. The limited human data on such agents suggest they are more toxic than most of the pesticides in our study [29]. It is likely that any country developing a policy based upon including pesticides of minimum risk in acute exposure would first attempt to regulate these class 1 agents.

Another potential limitation is that these data on deaths and poisonings were recorded from secondary referral hospitals. Deaths at home, in primary hospitals, and during transfers will affect both the numerator and denominator of the observed case fatality. Surviving patients not transferred will only reduce the denominator. Data collected for a previous study of all injury in the province identified only 3.8% of deaths from pesticides occurring outside the health system [32]. Our data would not include patients who took trivial nontoxic ingestions of agrochemicals and did not subsequently present for medical treatment. If this occurred it should be more common with the least toxic pesticides and thus to reduce differences observed between agents. It thus could not explain the very large differences in relative toxicity we observed.

We examined primary hospital mortality within two subsets of this cohort. In a small study of 260 patients done in 2002 from within this cohort, 80% of deaths occurred after transfer [12]. Of 471 patients presenting with pesticide poisoning to peripheral hospitals in a 6-mo period in 2005, just three patients died in the peripheral hospital compared to 32 patients dying after transfer. 77% of organophosphate, 84% of carbamate, and 90% of paraquat poisoned patients were transferred to the study hospitals [13].

We prospectively examined all poisonings presenting to all primary hospitals (*n*=30) and referral hospitals between September 2008 and December 2009 as part of an RCT of primary hospital educational intervention (ISRCTN73983810). 1,158 people with pesticide poisoning presented to the primary rural hospitals; 77% of these patients were transferred to the referral hospitals. A total of 72 deaths occurred within this group, nine deaths were in the primary hospital, and 63 deaths in referral hospital.. Median time to presentation in this study was 55 min (IQR 30–110).

As most deaths occur following referral it is unlikely that patients kept in primary hospitals and not referred would substantially change the overall or relative case fatality. Any bias from nonreferral of less severely poisoned patients would lead to overestimation of toxicity for the least toxic pesticides. None of the data presented suggests any systematic difference in pesticides causing death in the referral hospital compared with prereferral (primary hospitals and home). Thus this potential referral bias could not explain the very large differences in case fatality between pesticides that we found.

Future research

It is possible that other pesticides with apparently low case fatality based on small numbers may later emerge as important agents in poisoning as their agricultural use in rural Asia increases [20]. This possibility mandates a need for ongoing "toxico-vigilance" studies to follow any change in regulation. It is possible that examination of other important but nonfatal clinical outcomes may also help provide better estimates of the likely human fatal toxicity for these agents. While it is intuitive that a poisoning that never causes symptoms is less likely to be lethal than one that has caused major complications, but no deaths, the methodology for quantifying this hypothesis has not been developed.

CONCLUSION

There is marked variation in human lethality from acute poisoning within the existing pesticide classifications. Accounting for this in promotional, regulatory, and clinical decision making is likely to have a major impact upon overall mortality from suicide with pesticides and global suicide numbers.

REFERENCES

1. Gunnell D, Eddleston M, Phillips MR, Konradsen F (2007) The global distribution of fatal pesticide self-poisoning: systematic review. BMC Public Health 7: 357.
2. Gunnell D, Eddleston M (2003) Suicide by intentional ingestion of pesticides: a continuing tragedy in developing countries. Int J Epidemiol 32: 902–909.
3. Bertolote JM, Fleischmann A, Eddleston M, Gunnell D (2006) Deaths from pesticide poisoning: a global response. Br J Psychiatry 189: 201–203.
4. Eddleston M, Karunaratne A, Weerakoon M, Kumarasinghe S, Rajapakshe M, et al. (2006) Choice of poison for intentional self-poisoning in rural Sri Lanka. Clin Toxicol (Phila) 44: 283–286.
5. Eddleston M, Buckley NA, Gunnell D, Dawson AH, Konradsen F (2006) Identification of strategies to prevent death after pesticide self-poisoning using a Haddon matrix. Inj Prev 12: 333–337.
6. FAO (2003) International code of conduct on the distribution and use of pesticides. Rome: FAO. 9251049149 9251049149.
7. 7.Gunnell D, Fernando R, Hewagama M, Priyangika WD, Konradsen F, et al. (2007) The impact of pesticide regulations on suicide in Sri Lanka. Int J Epidemiol 36: 1235–1242.
8. Dawson A, Buckley N (2007) Integrating approaches to paraquat poisoning. Ceylon Med J 52: 45–47.
9. Eddleston M, Karalliedde L, Buckley N, Fernando R, Hutchinson G, et al. (2002) Pesticide poisoning in the developing world–a minimum pesticides list. Lancet 360: 1163–1167.
10. Wrighton SA, Stevens JC (1992) The human hepatic cytochromes P450 involved in drug metabolism. Crit Rev Toxicol 22: 1–21.
11. Tang J, Cao Y, Rose RL, Brimfield AA, Dai D, et al. (2001) Metabolism of chlorpyrifos by human cytochrome P450 isoforms and human, mouse, and rat liver microsomes. Drug Metab Dispos 29: 1201–1204.
12. Eddleston M, Sudarshan K, Senthilkumaran M, Reginald K, Karalliedde L, et al. (2006) Patterns of hospital transfer for self-poisoned patients in rural Sri Lanka: implications for estimating the incidence of self-poisoning in the developing world. Bull World Health Organ 84: 276–282.
13. Senarathna L (2006) How the level of resources and hospital staff attitude in primary care hospitals in rural Sri Lanka affect poisoning patient outcome. University of Newcastle. Available: http://www.sactrc.org/thesis.html Accessed 15 July 2010.
14. Eddleston M, Dawson A, Karalliedde L, Dissanayake W, Hittarage A, et al. (2004) Early management after self-poisoning with an organophosphorus or carbamate pesticide - a treatment protocol for junior doctors. Crit Care 8: R391–397.
15. Dean AGSK, Soe MM (2008) OpenEpi: open source epidemiologic statistics for public health, version 2.2.1. www.OpenEpi.com. 2.2.1 ed. Accessed 10 August 2009.
16. Eddleston M, Eyer P, Worek F, Mohamed F, Senarathna L, et al. (2005) Differences between organophosphorus insecticides in human self-poisoning: a prospective cohort study. Lancet 366: 1452–1459.
17. Srinivas Rao C, Venkateswarlu V, Surender T, Eddleston M, Buckley NA (2005) Pesticide poisoning in south India: opportunities for prevention and improved medical management. Trop Med Int Health 10: 581–588.
18. WHO (2005) The WHO recommended classification of pesticides by hazard and guidelines to classification 2004. Geneva: World Health Organisation.
19. Konradsen F, van der Hoek W, Gunnell D, Eddleston M (2005) Missing deaths from pesticide self-poisoning at the IFCS Forum IV. Bull World Health Organ 83: 157–158.
20. Roberts DM, Karunarathna A, Buckley NA, Manuweera G, Sheriff MH, et al. (2003) Influence of pesticide regulation on acute poisoning deaths in Sri Lanka. Bull World Health Organ 81: 789–798.
21. Manuweera G, Eddleston M, Egodage S, Buckley NA (2008) Do targeted bans of insecticides to prevent deaths from self-poisoning result in reduced agricultural output? Environ Health Perspect 116: 492–495.
22. Wilks MF, Fernando R, Ariyananda PL, Eddleston M, Berry DJ, et al. (2008) Improvement in survival after paraquat ingestion following introduction of a new formulation in Sri Lanka. PLoS Med 5: e49. doi:10.1371/journal.pmed.0050049.
23. Senarathna L, Adams J, De Silva D, Buckley NA, Dawson AH (2008) Personal and professional challenges in the management of deliberate self-poisoning patients in rural Sri Lanka: a qualitative study of rural hospital doctors' experiences and perceptions. BMC Public Health 8: 373.
24. Eddleston M, Rajapakshe M, Roberts D, Reginald K, Rezvi Sheriff MH, et al. (2002) Severe propanil [N-(3,4-dichlorophenyl) propanamide] pesticide self-poisoning. J Toxicol Clin Toxicol 40: 847–854.
25. Eddleston M, Haggalla S, Reginald K, Sudarshan K, Senthilkumaran M, et al. (2007) The hazards of gastric lavage for intentional self-poisoning in a resource poor location. Clin Toxicol (Phila) 45: 136–143.
26. Eddleston M, Wilks MF, Buckley NA (2003) Prospects for treatment of paraquat-induced lung fibrosis with immunosuppressive drugs and the need for better

prediction of outcome: a systematic review. QJM 96: 809–824.

27. Eddleston M, Buckley NA, Eyer P, Dawson AH (2008) Management of acute organophosphorus pesticide poisoning. Lancet 371: 597–607.

28. Roberts DM, Aaron CK (2007) Management of acute organophosphorus pesticide poisoning. BMJ 334: 629–634.

29. Lin TJ, Walter FG, Hung DZ, Tsai JL, Hu SC, et al. (2008) Epidemiology of organophosphate pesticide poisoning in Taiwan. Clin Toxicol (Phila) 46: 794–801.

30. Joshi PK, Gulati A, Birthal PS, Tewari L (2003) Agriculture diversification in South Asia: patterns, determinants, and policy implications. Econ Polit Wkly 39: 2457–2467.

31. Gunnell D, Fernando R, Hewagama M, Priyangika W, Konradsen F, et al. (2007) The impact of pesticide regulations on suicide in Sri Lanka. Int J Epidemiol 36: 1235–1242.

32. Eddleston M, Udayakumara N, Adhikari S, de Silva D, Sheriff MH, et al. (2007) The importance of poisoning vs. road traffic injuries as a cause of death in rural Sri Lanka. PLoS One 2: e599. doi:10.1371/journal.pone.0000599.

CHAPTER 27

DIFFERENTIAL EFFECTS OF METHYL-4-PHENYLPYRIDINIUM ION, ROTENONE, AND PARAQUAT ON DIFFERENTIATED SH-SY5Y CELLS

Martins JB, Bastos Mde L, Carvalho F, Capela JP.

INTRODUCTION

Parkinson's disease (PD) is considered the second most common neurodegenerative disorder worldwide, affecting 0.5 to 1% of the population aged between 65 and 69 years and 1 to 3% of the population over 80 years [1]. PD develops from a loss of nigrostriatal neuromelanin-containing dopaminergic neurons, whose cell bodies lay in the substantia nigra pars compacta (SNpc) [2]. This nigrostriatal pathway is essential for a normal motor function and movement control. PD is thought to have a multifactorial etiology, frequently including genetic and environmental factors [2, 3]. Several neurotoxic chemicals to dopaminergic neurons leading to PD-like symptoms have been used to study this disease. The synthetic compounds 1-methyl-4-phenyl-1,2,3,6-tetrahydropyridine (MPTP) and 1-methyl-4-phenyl-4-propionoxy-piperidine (MPPP) were the first to be associated with PD symptoms, as described by Langston and Ballard [4]. MPTP enters the blood-brain barrier and is metabolized in glial cells by monoamine oxidases to 1-methyl-4-phenyl-2,3-dihydropyridium ($MPDP^+$), which is subsequently oxidized to MPP^+ [5]. Next, MPP^+ enters the dopaminergic cell via dopamine transporter (DAT) [5], accumulates inside the mitochondria, and interferes with complex I of mitochondrial transport chain, inhibiting its activity [6]. This reduces ATP cellular stores, promoting reactive oxygen species (ROS) formation and consequentially leading to neuronal death [5]. Another substance known to promote Parkinsonism is the organic pesticide rotenone (ROT), which is used worldwide as an insecticide and to eliminate nuisance fish populations, in lakes and reservoirs [3]. It is used to study PD given its ability to cross biological membranes, not depending on transporters, inhibiting mitochondrial complex I [7] which increases the rate of mitochondrial ROS release, leading to cell apoptosis [3, 8]. Despite their use as PD models, neither ROT nor MPP^+ were correlated with the sporadic occurrence of PD [8]. These two neurotoxicants are currently used to study PD by means of in vivo and in vitro approaches; however, none of these substances reproduces completely all the clinical features observed in PD [8, 9].

The lack of adequate cellular and/or animal models of PD has prompted the screening of many putative neurotoxic compounds. Paraquat (PQ) has received recently a wide attention as a possible inducer of PD. In fact, occupational exposure, especially in farming, has been associated with Parkinsonism [10] and also, it was demonstrated that patients who died from PQ poisoning had severe brain damage [11].

Citation: João Barbosa Martins, Maria de Lourdes Bastos, Félix Carvalho, and João Paulo Capela, "Differential Effects of Methyl-4-Phenylpyridinium Ion, Rotenone, and Paraquat on Differentiated SH-SY5Y Cells," Journal of Toxicology, vol. 2013, Article ID 347312, 10 pages, 2013. doi:10.1155/2013/347312

This was corroborated by studies, in animals, where besides the affection of the lung which is the main target organ for PQ toxicity, it was also demonstrated to be toxic to dopaminergic neurons [12, 13]. Several mechanisms have been postulated for PQ-induced neurotoxicity, including increase in ROS formation, excitotoxicity, and mitochondrial complex I inhibition [14–16]. Nonetheless, the mechanisms by which PQ promotes neurotoxicity still remain to be fully elucidated.

The present work aimed to study the differences in terms of dopaminergic neurotoxic profile among PQ, ROT, and MPP^+ in a cell culture model with a dopaminergic phenotype. Also, we intended to provide further insights into the mechanism of PQ-induced neurotoxicity. For that purpose, human dopaminergic SH-SY5Y-differentiated cells were used.

MATERIALS AND METHODS

Materials

The reagents for cell culture were obtained from Gibco (Invitrogen, Paisley, UK): Dulbecco's Modified Eagle Medium (D-MEM), nonessential amino acids (NEAA), phosphate-buffered saline (PBS), trypsin/EDTA, and penicillin/streptomycin. 48 Multiwell plates and 35 mm plates were obtained from Corning Costar (Corning, NY, USA). 25 cm^3 flasks were obtained from TPP (Trasadingen, Switzerland); Fuchs-Rosenthal Counting Chamber was obtained from Carl-Rhode (Germany). Other reagents, namely, trypan blue solution (0.4%), dimethyl sulfoxide (DMSO), retinoic acid (RA), 12-O-tetradecanoyl-phorbol-13-acetate (TPA), 3-[4,5-dimethylthiazol]-2,5-diphenyltetrazolium (MTT), sodium dodecyl sulfate (SDS), enzyme-standard for kinetic lactate dehydrogenase (LDH)-assay, β-nicotinamide adenine dinucleotide reduced form (β-NADH), 1,1′-dimethyl-4,4′-bipyridinium dichloride (Paraquat or PQ), rotenone (ROT), 1-methyl-4-phenyl-pyridinium ion (MPP^+), N-acetylcysteine (NAC), tiron (TIR), 1-(2-[bis(4-fluorophenyl)methoxy]ethyl)-4-(3-phenyl-propyl)piperazine (GBR 12909), cycloheximide (CHX), 2-hydroxybenzoic acid sodium salt (NaSAL), and N_ω-nitro-L-arginine methyl ester hydrochloride (L-NAME), were obtained from Sigma-Aldrich (St Louis, MO, USA).

Cell Line and Culture Conditions

Human neuroblastoma SH-SY5Y cells (ATCC, Manassas, VA, USA) were used. Through differentiation (see protocol below), SH-SY5Y cells are able to express dopaminergic markers, as well as tyrosine hydroxylase, DAT, and higher ability to accumulate dopamine and exhibit extended neurites [17, 18]. In this way, the cells are no longer immature, mitosis rate is reduced, and also differentiation agents can mimic factors secreted by astrocytes in a the natural brain environment. In other words, differentiation can provide a cellular model more similar to dopaminergic neurons [17, 18]. The cells were grown in D-MEM containing 4.5 mg/L D-glucose, 2 mM L-glutamine, 110 mg/L sodium pyruvate, phenol red supplemented with 10% fetal bovine serum, 100 µg/mL penicillin, 100 µg/mL streptomycin, and 1% NEAA, under an atmosphere of 5% CO_2/95% air at 37°C.

Experimental Protocol

Stock cultures of SH-SY5Y cells (passages 20 to 45) were maintained in 25 cm^3 flasks and grown until confluence (70–80% confluence). Cells were washed with PBS, trypsinized (trypsin/EDTA 0.05/0.02% w/v), counted by trypan blue exclusion, using a Fuchs-Rosenthal counting chamber, and subcultured at the density of 25 000 cells/cm^2 in 48-well culture plates. SH-SY5Y cells were differentiated, in order to enhance the dopaminergic phenotype, by the addition of 10 µM RA to the medium for 3 days, after which the medium was added with 70 nM TPA and kept for another 3 days, in accordance with previous works [17, 18]. Finally, the medium was removed and replaced with 250 µL fresh medium alone or with the drugs: PQ (100, 500, and 1000 µM), MPP^+ (100, 500, and 1000 µM) and ROT (1, 10, and 100 µM). Concentrations of the neurotoxicants were selected in accordance with previous studies [19–24]. The cells were exposed to the drugs for different time periods (24, 48, and 72 h). ROT was initially prepared in DMSO and then diluted in medium in order to obtain a final concentration of 0.1% of DMSO in the culture medium, which was not toxic to cells. To avoid variations among cell cultures that could interfere in the toxicity outcome, results for the concentration-toxicity curves of the 3 toxins were obtained from several cell cultures resulting from different passages and were seeded in different days. Cell culture procedures and validation of the differentiation protocol of SH-SY5Y cells were previously published by our group [18]. After selecting the concentration and time of exposure through screening experiments, the antioxidants NAC (1 mM) [25], and TIR (100 µM and 1 mM) [26], the specific DAT inhibitor GBR 12909 (1 µM) [23], the protein synthesis inhibitor CHX (1.8 nM) [27], the radical scavenger NaSAL (100 µM and 1 mM) [28], and the nonselective nitric oxide synthase (NOS) inhibitor L-NAME (1 µM) [29] were added 30 minutes before exposure of cells to PQ. These concentrations of the pharmacological antagonists were selected according to the drug selectivity to the target and also taking into account previous cell culture studies mentioned above.

Life-Death Assays

Cell cultures were assessed morphologically by phase contrast microscopy at 3 different time points (24, 48, and 72 h). Cell damage was assessed quantitatively by the measurement of LDH release into the medium (as a measure of cell membrane integrity) using a kinetic measurement assay. Also, mitochondrial dysfunction was assessed by the measurement of MTT salt metabolism assay.

Lactate Dehydrogenase Kinetic Assay

The quantification of LDH activity was made by a colorimetric method, which is based on the reversible reduction of pyruvate to lactate in the presence of β-NADH, as described by Capela et al., 2006. After exposure to drugs, two aliquots (50 µL each) of the medium were removed, to which a previously prepared 0.15 mg/mLβ-NADH solution was added, at room temperature, in a 96-well microplate. Finally, pyruvate 22.7 mM was added to start the reaction. NADH oxidation to NAD^+ was measured at 340 nm, using a colorimetric 96-well plate reader (BioTek Instruments, VT, USA). The delta increase in LDH release into the medium was calculated by subtraction of the respective controls, which were untreated cells cultured alongside the treated cells. LDH values are expressed in units per liter (U/L), calculated based on a LDH standard solution activity of 500 U/L [29].

MTT Assay

This colorimetric assay relies on the ability of viable, but not dead cells to convert a soluble yellow tetrazolium dye, MTT, into an insoluble blue formazan product that can be measured at 550 nm. Given the removal of 100 µL of culture medium used for the LDH assay, each well was added 50 µL fresh medium to obtain 200 µL of cell medium per well, to which the MTT solution was added (final concentration of MTT 500 µg/mL). Subsequently, cells were incubated at 36.5°C for 3 hours. The reaction was stopped by adding an equal volume of 10% SDS in 0.01 M hydrochloric acid solution followed by an overnight incubation at 36.5°C. Finally, formazan was detected at 550 nm using a colorimetric 96-well plate reader, as previously described [29]. The viability of untreated control cells was set to 100%, and the effects resulting from toxicant exposure were expressed as the percentage of the respective controls.

Statistical Analysis

Results are presented as mean ± S.E.M., from at least 3 different independent experiments. The means for concentration/time graphics were compared using the two-way ANOVA, followed by the Bonferroni post hoc test, once a significant P had been obtained. The means for the tested neuroprotectors were compared using the one-way ANOVA, followed by Student-Newman-Keuls post hoc test, once a significant P had been obtained. Details of the statistical analyses are described in each figure legend. Significance was accepted when P was less than 0.05.

RESULTS

Paraquat Was Toxic to SH-SY5Y Cells in a Concentration- and Time-Dependent Manner

The exposure of differentiated SH-SY5Y cells to PQ (100 µM, 500 µM and 1000 µM) for 24 h, did not result in elevation of LDH release at any concentration tested (data not shown). However, at 48 h there was a significant LDH release with 500 µM, which was even more marked with 1000 µM exposure. As expected, LDH release into the medium was more pronounced at 72 h, for 500 and 1000 µM. Thus, the loss of cellular viability occurred in a concentration- and time-dependent manner (Figure 1(a)). Mitochondrial dysfunction was assayed by the MTT assay. In contrast to cellular death evaluated by the LDH release, mitochondrial dysfunction was already visible at the 24 h time-point for the 500 µM and 1000 µM concentrations. For the 100 µM concentration, PQ decreased significantly MTT reduction at 48 h but especially at 72 h. Therefore, it could be clearly observed that mitochondrial dysfunction also occurred in a concentration- and time-dependent manner (Figure 1(b)).

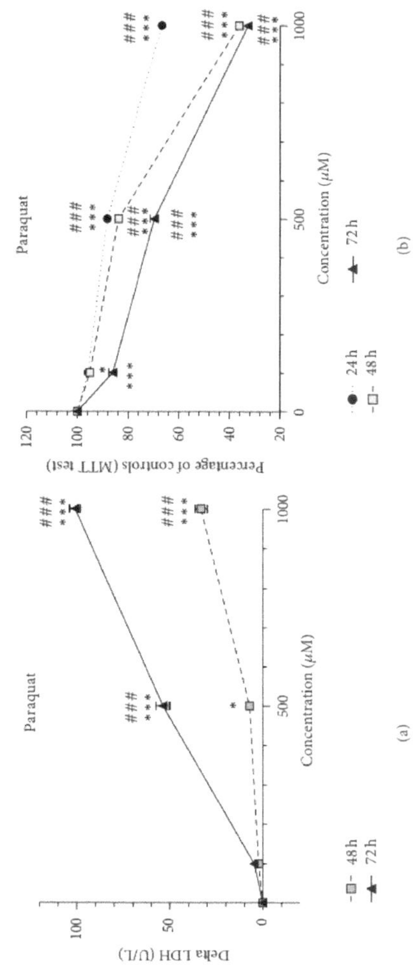

Figure 1: PQ toxicity occurred in a concentration- and time-dependent manner in differentiated SH-SY5Y cells. Cells were incubated with 100, 500 and 1000 µM of PQ for 24, 48 and 72 h. (a) Increase in LDH release into the medium in differentiated SH-SY5Y cells. The delta increase in LDH release in units per liter (U/L) into the medium was calculated by subtraction of the respective controls (results were pooled from 3 different experiments, each experiment having 6 different culture wells per condition). (b) Mitochondrial dysfunction in differentiated SH-SY5Y cells evaluated by the MTT test. The viability of untreated control cells was set to 100%, and all treatments were expressed as the percentage of the respective controls (results were pooled from 3 different experiments, each experiment having 6 different culture wells per condition). The means were compared using the two-way ANOVA test, followed by the Bonferroni post hoc test ($^{*}P < 0.05$, $^{***}P < 0.001$ concentration versus control; $^{\#\#\#}P < 0.001$ concentration versus concentration).

MPP$^+$-Induced Mitochondrial Dysfunction in SH-SY5Y Cells

Following exposure of SH-SY5Y cells to MPP$^+$ (100 µM, 500 µM, and 1000 µM), there was no increase in cell injury at any time-point or concentration tested, as assessed by the LDH release into the medium (data not shown). On the other hand, MPP$^+$ proved to induce mitochondrial dysfunction (Figure 2). In fact, there was significant mitochondrial dysfunction already after 24 h of exposure to 500 µM, and 1000 µM concentrations. There was no apparent increase in the toxicity by extending the exposure period to 48 h. However, at 72 h MTT metabolism decreased significantly for all concentrations tested, especially for 1000 μM. Only at this point the toxicity of 1000 μM was significantly higher than 500 μM (Figure 2). Thus, only longer periods of exposure resulted in a concentration-dependent effect.

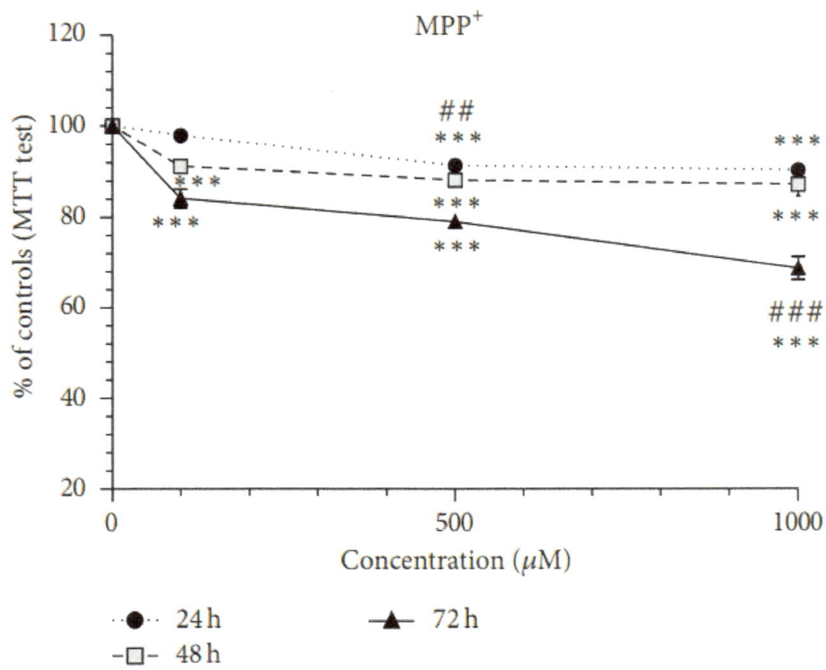

Figure 2: MPP^+-induced mitochondrial dysfunction in differentiated SH-SY5Y. The cells were incubated with 100, 500, and 1000 μM of MPP^+, and the MTT test was performed at 24, 48, and 72 h time-points. Mitochondrial dysfunction in differentiated SH-SY5Y cells evaluated by the MTT test. The viability of untreated control cells was set to 100%, and all treatments were expressed as the percentage of the respective controls (results were pooled from 3 different experiments, each experiment having 6 different culture wells per condition). The means were compared using the two-way ANOVA, followed by the Bonferroni post hoc test ($^{***}P < 0.001$ concentration versus control $^{\#\#}P < 0.01$, $^{\#\#\#}P < 0.001$ concentration versus concentration).

Rotenone Induced a Biphasic Pattern of Neurotoxicity in SH-SY5Y Cells

Exposure of SH-SY5Y cells to ROT (1 μM, 10 μM, and 100 μM) did not result in LDH release into the medium, at the 24 h time-point (data not shown). Interestingly, ROT exhibited a biphasic pattern of cellular lyses, at the 48 h time-point (Figure 3(a)). At this time-point, 1 μM ROT led to a significant reduction of LDH release into the medium, to levels below those of controls. Meanwhile, the 10 μM concentration elicited an increase in LDH release, which was significantly higher than that observed for 100 μM. Thus, cell injury occurred in a concentration-independent manner. After 72 h exposure there was a concentration-dependent toxicity. Curiously, values for LDH release at 48 h and 72 h for the 10 μM concentration were very similar (Figure 3(a)).

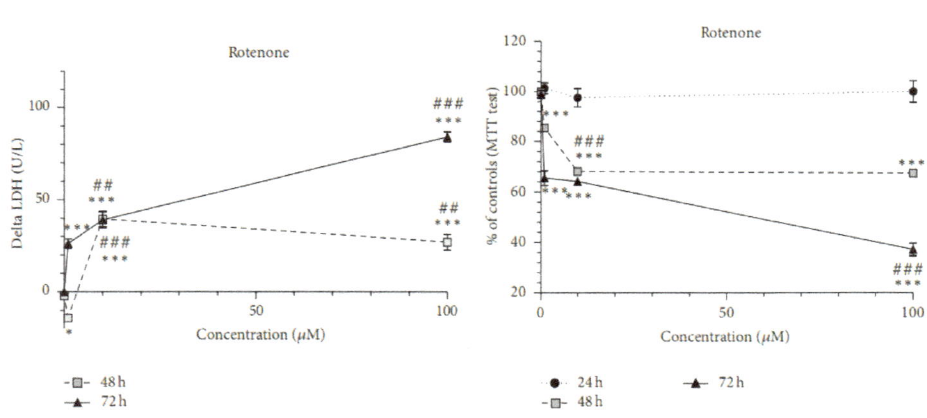

Figure 3: ROT-induced neurotoxicity showed a biphasic pattern with mitochondrial dysfunction and cell death in differentiated SH-SY5Y cells. The cells were incubated with 1, 10, and 100 μM of ROT, and then MTT and LDH tests were performed at 24, 48, and 72 h time points. (a) Increase in LDH release in units per liter (U/L) into the medium in differentiated SH-SY5Y cells. The delta increase in LDH release into the medium was calculated by subtraction of the respective controls (results were pooled from 3 different experiments, each experiment having 6 different culture wells per condition). (b) Mitochondrial dysfunction in differentiated SH-SY5Y cells evaluated by the MTT test. The viability

of untreated control cells was set to 100%, and all treatments were expressed as the percentage of the respective controls (results were pooled from 3 different experiments, each experiment having 6 different culture wells per condition). The means were compared using the two-way ANOVA, followed by the Bonferroni post hoc test ($^{***}P < 0.001$ concentration versus control; $^{\#\#}P < 0.01$, $^{\#\#\#}P < 0.001$ concentration versus concentration).

Exposure for 24 h to 10 μM, and 100 μM ROT did not induce mitochondrial dysfunction (Figure 3(b)). After 48 h exposure there was an increase of mitochondrial dysfunction from 1 μM to 10 μM, in which values were similar to those of the 100 μM concentration. However, after 72 h exposure there was a concentration-dependent toxicity, with the highest levels of mitochondrial dysfunction attaining values below 50% at 100 μM. Comparing the exposure during 24 or 48 h, mostly 10 μM and 100 μM ROT induced a time-dependent increase in mitochondrial dysfunction (Figure 3(b)).

Tiron and Sodium Salicylate Provided Protection against Paraquat Neurotoxicity

To carry out neuroprotective experiments in human neuroblastoma-differentiated SH-SY5Y cells, we selected the 500 μM PQ concentration and the 72 h exposure period, since under these conditions mitochondrial dysfunction reached about 50% of controls and cell injury was significant. The cells were preincubated with NAC (1 mM), TIR (100 μM and 1 mM), and NaSAL (100 μM, 1 mM, and 10 mM) 30 minutes before exposing cells to PQ. Putative protective drugs alone were also tested for their respective toxicities (Figure 4).

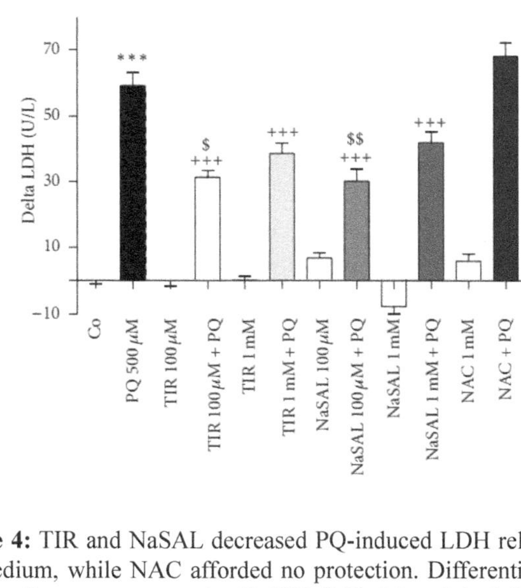

Figure 4: TIR and NaSAL decreased PQ-induced LDH release into the medium, while NAC afforded no protection. Differentiated SH-SY5Y cells were pretreated with TIR (100 μM and 1 mM), NaSAL (100 μM, 1 mM), and NAC (1 mM) 30 minutes prior to cultures exposure to PQ for 72 h. The delta increase in LDH release in units per liter (U/L) into the medium was calculated by subtraction of the respective controls (results were pooled from 3 different experiments, each experiment having 6 different culture wells per condition). The means were compared using one-way ANOVA, followed by Student-Newman-Keuls post hoc test ($^{***}P < 0.001$ PQ versus control; $^{+++}P < 0.001$ PQ versus PQ plus protector; $^{\$}P < 0.05$, $^{\$\$}P < 0.01$ PQ plus protector low concentration versus PQ plus protector high concentration).

TIR and NaSAL, both antioxidants, provided partial protection against 500 μM PQ neurotoxicity, as revealed by the LDH assay (Figure 4). The protective action of the referred compounds was only detected in cell injury, revealed by the LDH assay, since these compounds did not offer any protection against mitochondrial dysfunction, as revealed by the MTT assay (data not shown). For both TIR and NaSAL, the protective effect was higher at 100 μM of both protectors comparatively to the 1 mM concentration (Figure 4). Interestingly, NaSAL alone at the 1 mM concentration showed lower LDH release than controls, seemingly to reduce cell death occurring in untreated cells (Figure 4).

NAC, an antioxidant and glutathione precursor, did not provide any protection against PQ-induced toxicity as revealed both by LDH and MTT assays (Figure 4).

GBR 12909, Cycloheximide, and L-NAME Provide Protection against Paraquat Neurotoxicity

GBR 12909 (1 μM), a dopamine transporter blocker, CHX (1.8 nM), a protein synthesis inhibitor, and L-NAME (1 μM), a NOS inhibitor, provided significant protection against PQ neurotoxicity, as revealed by the LDH assay (Figure 5). CHX proved to be the most effective. On the other hand, none of the tested drugs proved protection against mitochondrial dysfunction induced by PQ (data not shown).

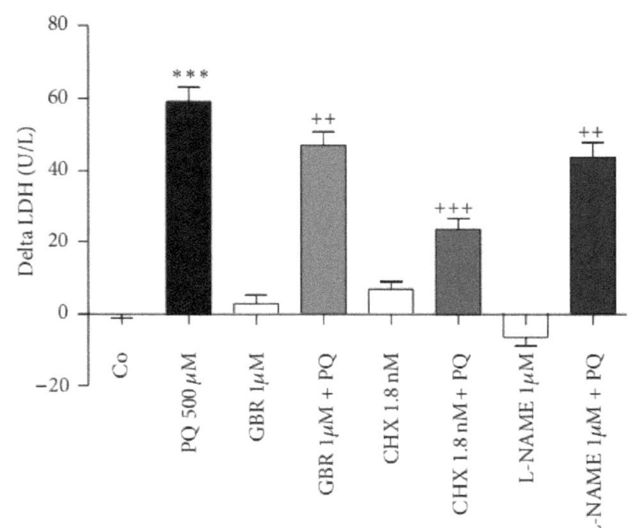

Figure 5: CHX, GBR 12909, and L-NAME decreased PQ-induced LDH release into the medium. Differentiated SH-SY5Y cells were pretreated with GBR 12909 (1 μM), CHX (1,8 nM), and L-NAME (1 μM) 30 minutes prior to cultures exposure to PQ for 72 h. The delta increase in LDH release in units per liter (U/L) into the medium was calculated by subtraction of the respective controls (results were pooled from 3 different experiments, each experiment having 6 different culture wells per condition). The means were compared using one-way ANOVA, followed by Student-Newman-Keuls post hoc test ($^{***}P < 0.001$ PQ versus control; $^{++}P < 0.01$, $^{+++}P < 0.001$ PQ versus PQ plus protector).

DISCUSSION

The key findings of our study conducted in differentiated dopaminergic SH-SY5Y cells were as follows: (1) PQ-induced neurotoxicity was concentration and time dependent, promoting a delayed type of cell death with an early mitochondrial dysfunction; (2) MPP^+ promoted mitochondrial dysfunction, especially at higher times of exposure, but not cellular lyses;

(3) ROT-induced neurotoxicity showed a biphasic pattern promoting a delayed type of cell death at later time-points of exposure and higher concentrations; (4) PQ neurotoxicity could be partially prevented by antioxidants, DAT inhibitors, NOS inhibitors, and protein synthesis inhibitors.

MPP^+, ROT, and PQ are viewed as experimental toxicants to study PD mechanisms in vitro [9, 30]. MPP^+ and ROT are commonly used instead of PQ, because of their well-known mechanisms of toxicity. In addition, studies using MPP^+ and ROT have already given significant insights into the molecular mechanisms of dopaminergic neuronal death [24, 31]. However, there is a need for more reliable cultured cell models of PD. Several studies using SH-SY5Y cells with these neurotoxicants have been published, without ever having fully elucidated their differential effects, concerning to cell death and optimal concentrations. In the present study, we compared the neurotoxicity of PQ with that of ROT and MPP^+ using differentiated dopaminergic SH-SY5Y cells. Our data demonstrated that PQ toxicity involved mitochondrial dysfunction and cell death. The increase in LDH release and mitochondrial dysfunction after PQ exposure occurred in a concentration and time dependent manner and was more pronounced at late times of exposure. We verified the existence of two events, an earlier damage to the mitochondrial electronic transport chain that may precede a later membrane burst, typical of cellular lyses. This cellular membrane disruption may be also promoted by external aggressions or other unknown mechanisms promoted by PQ. Our results are in accordance with our analysis, since mitochondrial dysfunction occurred at 24 h and LDH was not measurable at this time point. At higher PQ concentrations and times of exposure, once cells are not intact, the mitochondrial chain is not functional, thus leading to low MTT metabolism.

When compared to MPP^+, PQ induced a more pronounced mitochondrial dysfunction and cell injury for the same concentrations and time of exposure. Mitochondrial dysfunction may corroborate the hypothesis that PQ, like MPP^+, inhibits the complex I of the mitochondrial chain [6, 23]. Our study showed that in the same concentration range (100 to 1000 μM) PQ, but not MPP^+, induced cell lyses and LDH release. This event occurred several hours after mitochondrial dysfunction, since LDH release became only evident after 48 h exposure. In fact, MPP^+ exposed cells might have lost their metabolic capacity but yet not their membrane integrity, suggesting delayed cell death. Not only SH-SY5Y-differentiated cells seem to be more susceptible to PQ but also PQ is more stable in solution than MPP^+, which is photosensitive and may lose activity when in solution with longer exposure periods. Therefore, PQ may represent several advantages over MPP^+ to study Parkinson's mechanisms in vitro, namely, when using cultured cells.

Concerning ROT, a widely used toxicant to promote dopaminergic toxicity, it showed a biphasic pattern of neurotoxicity. Our results are not in agreement with those presented by Molina-Jimenez [19], who observed that ROT caused a proportional time- and dose-dependent decrease in SH-SY5Y cellular viability. This can be explained by a different cell culture protocol, namely, their FBS removal and lower cellular density. Herein, ROT, at 1 μM for 48 h, reduced cell lyses and promoted lower LDH leakage compared to control cells, an effect no longer seen at latter times of exposure. On the other hand, the MTT assay proved mitochondrial dysfunction after 48 h exposure to 1 μM. This may be connected to a late death pattern, as ROT is postulated to be a high affinity complex I inhibitor [7] and to induce apoptosis via activation of caspase 3 apoptosis pathway [20]. In fact, ROT binds near to the quinone-binding site and blocks electron transport, preventing NADH from being converted to ATP; in this way the proton pumping is compromised, which culminates in increased superoxide generation, and consequent cell death [32]. Cell membrane rupture occurs several hours after compromising the metabolic activity at lower concentrations, though at higher concentrations it may demonstrate toxicity by other means [8]. Other studies showed that ROT causes apoptosis at low doses and necrosis when applied at high doses, thus corroborating our results [33]. We demonstrated in SH-SY5Y cells that PQ promoted a more defined pattern of time-concentration-dependent cell death; meanwhile, ROT induced a biphasic pattern of toxicity. Moreover, PQ chloride salt is water soluble, while ROT has to be prepared in DMSO, which is an hazardous substance. Therefore, PQ may represent advantages over ROT to study Parkinson's mechanisms in vitro, at least in SH-SY5Y-differentiated cells.

Comparing the toxicity of ROT and MPP^+ in SH-SY5Y-differentiated cells, one can conclude that ROT promoted a higher grade of mitochondrial dysfunction and cell injury than MPP^+. In fact, 10 times lower concentrations of ROT and shorter exposure times were required for achieving the degree of toxicity seen with MPP^+. One possible explanation may be that ROT does not need a transporter to enter the cells as it crosses membranes by diffusion [7]. Our results are in accordance with Richardson and collaborators who demonstrated that higher MPP^+ concentrations were required to achieve the same degree of complex I inhibition, showing that ROT has a higher complex I affinity [8]. In contrast to ROT, the concentrations of MPP^+ used in our SH-SY5Y-differentiated cells did not result in cell lyses during the 72 h of exposure. Other studies using SH-SY5Y have reported cell death using higher concentrations of MPP^+, up to 10 mM [22, 34,35]. Moreover, differentiated SH-SY5Y cells have an enhanced resistance towards neurotoxins. Our group recently showed that differentiation of SH-SY5Y cells with RA and TPA led to SH-SY5Y neurons with higher ability to accumulate dopamine and higher resistance towards dopamine neurotoxicity [18]. Importantly, a study by Cheung and coauthors demonstrated that differentiation of SH-SY5Y cells with RA conferred higher resistance towards MPP^+ toxicity [36]. Thus, using higher concentrations of MPP^+ and longer periods of exposure should be necessary to obtain significant cell lyses.

Our study demonstrated that several compounds could partially prevent or slow PQ-induced toxicity. NaSAL is known to prevent PQ-induced apoptosis in the rat lung [37]. In fact, one of the proposed mechanisms of PQ neurotoxicity is oxidative stress by producing ROS such as superoxide anion ($O_2^{\bullet -}$), hydroxyl radicals ($OH^\bullet$), and hydrogen peroxide (H_2O_2), which increase lipid peroxidation, increase oxidation of proteins, DNA and iron content and promote a marked decrease in reduced glutathione (GSH) and GSH/glutathione disulfide ratio [23, 38]. Oxidative stress is also a typical feature of PD brains [39]. Salicylates are important $HO^\bullet$ scavengers and therefore reduce PQ toxicity [37]. On the other hand, salicylates may also form stable complexes with PQ [40]. These two proposed mechanisms may be the explanation of the neuroprotection obtained by us with NaSAL against PQ-induced injury. Interestingly, NaSAL did not prevent mitochondrial dysfunction. On the other hand, LDH values were reduced, possibly because direct cellular membrane damage was prevented, either by complex forming or oxidative radical reduction. Still PQ may promote toxicity by other means, once neurotoxicity was not fully prevented.

Another antioxidant used, TIR, partially prevented PQ-induced neurotoxicity. TIR is a known scavenger of $O_2^{\bullet-}$, acting both at extracellular and intracellular levels. $O_2^{\bullet-}$ that originated from PQ redox cycle can be scavenged by TIR, therefore affording protection. Also, $O_2^{\bullet-}$ can be converted further to H_2O_2 and to $HO^{\bullet}$through Fenton-type reactions, using Fe^{2+}, promoting more oxidative stress [41]. However, TIR only partially prevented cell lyses and not mitochondrial dysfunction promoted by PQ, which may indicate that its neurotoxicity occurred by additional mechanisms.

PQ-induced cell death might occur through the formation of reactive nitrogen species (RNS), which also promote oxidative stress. The NOS inhibitor L-NAME also attenuated PQ toxicity. Nitric oxide produced by NOS forms peroxynitrite anion, by reacting with $O_2^{\bullet-}$ produced in the redox-cycle of PQ, crosses membranes, and can easily oxidize proteins, lipids, RNA, and DNA [42]. Overall the protective effects of the two antioxidants and the NO synthesis inhibitor corroborate the hypothesis that oxidative stress is a major mechanism of PQ neurotoxicity [23, 42, 43].

Our study revealed that CHX, a protein synthesis inhibitor, protected against PQ-induced neurotoxicity. Therefore, PQ-induced cell death might involve proteins, whose synthesis is prevented by CHX. Protein synthesis is involved in many processes of programmed and nonprogrammed cell death, and therefore PQ-induced dopaminergic death might involve those processes [44].

GBR 12909 conferred partial protection against PQ-induced neurotoxicity revealing that PQ entrance into the dopaminergic neuron might occur through the DAT transporter, which is corroborated by Yang and Tiffany-Castiglioni [23]. Since PQ is structurally very similar to MPP^+, it may as well use dopamine transporters [45], though this still remains a controversial issue, as there are contrary opinions like that of Richardson and collaborators [8], who claim that PQ toxicity is independent of DAT expression or Ramachandiran and coauthors [46], who claim that PQ does not require a functional dopamine transporter for dopaminergic toxicity. In fact, we found that despite DAT blocking, PQ still exerts neurotoxicity, so it is suggested that it may nevertheless enter the cell or exert toxic effects on the outside leading to cellular lyses.

Other studies have evaluated the effects of the pharmacological agents that we used against PQ neurotoxicity to circumvent MPP^+ or ROT neurotoxicity. L-NAME did not present any significant protection to MPP^+ toxicity in SH-SY5Y cells [47], whereas GBR 12909 blocked its neurotoxic effects [17]. Meanwhile, CHX reduced proapoptotic proteins production in response to MPP^+-induced toxicity [48], and also CHX blocked MPP^+-induced cell death in the dopaminergic cell line MN9D [49]. In rats, NaSAL significantly attenuated striatal dopamine depletion caused by intrastriatal MPP^+ infusion [50]. In what concerns ROT, CHX was demonstrated to reduce cell death in cultured cortical neurons [51]. In another study, GBR 12909 significantly prevented the ROT-induced decrease of cell viability in PC12 cells [52]. In rats, NaSAL demonstrated neuroprotective efficacy against ROT toxicity [53]. Also, in oral cancer cell lines ROT-induced apoptosis was inhibited by TIR [54].

CONCLUSIONS

The results obtained in the present study showed that PQ promoted a diverse profile of toxicity when compared to MPP^+ and ROT and could present advantages over those two toxicants for modelling PD in vitro. In fact, PQ in differentiated dopaminergic SH-SY5Y cells promoted a concentration- and time-dependent toxicity, promoting a delayed type of cell death with mitochondrial dysfunction leading to cellular lyses. We further studied the mechanisms of PQ-induced toxicity and demonstrated that antioxidants, NOS inhibitors, DAT inhibitors, and protein synthesis inhibitors could be useful tools in preventing dopaminergic toxicity, at least in vitro.

CONFLICT OF INTERESTS

The authors declare no conflict of interests.

ACKNOWLEDGMENTS

This work received financial support from "Fundacão para a Ciência e Tecnologia," Portugal (Project PTDC/SAU-FCF/102958/2008), under the frame of "Programa Operacional Temático Factores de Competitividade (COMPTE) do Quadro Comunitário de Apoio III" and "Fundo Comunitário Europeu (FEDER) (FCOMP-01-0124-FEDER-011079)." J. P. Capela was the recipient of a Postdoc grant from "Fundação para a Ciência e a Tecnologia," Portugal (SFRH/BPD/30776/2006).

REFERENCES

1. L. M. de Lau and M. M. Breteler, "Epidemiology of Parkinson's disease," The Lancet Neurology, vol. 5, no. 6, pp. 525–535, 2006.
2. P. Piccini, D. J. Burn, R. Ceravolo, D. Maraganore, and D. J. Brooks, "The role of inheritance in sporadic Parkinson's disease: evidence from a longitudinal study of dopaminergic function in twins," Annals of Neurology, vol. 45, no. 5, pp. 577–582, 1999.
3. R. Betarbet, T. B. Sherer, G. MacKenzie, M. Garcia-Osuna, A. V. Panov, and J. T. Greenamyre, "Chronic systemic pesticide exposure reproduces features of Parkinson's disease," Nature Neuroscience, vol. 3, no. 12, pp. 1301–1306, 2000.
4. J. W. Langston and P. A. Ballard Jr., "Parkinson's disease in a chemist working with 1-methyl-4-phenyl-1,2,5,6-tetrahydropyridine," The New England Journal of Medicine, vol. 309, no. 5, article 310, 1983.
5. R. J. Smeyne and V. Jackson-Lewis, "The MPTP model of Parkinson's disease," Molecular Brain Research, vol. 134, no. 1, pp. 57–66, 2005.
6. K. Suzuki, Y. Mizuno, and M. Yoshida, "Effects of 1-methyl-4-phenyl-1,2,3,6-tetrahydropyridine (MPTP)-like compounds on mitochondrial respiration," Advances in Neurology, vol. 53, pp. 215–218, 1990.
7. J. T. Greenamyre, R. Betarbet, and T. B. Sherer,

"The rotenone model of Parkinson's disease: genes, environment and mitochondria," Parkinsonism and Related Disorders, vol. 9, supplement 2, pp. S59–S64, 2003.

8. J. R. Richardson, Y. Quan, T. B. Sherer, J. T. Greenamyre, and G. W. Miller, "Paraquat neurotoxicity is distinct from that of MPTP and rotenone," Toxicological Sciences, vol. 88, no. 1, pp. 193–201, 2005.
9. J. Bové, D. Prou, C. Perier, and S. Przedborski, "Toxin-induced models of Parkinson's disease," NeuroRx, vol. 2, no. 3, pp. 484–494, 2005.
10. J. M. Gorell, C. C. Johnson, B. A. Rybicki, E. L. Peterson, and R. J. Richardson, "The risk of Parkinson's disease with exposure to pesticides, farming, well water, and rural living," Neurology, vol. 50, no. 5, pp. 1346–1350, 1998.
11. J. T. Hughes, "Brain damage due to Paraquat poisoning: a fatal case with neuropathological examination of the brain," NeuroToxicology, vol. 9, no. 2, pp. 243–248, 1988.
12. M. J. Kang, S. J. Gil, and H. C. Koh, "Paraquat induces alternation of the dopamine catabolic pathways and glutathione levels in the substantia nigra of mice," Toxicology Letters, vol. 188, no. 2, pp. 148–152, 2009.
13. L. McCormack, M. Thiruchelvam, A. B. Manning-Bog et al., "Environmental risk factors and Parkinson's disease: selective degeneration of nigral dopaminergic neurons caused by the herbicide paraquat," Neurobiology of Disease, vol. 10, no. 2, pp. 119–127, 2002.
14. K. Shimizu, K. Matsubara, K. Ohtaki, S. Fujimaru, O. Saito, and H. Shiono, "Paraquat induces long-lasting dopamine overflow through the excitotoxic pathway in the striatum of freely moving rats," Brain Research, vol. 976, no. 2, pp. 243–252, 2003.
15. T. Tawara, T. Fukushima, N. Hojo et al., "Effects of paraquat on mitochondrial electron transport system and catecholamine contents in rat brain," Archives of Toxicology, vol. 70, no. 9, pp. 585–589, 1996.
16. D. Bagchi, M. Bagchi, E. A. Hassoun, and S. J. Stohs, "In vitro and in vivo generation of reactive oxygen species, DNA damage and lactate dehydrogenase leakage by selected pesticides," Toxicology, vol. 104, no. 1–3, pp. 129–140, 1995.
17. S. P. Presgraves, T. Ahmed, S. Borwege, and J. N. Joyce, "Terminally differentiated SH-SY5Y cells provide a model system for studying neuroprotective effects of dopamine agonists," Neurotoxicity Research, vol. 5, no. 8, pp. 579–598, 2003.
18. P. S. Ferreira, T. B. Nogueira, V. M. Costa et al., "Neurotoxicity of "ecstasy" and its metabolites in human dopaminergic differentiated SH-SY5Y cells," Toxicology Letters, vol. 216, no. 2-3, pp. 159–170, 2013.
19. M. F. Molina-Jimenez, M. I. Sanchez-Reus, and J. Benedi, "Effect of fraxetin and myricetin on rotenone-induced cytotoxicity in SH-SY5Y cells: comparison with N-acetylcysteine," European Journal of Pharmacology, vol. 472, no. 1-2, pp. 81–87, 2003.
20. T. Pan, P. Rawal, Y. Wu, W. Xie, J. Jankovic, and W. Le, "Rapamycin protects against rotenone-induced apoptosis through autophagy induction," Neuroscience, vol. 164, no. 2, pp. 541–551, 2009.
21. K. Y. Chau, L. V. P. Korlipara, J. M. Cooper, and A. H. V. Schapira, "Protection against paraquat and A53T alpha-synuclein toxicity by cabergoline is partially mediated by dopamine receptors," Journal of the Neurological Sciences, vol. 278, no. 1-2, pp. 44–53, 2009.
22. J. R. Mathiasen, B. A. W. McKenna, M. S. Saporito et al., "Inhibition of mixed lineage kinase 3 attenuates MPP^+-induced neurotoxicity in SH-SY5Y cells," Brain Research, vol. 1003, no. 1-2, pp. 86–97, 2004.
23. W. Yang and E. Tiffany-Castiglioni, "The bipyridyl herbicide paraquat produces oxidative stress-mediated toxicity in human neuroblastoma SH-SY5Y cells: relevance to the dopaminergic pathogenesis,"Journal of Toxicology and Environmental Health—Part A, vol. 68, no. 22, pp. 1939–1961, 2005.
24. H. An, I. S. Kim, S. Koppula et al., "Protective effects of Gastrodia elata Blume on MPP^+-induced cytotoxicity in human dopaminergic SH-SY5Y cells," Journal of Ethnopharmacology, vol. 130, no. 2, pp. 290–298, 2010.
25. J. P. Capela, C. Macedo, P. S. Branco et al., "Neurotoxicity mechanisms of thioether ecstasy metabolites,"Neuroscience, vol. 146, no. 4, pp. 1743–1757, 2007.
26. J. Yamada, S. Yoshimura, H. Yamakawa et al., "Cell permeable ROS scavengers, Tiron and Tempol, rescue PC12 cell death caused by pyrogallol or hypoxia/reoxygenation," Neuroscience Research, vol. 45, no. 1, pp. 1–8, 2003.
27. M. A. Lopes, A. Meisel, U. Dirnagl, F. D. Carvalho, and M. D. L. Bastos, "Doxorubicin induces biphasic neurotoxicity to rat cortical neurons," NeuroToxicology, vol. 29, no. 2, pp. 286–293, 2008.
28. J. T. Bau and E. U. Kurz, "Sodium salicylate is a novel catalytic inhibitor of human DNA topoisomerase II alpha," Biochemical Pharmacology, vol. 81, no. 3, pp. 345–354, 2011.
29. J. P. Capela, K. Ruscher, M. Lautenschlager et al., "Ecstasy-induced cell death in cortical neuronal cultures is serotonin 2A-receptor-dependent and potentiated under hyperthermia," Neuroscience, vol. 139, no. 3, pp. 1069–1081, 2006.
30. K. Nakamura, D. Tsuchiya, M. Inden, and T. Taniguchi, "In vitro neurodegeneration model: dopaminergic toxin-induced apoptosis in human SH-SY5Y cells," International Congress Series, vol. 1260, pp. 287–290, 2004.
31. D. V. G. De Andrade, D. Madureira de Oliveria, G. Barreto et al., "Effects of the extract of Anemopaegma mirandum (Catuaba) on Rotenone-induced apoptosis in human neuroblastomas SH-SY5Y cells," Brain Research, vol. 1198, pp. 188–196, 2008.
32. J. Lambert and M. D. Brand, "Inhibitors of the quinone-binding site allow rapid superoxide production from mitochondrial NADH:ubiquinone oxidoreductase (complex I)," The Journal of Biological Chemistry, vol. 279, no. 38, pp. 39414–39420, 2004.

33. Hartley, J. M. Stone, C. Heron, J. M. Cooper, and A. H. V. Schapira, "Complex I inhibitors induce dose-dependent apoptosis in PC12 cells: relevance to Parkinson's disease," Journal of Neurochemistry, vol. 63, no. 5, pp. 1987–1990, 1994.

34. K. E. Beck, L. A. De Girolamo, M. Griffin, and E. E. Billett, "The role of tissue transglutaminase in 1-methyl-4-phenylpyridinium (MPP^+)-induced toxicity in differentiated human SH-SY5Y neuroblastoma cells," Neuroscience Letters, vol. 405, no. 1-2, pp. 46–51, 2006.

35. P. Fall and J. P. Bennett, "Characterization and time course of MPP^+-induced apoptosis in human SH-SY5Y neuroblastoma cells," Journal of Neuroscience Research, vol. 55, no. 5, pp. 620–628, 1999.

36. Y. T. Cheung, W. K. W. Lau, M. S. Yu et al., "Effects of all-trans-retinoic acid on human SH-SY5Y neuroblastoma as in vitro model in neurotoxicity research," NeuroToxicology, vol. 30, no. 1, pp. 127–135, 2009.

37. R. J. Dinis-Oliveira, C. Sousa, F. Remião et al., "Sodium salicylate prevents paraquat-induced apoptosis in the rat lung," Free Radical Biology and Medicine, vol. 43, no. 1, pp. 48–61, 2007.

38. M. P. Mattson, "Neuronal life-and-death signaling, apoptosis, and neurodegenerative disorders," Antioxidants and Redox Signaling, vol. 8, no. 11-12, pp. 1997–2006, 2006.

39. P. Jenner, "Oxidative stress as a cause of Parkinson's disease," Acta Neurologica Scandinavica, Supplement, vol. 84, no. 136, pp. 6–15, 1991.

40. R. J. Dinis-Oliveira, P. G. de Pinho, A. C. S. Ferreira et al., "Reactivity of paraquat with sodium salicylate: formation of stable complexes," Toxicology, vol. 249, no. 2-3, pp. 130–139, 2008.

41. R. Franco, S. Li, H. Rodriguez-Rocha, M. Burns, and M. I. Panayiotidis, "Molecular mechanisms of pesticide-induced neurotoxicity: relevance to Parkinson's disease," Chemico-Biological Interactions, vol. 188, no. 2, pp. 289–300, 2010.

42. M. J. La Voie and T. G. Hastings, "Peroxynitrite- and nitrite-induced oxidation of dopamine: implications for nitric oxide in dopaminergic cell loss," Journal of Neurochemistry, vol. 73, no. 6, pp. 2546–2554, 1999.

43. W. L. Yang and A. Y. Sun, "Paraquat-induced free radical reaction in mouse brain microsomes," Neurochemical Research, vol. 23, no. 1, pp. 47–53, 1998.

44. Harms, M. Lautenschlager, A. Bergk et al., "Differential mechanisms of neuroprotection by 17 β-estradiol in apoptotic versus necrotic neurodegeneration," Journal of Neuroscience, vol. 21, no. 8, pp. 2600–2609, 2001.

45. B. K. Barlow, M. J. Thiruchelvam, L. Bennice, D. A. Cory-Slechta, N. Ballatori, and E. K. Richfield, "Increased synaptosomal dopamine content and brain concentration of paraquat produced by selective dithiocarbamates," Journal of Neurochemistry, vol. 85, no. 4, pp. 1075–1086, 2003.

46. S. Ramachandiran, J. M. Hansen, D. P. Jones, J. R. Richardson, and G. W. Miller, "Divergent mechanisms of paraquat, MPP^+, and rotenone toxicity: oxidation of thioredoxin and caspase-3 activation," Toxicological Sciences, vol. 95, no. 1, pp. 163–171, 2007.

47. H. S. Lee, C. W. Park, and Y. S. Kim, "MPP^+ increases the vulnerability to oxidative stress rather than directly mediating oxidative damage in human neuroblastoma cells," Experimental Neurology, vol. 165, no. 1, pp. 164–171, 2000.

48. J. Dennis and J. P. Bennett, "Interactions among nitric oxide and Bcl-family proteins after MPP^+exposure of SH-SY5Y neural cells II: exogenous NO replicates MPP^+ actions," Journal of Neuroscience Research, vol. 72, no. 1, pp. 89–97, 2003.

49. W. S. Choi, L. M. T. Canzoniero, S. L. Sensi et al., "Characterization of MPP^+-induced cell death in a dopaminergic neuronal cell line: role of macromolecule synthesis, cytosolic calcium, caspase, and Bcl-2-related proteins," Experimental Neurology, vol. 159, no. 1, pp. 274–282, 1999.

50. K. Sairam, K. S. Saravanan, R. Banerjee, and K. P. Mohanakumar, "Non-steroidal anti-inflammatory drug sodium salicylate, but not diclofenac or celecoxib, protects against 1-methyl-4-phenyl pyridinium-induced dopaminergic neurotoxicity in rats," Brain Research, vol. 966, no. 2, pp. 245–252, 2003.

51. W. Pei, A. K. Liou, and J. Chen, "Two caspase-mediated apoptotic pathways induced by rotenone toxicity in cortical neuronal cells," The FASEB Journal, vol. 17, no. 3, pp. 520–522, 2003.

52. Y. Sai, Q. Wu, W. Le, F. Ye, Y. Li, and Z. Dong, "Rotenone-induced PC12 cell toxicity is caused by oxidative stress resulting from altered dopamine metabolism," Toxicology in Vitro, vol. 22, no. 6, pp. 1461–1468, 2008.

53. P. Thakur and B. Nehru, "Anti-inflammatory properties rather than anti-oxidant capability is the major mechanism of neuroprotection by sodium salicylate in a chronic rotenone model of Parkinson's disease," Neuroscience, vol. 231, pp. 420–431, 2013.

54. J. Lee, M. S. Huang, I. C. Yang et al., "Essential roles of caspases and their upstream regulators in rotenone-induced apoptosis," Biochemical and Biophysical Research Communications, vol. 371, no. 1, pp. 33–38, 2008.

CHAPTER 28 THE NATURAL PESTICIDE DIHYDROROTENONE

Zhang J, Tang J, Cao B, Zhang Z, Li J, Schimmer AD, He S, Mao X.

INTRODUCTION

Organic food is becoming more and more popular in today's green living style. Because utilization of synthetic pesticide, plant growth hormone, and chemical fertilizers are prohibited from organic produces, natural alternatives such as rotenone become the choice. Rotenone is a natural product extracted from the seeds and stems of several plants, such as the jicama vines. Rotenone could be quickly transformed into several major metabolites, one of which is dihydrorotenone (DHR). DHR is produced by the catalytic hydrogenation of the side chain of rotenone with elimination of the double bond. Like rotenone, DHR is also active as a pesticide but is much less toxic. The oral LD_{50} of rotenone is 300–500 mg/kg for rats, while it is more than 2.5 g/kg for DHR [1]. Mechanistic investigations suggested that DHR bound to and inhibited the complex I in the electron transport chain, thus inhibiting mitochondrial function and decreasing ATP production [2]. Inhibition of mitochondrial function and disruption of the energy supply lead to insect death. Although DHR is non-toxic in rats, it induces Parkinsonian syndrome in the long-term treated mice [1], which suggesting DHR is toxic to neural cells. However, whether DHR is toxic to other types of cells is not clear.

The blood system is the major target of most xenobiotics and blood cells have been developed as an efficient tool to evaluate the safety of xenobiotics. For example, gene expression profiling in monocytes exposed to xenobiotics has been proposed as a potential prediction method to evaluate toxicity of chemicals [3]. B cells and immune systems are sensitive to foreign substances, thus B cells are the major subjects for immunotoxicity study. Primary human B cell models have been established to assess the sensitivity of antibody responses to modulation by xenobiotics [4]. In the present study, we evaluated the cytotoxicity of DHR on human plasma cells, and explored the underlying molecular mechanisms. It demonstrated that DHR induced plasma cell apoptosis which was probably resulted from mitochondrial dysfunction and endoplasmic reticulum (ER) stress via activating the p38 MAP kinase. This study demonstrated that DHR is toxic to human plasma cells. Because plasma cells are a key player in the immune system and more exposure to DHR is expected with the increasing need of organic produces, caution should be taken in the assessment of DHR safety.

Citation: Zhang J, Tang J, Cao B, Zhang Z, Li J, Schimmer AD, et al. (2013) The Natural Pesticide Dihydrorotenone. PLoS ONE 8(7): e69911. doi:10.1371/journal.pone.0069911.

MATERIALS AND METHODS

Cells and Reagents

Human plasma cell lines (KMS11, OPM2) were originally derived from patients of plasma cell neoplasm (multiple myeloma), and were generously provided by Dr. Keith Stewart, Mayo Clinic, Scottsdale, Arizona)[5]–[7]. LP1, RPMI-8226, U266 cell lines were purchased from American Type Culture Collection (ATCC). All cells were grown in Iscove's Modified Dulbecco's medium (IMDM, Thermo Scientific HyClone) supplemented with 10% fetal bovine serum (Invitrogen), penicillin (100 units/ml), and streptomycin (100 μg/ml) in an incubator humidified with 95% air and 5% CO_2 at 37°C. DHR was purchased from Maybridge Chemicals, UK. SB203580 and z-VAD-fmk were purchased from Beyotime Biotechnology Institute, Nantong, China.

Analysis of Apoptotic Cells by Flow Cytometry

Plasma cell lines LP1, KMS11, OPM2, and U266 were plated in 24-well plates (Wuxi Nest Biotechnology Co., Ltd, Wuxi, China), and treated with DHR for 24 h followed by staining with Annexin V-fluorescein isothiocyanate (Annexin V-FITC) and propidium iodide (PI, Biouniquer, Nanjing, China) according to the manufacturer's instructions. Cells were then incubated for 10 min in dark before being subject to analysis on a flow cytometer (FACSCalibur, Becton Dickinson) as reported previously [8]. To analyze whether caspase activation is involved in DHR-induced plasma cell apoptosis, KMS11 and LP1 cells were treated in the presence of pan-caspase inhibitor, followed by evaluation on caspase-3 activation by Western blotting and plasma cell apoptosis by Annexin V/PI double staining and flow cytometry.

Measurement of Mitochondrial Membrane Potential

LP1 cells were treated with DHR for 0, 10 or 20 μM for 24 h, or 10 μM for 0.5 to 24 h. Cells were then washed in phosphate buffered saline (PBS) and incubated with 25 nM tetramethylrhodamine methyl ester (TMRM, Promega) or co-incubated with 25 nM TMRM and 20 μg/ml Annexin V-FITC (Roche) in IMDM for 15 min at 37°C. The TMRM and Annexin V-FITC fluorescence were analyzed by flow cytometry.

Immunoblotting

After treatment, human plasma cells were washed in cold PBS and lysed in a cell lysis buffer containing 50 mM Tris-HCl, pH 7.4, 1% NP-40, 0.5% Na-deoxycholate, and 0.1% SDS, 150 mM NaCl, 2 mM EDTA, and 50 mM NaF. For the detection of phosphoproteins, 1 mM sodium orthovanadate was added to the lysis buffer. The lysates were then sonicated followed by centrifugation at 13,000×g at 4°C for 20 min. The supernatants were collected and subject for protein concentration determination by the BCA Protein Assay Kit (Beyotime). Equal amount of proteins were fractionated by SDS–polyacrylamide gel electrophoresis. Proteins were then transferred onto a PVDF membrane (Millipore). The membranes were blocked with 5% non-fat milk or 5% bovine serum albumin (BSA) in Tris-buffered saline-Triton X-100 (TBST) for 1 h at room temperature and subsequently incubated with primary antibodies overnight at 4°C. After wash with TBST, the blots were incubated with a horseradish peroxidase conjugated secondary antibody for 1 h followed by washing with TBST. The blots were visualized by an enhanced chemoluminescence (ECL) detection system (Beyotime). Primary antibody against GRP78 was purchased from Santa Cruz Biotechnology Inc.; ATF4 antibody was purchased from BD Pharmagin; Bcl-2, Mcl-1, p-p38, p-JNK, and CHOP were purchased from Cell Signaling Technology (CST). Caspase-3, -8, -9 and -12, β-actin, and anti–mouse immunoglobulin G (IgG) and anti–rabbit IgG horseradish peroxidase conjugated antibody were purchased from R&D Systems. Bim and PARP were purchased from Abcam, China. GAPDH was purchased from Abgent, China.

Statistical Analysis

All experiments were repeated at least 3 times. Significant analysis was performed by Student's *t* test. Statistical significance was defined with a p value <0.05.

RESULTS

DHR Induces Apoptosis of Human Plasma Cells

To investigate whether DHR induces human plasma cell apoptosis, human plasma cell lines LP1, OPM2, KMS11, and U266 were treated with DHR for 24 h, followed by flow cytometric analysis after being stained with Annexin V-FITC and PI. Annexin V specifically binds to the exposed phosphatidylserine on the apoptotic cell surface while PI can penetrate into dead cells and intercalates with nucleic acid. The Annexin V and PI positive fraction of all four cell lines were raised in a concentration-dependent manner (Figure 1). For example, apoptotic cells (Annexin V+) were increased from 11.2% and 11.15% in DMSO-treated control group to 47.19% and 23.91% (15 μM DHR), 58.21% and 51.64% (30 μM DHR), in LP1 and OPM2, respectively (Figure 1). Caspase-associated apoptotic pathway was then analyzed. As shown in Figure 2A, DHR activated both initiative apoptotic enzymes (caspase-8 and caspase-9) and, the executive apoptotic enzyme (caspase-3). All cleaved forms from three enzymes were increased upon DHR treatment in a concentration-dependent manner in both KMS11 and LP1 cells (Figure 2A). Because caspase activation is critical for cell apoptosis [9], to find out whether caspase activation is involved in DHR-induced apoptosis, KMS11 and LP1 cells were treated with DHR in the absence or presence of the pan-caspase inhibitor-z-VAD-fmk. Western blotting showed that DHR induced caspase-3 activation in a concentration dependent manner, but cleaved caspase-3 fragments were decreased by z-VAD-fmk (Figure 2B). Next, we evaluated cell apoptosis by Annexin-V and PI staining followed by flow cytometric analysis. It turned out that DHR increased the fraction of Annexin-V positive cells, but this fraction was significantly decreased by the addition of z-VAD-fmk (Figure 2C). For example, apoptotic cells in LP1 cell line were 43.71% induced by DHR, but it was decreased to 25.46% in the presence of z-VAD-fmk (Figure 2C). This finding was consistent with previous studies on z-VAD [10],[11]. All of these thus clearly demonstrated that caspase activation is important for DHR-induced plasma cell apoptosis.

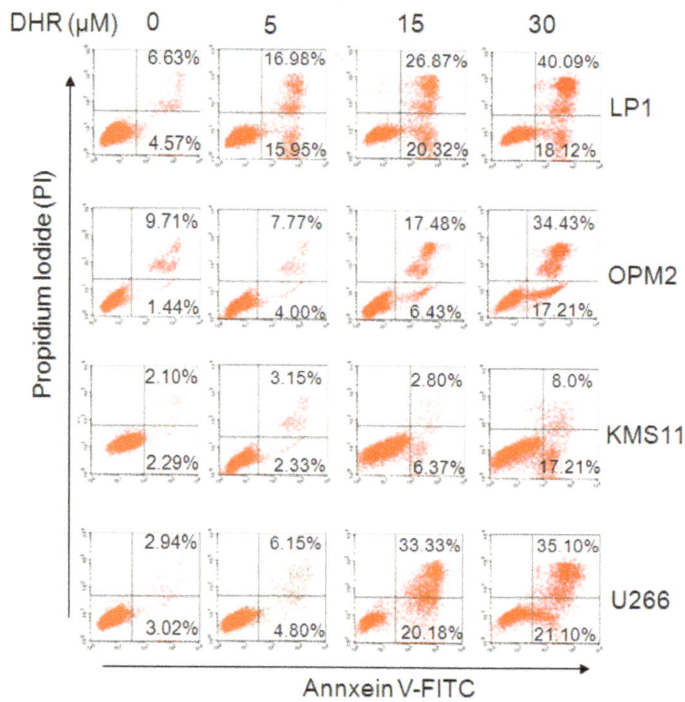

Figure 1: DHR induces human plasma cell apoptosis. Human plasma cell lines LP1, OPM2, KMS11 and U266 were treated with DHR for 24 h. Induction of apoptosis in human plasma cells by DHR was assessed by Annexin V-FITC and propidium iodide (PI) double staining followed by analysis on a flow cytometer. http://dx.doi.org/10.1371/journal.pone.0069911.g001

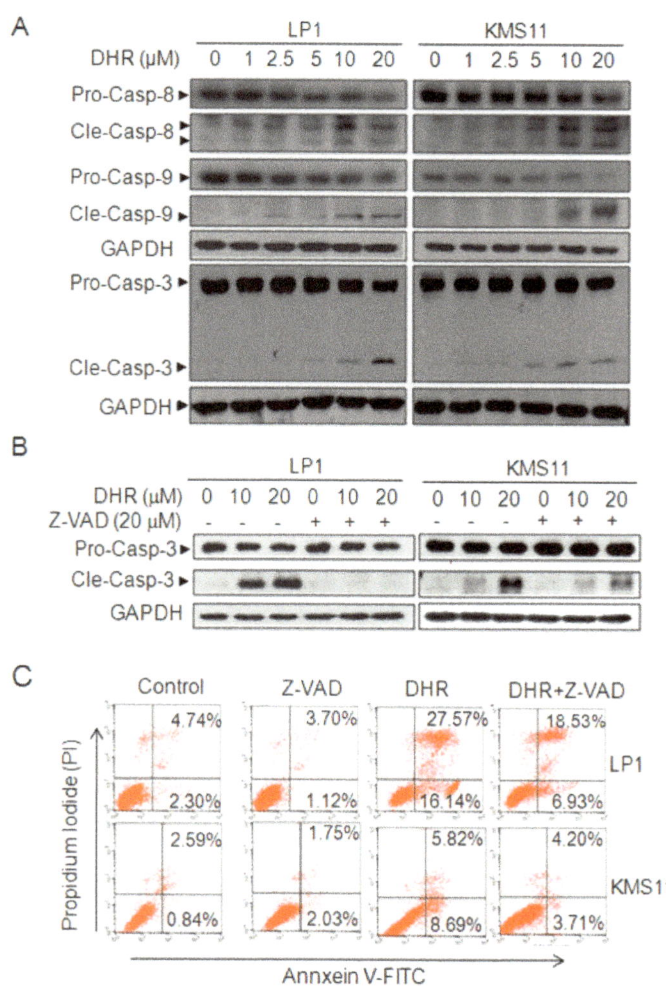

Figure 2: DHR induces human plasma cell death by activating apoptotic pathway. **A**, Human plasma cells LP1 and KMS11 were treated with DHR at the indicated concentrations for 24 h. Cell lysates were then prepared and subject to immunoblotting assay against apoptosis-

associated proteins caspase-3, -8 and -9. GAPDH were used as a loading control. B, LP1 and KMS11 cells were treated for 24 h with DMSO, DHR, z-VAD-fmk or DHR+Z-VAD-fmk, followed by caspase-3 analysis by Western blotting. C, LP1 and KMS11 cells were treated for 24 h with DMSO, DHR, z-VAD-fmk or DHR+Z-VAD-fmk, followed by Annexin-V-FITC/PI staining and flow cytometric analyses. Pro-casp: pro-caspase; Cle-casp: cleaved caspase. http://dx.doi.org/10.1371/journal.pone.0069911.g002

The Bcl-2 family proteins are critical regulators of apoptosis and these proteins can be divided into two main groups, anti-apoptotic (such as Bcl-2 and Mcl-1) and pro-apoptotic (such as Bim and Bax) [12]. As shown in Figures 3, pro-apoptotic Bim (Figure 3A) was induced while anti-apoptotic Bcl-2 (Figure 3B) and Mcl-1 (Figure 3C) were down-regulated in a concentration-dependent manner by DHR. Therefore, these studies suggested that DHR induced human plasma cell apoptosis.

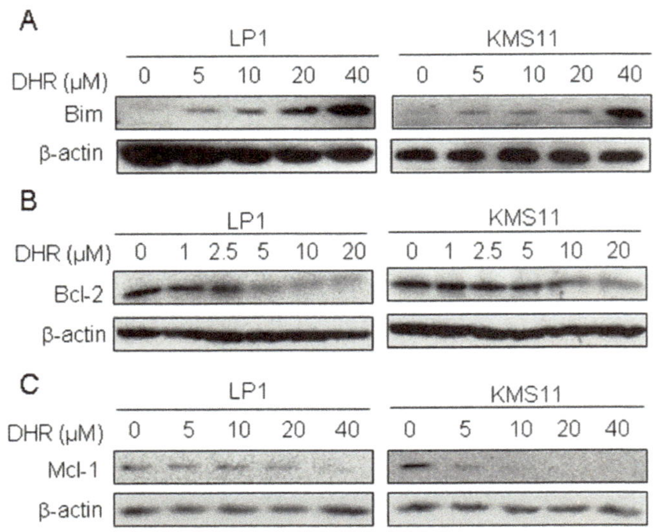

Figure 3: DHR dysregulates mitochondrial resident proteins in human plasma cells. Human plasma cell lines LP1 and KMS11 were treated with DHR at the indicated concentrations for 24 h. Cell lysates were then prepared and subject to immunoblotting assay against Bim (A), Bcl-2 (B) and Mcl-1 (C).β-actin was used as a loading control. http://dx.doi.org/10.1371/journal.pone.0069911.g003

DHR Induces Loss of the Mitochondrial Membrane Potential in Human Plasma Cells

It is reported that DHR could bind to and inhibit the Complex I (NADH:ubiquinone oxidoreductase) in the mitochondrial respiratory chain by which it blocks the electron transfer from NADH to O_2 via the transfer of H^+ ions (protons) across the inner mitochondrial membrane [2]. This blockade results in an insufficient proton gradient across the mitochondrial membrane, or mitochondrial membrane potential ($\Delta\psi$), a sensitive marker of mitochondrial insult and its reduction has been associated with mitochondrial insult. To view this change induced by DHR, LP1 cells were treated with 10 or 20 μM of DHR for 24 h, followed by staining with tetramethylrhodamine methyl ester (TMRM), a monovalent cationic fluorescent dye widely used for measuring $\Delta\psi$. Flow cytometric analysis revealed that $\Delta\psi$ was rapidly collapsed in response to DHR, where the potential staining cells (TMRM positive) were left-shifted (Figure 4A). Next, LP1 cells were treated for 24 h by DHR (10 or 20 μM) and co-stained with Annexin V-FITC and TMRM followed by flow cytometric analysis. As shown in 4B, addition of DHR led to increased fractions of TMRM-negative cells, especially those Annexin-V positive cells. Because TMRM is a sensitive biomarker of mitochondrion insult, to find out the time-course and relationship between mitochondrial damage and cell apoptosis, LP1 cells were incubated with 10 μM of DHR for 0.5 to 24 h followed by TMRM and Annexin V-FITC staining. Flow cytometric analysis indicated that the fractions of TMRM-negative cells were increased upon extension of incubation as shown in Figure 4C. The significant changes occurred at 8 h after DHR treatment. Interestingly, not all MMP-lost cells were Annexin V positive, suggesting mitochondrial damage was probably earlier than apoptosis.

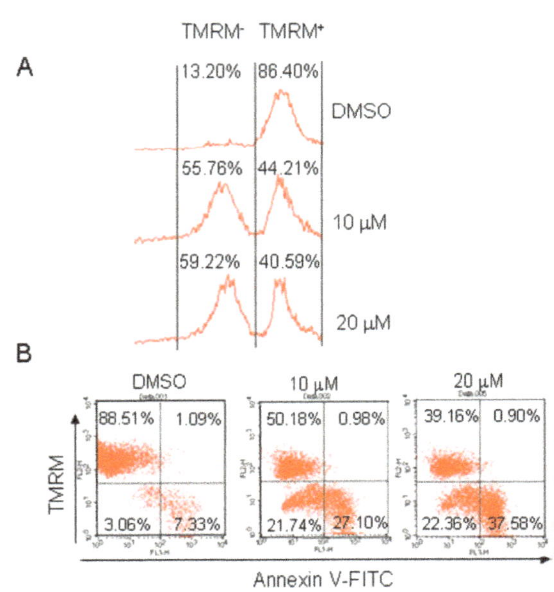

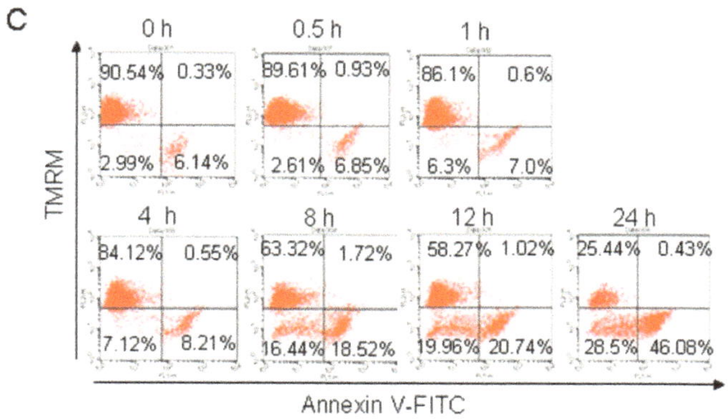

Figure 4: DHR leads to mitochondrial membrane potential collapse in human plasma cells. LP1 cells were treated with DMSO, 10 or 20 µM of DHR for 24 h, stained by TMRM alone (A) or in combination with Annexin V-FITC (B) followed by flow cytometric analysis. (C) LP1 cells were treated with 10 µM of DHR for indicated time periods, followed by TMRM and Annexin V-FITC staining and flow cytometric analysis. http://dx.doi.org/10.1371/journal.pone.0069911.g004

DHR Induces Unfolded Protein Response and Endoplasmic Reticulum Stress in Human Plasma Cells

The endoplasmic reticulum (ER) contains the majority of cytochrome P450 enzymes involved in xenobiotic metabolism, as well as a number of conjugating enzymes, thus ER is involved in an array of cellular functions and plays important roles in xenobiotic metabolism and toxicity[13]. Rotenone has been found to induce ER stress in multiple cell models [14] which is proposed to be responsible for cell death [15]. As shown in the above studies, DHR was able to induce human plasma cell apoptosis which is possibly associated with mitochondrial dysfunction. But its association with ER stress is not known. To evaluate whether DHR insults endoplasmic reticulum and triggers unfolded protein response (UPR) in human plasma cells, LP1 and OPM2 were treated by DHR at increasing concentrations, followed by evaluation of the hallmarks of UPR and ER stress. We first examined glucose-regulated protein 78 (GRP78), the sensor of UPR and ER stress and a resident protein on ER membrane, which is induced when UPR is initiated. Immunoblotting analysis indicated that GRP78 was induced by DHR in a concentration-dependent manner and the highest expression level was seen at the treatment with 40 µM of DHR (Figure 5A). We next evaluated other ER stress-associated signal proteins such as ATF4 and CHOP. Western blotting analyses revealed that these two proteins were increased by DHR in both time- and concentration-dependent manners (Figures 5B and 5C). Caspase-12, the enzyme specifically responsible for the ER stress-induced apoptosis, was also decreased (Figure 5D), further suggesting that DHR induces ER stress in human plasma cells.

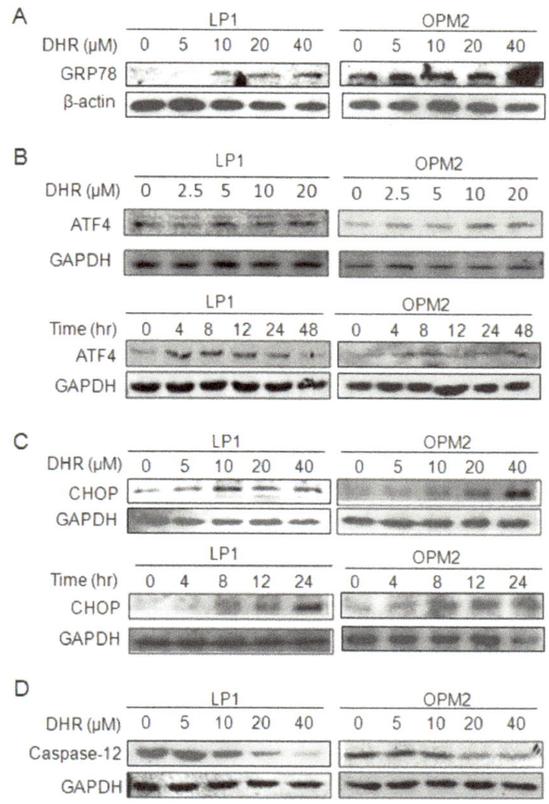

Figure 5: DHR activates the ER stress signaling in human plasma cells. A, LP1 and OPM2 cells were treated with DHR for 24 h, the expression of GRP78 was then detected by immunoblotting. (B) and (C) LP1 and OPM2 cells were treated DHR for different concentrations and time periods before subject to ATF4 and CHOP analysis. (D) ER-associated caspase-12 was evaluated after exposed to DHR at indicated concentrations for 24 h. http://dx.doi.org/10.1371/journal.pone.0069911.g005

DHR Activates p38 but not the c-Jun N-terminal Kinase in Human Plasma Cells

ER stress is highly associated with p38 and JNK signals [16], [17]. To find out the effects of DHR on these kinases associated with ER stress in human plasma cells, LP1 and OPM2 cells were treated with DHR for 24 h followed by immunoblotting using specific antibodies. As shown in Figure 6, DHR markedly induced phosphorylation of p38, but not JNK in both examined cell lines. In contrast, DHR suppressed the activation of JNK. This finding was differently from previous reports where both JNK and p38 were activated in rotenone-induced ER stress [18], suggesting that DHR probably acted in its own manner in human plasma cells.

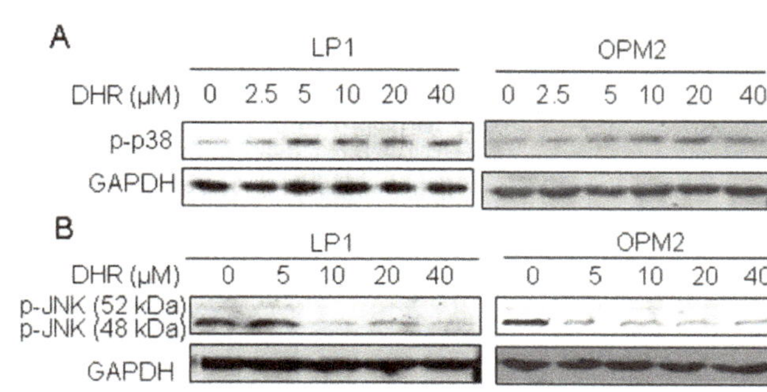

Figure 6: DHR activates p38 MAP kinase but suppresses JNK

kinase in human plasma cells. LP1 and OPM2 cells were treated with DHR at indicated concentrations followed by immunoblotting analyses for p38 (A) and JNK (B) against specific antibodies. GAPDH was used as an internal loading control. http://dx.doi.org/10.1371/journal.pone.0069911.g006

The p38 MAP Kinase Contributes to DHR-induced Human Plasma Cell Apoptosis

To further evaluate the effect of p38 activation on DHR-induced human plasma cell apoptosis, LP1, OPM2, RPMI-8226, and U266 cells were treated with DHR for 30 or 60 min, followed by detection of p38 activation using specific antibody against phosphorylated p38. It showed that p38 was activated by DHR in all examined cell lines (Figure 7A). DHR induced p38 phosphorylation was time-dependent. As shown in Figure 7B, activated p38 signal was detected at 5 min after DHR treatment, and the highest level was seen at 240 min. Next, we evaluated the effects of DHR on cell death when p38 activation was blocked by SB203580, a specific inhibitor of p38. Pre-treatment with SB203580 attenuated activation of p38 by DHR (Figure 7C). To further evaluate the effect of p38 activation on plasma cell apoptosis, LP1 and OPM2 cells were pre-treated with SB203580 for 30 min, followed by DHR for 12 or 24 h. Immunoblotting assay demonstrated that both cleavage of PARP and caspase-3 were partly attenuated by SB203580 (Figure 7D). Because PARP and caspase-3 are key apoptotic markers [9], these results confirmed that p38 MAP kinase pathway contributed to DHR-induced plasma cell apoptosis.

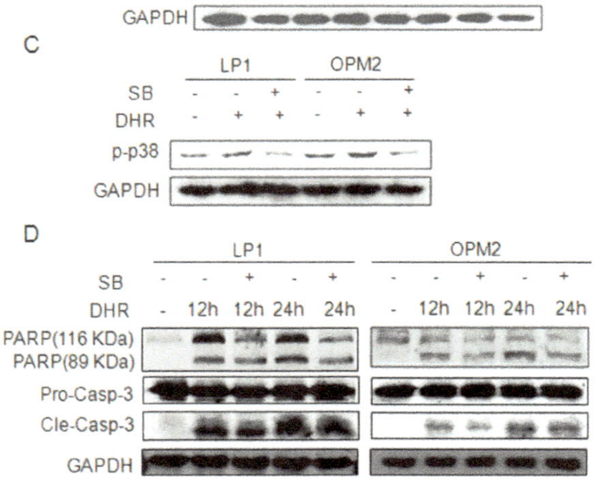

Figure 7: DHR activates p38 phosphorylation which is important for DHR-induced human plasma cell apoptosis. (A) Human plasma cell lines LP1, OPM2, RPMI-8226, and U266 were treated with 10 μM of DHR for 30 or 60 min, followed by p38 phosphorylation analysis. The relative phosphorylated level of p38 to GAPDH was calculated by Quality One software. (B) LP1 cells were treated by DHR at indicated time points to examine p38 activation. (C) LP1 and OPM2 were pre-treated with p38 inhibitor SB203580 (2 μM) for 30 min, followed by DHR (20 μM) for 30 min. (D) LP1 and OPM2 were pretreated with SB203580 (2 μM) for 30 min, followed by DHR (20 μM) for 12 or 24 h. Cell lysates were analyzed by specific antibodies. GAPDH was used as an internal loading control. Pro-casp-3: pro-caspase-3; Cle-casp-3: cleaved caspase-3. http://dx.doi.org/10.1371/journal.pone.0069911.g007

DISCUSSION

In the above studies, we investigated the effects on DHR on human plasma cell apoptosis and underlying mechanisms. DHR is the catalytic reduction product of rotenone at the isopropylene side chain by *C. blakesleeana* [19]. Although several compounds can be isolated from rotenone metabolites, DHR is the only active one in killing pests and insects by inhibiting the electron transport chain [20]. DHR is less toxic than rotenone in the acute toxicity evaluation in rats by oral administration [1], but it also induces Parkinson's syndrome, which suggested that DHR might be toxic in chronic exposure [1]. Because mitochondrial insult is a major factor in induction of cell death, there is no wonder that DHR can induce human plasma cell apoptosis as demonstrated in Figure 1. This apoptosis induced by DHR in human plasma cells is associated with downregulation of pro-survival proteins (such as Bcl-2 and Mcl-1) and upregulation of pro-apoptotic proteins such as Bim. Because these proteins are critical for maintenance of mitochondrial membrane integrity and membrane potential, thus DHR-induced MMP collapse further demonstrated that DHR was toxic to mitochondria.

In addition to mitochondria, ER is also an important organelle in regulating cell apoptosis. Mitochondria and ER interact both physically and functionally via the mitochondria-associated ER membrane, a linkage between the duo [21]. Mitochondria dysfunction is believed to induce UPR and ER stress featured with induced expression of GRP78 and CHOP [22]. This was also observed in DHR-treated human plasma cells. After treatment with DHR, ER stress hallmarks including GRP78, ATF4, and CHOP were induced in a concentration-dependent manner. GRP78, an ER resident molecular chaperone, binds to newly-synthesized proteins as they are translocated into the ER, and maintains them in a state competent for subsequent folding and oligomerization. Therefore, GRP78 is a central regulator of ER homeostasis and a sensor of ER stress. When unfolded or misfolded proteins are overloaded, the interaction between GRP78 and their partners is destabilized thus inducing UPR. In this study, GRP78 was markedly induced in both LP1 and OPM2 cells exposed to DHR, suggesting ER stress was initiated by DHR. Under ER stress, all PERK, ATF6 and Ire1 signals converge to induced transcription of CHOP [23], a central transcription factor in ER stress. Increased concentrations or extended treatment periods lead to more expression of CHOP by DHR (Figure 5B). We also found that DHR activated caspase-12, an initiating apoptotic enzyme responsible for ER stress-induced cell apoptosis [24]. This finding further demonstrated that ER stress was involved in DHR-induced cell death.

The mitogen-activated protein kinases (MAPKs) mainly including ERK, p38 and JNK, are involved in the development and progression of cancer and are also associated with ER stress. ERK1/2 are activated by growth factors, while p38 and JNK are mainly activated by cellular stresses [25]. The present results showed that DHR-induced activation of p38 (Figure 7), and the inhibition of p38 by SB203580 led to an ablation of

DHR-induced apoptosis (Figure 7D). These results revealed a strong correlation between the level of p38 activation and sensitivity to DHR toxicity. However, DHR failed to activate the JNK signaling pathway in human plasma cells which is critical for rotenone [18], suggesting that DHR induces ER stress in a manner different from rotenone. However, activation of p38 and inactivation of JNK are possibly equally important for DHR-induced human plasma cell death because these two pathways also have antagonistic effects [26]. Recently, p38-dependent Fas-mediated apoptosis was found to be potentiated by the inhibition of JNK1/2 [27]. Down-regulation of JNK activity associated with ER stress was observed in dexamethasome-treated OCI-MY5 cells in which dexamethasome-induced apoptosis does not involve activation of JNK [28]. Therefore, the lack of activation of JNK by DHR in human plasma cells suggests that antagonistic effect of p38 and JNK in DHR-induced apoptosis.

In summary, this study demonstrated that DHR exposure leads to human plasma cell death in association with mitochondrial dysfunction, ER stress and p38 signaling. Because plasma cells are an important component of the immune system, the present study suggested that DHR probably interferes with the immune system. With the emerging need of the organic produces, exposure to DHR is also increasing, therefore, safety assessment of DHR and other rotenoids should be cautious.

REFERENCES

1. Ambrose AM, Christensen HE, Rather LJ (1953) Toxicological and pharmacological studies on dihydrorotenone. J Am Pharm Assoc Am Pharm Assoc (Baltim) 42: 364–366. doi: 10.1002/jps.3030420615
2. Talpade DJ, Greene JG, Higgins DS Jr, Greenamyre JT (2000) In vivo labeling of mitochondrial complex I (NADH:ubiquinone oxidoreductase) in rat brain using [(3)H]dihydrorotenone. J Neurochem 75: 2611–2621. doi: 10.1046/j.1471-4159.2000.0752611.x
3. Arkusz J, Stepnik M, Sobala W, Dastych J (2010) Prediction of the contact sensitizing potential of chemicals using analysis of gene expression changes in human THP-1 monocytes. Toxicol Lett 199: 51–59. doi: 10.1016/j.toxlet.2010.08.005
4. Lu H, Crawford RB, North CM, Kaplan BL, Kaminski NE (2009) Establishment of an immunoglobulin m antibody-forming cell response model for characterizing immunotoxicity in primary human B cells. Toxicol Sci 112: 363–373. doi: 10.1093/toxsci/kfp224
5. Namba M, Ohtsuki T, Mori M, Togawa A, Wada H, et al. (1989) Establishment of five human myeloma cell lines. In Vitro Cell Dev Biol 25: 723–729. doi: 10.1007/bf02623725
6. Tiedemann RE, Mao X, Shi CX, Zhu YX, Palmer SE, et al. (2008) Identification of kinetin riboside as a repressor of CCND1 and CCND2 with preclinical antimyeloma activity. J Clin Invest 118: 1750–1764. doi: 10.1172/jci34149
7. Katagiri S, Yonezawa T, Kuyama J, Kanayama Y, Nishida K, et al. (1985) Two distinct human myeloma cell lines originating from one patient with myeloma. Int J Cancer 36: 241–246. doi: 10.1002/ijc.2910360217
8. Mao X, Liang SB, Hurren R, Gronda M, Chow S, et al. (2008) Cyproheptadine displays preclinical activity in myeloma and leukemia. Blood 112: 760–769. doi: 10.1182/blood-2008-02-142687
9. Miller DK (1997) The role of the Caspase family of cysteine proteases in apoptosis. Semin Immunol 9: 35–49. doi: 10.1006/smim.1996.0058
10. Gao J, Liu X, Rigas B (2005) Nitric oxide-donating aspirin induces apoptosis in human colon cancer cells through induction of oxidative stress. Proc Natl Acad Sci U S A 102: 17207–17212. doi: 10.1073/pnas.0506893102
11. Slee EA, Zhu H, Chow SC, MacFarlane M, Nicholson DW, et al. (1996) Benzyloxycarbonyl-Val-Ala-Asp (OMe) fluoromethylketone (Z-VAD.FMK) inhibits apoptosis by blocking the processing of CPP32. Biochem J 315 (Pt 1): 21–24.
12. Sheridan C, Martin SJ (2010) Mitochondrial fission/fusion dynamics and apoptosis. Mitochondrion 10: 640–648. doi: 10.1016/j.mito.2010.08.005
13. Cribb AE, Peyrou M, Muruganandan S, Schneider L (2005) The endoplasmic reticulum in xenobiotic toxicity. Drug Metab Rev 37: 405–442. doi: 10.1080/03602530500205135
14. Chen YY, Chen G, Fan Z, Luo J, Ke ZJ (2008) GSK3beta and endoplasmic reticulum stress mediate rotenone-induced death of SK-N-MC neuroblastoma cells. Biochem Pharmacol 76: 128–138. doi: 10.1016/j.bcp.2008.04.010
15. Goncalves AP, Maximo V, Lima J, Singh KK, Soares P, et al. (2011) Involvement of p53 in cell death following cell cycle arrest and mitotic catastrophe induced by rotenone. Biochim Biophys Acta 1813: 492–499. doi: 10.1016/j.bbamcr.2011.01.006
16. Chen CL, Lin CF, Chang WT, Huang WC, Teng CF, et al. (2008) Ceramide induces p38 MAPK and JNK activation through a mechanism involving a thioredoxin-interacting protein-mediated pathway. Blood 111: 4365–4374. doi: 10.1182/blood-2007-08-106336
17. Park GB, Kim YS, Lee HK, Song H, Cho DH, et al. (2010) Endoplasmic reticulum stress-mediated apoptosis of EBV-transformed B cells by cross-linking of CD70 is dependent upon generation of reactive oxygen species and activation of p38 MAPK and JNK pathway. J Immunol 185: 7274–7284. doi: 10.4049/jimmunol.1001547
18. Deng YT, Huang HC, Lin JK (2010) Rotenone induces apoptosis in MCF-7 human breast cancer cell-mediated ROS through JNK and p38 signaling. Mol Carcinog 49: 141–151. doi: 10.1002/mc.20583
19. Sariaslani FS, Rosazza JP (1983) Microbial Transformations of Natural Antitumor Agents: Products of Rotenone and Dihydrorotenone Transformation by Cunninghamella blakesleeana. Appl Environ Microbiol 45: 616–621.
20. Higgins DS Jr, Greenamyre JT (1996) [3H]dihydrorotenone binding to NADH: ubiquinone reductase (complex I) of the electron transport chain: an

autoradiographic study. J Neurosci 16: 3807–3816.

21. Simmen T, Lynes EM, Gesson K, Thomas G (2010) Oxidative protein folding in the endoplasmic reticulum: tight links to the mitochondria-associated membrane (MAM). Biochim Biophys Acta 1798: 1465–1473. doi: 10.1016/j.bbamem.2010.04.009
22. Lee JW, Kim WH, Yeo J, Jung MH (2010) ER stress is implicated in mitochondrial dysfunction-induced apoptosis of pancreatic beta cells. Mol Cells 30: 545–549. doi: 10.1007/s10059-010-0161-5
23. Szegezdi E, Logue SE, Gorman AM, Samali A (2006) Mediators of endoplasmic reticulum stress-induced apoptosis. EMBO Rep 7: 880–885. doi: 10.1038/sj.embor.7400779
24. Szegezdi E, Fitzgerald U, Samali A (2003) Caspase-12 and ER-stress-mediated apoptosis: the story so far. Ann N Y Acad Sci 1010: 186–194. doi: 10.1196/annals.1299.032
25. Keshet Y, Seger R (2010) The MAP kinase signaling cascades: a system of hundreds of components regulates a diverse array of physiological functions. Methods Mol Biol 661: 3–38. doi: 10.1007/978-1-60761-795-2_1
26. Ichijo H (1999) From receptors to stress-activated MAP kinases. Oncogene 18: 6087–6093. doi: 10.1038/sj.onc.1203129
27. Tourian L Jr, Zhao H, Srikant CB (2004) p38alpha, but not p38beta, inhibits the phosphorylation and presence of c-FLIPS in DISC to potentiate Fas-mediated caspase-8 activation and type I apoptotic signaling. J Cell Sci 117: 6459–6471. doi: 10.1242/jcs.01573
28. Chauhan D, Pandey P, Ogata A, Teoh G, Treon S, et al. (1997) Dexamethasone induces apoptosis of multiple myeloma cells in a JNK/SAP kinase independent mechanism. Oncogene 15: 837–843. doi: 10.1038/sj.onc.1201253

CHAPTER 29

A COMPARATIVE STUDY OF ALLOWABLE PESTICIDE RESIDUE LEVELS ON PRODUCE IN THE UNITED STATES

Roni A Neff, Jennifer C Hartle, Linnea I Laestadius, Kathleen Dolan, Anne C Rosenthal and Keeve E Nachman

Keywords: Pesticides Agriculture International Trade Policy Food Safety

BACKGROUND

Since the 1980's, fruit and vegetable consumption has risen across the U.S. About half of the increased demand for fresh fruit and a quarter of the demand for fresh vegetables has been met by imports. Since NAFTA was signed in 1992, fruit and vegetable importation to the U.S. from trade partners has nearly quadrupled [1]. The primary drivers of U.S. consumer demand include the desire to eat off-season and tropical fruit items, promotion of produce-rich diets, and lower prices available from other countries, particularly when supported by favorable terms in trade agreements [1, 2]. The U.S. Department of Agriculture indicates that 48.8 percent of fresh fruits and 25 percent of fresh vegetables consumed in the U.S. in 2010 were grown abroad. This reflects a significant increase from 1990, when only 40.4 percent of fresh fruits and 9.9 percent of fresh vegetables were imported (Glaser, L., USDA, personal communication, October 24, 2011). For some produce items, importing is relatively consistent year round; others vary seasonally.

Citation: Roni A NeffEmail, Jennifer C Hartle, Linnea I Laestadius, Kathleen Dolan, Anne C Rosenthal and Keeve E Nachman, A comparative study of allowable pesticide residue levels on produce in the United States, DOI: 10.1186/1744-8603-8-2

Countries exporting produce to the U.S. are required to adhere to U.S. pesticide tolerance limits, defined as the amount that may legally remain on food post-production. U.S. agencies perform fairly low levels of testing on these imports, as will be described; information thus remains limited on the extent to which these imports may expose U.S. consumers to elevated levels of pesticide residues or other contaminants, relative to domestically grown produce. This analysis aims to gain insight into that gap, and to highlight needs in policy, oversight, and monitoring.

We examine quantities of pesticide residues that could enter the U.S. on top imported produce items, under the scenario that exporters comply with the maximum limits of their own domestic regulations, and not with those of the U.S. In the absence of "negative regulatory feedback" -- frequent inspections and strong enforcement -- there may be little incentive for exporters to comply with U.S. tolerance limits; in some cases, they may even have little awareness of such limits [3]. Accordingly, factors including originating-country regulations might play a stronger role in driving practices and norms than U.S. policy.

There is a complex interplay of factors affecting farmer, intermediary and exporter practice, and affecting pesticide residue levels. It is possible that those exporting to the U.S. fail to comply even with their own nations' residue policies, particularly in developing economies with limited enforcement capacity. Alternately, there is evidence from some countries that farmers may comply with regulations in the top countries to which they export - *in* products for export - but apply lower standards for products for domestic markets [4]. Regardless, farmers are unlikely to apply all allowable pesticides to the maximum limit in all crops, and the level of residues remaining will vary in mixed ways by weather, crop, time of application, and other factors.

Pesticides and their Health Impacts

Pesticides are defined by the U.S. Environmental Protection Agency (EPA) as "any substance or mixtures of substances intended for preventing, destroying, repelling, or mitigating any pest" [5]. The category includes insecticides, herbicides, and fungicides [5]. Over 20 700 pesticide products were registered for use in the U.S. in 1998, the most recent year for which data are available; these contained approximately 891 active ingredients [6, 7]. In 2007, an estimated 498 951 607 kg of pesticides were used in the U.S., and 2 358 680 324 kg were used globally [8]. This estimate includes both synthetic pesticides and other chemicals used as pesticides, such as sulfur and petroleum oil. Residues from these pesticides often remain on or in produce, thus creating a source of human exposure when treated produce items are ingested.

Pesticides work through mechanisms of action intended either to kill pests or render them ineffective [9]. Accordingly, they can also act upon unintended organisms, such as humans. Children in particular may be susceptible to adverse neurological, developmental and other effects from pesticide exposures [6, 10]. Despite an extensive literature, the potential adverse health consequences stemming from dietary exposures to a number of routinely-used pesticides remain poorly characterized. Even less well characterized are the cumulative toxicological effects of the complex *mixtures* of pesticide residues and other substances to which we are exposed [11]. Beyond dietary exposures, there are well documented health effects of occupational and residential exposures related to pesticide application to food and other crops. Vulnerable populations including children and pregnant women may face particular risk from such exposures [12, 13].

Pesticide Policy in the U.S. and Abroad

While the U.S. Food and Drug Administration (FDA) is charged with inspecting domestic and imported produce for food safety purposes, the EPA is responsible for monitoring the use of pesticides in domestic food production and establishing limits on the amount of pesticide residue that can remain in or on foods sold. The EPA's pesticide work has traditionally been driven by three main statutes:

1) The Federal Food, Drug, and Cosmetic Act (FFDCA), which establishes maximum residue limits (MRLs) for pesticides on food in interstate commerce, including imports [14];
2) The Federal Insecticide, Fungicide, and Rodenticide Act (FIFRA), which governs the sale and use of pesticide products in the U.S. through registrations. Only these registered pesticides are allowable on imports [15]; and
3) The Food Quality Protection Act (FQPA), passed in 1996, which amended both FFDCA and FIFRA, including mandating a "reasonable certainty of no harm" standard for pesticide safety [16]. It also required that in setting MRLs, the EPA must consider child health, the aggregate risks of exposure to a pesticide in multiple products, and cumulative risks from exposures to multiple pesticides with similar mechanisms of action.

Internationally, many exporters to the U.S. follow either Codex Alimentarius, European Union, or U.S. MRLs. The Codex Alimentarius Commission, established jointly by the United Nations' Food and Agriculture Organization and the World Health Organization in 1963, sets non-binding consensus-based MRLs, as well as other food standards to protect health and ensure fair trade practices [17]. The European Union (E.U.) maintains its own set of standards, which became harmonized across member states in 2008, while Mexico defaults to U.S. MRLs [18, 19]. Other countries, including Japan, Canada, Brazil, and Argentina, maintain their own standards. The World Trade Organization's Agreement on the Application of Sanitary and Phytosanitary Measures requires that pesticide standards be based upon "an assessment, as appropriate to the circumstances, of the risks to human, animal or plant life or health" and encourages compliance with the Codex [20, 21].

Table 1 illustrates the diversity of MRLs for one commodity across a sample of different pesticides and markets.

Table 1: Apple maximum residue limits (MRLS) for selected pesticides and markets, 2008

Pesticide*	U.S. MRL	Codex MRL	E.U. MRL	Canadian MRL
Azinphos-methyl	1.5	2	0.5	2
Inorganic bromide resulting from fumigation	5	20	0.05	---
Metalaxyl	0.2	1	1	1
Methidathion	0.05	0.5	0.05	0.5
Methomyl	1	99**	99**	0.5
Methoxyfenozide	1.5	2	2	1.5
Novaluron	2	3	---	2
Permethrin	0.05	2	0.05	1
Tebuconazole	0.05	0.5	1	---

Thiophanate-methyl	2	3	0.5	5

All units parts per million (ppm).

*Pesticides selected to demonstrate differentials between U.S. and Codex MRLs for apples.

** Established for the sum of methomyl and thiodicarb.

"---" means no MRL for apples was established.

Data: http://www.mrldatabase.com/

Imported Produce and Pesticide Inspection

The FDA selects import shipments for screening using a "focused sampling" method, which aims to target items at highest risk of exceeding residue tolerances. The FDA may prioritize inspection of specific food types and/or the inspection of imported produce from specific countries based on: past findings; intelligence information; dietary significance; volume imported and domestically produced; and potential pesticide hazards [21]. The FDA's Office of Regulatory Affairs also conducts inspections of domestic and foreign food processing facilities to ensure compliance with the FFDCA [22]. Numbers are low, however; inspections of foreign food processing facilities decreased from 211 inspections in 2001 to 153 in 2008 [23]. The FDA's Office of International Programs has established permanent offices in China, India, Europe, and Latin America in an effort to help build local regulatory capacity and strengthen the FDA's ability to perform timely inspections [24].

According to an analysis by the U.S. Government Accountability Office (GAO), the FDA inspected approximately 1 in every 129 shipments (0.77%) of imported produce during fiscal years 2000-2007. Laboratory analysis was performed on about 1 in 455 shipments (0.22%) [calculated] [25]. In 2009, the FDA employed 272 full time field personnel conducting inspections of imported foods [23]. Current FDA testing protocols cover only about half of pesticides with U.S. MRLs, and exclude many pesticides that are legal internationally but not in the U.S. [21, 26]. Further increasing the challenge of detecting violative shipments, importers are known to "shop ports," aiming for ports with lower inspection rates. Overall, FDA capacity to detect instances of excess pesticide residue on imported produce is limited; the agency itself has noted that it neither has, nor will have, "the resources to adequately keep pace with the pressures of globalization" [27].

When FDA tests reveal pesticide residues above EPA tolerances, or residues of pesticides disallowed in the U.S., the entire shipment should be removed from commerce (although this may not always occur) and the relevant exporting companies and originating nations may face an increased likelihood of future scrutiny [28]. An examination of import shipments the U.S. rejected between 1998 and 2004 found that vegetables and vegetable products were the top category of food rejected, with pesticide violations the most frequent cause, reflecting 26.6 percent of rejections of vegetable shipments [calculated] [28].

Pesticide Residue Monitoring Data

Beyond examining results of enforcement-related screening, we can also gain insights into the relative portion of imports and domestic products with detectable pesticide levels by examining data from governmental monitoring programs aimed at characterizing risks. Two main government programs compile such monitoring data:

The FDA Pesticide Monitoring Program (PMP) annually inspects imported produce at the point of entry to the U.S., as well as domestic produce. In 2008, the agency analyzed 3,656 fruit and vegetable samples [29]. Of these, 4.4% of imported vegetables had violative pesticide residues, compared to 1.7% of domestic vegetables. For fruits, the percentages were 4.8% and 0% respectively (calculated) [29].

The United States Department of Agriculture (USDA) Pesticide Data Program (PDP) conducts tests on agricultural commodities available for consumption in the U.S., with a focus on items commonly consumed by infants and children [29]. In 2009, 9,231 fresh fruit and vegetable samples were tested, covering 14 items [30]. While significant quantities of imports are tested, the 2009 report only presents comparison data on pesticide residues for cucumbers (U.S. vs. Mexico) and grapes (U.S. vs. Chile), and only for pesticides where residues were detected in at least 10 percent of samples. Averaging percent of samples with residue detections for each pesticide, U.S. cucumbers averaged 14.7 percent, compared to 24.1 percent for Mexico. For grapes, the average was 25.6 for U.S. samples, vs. 38.6 percent for Chile [30](Appendix I, calculated). The EPA uses PDP data to calculate a Dietary Risk Index for different commodities, and compares imported and domestic produce items [31].

A broader assessment across markets, produce items and pesticides remains needed.

Study Purpose

This analysis aims to provide an additional perspective by estimating quantities of pesticide residues to which U.S. consumers could be exposed. Specifically, it models the amount of excess pesticides that could remain on the top U.S. imported produce items if exporters adhered to the maximum allowable application rates based on their own market guidelines rather than those of the U.S. It further aims to present the known health effects associated with low level exposure to the pesticides of concern that we modeled. Finally, it aims to suggest commodity-market-pesticide combinations that should be prioritized for oversight.

This study focuses on examining situations where pesticide residues on imports may pose an excess risk relative to domestic produce, so data on the situations where importation may be protective were not examined in detail. While there may be interest in examining which of these situations dominates, we consider it more useful to consider them separately, each implying a distinct set of concerns and policy responses. The large volumes of produce imports mean significant quantities of excess pesticide residues are introduced into the U.S. food supply, and also suggests environmental and occupational risks internationally, generated by U.S. consumption. Instances where importation could be protective do not "cancel out" these risks. Additionally, modeling these excesses helps identify specific targets for increased scrutiny, thus contributing to the potential for intervention.

METHODS

Identifying commodities, markets, and pesticides for examination

The analysis relies on the United States Foreign Agricultural Service Maximum Residue Limit (FAS MRL) database for allowable MRLs by commodity, market, and pesticide [32]. This database also indicates which countries subscribe to Codex, European Union or U.S. standards. The database was made public in 2008; it is updated as often as weekly. We downloaded data in August, 2008, and updated data for the E.U. on September 8, 2008 due to widespread changes in standards that had occurred. To prioritize the investigation of potential exposures, the following selections were made:

Commodity Selection

Produce items were selected based on a combination of the greatest quantities imported to the U.S., and the greatest overall consumption levels in the U.S. USDA disappearance data, a proxy for consumption, reflects the summed quantities of imports, annual production, and initial stocks of an item minus the total value of exports, non-food uses, and remaining stock of that item per year, on a national level. We used data on retail weight of food disappearance, even though in some cases such as peeled produce, the weight of food as consumed may differ from retail weight. We derived data on both imports and disappearance from the USDA Economic Research Service's (ERS) *Food Availability (Per Capita) Data System*[33]. Fruits and vegetables were ranked by quantities imported and retail disappearance per capita. For each commodity, we summed the two sets of ranks, selecting for analysis the top ten fruits and ten vegetables. (Table 2).

Table 2: Top 20 commodities based on import and consumption data, 2007

		Imports, thousand kg (Rank)	**Consumption, thousand kg (Rank)**	**Composite Rank**
Vegetables	Tomato	1 071 (1)	2 780 (3)	2
	Potato	502 (2)	5 371 (1)	1
	Cucumber	459 (3)	864 (7)	4
	Onion	418 (4)	2 971 (2)	3
	Bell pepper	329 (5)	926 (6)	5
	Squash**	257 (6)	611 (8)	7
	Garlic	225 (7)	405 (9)	9
	Artichoke	166 (8)	221 (10)	10
	Carrot	112 (9)	1 227 (4)	6
	Head lettuce	70 (10)	2 774 (5)	8
Fruits	Banana	3 543 (1)	3 552 (2)	1
	Melon	953 (2)	3 851 (1)	1
	Pineapple*	697 (3)	688 (7)	3
	Grape	569 (4)	1 103 (4)	2
	Lime *	328 (5)	326 (10)	6
	Avocado	302 (6)	471 (8)	5
	Apple	173 (7)	2 262 (3)	3
	Orange	112 (8)	1 021 (5)	4
	Pear	86 (9)	425 (9)	8
	Strawberry	72 (10)	882 (6)	7

Items listed in order of combined ranks for imports and consumption. Consumption measured as "Disappearance." Data:http://www.ers.usda.gov/Data/FoodConsumption/FoodAvailSpreadsheets.htm#fruitveg

* In a few cases, imports exceed disappearance due to re-exportation.

**Squash: No breakdowns could be obtained to specify relative quantities imported of summer, winter, and non-specified squashes, to parallel available data in the MRL database.

Market Selection

For each commodity, we included all markets (countries) that supplied at least 453 592 kg annually to the U.S. in 2007, as calculated from the USDA FAS trade database[1] (Patrick Woodall, personal communication, July 2008) [34].

Pesticide Selection

We used all pesticides included in the FAS MRL database for the relevant country/market combinations. The FAS MRL database only includes pesticides with established EPA tolerances, and only shows pesticide standards when the exporting country has them.

Health Effects Identification

To identify potential human health effects and corresponding toxicity values, we located risk assessment documents for each included pesticide. We employed a two-tiered search process: first, we examined the EPA's database of pesticide Reregistration Eligibility Decision (RED) documents for updated toxicity assessments. For pesticides first registered after 1984, we consulted the federal database of government regulations and related documents http://www.regulations.gov. We identified the most recent risk assessment containing chronic toxicity evaluations and abstracted toxicity values.

We also abstracted non-cancer chronic toxicity values for pesticides, preferably in the form of chronic population adjusted doses [cPADs], and cancer slope factors, as well as qualitative carcinogenicity classifications. Where cPADs were not listed, we calculated them from non-cancer reference doses (RfDs). The EPA defines the cPAD as the highest dose at which a person could be exposed over the course of a lifetime, with no expected adverse health effects [35]. This dose is intended to correspond to the most sensitive health effect that occurs as a result of exposure to the pesticide of interest (known as the critical effect), and as a result, is believed to be protective against additional health effects that may be expected to occur at higher doses. We considered acute toxicity values, intended to address high-level exposures such as those potentially incurred by pesticide applicators, to be outside of the scope of this effort.

We identified and categorized the critical effects related to the selected pesticides in a framework primarily based on the work of Fox et al (2004) [36]. Categories were: blood, body weight, bone marrow, cardiac, CNS, developmental, endocrine, GI, kidney, liver, mortality, musculoskeletal, ocular, reproductive, respiratory, spleen, and vascular.

Analysis

For every commodity-market-pesticide combination, we performed calculations to quantify the difference between MRLs in the originating-country market versus U.S. tolerances. We multiplied differences in MRLs by quantity imported, as a way to model the potential increased or decreased quantity of pesticide residue that could be entering the U.S. food supply, above that allowable on domestic produce. We refer to these combinations as "excess residue" (more residue would enter the U.S. because the originating country has a higher MRL than the U.S); and "reduced residue" (less residue would enter the U.S. because the originating country has a lower MRL than the U.S). To illustrate the MRL analysis process, Chile has an MRL of 5 parts per million (ppm) for the application of the pesticide Ferbam to grapes. The U.S. has a more restrictive MRL of 4 ppm. The U.S. imported 427 601 527 kg of Chilean grapes in 2007. The modeling would thus show that, 427.60 kg of *excess* Ferbam residue could have entered the U.S. food supply. [1 part/million × 427 601 527 kg.] While not discussed here, the model more broadly suggests that a *total* 2 138.01 kg of Ferbam residue could enter the U.S. on Chilean grapes. [5 parts/million × 427 601 527 kg]

This model has important sources of both potential overestimation and underestimation of excesses. Overestimation may be caused by the fact that producers do not generally apply all allowable pesticides at once or in the maximum allowed quantities, and that they may be particularly inclined to follow U.S. regulations in products designated for export. A key source of underestimation is the fact that many producers may exceed their own countries› tolerance limits, and may also apply pesticides banned in produce imported to the U.S. and therefore not included in the model used here [3, 4]. The inability to include factors such as weather conditions and the length of time that passes between pesticide application and harvesting, both of which influence the actual residue levels on produce, is also a limitation of the model.

RESULTS

Across the entire sample, the model suggested that a total of 120 439 kg of excess pesticide residue could be imported into the U.S. if every exporter to the U.S. followed their originating country but not U.S. tolerances. This figure is over and above the allowable residue based on domestic U.S. tolerances. Although it is not the focus of this paper, the modeling also suggested that in items for which foreign regulations were more stringent than those in the U.S., importation could reduce 142 408 kg of pesticide residues.

Table 3 shows the top five pesticides, commodities, and markets, by excess residue modeled to be imported into the U.S. The top produce item, market, and pesticide of concern, respectively, were oranges, Chile, and Zeta-Cypermethrin.

Table 3: Top 5 pesticides, produce items, markets (based on modeling as described in methods)

	PESTICIDE	MODELED EXCESS RESIDUE (kg)
1	Zeta-Cypermethrin	23 502
2	Inorganic bromide resulting from fumigation	22 719
3	Methomyl	18 888

4	Thiabendazole	8 132
5	Chlorpyrifos	7 589
	PRODUCE ITEM	**MODELED EXCESS RESIDUE (kg)**
1	Orange	19 883
2	Cucumber	18 702
3	Apple	16 660
4	Melon	16 632
5	Banana	15 564
	IMPORTING MARKET	**MODELED EXCESS RESIDUE (kg)**
1	Chile	24 530
2	Costa Rica	19 980
3	Spain	16 978
4	Netherlands	13 449
5	Guatemala	12 359

Table 4 provides a detailed look at the top commodity/market combinations with the highest modeled pesticide residue levels. For each commodity/market combination, the table shows the top pesticides contributing to the modeled burden.

Table 4: Top commodity/market combinations, and key associated pesticides

Commodity and Market	Total Modeled Excess Pesticides Above U.S. MRLs (Kg)	Pesticide (excesses only)	Potential Pesticide Residues in Excess of U.S. MRLs (Kg)***
Oranges from Spain *	15 169	Abamectin	2 262
		Carfentrazone-ethyl	2 260
		Aldicarb	2 256
		Zeta-Cypermethrin	2 255
		Fenamiphos	2 249
		Oxamyl	2 194
		Fosetyl-Al	1 600
Apples from Chile **	14 846	Methomyl	12 079
		Inorganic bromide resulting from fumigation	1 849
Bell peppers from Netherlands *	11 178	Carfentrazone-ethyl	1 600
		Metolachlor	1 600
		S-metolachlor	1 600
		Methomyl	1 598
		Quinoxyfen	1 596
		Acibenzolar-S-methyl	1 585
		Fenamidone	1 585
Cucumbers from Costa Rica **	11 106	Inorganic bromide resulting from fumigation	9 999
		Propamocarb hydrochloride	500
Grapes from Chile **	7 852	Fenhexamid	4 694
		Boscalid	640
		Quinoxyfen	598
Melons from Guatemala **	7 406	Zeta-Cypermethrin	7 082
Cucumbers from Dominican Republic **	5 972	Inorganic bromide resulting from fumigation	5 377

Melons from Honduras **	4 361	Zeta-Cypermethrin	4 170
Bananas from Guatemala **	4 283	Thiabendazole	2 182
		Chlorpyrifos	2 072
Oranges from Italy *	4 086	Abamectin	610
		Carfentrazone-ethyl	609
		Aldicarb	608
		Zeta-Cypermethrin	608
		Fenamiphos	606
		Oxamyl	591
Bananas from Costa Rica **	4 061	Thiabendazole	2 070
		Chlorpyrifos	1 966
Bananas from Ecuador **	3 641	Thiabendazole	1 855
		Chlorpyrifos	1 762
Melons from Costa Rica **	2 644	Zeta-Cypermethrin	2 529
Tomatoes from Netherlands *	2 270	Fosthiazate	508
		Carfentrazone-ethyl	508
		S-metolachlor	508
Bananas from Honduras **	1 891	Thiabendazole	963
		Chlorpyrifos	915
Bell peppers from Spain *	1 597	Carfentrazone-ethyl	229
		Metolachlor	229
		S-metolachlor	229
		Methomyl	229
		Quinoxyfen	228
		Acibenzolar-S-methyl	226
		Fenamidone	226
Cucumbers from Honduras **	1 531	Inorganic bromide resulting from fumigation	1 378
Bananas from Colombia **	1 478	Thiabendazole	753
		Chlorpyrifos	715
Squash from Costa Rica **	1 340	Methomyl	659
		Zeta-Cypermethrin	659
Melons from Panama **	1 276	Zeta-Cypermethrin	1 221

* EU

** Codex

*** Reflects only pesticides modeled to be imported at levels greater than 1000 lb [454 kg] excess. (In case of bell peppers from Spain, no one pesticide was modeled at > 1000 l b so pesticides at lower levels are reported.)

Examining Table 4 it is notable that all of the produce items with modeled residues high enough to be included in the table originated in markets governed by E.U. or Codex rules. Possible explanations will be considered in the discussion section. The table also highlights the divergence in pesticide standards present even between developed nations.

Table 5 shows the top twenty pesticides based on overall excess pesticide residue, their associated health effects, and the critical effects level identified for each. The table notes the health effects corresponding to chronic, low level dietary exposures to these pesticides, with cPADs listed in corresponding health effect columns. A lower cPAD indicates that a lesser exposure is needed to induce a toxic effect. Additionally, higher levels of exposure or exposures to multiple pesticides may result in additional health effects not noted here. We reviewed toxicity assessments for the top 100 pesticides (by kg excess), finding that body weight and liver effects were the most common health effect categories. Effects on blood, endocrine system, kidneys and central nervous system were also found for at least fifteen pesticides each, while reproductive and developmental endpoints were of concern for seven pesticides each. We do not note carcinogenicity status in the table, as only one among the top twenty pesticides was identified as a probable or known human carcinogen (Captan is a B2 probable human carcinogen). Sixteen of the top 100 pesticides, however, were identified either as known or probable human carcinogens. It should be noted that pesticide toxicity assessments, depending on date, use slightly varying terminology to classify carcinogenicity status. Our approach to classifying for the purpose of this manuscript was to highlight either known or probable human carcinogens.

Table 5: Top 20 pesticides and their sensitive health effects ("critical effects")

Pesticide	Excess (kg)	Body Weight[1]	Liver[1]	Blood[1]	**Endocrine[1]**	**Kidney[1]**	**CNS[1]**	**Reproductive[1]**	**Developmental[1]**
Zeta-Cypermethrin	10 683	0.06					0.06		
Inorganic bromide	10 327								
Methomyl	8 586					X			
Thiabendazole	3 696	0.10	0.10						
Chlorpyrifos	3 450			0.0003					
Carfentrazone-ethyl	2 468		0.03						
Fenhexamid	2 167			0.17	0.17				
Fenamiphos	1 324			0.0001					
Oxamyl	1 307								
Abamectin	1 307	0.0004							0.0004
Aldicarb	1 302								
Fosetyl-Al	1 201							2.50	
S-metolachlor	1 137	0.10							
Quinoxyfen	1 136	0.20				0.20			
Metolachlor	860	0.10							
Propamocarb hydrochloride	853	X							
Acibenzolar-S-methyl	852			0.25					
Fenamidone	852				0.0283				
Ferbam	653	0.015	0.015	0.015					
Captan	649	0.13							0.13

This table shows the top 20 pesticides modeled to have the highest excess levels when summed across all importing markets. For each, the table shows "critical effects," meaning the most sensitive non-cancer endpoint/s documented in EPA risk assessments.

[1] *Numbers in health effects column indicate the chronic population adjusted doses (cPADs) EPA identified, i.e. the highest dose to which a person could be exposed over the course of a lifetime with no expected adverse health effects. cPADs provided are provided in units of mg pesticide per kg bodyweight per day. Value of «X» in health effects column indicates that EPA did not quantitatively estimate a cPAD.*

DISCUSSION & CONCLUSIONS

Summary

This analysis models the quantity of excess pesticide residues that might be imported into the U.S. assuming exporters comply with originating country tolerances but not U.S. MRLs. The modeling focused on the top 20 produce items based on importation and consumption (disappearance) in the U.S. The model estimates that among those items, and based on the top markets exporting those items and top pesticides used, a total of over 120 202 kg of pesticides *in excess of* U.S. tolerances would enter the country annually, in addition to the maximum levels allowable on domestic produce.

Based on low level dietary exposures, the selected pesticides in this review are associated with health effects on thirteen organ systems, and several are associated with carcinogenic effects. These risks may be of special concern for children, given the prevalence of these foods in their diets, and their smaller size and heightened vulnerability to chemical exposure as a result of developmental processes. It is also critical to note that there are common targets of action for many of the modeled pesticides (Table 6). We emphasize, however, that the pesticide health effects are presented for context only. The analysis lacks data to suggest the extent to which these might be experienced in the population due to food imports.

Table 6: Common targets of action for pesticides included in this analysis

Organ System	# of pesticides for which critical effect corresponds to organ system
Body Weight	31
Liver	30
Blood	23
Endocrine	19
Kidney	15
CNS	15
Reproductive	7
Developmental	7
Spleen	4
GI	3
Ocular	3
Respiratory	2
Vascular	2
Unspecified	1
Carcinogens	16

Targets of action were identified based on EPA cpad.

Methods: Modeling

By its nature, this analysis cannot provide insight into real-world practice; rather, its aim is to model the differences in potential residues based on U.S. and exporting country law. There are no available comprehensive data on the extent to which exporting countries comply with either their own or U.S. MRLs.

Many producers apply pesticides in excess of their domestic tolerances, and some also apply pesticides that are disallowed in the U.S. [3, 4] Intermediaries and exporters may also fail to assure compliance. If farmers are not following their own domestic MRLs, the volume of pesticide residues imported in excess of U.S. MRLs might be higher than anticipated by this modeling. Residues on imported produce could also be lower than predicted. Evidence suggests pesticide use in developing nations may diverge by market orientation, with farmers producing for export markets using less toxic (although still not necessarily safe) pesticides relative to farmers producing for national markets, due in large part to increased regulatory pressure from outside countries [37]. Galt (2009) found that gaps in testing and enforcement caused many Costa Rican farmers to feel unrestricted by domestic pesticide standards when producing for their open national markets [4]. Farmers are also unlikely to use every allowable pesticide to the maximum allowable level on each crop. The model is further unable to take into account factors influencing the actual residue levels on produce, such as weather conditions and the length of time that passes between pesticide application and harvesting.

In the years before the U.S. government had solid data on actual pesticide residues in foods, the National Academies of Sciences and others performed modeling analyses similar in concept to ours, examining potential population pesticide exposures based on allowable rather than actual application rates [37]. Industry advocates and others criticized these methods, because existing residue tests showed far lower residue levels. These analyses, and the risk assessments on which they were based, also often used the assumption that everyone consumed every food at the high end of population consumption [38]. While potentially overstating risk for these reasons, the risk assessments also did not yet take account of vulnerable subgroups and of cumulative risk, thus potentially understating other risks. Improved dietary survey data and Monte Carlo analysis methods eventually enabled more realistic risk assessments, as currently required under the Food Quality Protection Act [16] (although further improvement remains needed).

Modeling analyses based on policy, such as this one, are still needed for several reasons. First, these methods provide a relatively inexpensive way to help identify pesticides, foods, or importing markets of potential concern for further followup. If significant policy gaps are identified for widely consumed foods, the case may be made for additional inspection resources. Second, analyses like this one highlight tolerance policy differentials between markets, which may be key targets for future attention or harmonization. As noted in Table 1 there is substantial divergence in pesticide standards present even between developed nations. Finally, the lack of sufficient import laboratory testing means that data simply do not exist to perform the needed analyses in a more rigorous way at this time.

Methods: "Excess" vs. "reduced" residues

In this model, importing the top 20 produce items was slightly more likely to be "protective" due to more stringent tolerances in originating countries than in the U.S. for the examined commodity-market-pesticide combinations. However, we emphasize the benefits of considering the "excess" and "reduced" categories separately, as their impacts are not additive. An exposure prevented does not minimize the impact of another exposure that exists.

This analysis focused on the excess residues, for three primary reasons. First, there remains a large volume of excess pesticides imported into the U.S. on produce, with potential public health ramifications in this country. Second, these "excesses" may reflect environmental and occupational health threats affecting exporting countries, generated by global trade. Third, focusing on excess residues is helpful for highlighting products potentially in need of increased governmental screening.

By contrast, a study examining areas where importation is protective might be useful for discussion of questions about the strength of U.S. tolerance assessments relative to those internationally. Indeed, we note that while U.S. tolerances served as the baseline for the model, neither their protectiveness nor domestic levels of compliance with these standards was examined.

Methods: Exposure and Risk

The model considers potential pesticide exposures and risks in only the most basic way. Exposure is expressed in terms of how much excess residue may be entering the food supply. The analysis does not account for population variation in diet, "dose" or varying food consumption in vulnerable populations. We note that many of the produce items we identified as having the largest excess pesticide residues also have skins or outer shells that consumers do not consume; the removal of skins and shells will significantly reduce pesticide residue exposure risk. These produce items remain important, however, because while most pesticide may be on the skin, some may penetrate skins and/or be absorbed through roots to permeate the item. Dermal exposure is also a potential concern.

Risk too is characterized in a basic way for this model. EPA's approach used to derive cPADs accounts only for the individual impact of a single chemical on a single health endpoint. Many of the studied pesticides, however, when acting alone, can act on multiple organ systems. Even under circumstances when an exposure to a single chemical may be insufficient to elicit an adverse effect, the cumulative impact of multiple pesticides may be additive or synergistic; thus, simultaneous exposure to numerous chemicals may result in toxicological effects. This suggests that existing residue tolerances may be inadequate to protect public health. These concerns exist independently of international differences in pesticide tolerances, and stem from the antiquated approach of evaluating pesticides on a single chemical basis.

Context: Top Items of Concern Identified by Others

It is useful to consider how the findings from this analysis compare to those from monitoring and other assessments. Table 7 shows the top produce items of concern identified by the FDA Pesticide Monitoring Program, EPA Dietary Risk Index, the nonprofit Environmental Working Group (EWG), and this analysis. EWG annually presents a "dirty dozen" produce items, based on data from both the USDA and FDA testing programs. Their compilation does not create distinct lists of domestic and imported produce, but rather highlights those items it finds to be of most concern regardless of origin.

Table 7: Top produce items of concern, 2007

FDA Pesticide Monitoring Program* (imported commodities)	EPA Dietary Risk Index** **(imported commodities)**	**Environmental Working Group's "Dirty Dozen" (imported and domestic commodities)*****	**Top 10 Items of Concern (based on excess residue modeling as described in methods)**
Fruits and Vegetables	***Fruits***	***Fruits and Vegetables***	***Fruits and Vegetables***
Berries, dried or paste	Grapes	Peaches	Oranges
Ginseng, herbal and botanical, other than tea	Peaches	Apples	Cucumbers
Snow peas	Cantaloupe	Sweet bell peppers	Apples
Mango, dried or paste	Apples	Celery	Melons
Celery, dried or paste		Nectarines	Bananas
Chinese okra (luffa)		Strawberries	Bell peppers
Chinese/Thai eggplant	***Vegetables***	Cherries	Grapes
Red beet	Lettuce	Kale	Summer Squash
Pear	Peppers	Lettuce	Tomatoes
Chutney	Cucumbers	Grapes (imported)	Winter Squash
Papaya	Celery	Carrots	
Spinach	Tomatoes	Pears	
Blackberries			

*The FDA Pesticide Monitoring Program annually samples imported produce at the point of entry to the U.S.

** The EPA Dietary Risk Index is based on data from the USDA Pesticide Data Program, which conducts tests on agricultural commodities available for consumption in the U.S.

*** Environmental Working Group's "dirty dozen" reflects an analysis of data from both USDA and FDA testing.

As can be seen in Table 7 there is substantial variation in the top produce items of concern. This may be significantly explained by different criteria for inclusion. The FDA list of items of concern may have been driven by particular outlier findings in compliance inspections rather than reflecting the full spectrum of food shipments - a possibility suggested by the relative rarity in the food supply of many of the highlighted items. The EPA Dietary Risk Index (2006) is a function of the percent of positive tests in the USDA's Pesticide Data Program, and the level of potential risk (which includes pesticide toxicity, children's consumption levels, and residue levels.) [31], and thus takes into account a broader range of data; the EPA report only covered a small number of produce items altogether, and did not indicate how these were chosen. The EWG compiles its report based on a composite index score reflecting six measures of pesticide contamination [39]. Of EWG's so-called "dirty dozen," only seven met the criteria to be included in our model (apples, sweet bell peppers, strawberries, lettuce, imported grapes, carrots, and pears) based on quantities imported and importing markets. Further, no data from strawberries impacted our models, because only Mexico exported enough strawberries to the U.S. to be included in the model, and Mexico uses U.S. pesticide tolerances. The findings from all of these different types of analyses should be considered, as inspection and monitoring priorities are determined.

Context: International Production Practices

The analysis found that the 20 commodity-market combinations with the highest modeled pesticide residues all followed E.U or Codex regulations. Perhaps this finding is to be expected. Wealthier countries such as those in the E.U. may have more pesticides registered than less wealthy countries, because manufacturers may target them for marketing. Even if such countries were more stringent than the U.S. for half the pesticides and less stringent for the other half, that would mean half their pesticides would enter our modeling calculations. With more pesticides counted, as well as high trade volumes, it makes sense that wealthier countries would rate high in this model. Countries following Codex standards may be overrepresented for a different reason: Codex standards are developed through a representative international process, and as such, might be pushed to a lower level than those in the U.S in order to succeed in obtaining broad support [40]. Verifying this possibility is beyond the scope of this analysis.

It is also important to note that the top five markets of concern identified in this analysis include both developing and developed nations. While one might anticipate that developed nations would be more likely to export crops that meet U.S. MRLs even if their own MRL is less stringent, there is evidence that illegally high levels of pesticide residue are not limited to developing nations [41], although the top causal factors underlying violations will vary by economic and other factors. Spain, for example, has a high rate of illegal pesticide residue levels relative to the number of FDA samples taken. Arguably, this is because Spain's primary export market is the E.U., thus reducing the incentive to adapt practices for U.S. markets [41].

There remains little U.S. oversight of how imported produce is grown or of the working conditions that farmers face. While export production may yield economic benefits, it can also mean prime agricultural resources are diverted to producing for export rather than for domestic consumption, with impacts on food security in exporting countries. Further, in order to bolster exports, some farms may turn to monocropping systems and the use of genetically modified seeds that can result in increased pesticide use. Financial pressures arising from low farm prices may also encourage the application of illegal levels of pesticides in order to cut costs and boost production [41]. As one of the larger produce importers in the world, the U.S. bears some responsibility for these negative outcomes.

Proper enforcement of U.S. tolerances could help encourage exporting farmers to limit their pesticide use to prevent produce from being turned away by U.S. inspectors, which could in turn lead to a farmer losing future business with export firms. In developing nations without strong enforcement of domestic MRLs, U.S. tolerances can indeed represent a key means of improving production standards. A number of studies have documented the beneficial impacts that outside standards, when clearly enforced, can have on production practices in developing nations [3, 42, 43]. It should be noted, however, that farmers may also seek to avoid residue violations through the use of pesticides that break down rapidly rather than pesticides that actually comply with U.S. standards [3]. It should also be stressed that U.S. standards are not necessarily safe even if they do represent an improvement on many developing nation standards, as they too are subject to limitations and political pressures [38]. Finally, given the practice of "pesticide divergence by market orientation," it is unlikely that U.S. standards will impact pesticide use among farmers producing for their own domestic markets [42].

Strengths and Limitations

The strength of this analysis is that it uses a newly available database to help understand the public health implications of pesticide levels on imported food. As discussed above, limitations include the artificiality of assumptions and the inability to model real world scenarios of pesticide application, produce consumption, and potential health effects. This analysis is not intended to provide such information; rather, it aims to model the differences in potential residues based on U.S. and importing country law. An additional limitation is that we did not verify the quality of the underlying data provided on governmental websites.

Implications for Policy

These results demonstrate the need for increased efforts to characterize the levels of actual pesticide residues on imported produce that may be entering the U.S. The Food Safety Modernization Act of 2010 (FSMA) represents an important step forward. Under the FSMA, importers of foreign foods (those who own shipments at the time of U.S. entry) must establish foreign supplier verification programs to ensure that the foods they are importing are produced in compliance with specified provisions, including a mandate that producers evaluate and take action to minimize or prevent any reasonably foreseeable hazards from pesticides in use at a facility. The FDA must also establish additional offices in foreign countries to aid agencies there in ensuring the safety of foods exported to the U.S., and may now make agreements with foreign governments regarding inspection of foreign food facilities. The FDA can also refuse shipments from facilities or countries that do not allow inspections. Within the first year of enactment, at least 600 foreign food facilities must be inspected, with that number doubling every year for a period of five years. However, the FDA has noted that this will quickly become impossible without significantly more resources or substantial restructuring of FDA operations [27]. Indeed, the sheer volume of imports to the U.S. suggests that FSMA may not be able to significantly address the challenge at hand, particularly if the legislation is not fully funded.

In June 2011, the FDA declared a new strategic focus on international partnerships and data sharing with foreign agency counterparts in an effort to ensure a safer food supply in the face of limited resources and an ever growing number of imports. As a part of this strategy, the FDA will also focus increasingly on risk analytics and targeting surveillance efforts on risk-based priorities, as well as greater use of public and private third-party auditors [27]. The implications of this strategy for pesticide inspection have yet to be seen, however, it may represent a significant departure from the current model of operations.

Overall, the uncertainties highlighted in this investigation reinforce the message that the U.S. produce import inspection system needs strengthening. Failure to enforce U.S. regulations can mean increased exposures to pesticides not only for U.S. consumers, but also for exporting country farmers and communities where domestic enforcement may be lacking [3]. Following are a set of policy responses that would help address these concerns.

1) Appropriate full funding for the FSMA and ensure that provisions for increased import inspections and international food safety capacity building are fully implemented.

Continue to improve assessments of exporting country oversight and provide technical assistance and support for improving oversight effectiveness.

Work to ensure that farmers and exporters have adequate information about U.S. regulations and food production methods that minimize pesticide usage.

Require unique identifiers for food importers, to enable improved inspection targeting and an improved incentive for importers to ensure regulatory compliance. While the FSMA mandates a study of unique identifiers, the law contains no requirement for their establishment.

2) Improve FDA pesticide inspections and develop additional programs beyond current requirements.

Increase funding for FDA import inspections and laboratory testing, including pesticide screening.

Specifically address pesticide inspections in new efforts to promote FDA collaboration with third-party auditors and foreign agency counterparts.

Strengthen FDA standards governing expectations for the frequency of import shipment screening and laboratory testing. The standards should specify an expanded list of pesticides for screening based on on-the-ground investigation of the most commonly used pesticides for particular items in top exporting markets. On a pilot basis, enhance inspections of the items identified in this modeling.

When legally appropriate and feasible, destroy tainted shipments to assure that increased inspections do not lead to shipments entering the food supplies of other countries.

Improve transparency in FDA inspection records, such as by establishing a publicly accessible database.

Address gaps in Country of Origin Labeling (COOL) policy. The U.S. requires COOL labels on most fruits and vegetables (as well as some other products), but labels are still not required for items such as processed fruits and vegetables, and fruit juices [44]. Such labels can help consumers make informed purchasing choices.

3) Re-examine U.S. tolerances for pesticides where other countries have more stringent requirements.

4) Expand USDA and FDA pesticide residue monitoring programs to include a greater number of samples analyzed annually, with a particular emphasis on imported produce. Develop a cross-agency complementary strategy to avoid duplication.

5) Pause trade negotiations pending improvements in oversight capacity. As described above, a significant portion of the increase in fruit and vegetable imports may relate to the reduced tariffs negotiated through trade agreements. The U.S. inspection system is currently unable to absorb further increases in imports through new trade agreements.

CONCLUSION

The U.S. imports a significant and rising portion of its fruits and vegetables, and the impacts of this practice on domestic pesticide exposure have yet to be characterized. Based on the limited extent of pesticide residue screening and the potential for increased exposures, a more rigorous hazard evaluation is warranted. The commodity-market-pesticide combinations identified in this analysis are worthy of attention. Without strict enforcement of pesticide residue regulations, exporters have little reason to meet pesticide tolerance levels for the U.S. or their home country. There is a critical need for increased produce inspection and pesticide residue screening. Filling this information gap is a necessary step to improve food safety.

ENDNOTE

[1]Calculations were performed initially in lbs rather than kg, and thus the original cutoff value was 1 million lbs.

DECLARATIONS

Acknowledgements

Thanks to Patrick Woodall, Research Director and Senior Policy Advocate at Food and Water Watch, for sharing his import data calculations from the USDA FAS trade database, and for his expertise. Thanks to Juan Pablo Gomez for assistance with analyses. Thanks to the anonymous reviewers for their insightful feedback.

Competing interests

The authors declare that they have no competing interests.

Authors' contributions

All authors read and approved the final manuscript. RN designed most of the study and analysis, managed the project, participated in data management and analysis, and participated in drafting and revising the manuscript. JH participated in data analysis and in drafting and revising the manuscript. LL participated in drafting and revising the manuscript. KD participated in data analysis and in drafting and revising the manuscript. AR participated in data analysis. KN designed parts of the study and analysis, and participated in data analysis and in drafting and revising the manuscript.

REFERENCES

1. Huang S, Huang K: Increased U.S. Imports of Fresh Fruit and Vegetables. Economic Research Service/ USDA. 2007, Washington, DC
2. Food and Water Watch: The poisoned fruit of American trade policy. Food and Water Watch. 2008, Washington, DC

3. Galt RE: Regulatory risk and farmers' caution with pesticides in Costa Rica. Transactions of the Institute of British Geographers. 2007, 32 (3): 377-394. 10.1111/j.1475-5661.2007.00256.x.
4. Galt RE: "It just goes to kill Ticos": national market regulation and the political ecology of farmers' pesticide use in Costa Rica. Journal of Political Ecology: Case Studies in History and Society. 2009, 16: 1-33.
5. U.S. EPA: What is a Pesticide?. [http://www.epa.gov/opp00001/about/]
6. Weiss B, Amler S, Amler RW: Pesticides. Pediatrics. 2004, 113 (4 Suppl): 1030-1036.
7. Aspelin A, Grube A: Pesticides Industry Sales and Usage: 1996 and 1997 Market Estimates. 1999
8. U.S. Environmental Protection Agency: 2006-2007 Pesticide Market Estimates: Usage. [http://www.epa.gov/opp00001/pestsales/07pestsales/usage2007.htm#3_1]
9. Casida JE: Pest toxicology: the primary mechanisms of pesticide action. Chem Res Toxicol. 2009, 22 (4): 609-19. 10.1021/tx8004949.
10. Committee on Pesticides in the Diets of Infants and Children: Pesticides in the Diets of Infants and Children:. 1993, Washington, DC.: National Research Council
11. Boobis AR, Ossendorp BC, Banasiak U, Hamey PY, Sebestyen I, Moretto A: Cumulative risk assessment of pesticide residues in food. Toxicol Lett. 2008, 180 (2): 137-50. 10.1016/j.toxlet.2008.06.004.
12. Bouchard MF, Chevrier J, Harley KG, Kogut K, Vedar M, Calderon N, Trujillo C, Johnson C, Bradman A, Barr DB, Eskenazi B: Prenatal exposure to organophosphate pesticides and IQ in 7-year-old children. Environmental health perspectives. 2011, 119 (8): 1189-95. 10.1289/ehp.1003185.
13. Grandjean P, Landrigan PJ: Developmental neurotoxicity of industrial chemicals. Lancet. 2006, 368 (9553): 2167-78. 10.1016/S0140-6736(06)69665-7.
14. USC (United States Code): Federal Food, Drug and Cosmetics Act (FFDCA). 21 USC, Chapter 9, Section 346a.
15. USC (United States Code): Federal Insecticide, Fungicide, and Rodenticide Act. U.S. Code Title 7, Chapter 6, Section 136a.
16. U.S. Environmental Protection Agency: Food Quality Protection Act; 1996, Public Law 104-170.
17. Food and Agriculture Organization of the United Nations and World Health Organization: FAO/WHO Food Safety Standards. Codex Alimentarius. [http://www.codexalimentarius.net]
18. European Commission: Plant Protection - Pesticide Residues. [http://ec.europa.eu/food/plant/protection/pesticides/index_en.htm]
19. Gonzalez C, Hernandez G: Mexico Food and Agricultural Import Regulations and Standards Mexico's Maximum Residue Limit (MRL) Policy 2005. GAIN Report. 2005, USDA Foreign Agricultural Service
20. World Trade Organization: The WTO Agreement on the Application of Sanitary and Phytosanitary Measures (SPS Agreement). [http://www.wto.org/english/tratop_e/sps_e/spsagr_e.htm]
21. U.S. Food & Drug Administration: Pesticide Monitoring Program FY 2007. 2009, U.S. FDA. Washington, DC
22. U.S. Food & Drug Administration: ORA Field Management Directive No. 13. [http://www.fda.gov/ICECI/Inspections/ForeignInspections/ucm110656.htm]
23. Shames L: Testimony Before the Subcommittee on Oversight and Investigations, Committee on Energy and Commerce, House of Representatives. FDA Could Strengthen Oversight of Imported Food by Improving Enforcement and Seeking Additional Authorities. 2010, U.S. Government Accountability Office
24. U.S. Food & Drug Administration: Office of International Programs - Overview. [http://www.fda.gov/AboutFDA/CentersOffices/OfficeofGlobalRegulatoryOperationsandPolicy/OfficeofInternationalPrograms/ucm236581.htm]
25. U.S. Government Accountability Office: Food Safety: Improvements Needed in FDA Oversight of Fresh Produce. 2008, U.S. Government Accountability Office. Washington, DC
26. Galt RE: Overlap of US FDA residue tests and pesticides used in imported vegetables: Empirical findings and policy recommendations. Food Policy. 2009, 34: 468-476. 10.1016/j.foodpol.2009.05.005.
27. U.S. Food & Drug Administration: Pathway to Global Product Safety and Quality. 2011
28. Buzby JC, Unnevehr LJ, Roberts D: Food Safety and Imports: An Analysis of FDA Food-Related Import Refusal Reports. 2008, USDA. Washington, DC
29. USDA AMS: Pesticide Data Program: Annual Summary, Calendar Year 2007. 2008
30. U.S. Department of Agriculture and Agricultural Marketing Service: Pesticide data program: Annual summary calendar year 2009. 2011, USDA. Washington, DC
31. U.S. EPA: Supplemental Report: Details on Dietary Risk Data in Support of Report No. 2006-P-00028, "Measuring the Impact of the Food Quality Protection Act: Challenges and Opportunities". 2006, U.S. EPA. Washington, DC
32. USDA Foreign Agricultural Service: International Maximum Residue Level Database. [http://www.mrldatabase.com/]
33. USDA Economic Research Service: Food availability, spreadsheets. "Fresh Fruits" and "Fresh Vegetables", 2007. 2009
34. USDA Foreign Agricultural Service: Trade database. Harmonized tariff schedule 2-digit imports for HS-7 (fresh vegetables) and HS-8 (fresh fruit). [http://www.fas.usda.gov/ustrade.asp]
35. U.S. EPA: Report of the Food Quality Protection Act (FQPA) Tolerance Reassessment Progress and Risk Management Decision (TRED) for Bitertanol. [http://www.epa.gov/oppsrrd1/REDs/bitertanol_tred.pdf]
36. Fox MA, Tran NL, Groopman JD, Burke TA:

Toxicological resources for cumulative risk: an example with hazardous air pollutants. Regulatory Toxicology and Pharmacology. 2004, 40 (3): 305-311. 10.1016/j.yrtph.2004.07.008.

37. Committee on Scientific and Regulatory Issues Underlying Pesticide Use Patterns and Agricultural Innovation, National Research Council: Regulating Pesticides in Food: The Delaney Paradox. 1987, Washington, D.C.: National Academies Press, online

38. Wargo J: Our children's toxic legacy: How science and law fail to protect us from pesticides. 1998, New Haven: Yale University Press, 2

39. Environmental Working Group: Shopper's guide to pesticides. [http://www.foodnews.org/walletguide.php]

40. Winickoff DE, Bushey DM: Science and Power in Global Food Regulation: The Rise of the Codex Alimentarius. Science Technology Human Values. 2010, 35 (3): 356-381. 10.1177/0162243909334242.

41. Galt RE: Scaling Up Political Ecology: The Case of Illegal Pesticides on Fresh Vegetables Imported into the United States, 1996-2006. Ann Assoc Am Geogr. 2010, 100 (2): 327-355. 10.1080/00045601003595388.

42. Galt RE: Beyond the circle of poison: significant shifts in the global pesticide complex, 1976-2008. Global Environmental Change. 2008, 18 (4): 786-799. 10.1016/j.gloenvcha.2008.07.003.

43. Okello J, Okello R: Do EU pesticide standards promote environmentally-friendly production of fresh export vegetables in developing countries? The evidence from Kenyan green bean industry. Environ Dev Sustainability. 2010, 12 (3): 341-355. 10.1007/s10668-009-9199-y.

44. USDA Agricultural Marketing Service: Country of Origin Labeling. [http://www.ams.usda.gov/AMSv1.0/cool]

INDEX

G

H

I

L

M

N

O

P

Q

R

S

T

U

V

W